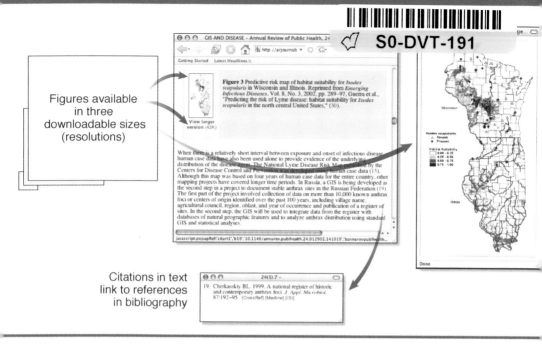

Figures available in three downloadable sizes (resolutions)

Citations in text link to references in bibliography

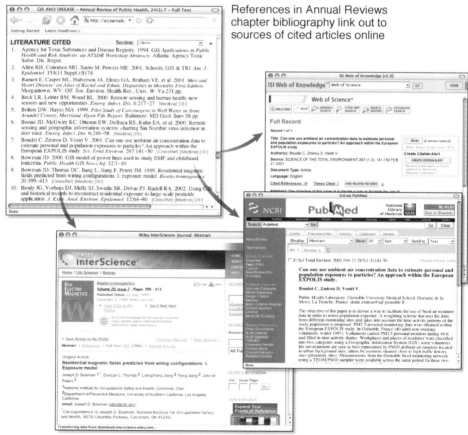

References in Annual Reviews chapter bibliography link out to sources of cited articles online

ANNUAL REVIEW OF PUBLIC HEALTH

ANNUAL REVIEW OF
PUBLIC HEALTH

VOLUME 26, 2005

JONATHAN E. FIELDING, *Editor*
University of California at Los Angeles

ROSS C. BROWNSON, *Associate Editor*
Saint Louis University

NOREEN M. CLARK, *Associate Editor*
University of Michigan

www.annualreviews.org   science@annualreviews.org   650-493-4400

ANNUAL REVIEWS
4139 El Camino Way • P.O. Box 10139 • Palo Alto, California 94303-0139

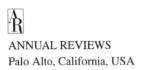

ANNUAL REVIEWS
Palo Alto, California, USA

International Standard Serial Number: 0163-7525
International Standard Book Number: 0-8243-2726-8

TYPESET BY TECHBOOKS, FAIRFAX, VA
PRINTED AND BOUND BY MALLOY INCORPORATED, ANN ARBOR, MI

PREFACE: AND THEN AGAIN...

How important is it to update regularly the critical reviews in the *Annual Review of Public Health*? Of course the only correct answer is, "It depends." Some reviews would cover the same issues and come to the same conclusions about our state of knowledge a decade or more after the previous review. In these situations, for an important topic area, the Editorial Advisory Committee may commission another review anyway because readers often want a more current piece with the latest references, even if the prior review is a classic.

For some topics, new knowledge requires a fresh look, sometimes even on the heels of the prior review. The argument for a topic re-review is strengthened when the recommendations carry important implications. A telling illustration of this principle is the two reviews of a controversial subject, hormone replacement therapy (HRT). The first review appeared in Volume 19 (1998), whereas the second appears is this volume, seven years later. The 1998 Barrett-Connor review is one of the most highly cited reviews in the history of the *Annual Review of Public Health*.

Both reviews were authored by Elizabeth Barrett-Connor and Deborah Grady; Marcia Stefanick is a coauthor on the second review. The first review was undertaken during a period of time in which there was much positive publicity about the value of both postmenopausal estrogen and estrogen-progesterone preparations in reducing the risk of acquired coronary heart disease. Although Barrett-Connor & Grady found that the results of the observational studies were, at that time, "strong and consistent," they concluded that HRT should not be recommended for all postmenopausal women because "most of the known biases would tend to exaggerate estrogen's benefit," and long-term use increased the risk of endometrial cancer, venous thrombosis, gallbladder disease, and probably also breast cancer. Despite these concerns by our authors, and other distinguished epidemiologists, millions of women continued to take these medications, including many who consulted with their own physician.

In the current volume, an updated review, broader in scope, chronicles the rise and fall of menopausal hormone therapy. The authors conclude that HRT can improve vasomotor symptoms and vaginal dryness in women with these symptoms and can improve sleep, with overall improvement in quality of life. Further, in the Women's Health Initiative clinical trials, it prevented bone loss and fractures. However, in this large study, neither estrogen nor estrogen-progesterone therapy reduced the risk of heart disease. Most important, the new studies found that these therapies significantly increased the risk of stroke and dementia, in addition to deep vein thrombosis. And estrogen-progesterone combination therapy, but not estrogen alone, increased the risk of breast cancer, while reducing colon cancer risk.

The Women's Health Initiative study results have caused many women to reevaluate their use of these medications, and the number of women using them has fallen precipitously. Still our authors remind us that good research often begets more nuanced questions. They posit that benefits might accrue on the basis of subgroup and/or exposure level. For example, the overall ratio of benefits to risk might be more favorable in younger women than in older women, and very low dose HRT might reduce bone loss without increasing other observed risks seen with standard therapy.

These reviews richly illustrate a growing problem for the public and for medical practitioners: how to interpret complicated studies in ways that facilitate decisions by consumers and by the physicians expected to counsel them. And when there is this type of sea change in what the evidence shows, attendant attention both in the scientific community and in the popular press may lead to policy change. Practitioners change their recommendations, health insurance payers alter what is covered, manufacturers change what they offer for sale, and class-action lawyers litigate against makers.

Most medications can have serious adverse effects. When the condition for which they are prescribed is very serious, the perceived downside of adverse effects is diminished. However, when the condition for which they are prescribed is primarily a quality-of-life issue, such as the menopausal or postmenopausal symptoms, how should an individual construct a balance sheet to make a personal decision? The issue is not solved by constructing a ledger of benefits and risks because it is difficult to compare a very likely benefit with an incremental risk of a serious medical complication in the order of 1 in 100 or 1 in 100,000. And what are physicians to counsel? Do most physicians have the time and knowledge to help each patient make risk/benefit decisions about each recommended therapy?

Development of better decision-aiding tools for physicians, patients, and policy makers remains a high priority, and is thus an apt topic for critical reviews.

Jonathan E. Fielding

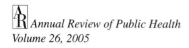 *Annual Review of Public Health*
Volume 26, 2005

CONTENTS

ERRATA

An online log of corrections to *Annual Review of Public Health*
chapters may be found at http://publhealth.annualreviews.org/

RELATED ARTICLES

From the *Annual Review of Genomics and Human Genetics*, Volume 5 (2004)

Genetic Testing in Primary Care, Wylie Burke

Genetic Screening: Carriers and Affected Individuals,
   Edward R.B. McCabe and Linda L. McCabe

Genetics of Atherosclerosis, Aldons J. Lusis, Rebecca Mar,
   and Paivi Pajukanta

From the *Annual Review of Medicine*, Volume 56 (2005)

Genetics of Longevity and Aging, Jan Vijg and Yousin Suh

Progress Toward an HIV Vaccine, Norman L. Letvin

Severe Acute Respiratory Syndrome (SARS): A Year in Review,
   Danuta M. Skowronski, Caroline Astell, Robert C. Brunham,
   Donald E. Low, Martin Petric, Rachel L. Roper, Pierre J. Talbot,
   Theresa Tam, and Lorne Babiuk

From the *Annual Review of Nutrition*, Volume 25 (2005)

Developmental Determinants of Blood Pressure in Adults,
   Linda S. Adair and Darren Dahly

*Pediatric Obesity and Insulin Resistance: Chronic Disease Risk
   and Implications for Treatment and Prevention Beyond Body Weight
   Modification*, M.L. Cruz, G.Q. Shaibi, M.J. Weigensberg,
   D. Spruijt-Metz, G.D.C. Ball, and M.I. Goran

From the *Annual Review of Sociology*, Volume 31 (2005)

*Macro-Structural Analyses of Race, Ethnicity, and Violent Crime:
   Recent Lessons and New Directions for Research*, Ruth D. Peterson
   and Lauren J. Krivo

The Social Psychology of Health Disparities, Jason Schnittker
   and Jane D. McLeod

Annu. Rev. Public Health 2005. 26:1–35
doi: 10.1146/annurev.publhealth.26.021304.144505

A LIFE COURSE APPROACH TO CHRONIC DISEASE EPIDEMIOLOGY

John Lynch[1] and George Davey Smith[2]

[1]Center for Social Epidemiology and Population Health, Department of Epidemiology,
University of Michigan, Ann Arbor, Michigan 48104-2548; email: jwlynch@umich.edu
[2]Department of Social Medicine, University of Bristol, BS8 2PR, Bristol,
United Kingdom; email: Zetkin@bristol.ac.uk

Key Words time, risk factor, population

■ **Abstract** A life course approach to chronic disease epidemiology uses a multidisciplinary framework to understand the importance of time and timing in associations between exposures and outcomes at the individual and population levels. Such an approach to chronic diseases is enriched by specification of the particular way that time and timing in relation to physical growth, reproduction, infection, social mobility, and behavioral transitions, etc., influence various adult chronic diseases in different ways, and more ambitiously, by how these temporal processes are interconnected and manifested in population-level disease trends. In this review, we discuss some historical background to life course epidemiology and theoretical models of life course processes, and we review some of the empirical evidence linking life course processes to coronary heart disease, hemorrhagic stroke, type II diabetes, breast cancer, and chronic obstructive pulmonary disease. We also underscore that a life course approach offers a way to conceptualize how underlying socio-environmental determinants of health, experienced at different life course stages, can differentially influence the development of chronic diseases, as mediated through proximal specific biological processes.

INTRODUCTION

A life course approach to chronic disease epidemiology explicitly recognizes the importance of time and timing in understanding causal links between exposures and outcomes within an individual life course, across generations, and on population level disease trends. The importance of time is illustrated by the fact that chronic conditions such as cancers and cardiovascular diseases have long latency periods—i.e., they develop over time (166). Time lags between exposure, disease initiation, and clinical recognition (latency period) suggest that exposures early in life are involved in initiating disease processes prior to clinical manifestations. Similarly, many important adult risk factors for chronic diseases (poverty, smoking, diet, physical activity) have their own natural histories, e.g., what people eat or do not eat in adulthood may be sensitive to the dietary habits they established in

0163-7525/05/0421-0001$20.00

early life. The importance of timing is illustrated by knowledge that the particular stage of life when an exposure occurs can be important in understanding its later effects. For example, evidence is mounting that human papilloma virus (HPV) is a necessary cause of cervical cancer (148). The infection is acquired through sexual intercourse, and there is some evidence that younger age at sexual debut increases the effect of infection on the risk of developing cervical cancer (169).

Adopting a life course approach should not be construed as suggesting that the recognition of important early-life influences on chronic diseases implies deterministic processes that negate the possibility of later-life intervention (196). One illustration is that *Helicobacter pylori* infection, which is acquired mainly in early life (81), has relatively recently been confirmed as the predominant cause of cardia and noncardia gastric cancer (1, 20)—a disease that is rare below age 50. Gastric (stomach) cancer was the single leading cause of cancer mortality in the United States and many industrialized countries through the 1940s and is still a leading cause of cancer death in Asia. The recent identification of this crucial early-life exposure has lead to successful treatment in adulthood, which helps eradicate *H. pylori* infection and dramatically reduces the risk of developing stomach cancer (29, 187). This also provides additional justification for what we already know about ensuring adequate housing and hygiene conditions, especially for poor children. The bulk of adult chronic diseases is unlikely to be explained as the predetermined outcome of inevitable trajectories of exposures in utero or infancy, but rather as longer-term consequences of the albeit complex accumulation and interaction, across generations, of early and later-life exposures. The relative importance, however, of early and later-life exposures will differ by health outcome (34).

A life course perspective on chronic disease epidemiology relies on a multidisciplinary framework for understanding how early- and later-life biological, behavioral, social, and psychological exposures affect adult health (16). However, although general theorizing about these interconnected and multi-faceted processes is important (87), a life course approach to chronic disease epidemiology is enriched by specification of the particular way that time and timing in relation to physical growth, reproduction, infection, social mobility, and behavioral transitions, etc., influence various adult chronic diseases in different ways (112), and by how these temporal processes are interconnected within the life course of one cohort. More ambitiously, a life course approach also attempts to understand how such temporal processes across the life course of one cohort occur in previous and subsequent birth cohorts and are manifested in disease trends that are observed over time at the population level.

THE DEVELOPMENT OF A LIFE COURSE APPROACH IN EPIDEMIOLOGY

The appreciation of life course processes is hardly a new idea. In 1667, Milton wrote in *Paradise Lost*,

"The childhood shows the man,
As the morning shows the day." (144a, lines 220–21)

Life course thinking has been prominent in disciplines such as psychology, sociology, neurodevelopment, and anthropology (113), and there are important historical examples in epidemiology. For instance, in 1934, Kermack (107) showed cohort patterns in mortality declines in Britain between 1850 and the 1930s (Figure 1), which suggests that each successive generation carried with it, from birth, the potential for a longer life (44). In a study of Maryland school children, Ciocco commented in 1941 that "disease in adulthood is often brought about by the cumulative effects over a long period of time of many pathological conditions, many incidents, some of which take place and are even perceived in infancy" (26, p. 2375). In the 1960s there were papers on the role of early-life influences on chronic diseases (96), and Dubos discussed the long-lasting effects of early environmental exposures under the intriguing title of biological Freudianism (54). Even in the 1970s, there was recognition by chronic disease epidemiologists of the importance of early-life influences on coronary heart disease (CHD) (104). Nevertheless, from the 1960s, chronic disease epidemiology came increasingly to focus on adult lifestyles, and interest in the childhood origins of disease understandably waned with the identification, among adults, of the major CHD risk factors of

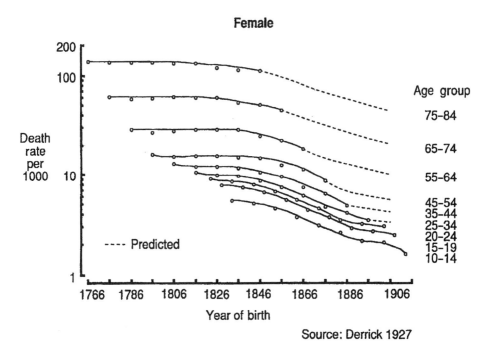

Figure 1   Changes in generation mortality (England and Wales). An example of birth cohort effects in female mortality declines in Britain (106).

smoking, hypertension, and cholesterol. The revival of life course approaches to chronic diseases was stimulated by the work of Forsdahl beginning in the early 1970s (68). Forsdahl suspected that adverse environmental conditions in infancy and early childhood could increase the risk of CHD in adult life. He analyzed aggregate data from Norway and demonstrated that infant mortality rates early in the twentieth century correlated strongly with CHD mortality rates 70 years later (66). Forsdahl speculated that permanent damage may be caused by nutritional deficits in early life that rendered individuals less able to tolerate particular forms of fat in their adult diet, so early-life social disadvantage might interact with affluence in later life to increase CHD risk (67).

The most influential replication of this work was by Barker and colleagues in the United Kingdom (7). The Barker group interpreted their findings as indicating an influence of childhood nutrition, but the focus of their investigations quickly came to rest on exposures in the prenatal environment (8). From these initial observations, the now well-known fetal origins hypothesis was developed, which focused on the long-term effects of in utero biological programming associated with maternal and fetal undernutrition. A key problem with the initial studies in the fetal origins field was that when relating early-life exposures to health outcomes many decades later the intervening anthropometric, biological, behavioral, psychological, and social trajectories of individuals (which were largely unmeasured in the available data) were correlated with early-life exposures. Thus, because the processes affecting birth weight and postnatal growth may also influence subsequent weight in childhood, growth before puberty, and weight in adulthood, it was not clear whether early-life exposures were linked to adult disease only through their links with later-life exposures (14, 102, 130). After a decade of almost exclusive concentration on the independent effect of the prenatal period, studies by Barker and colleagues have also shown the importance of potentially modifying influences of experiences acting in later life (9, 59).

Research on early-life factors, in particular birth anthropometry, appeared against the backdrop of the huge amount of chronic disease epidemiology that was carried out during the second half of the twentieth century on adult behaviors (smoking, diet, exercise), physiological parameters (blood pressure, lipids, hemostatic factors), adult socioeconomic position (social class, income, occupation), and adult psychosocial factors (psychological dispositions, social networks, and work stress). The flurry of reports on the fetal origins of CHD during the 1990s produced somewhat polarized opinions; many epidemiologists emphasized the primacy of the already well-known adult risk factors (particularly as indicated by successful interventions on lowering blood pressure and cholesterol), whereas others focused almost exclusively on events happening very early during development. To counteract the increasing polarization of approaches that emphasized biological programming in utero and adult lifestyle approaches to chronic disease etiology, a partial synthesis under the rubric of life course epidemiology was built on the premise that various biological and social factors over the life course independently, cumulatively, and interactively influence health and disease in adult life (16, 113). Life course epidemiology does not deny the importance of conventional chronic disease risk factors, such as smoking, diet, and hypertension, which were successfully identified by the early postwar adult cohort studies. Rather, its purpose is to bridge the perinatal and adult period by studying the contribution of early-life factors jointly with later-life factors to identify risk and protective processes across the life course. The fetal origins hypothesis provided a stimulus for broader thinking about a range of influences acting from before birth and then right across the life course. In 1997 [(111); second edition published in 2004 (112)] a book edited by Kuh & Ben-Shlomo, *A Life Course Approach to Chronic Disease Epidemiology*, collected contributions from across the disciplinary and disease spectrum and, for many researchers, helped re-establish life course thinking as important to the epidemiological endeavor.

THEORETICAL MODELS OF LIFE COURSE PROCESSES

Life course epidemiology examines a range of potential processes through which exposures acting at different stages of life can, singly or in combination, influence disease risk.

The critical period model emphasizes the timing of exposure, such that an exposure at a specific period in the life course has long-lasting effects on anatomical structure or physiological function that may eventually result in disease. The term critical period is usually reserved for exposures occurring during known periods of unalterable biological development. This is well understood in a variety of situations, such as with prenatal infections or drug exposure, where during a particular period of fetal development these can lead to devastating permanent developmental changes, whereas if they were experienced just a few days earlier or later they would have no long-term impact. The fetal origins hypothesis in its original formulation took this critical period approach. Other examples of processes where outcomes may depend on the time window at which an exposure acts are

- limb development in relation to maternal thalidomide use;
- fracture across the epiphysis (growth plate) when bone is growing during childhood and adolescence;
- very early postnatal infection with Hepatitis B and risk of adulthood liver cancer;
- congenital infections and environmental lead exposure that result only in serious neurodevelopmental deficits if occurring in infancy and childhood; and
- absence of certain infections or exposure to dirt in childhood, which may increase the risk of asthma, hay fever, Hodgkin's disease, non-Hodgkin's lymphoma, and type I diabetes.

Additionally, there may also be sensitive periods where the effect of an exposure is magnified more than the effect of the same exposure in another time period (113) (e.g., poverty during periods of important childhood social transitions such as school entry) (55), or energy imbalance and overweight just prior to puberty (144). The influence of exposures acting during critical or sensitive periods of susceptibility may also be modified by later-life exposures. This seems to be the case for the associations of birth weight with some chronic diseases in which associations are stronger (or only evident) among those who become obese during adolescence or adulthood (61, 69, 71).

The other main class of life course processes are those represented in accumulation of risk models, which focus on the total amount and/or sequence of exposure. Such models suggest that effects accumulate over the life course, although they also allow for developmental periods during which susceptibility may be greater (16) so that the sequence or trajectory of accumulation may also be important. The simplest model is dose-response, where health damage increases with the duration and/or number of detrimental exposures. Studies have shown this in relation to poor socioeconomic conditions, where additive effects of experiencing low socioeconomic position across different stages of the life course influence risk of several adult health outcomes (40, 132). Accumulation of risk can also be due to clustering of exposures. For example, children from poorer socioeconomic backgrounds are also more likely to be of low birth weight, to have poorer diets, to be more exposed to passive smoking and some infectious agents, and to have fewer opportunities for physical activity. Additionally, life course exposures may form chains of risk so that one negative exposure increases the subsequent risk of another negative exposure. For example, becoming overweight in childhood may cause reduced physical activity in adolescence. Chronic diseases likely result from the complex interplay of critical and sensitive period, and trajectory and accumulation processes. Although these general conceptual models are simplistic representations of life course processes that are likely very complex, even such simple models may be difficult to distinguish empirically (88). See Table 1.

EVIDENCE FOR LIFE COURSE PROCESSES AND CHRONIC DISEASES

Different types of epidemiological evidence may indicate the importance of life course processes for adult chronic diseases (Table 2). Readers should see Lawlor et al. (120) for a more thorough discussion of the strengths and limitations of different types of evidence in regard to cardiovascular diseases (CVD). Table 2 illustrates the ways in which epidemiological insights into life course processes have been gained from a variety of study types. This process of triangulation is important in life course epidemiology because it attempts to integrate knowledge gained about life course processes at the individual, generational, and population levels.

TABLE 1   Conceptual life course models (16)

Critical period models
(focus on the importance of timing of exposure)
- with or without later-life risk factors
- with later-life effect modifiers

Accumulation of risk models
(focus on the importance of exposure over time and the sequence of exposure)
- with independent and uncorrelated insults
- with correlated insults
  - risk clustering
  - chains of risk with additive or trigger effects

LIFE COURSE RISK FACTORS FOR CHRONIC DISEASES

Table 3 summarizes putative life course exposures for CHD, hemorrhagic stroke, type 2 diabetes, breast cancer, and chronic obstructive pulmonary disease (COPD) by arranging known risk factors according to life course stage and including evidence for early-life exposures. Space limitations preclude full discussion of each of these, and readers should consult more comprehensive sources (34, 38, 45, 85, 111, 112, 115, 137, 150, 152). Additionally, it is important to recognize that many of the life course risk factors discussed here—birth weight, growth, nutrition, smoking, obesity, etc.—are socially patterned and are thus important mechanisms in generating social inequalities in adult health (11, 38, 46, 74). Table 3 is intended to be illustrative of the scope of research on the life course epidemiology of chronic diseases and underscores how early- and later-life processes may differentially contribute to different chronic diseases.

Coronary Heart Disease

CHD remains a major cause of death in many industrialized countries and is rising alarmingly in developing countries (197, 198). Adopting a life course approach to CHD prevention (82) may have some of its most important public health applications in developing countries (2). Here, we discuss CHD and ischemic stroke together because their associations with life course risk factors appear similar. Several lines of evidence converge around the idea that both early and later-life exposures are important in CHD and ischemic stroke. This begins with recognition that the precursors of atherosclerosis—fatty streaks—are already evident in the arteries of children (17, 18). Evidence from autopsy studies of young male U.S. war fatalities in the 1950s and 1960s demonstrated high prevalence of atherosclerosis and coronary artery narrowing (58, 143).

BIRTHWEIGHT AND GROWTH   There is now good evidence that early-life anthropometry and growth are linked to CHD in adulthood. In their review, Lawlor et al.

TABLE 2 Types of epidemiological evidence of life course processes*

Type of data	Evidence of life course processes
Birth cohort effects (107, 184) (for example see Figure 1)	Cohort effects in health trends have been used as indirect evidence for the importance of early-life exposures.
Historical, area-level infant and maternal mortality rates (10, 67, 126)	Because past infant and maternal mortality rates in an area may indicate childhood social conditions for those born at that time, associations between these historical rates and current chronic disease rates (net indicators of current social conditions) provide indirect evidence of early-life exposures and by examining differences in associations with different indicators (e.g., maternal mortality, perinatal mortality, or postneonatal mortality) may provide insight into more specific mechanisms.
Place of birth (63, 94)	When those who migrate (especially as children) have different adult disease rates than does the population into which they migrate, this may indirectly suggest the importance of early-life exposures, although such studies are hard to interpret because of selection and intervening behavioral, socioeconomic, and other adult differences in exposure among migrants.
Adult recall of events and circumstances at birth and in childhood (13, 28, 64)	Associations between recalled age at menarche, parental occupation, or adverse childhood experiences and chronic disease risk may implicate early-life exposures but are potentially subject to recall biases and greater measurement error.
Objectively measured events and circumstances at birth and in early childhood (27, 70, 146)	Indicators of social circumstances, such as socioeconomic position, family structure, number of siblings, and crowding measured in early life, when associated with disease risk in adulthood (net relevant adult risk factors), provide direct support for life course processes.
Anthropometry at birth and during childhood collected from objective sources such as birth, obstetric, school records, and childhood growth studies (71, 127, 153)	Weight and height taken from records collected at birth, postnatally, or in childhood associated with chronic diseases in adulthood provide direct evidence for early-life processes, but interpretation relies on the adequacy of control for adult risk factors.
Adult height and leg length (37, 85)	As adult height is largely attained by the end of adolescence, associations between height and chronic diseases in middle age reflect factors driving growth processes early in life. Leg length is a more specific measure of growth period as it is largely determined before puberty (76). Nevertheless, such studies are unable to capture the relative importance for later chronic diseases of the determinants of different stages and pace of growth in utero through adolescence.

(Continued)

TABLE 2   *(Continued)*

Type of data	Evidence of life course processes
Birth anthropometry of offspring (42, 160)	When birth anthropometry of offspring predicts similar or different maternal and paternal adult health outcomes, this may help distinguish between early-life intergenerational processes involving in utero environment and/or genetic effects.
Objective measurement of infectious, biological, behavioral, socioeconomic, and psychosocial risk factors at birth and during childhood and adolescence (4, 49, 109, 141, 149)	Associations between risk factors, such as blood pressure, lipid levels, socioeconomic position, or psychological disposition measured in early-life and adult chronic diseases (net of relevant adult risk factors) provide important evidence for early-life exposures. Many studies of this type, however, involve younger cohorts in which there are few cases of chronic diseases.

*Adapted from Lawlor et al. (120).

(120) found 11 studies that examined associations between birth size and CHD. They concluded that there was generally an inverse association between birth weight and CHD, but associations with other anthropometric measures, such as ponderal index (thinness) at birth, were not consistent (120). Furthermore, it is not birth size per se but rather growth rate in utero that seems most relevant (61, 127), and additionally, evidence is converging on the important role of postnatal growth, such that long-term effects of in utero growth retardation are modified by postnatal and childhood growth, or obesity in adulthood (61, 71). Associations between birth weight and CHD appear nonlinear so that higher CHD is associated with both lower and higher birth weights (127), suggesting different mechanisms of in utero nutritional influences for growth retardation but altered glucose metabolism and insulin resistance subsequent to gestational diabetes for babies of high birth weights (170).

It is important to distinguish maternal and fetal nutrition in considering influences on in utero growth retardation (89). There is relatively little human evidence on alterations to maternal nutrition during pregnancy and effects on later chronic diseases or risk factors (98). There have, however, been several studies of pregnant women who suffered severe nutritional deprivation during World War II (167, 178). These studies were able to examine the effects of maternal nutritional deprivation in different pregnancy trimesters on the basis of assumptions that most fetal length is gained in the second trimester, whereas weight is gained mainly in the third trimester. However, even this basic understanding of the tempo of in utero growth has been questioned recently (118); so in hindsight, it is perhaps less surprising that the results of these studies are inconsistent, especially when they are based on small numbers of events. The results of long-term follow-up of dietary trials during pregnancy will be especially important in better understanding the role of

TABLE 3 Putative life course risk factors for selected chronic diseases*

Life course stage	CHD	Hemorrhagic stroke	Type 2 diabetes	Breast cancer	COPD
Trans-generational	Parental history Maternal health, behavior, stress, and diet before pregnancy Low SEP	Parental history Maternal health, behavior, stress, and diet before pregnancy Low SEP	Parental history Maternal health, behavior, stress, and diet before pregnancy Low SEP Gestational diabetes	Parental history	Parental history
In utero	Maternal health, behavior, stress, and diet during pregnancy Growth retardation Low birth weight	Maternal health, behavior, stress, and diet during pregnancy Growth retardation Low birth weight	Maternal health, behavior, stress, and diet during pregnancy Low and high birth weight	High birth weight	Low birth weight
Infancy	Infant feeding Maternal attachment Catch-up growth Poor growth Low SEP	Infant feeding	Infant feeding Catch-up growth		Infections Crowding ETS
Childhood	Low SEP Poor growth Poor prepubertal growth Shorter leg length Diet Obesity Certain infections	Low SEP Poor growth High number of siblings	Low SEP Shorter leg length Adiposity rebound Obesity Insulin resistance Diet	High SEP Height velocity BMI velocity Longer leg length Calorie restriction	Low SEP Shorter leg length Crowding ETS Obesity Indoor/outdoor air quality

Adolescence	Low SEP Diet Physical activity Obesity Blood pressure Cholesterol Parity (women)	Low SEP Blood pressure	Low SEP Diet Physical activity Obesity Insulin resistance	Height velocity Early age at menarche Weight gain Calorie restriction	Low SEP Shorter leg length Smoking Obesity
Adulthood	Low SEP Short height Quitting smoking Diet Physical activity Obesity Cholesterol Blood pressure Binge drinking Insulin resistance Work factors Psychosocial factors Offspring birth weight	Low SEP Short height Quitting smoking Blood pressure Offspring birth weight Obesity Alcohol	Low SEP Short height Diet Physical activity Obesity Alcohol Insulin resistance Offspring birth weight Work factors Psychosocial factors	High SEP Greater height Obesity Later age at first birth Lower parity Contraceptive use Diet Alcohol Physical activity Later age at menopause Hormone replacement therapy	Low SEP Shorter height Quitting smoking Diet Obesity Physical activity Occupational exposures Indoor/outdoor air quality

*Abbreviation: SEP, socioeconomic position; ETS, environmental tobacco smoke.

maternal nutrition during pregnancy and later chronic diseases in her offspring (120).

The small number of studies that have examined offspring birth weight in relation to parents' CHD risk (42, 48) show both increased maternal and paternal CHD risk with lower offspring birth weight, although maternal risk seems somewhat more strongly associated (161). Although there are nongenomic mechanisms for intergenerational effects of in utero influences (53), these studies also provide some support for genetic mechanisms driving both growth retardation and CHD risk (33); definitive interpretation of these findings awaits further investigation.

Various studies have confirmed the inverse association between height and CHD in both men and women in countries that have experienced high rates of CHD (43, 165, 194). However, recent contradictory evidence from Korea—a low CHD country—suggests that associations between height and CHD risk depends on the presence of other factors, perhaps high levels of dietary fat (173). The association between height and CHD risk appears to be independent of birth weight (165), and the leg length component of total stature seems especially important (37). Leg length is particularly influenced by nutrition and possibly infection in infancy and prepubertal childhood (191).

MAJOR CHD RISK FACTORS   Several CHD risk factors are already present during childhood and adolescence. Cholesterol, blood pressure, and overweight measured at young ages track, albeit imperfectly, into adulthood (5, 117, 119, 134), but physical activity in childhood or adolescence is only modestly correlated with physical activity in adulthood (23, 186). For example, the Bogalusa Heart Study showed that 77% of obese children became obese adults with worse CHD risk factor profiles (73). In an extensive review (137), blood cholesterol, blood pressure, and body mass index (BMI) measurements taken in adolescence or early adulthood were found to be predictive of CHD up to 50 years later. The incidence of CHD over a 40-year follow-up of young men in the Johns Hopkins Precursor study showed gradients between cholesterol level measured at young ages and later incidence of CHD (109). Studies that measured cholesterol in childhood demonstrated that this predicts carotid artery intima-media thickness (a marker of atherosclerosis) at least as strongly as cholesterol measured in adulthood, and that the childhood measures remain predictors after adulthood measures are taken into account (158). Long-term exposure to circulating cholesterol is a stronger risk factor than are single measures in either childhood or adulthood (128). This observation is in accord with evidence from other sources. Rose (166) demonstrated that ecological correlations between cholesterol levels and CHD were stronger for cholesterol measured many years before CHD was assessed than if contemporaneous cholesterol measures were used (166). Additionally, clinical trial results have shown that the relative reduction in CHD risk among those allocated to cholesterol-lowering drugs increases with duration of treatment (93). Furthermore, evidence from Mendelian randomization approaches demonstrates that the lifetime differences in cholesterol levels generated by genetic polymorphisms are consistent with greater effects of lifetime cholesterol exposure than are seen with single cholesterol measures in adulthood (36). All this evidence suggests that accumulation over the life course of exposure to high levels of cholesterol is important in CHD risk. High fat diets and cholesterol seem to be the crucial risk factors for CHD (177) because there are no examples of CHD epidemics in countries that have low-fat diets.

For blood pressure, the situation is somewhat different. Although blood pressure measured in early adulthood predicts CHD risk 50 years later (138), the effects appear no greater than those seen for blood pressure measured in adulthood (145). Cholesterol measured during early life reflects long-term exposure that is not influenced by early stages of CHD. Thus, cholesterol measured in early life generally produces greater prediction than do such measurements taken in later life because they may reflect long-term accumulative atherosclerotic process. In contrast, blood pressure levels in early life, though influencing later disease, do not show the enhanced association seen for cholesterol.

The situation described for blood pressure is similar to that observed for smoking, where smoking among adolescent or young adults is strongly related to later disease risk but no more strongly than is adult smoking (142). The age at smoking cessation is the key to reducing risk, which declines fairly rapidly after cessation (51, 105, 154, 193). Whether earlier age of initiation and smoking intensity in early life strongly influence the amount smoked over the life course and age at quitting is unclear; but given the generally narrow age range of initiation compared with the much broader age range for quitting, adult factors that more directly influence earlier age at quitting seem to be most important.

STROKE   Stroke is a heterogeneous outcome comprising mainly ischemic and hemorrhagic subtypes, although accurate classification is uncertain using routinely collected death certificate data. Epidemiological investigations of stroke in Western industrialized countries are dominated by ischemic strokes ($\sim70\%$–80% of all strokes), which involve similar atherosclerotic/thrombotic processes as in ischemic/coronary heart disease. Thus, the associations of CHD and life course risk factors described above also apply largely to ischemic stroke. Many studies have identified shared adult risk factors for CHD and stroke, such as hypertension, obesity, smoking, lipids, etc., so they are often combined into a single category of CVD. There are several reasons, however, to distinguish different subtypes when considering etiology and the potential for life course exposures to influence stroke. There are generally weak international correlations between stroke and CHD such that Japan and Korea have high stroke rates (especially hemorrhagic) but low levels of CHD. Historical ecological studies show stronger correlations between infant mortality and stroke than with CHD 70 years later (126). Stroke and CHD have different epidemiological profiles; stroke has undergone continuous decline and CHD has shown an epidemic rise and fall over the course of the twentieth century. Lawlor and colleagues (121) showed that when the hemorrhagic component of total stroke was removed, trends in ischemic stroke parallel trends in CHD. A major difference in the epidemiology of ischemic and hemorrhagic stroke is that circulating cholesterol levels are positively related with the risk of ischemic stroke and are either unrelated or negatively related to hemorrhagic stroke (91). Similarly BMI shows a stronger and more consistent association with ischemic than with hemorrhagic stroke (175).

Regarding early-life factors, there is evidence that height, greater number of siblings, and early-life socioeconomic disadvantage are more strongly associated with hemorrhagic stroke than with ischemic stroke or CHD (90, 139, 173). Few studies have examined the role of birth anthropometry on stroke risk, but available evidence suggests that associations with low birth weight are stronger for hemorrhagic than ischemic stroke (99). Given that hemorrhagic strokes are more strongly linked to hypertension than are ischemic strokes (176), one hypothesis states that associations with birth weight reflect the influence of in utero and early-life growth and nutrition processes on the development of hypertension. Breast-feeding is associated with lower offspring blood pressure (136) and randomized controlled trials of restricting sodium intake in infants resulted in lower blood pressure at the age of 6 months (95) and at age 15 (75). Sodium levels are lower in breast milk than in most formula feeds, and the sodium content of formula feeds has decreased across the century. Although this is only one possible hypothesis, this individual-level mechanism is consistent with evidence from the population level, where hemorrhagic stroke has declined continuously over the twentieth century in the United States and United Kingdom; there have also been strong birth cohort declines in blood pressure (79, 138, 140). Additionally, there is intriguing evidence linking hemorrhagic stroke and stomach cancer, both ecologically and through their strong individual-level associations with numbers of siblings, and thus infection risk in early life. For stomach cancer, *H. pylori* is clearly key, but the same processes that lead to *H. pylori* infection could be related to other early-life infection (or *H. pylori* itself) that increases risk of hemorrhagic stroke. A recent systematic review of studies linking *H. pylori* to stroke unfortunately contained no useful data regarding hemorrhagic stroke (31). In summary, this evidence suggests that the hemorrhagic component of stroke is more directly sensitive to early-life conditions than is either ischemic stroke or CHD, which involve contributions from both early- and later-life exposures.

TYPE 2 DIABETES   Type 2 diabetes is an increasing public health problem in the United States (147), in other rich countries, and especially in parts of the developing world, where rates will likely double over the next two or three decades (108). It is a condition characterized by elevated levels of blood glucose, resulting from insufficient insulin production in the beta cells of the pancreas and/or from cellular (mainly muscle) resistance to insulin that controls glucose uptake. In the natural history of type 2 diabetes it appears that insulin resistance—with concomitant increased insulin secretion—proceeds an end-stage failure in insulin production and that early-life exposures are more strongly associated with the insulin resistance than with the insulin production mechanism (150). A premorbid condition, known as insulin resistance syndrome, is characterized by the clustering of adverse levels of blood pressure, triglycerides, lipids, insulin, glucose, and central obesity. Because these are also some of the main risk factors for CHD, insulin resistance syndrome has been proposed as the common patho-physiological disturbance behind both CHD and type 2 diabetes (162); thus some similar associations are observed between life course exposures and CHD and diabetes.

A systematic review identified 48 studies examining associations between birth weight and diabetes or impaired glucose tolerance (IGT) in young adulthood and later life (150). Overall there was consistent evidence, especially among middle-age cohorts, linking in utero growth to diabetes/IGT risk. Inverse associations between birth weight and risk of diabetes/IGT were found generally in populations where overall diabetes risk was relatively low. In the United States, where diabetes is more common, the largest study on U.S. nurses showed a U-shaped association between birth weight and type 2 diabetes that became linearly inverse after control for maternal diabetes history or adult obesity (164). Thus, associations between higher birth weight and increased diabetes/IGT risk may reflect the effects of higher birth weight on later-life obesity and/or the effects of an in utero environment affected by maternal gestational diabetes, which is itself linked to maternal low birth weight (100).

Both genetic and environmental mechanisms have been proposed to explain links between birth weight and diabetes/IGT risk. The thrifty phenotype hypothesis suggests that impaired in utero growth and later-life obesity may lead to insulin resistance (86). In contrast, the fetal insulin hypothesis suggests that because insulin promotes fetal growth, it is possible that a genetic mechanism generating resistance to insulin lies behind both reduced fetal growth and insulin resistance in later life (92). Evidence in support of this hypothesis comes from the fact that paternal type 2 diabetes risk and insulin resistance are associated with lower offspring birthweight (47, 192).

The results from studies of birth weight and IGT at younger ages underscore the importance of differential patterns of postnatal growth (65) including associations between lower leg: trunk length ratio (determined prepubertally) and higher insulin resistance (37, 122) and adiposity rebound (the age after infancy when body mass begins to rise) (60). Higher risk of IGT has been observed among children with low BMI until age 2 years, but who then experienced adiposity rebound at younger ages and sustained a higher rate of weight gain through childhood (19). According to current guidelines, only 3% of these individuals were overweight and none were obese at age 12; thus these findings from India reflect processes—the temporal dynamics of early growth—rather than simply the outcome of childhood overweight and obesity. In rich countries, where the whole distribution of BMI in children has a much higher mean, it is uncertain how growth processes like early adiposity rebound may affect later diabetes/IGT risk.

Recognition of the role of in utero factors on diabetes risk provides motivation to appreciate more broadly the importance of physical growth processes in utero, across infancy, childhood, adolescence, and into adulthood. Childhood and adult obesity are by far the most important risk factors for diabetes in rich countries such that very few cases of diabetes occur among nonoverweight adults. Thus, child and adulthood obesity and maternal gestational diabetes remain the most important avenues for public health interventions. Nevertheless, in utero, early-life growth processes and energy balance in childhood and adolescence are important pathways to the development of obesity and insulin resistance in later life.

BREAST CANCER   Breast cancer is one chronic disease for which the main established reproductive and menstrual risk factors are already considered within a temporal framework consistent with a life course approach. Although possibly differentially associated with pre- and postmenopausal breast cancer, the main risk factors—parental history, younger age at menarche, younger age at first birth, lower parity, and later age at menopause—are temporally consistent with the basic understanding that breast cancer is related to cumulative and/or interactive exposures over the years of active ovarian function (52). In a systematic review of early-life breast cancer risk factors (prior to age 25), Okasha and colleagues (152) examined birth weight, infant and childhood growth, peak height velocity, height, childhood obesity, diet, age at menarche, and exercise in relation to breast cancer risk. They concluded that there was some evidence for an association between higher birth weight and breast cancer risk, strong evidence for an association between increased height (and possibly leg length), and inconsistent evidence for the role of weight in childhood or adolescence (despite their inverse associations with age at menarche), physical activity, diet, smoking, or alcohol consumption, and later breast cancer risk. They argued that exposures in the period from age at menarche to first birth may be critical because of the susceptibility of rapidly differentiating breast cells to carcinogenic exposures that may enhance cell proliferation.

Results of recent studies not included in the review by Okasha and colleagues (152) may add weight to their conclusions. First, the largest study of the association between birth weight and breast cancer risk among more than 100,000 women shows a clear association between higher birth weight and higher breast cancer risk after control for age at first birth and parity (3). Second, a study using the 1946 U.K. birth cohort found that after adjustment for several confounders, height velocity from ages 4–7 and 11–15, and BMI velocity from ages 2–4, were associated with increased premenopausal breast cancer risk, especially among girls with age at menarche less than 12.5 years. Thus, faster childhood growth leading to earlier attainment of adult height among girls with earlier age at menarche magnified breast cancer risk (50). Finally, a Swedish study showed that women who had been hospitalized for anorexia nervosa before age 40 had a more than 50% reduced risk of breast cancer, and this effect was even stronger among parous women. This suggests the importance of early-life diet and caloric restriction and their potentially interactive effects with known risk factors such as parity (144).

Insulin-like growth factor-1 (IGF-1) and its binding proteins may be important in understanding some of the findings linking birth weight, growth, height, and diet to cancer risk (39). IGF-1 and its binding proteins are important mediators between growth hormone and growth and have been linked to prostate, colorectal, and premenopausal breast cancer (155, 163). Positive associations between height, leg length, childhood growth in relation to age at menarche, and breast cancer may reflect higher levels of IGF-1 and lower levels of binding proteins. Although adult height is not strongly linked to IGF-1 levels, it is associated with childhood growth (15, 103), and so childhood may be the period in which later cancer risk is increased. Additionally, childhood growth is influenced by diet, and both animal and human studies provide evidence that quality of diet and caloric restriction influence growth and cancer risk primarily through the action of IGF-1 (72). There are several possible pathways through which circulating IGF-1 levels could influence breast cancer risk. They could reflect activity of sex hormones, but this seems less likely because associations between IGF-1 and cancer are stronger than with directly measured sex hormones. As a growth promoter, IGF-1 levels may indicate greater cell proliferation and susceptibility to malignant transformation. Alternatively, IGF-1 may influence breast cancer risk through its negative effect on apoptosis.

Perhaps perversely, these same IGF-1 mechanisms may be implicated via greater height, leg length, etc. in decreased risk of cardiovascular diseases as noted above. Nevertheless, greater understanding of IGF-1 may provide insights into the growth mechanisms differentially linked to chronic diseases (39).

CHRONIC OBSTRUCTIVE PULMONARY DISEASE (COPD)   COPD is a heterogeneous outcome characterized by permanent airflow obstruction resulting from the destruction or remodeling of airways. Strachan & Sheikh (181) suggest that COPD results from a series of interacting processes potentially involving respiratory viral infections, atopic reactions (allergies), temporary airflow restrictions in response to irritants (asthma), and chronic secretion of mucous (bronchitis). Burrows and colleagues (22) argue that there are two major types of airway obstruction in adulthood: those related to smoking and those related to asthma and atopic allergy among nonsmokers. Clearly, the duration and intensity of smoking is the major cause of the population health burden of COPD at times when, and in countries where, smoking is common. However, COPD is sometimes prevalent in the absence of a large population smoking burden. For CHD or lung cancer, the age at smoking cessation was important in determining the extent to which disease risk declined over time (154). However, if COPD is related to early lung damage caused by smoking, then even lower levels of cumulative burden to the damaging effects of smoking may still be associated with poorer adult lung function many years later. Thus, the duration and intensity of smoking in early life may be more important for lung function in later life than it is for lung cancer or CHD (51, 80). Other influences over the life course such as birth weight (6), childhood respiratory infections (135), exposure to environmental tobacco smoke (30), outdoor and indoor air pollution (84), diet (97), physical activity and poorer socioeconomic circumstances (41, 101, 123, 135) in early and later life may also be important in COPD.

In terms of early-life influences, studies have suggested that low birth weight infants have an increased risk of respiratory disease in later life (6, 179), which could be owing to poor lung development in utero. Maternal but not paternal smoking has been associated with lower ventilatory function in adults; because maternal smoking during pregnancy is a strong predictor of birth weight, which could affect both in utero lung development as well as exposure to passive smoking in infancy (190). An interaction between maternal smoking and own smoking has been seen concerning adult lung function (189). Childhood respiratory infections of the chest especially before age 2 have been linked to poor adult lung function (135, 171), but these associations are difficult to interpret (180). Childhood chest infections may be associated with adult airflow obstruction for many reasons (181). Poor lung development in utero could increase susceptibility to both chest infections in childhood and adult respiratory disease, or childhood chest illness could cause lung damage, which then influences adult lung disease. Conversely, childhood chest illness and adult lung disease may be just a manifestation of an underlying asthmatic tendency, or both childhood and adult lung dysfunction may be related to the continuity of adverse exposures linked to poor socioeconomic circumstances.

Associations between life course exposures and obstructive airway disease in adulthood are further complicated by the possible role of early-life infections in allergic sensitization. Babies are born with immature immune systems and they develop responses partly on the basis of that to which they are exposed. Thus, there may be one or more critical periods in immune system development when exposure to certain infectious agents is important in programming an appropriate immune system response. Individuals who exhibit less allergic response tend to have greater thymus-derived helper 2 (Th2)–mediated responses, whereas those with atopy tend toward Th1-mediated responses (159) considered to be the normal response for bacterial and viral infections. In a recent review, Prescott (156) concluded that even though these processes affect immune system development, the effects are dependent on the timing of exposure, genetic factors, the nature of the infection, and possibly other factors in the prevailing environment (156). Although there is some support for this infectious-allergic response hypothesis, there is no direct evidence that reduced early-life infectious burden is responsible for documented increases in allergy and asthma (188, 195).

POPULATION LIFE COURSE PROCESSES

The life course approach may be useful when applied to considerations of population health. For example, Figure 2 demonstrates the strong correlation across countries between male stomach cancer mortality (1991–1993) and infant mortality 70 years earlier (126). It is difficult to understand why three countries—Japan, Russia, and Chile—should cluster together on this outcome. They share very little in terms of their current socio-environmental conditions, and historically they are very different countries culturally, economically, and socially. Yet they are

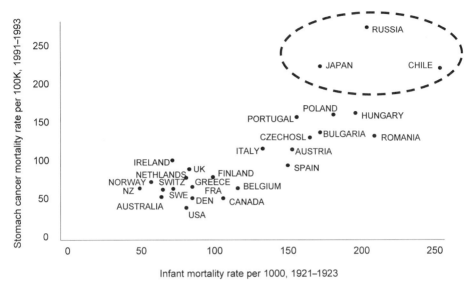

Figure 2   Infant mortality rate (1921–1923) and stomach cancer mortality rate (1991–1993) for men aged 65–74 (126).

all countries that had very high rates of infant mortality in the past, and the current generation dying of stomach cancer is that which, presumably, experienced the high rate of *H. pylori* infection, transmitted in the same way as the diarrheal diseases that killed infants in the past.

One of the more ambitious applications of a life course approach to chronic disease epidemiology is to integrate knowledge from individual level studies to help explain population-level trends in different diseases (32, 45, 116, 125). This means understanding how the array of life course risk factors, such as birth weight, height, diet, behaviors, etc., mentioned in Table 3 are configured across successive birth cohorts, and their long-term trends, and how these trends, given appropriate time lags, map onto trends in different diseases. For instance, if greater birth weight and height are both causally linked with lower CHD risk, then it is not simple to reconcile the consistent secular increases in birth weight and height over time, with the epidemic rise and fall of CHD observed in many countries during the twentieth century. If birth weight and height participate in causal mechanisms (168) sufficient to produce CHD, either these mechanisms must account for a relatively small number of cases or birth weight and height are complementary causes in other sufficient mechanisms involving major risk factors such as high blood lipid levels.

A counter example is smoking and lung cancer. We know that smoking is the most powerful risk factor for lung cancer, and in the United States we know the approximate birth cohort and age distribution of the uptake of smoking (62);

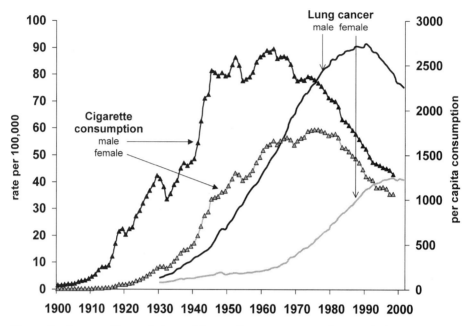

Figure 3   Sex-specific trends in smoking and lung cancer over the twentieth century in the United States.

we also know that the time lag between smoking and lung cancer is about 30–40 years. Although not by any means a perfect concordance, smoking explains most of the differences in lung cancer among individuals, between populations and within-population lung cancer trends (129). From individual-level U.S. data on sex-specific smoking prevalence by birth cohort (21, 62) and historical data on cigarette consumption, we have estimated sex-specific cigarette consumption trends over the twentieth century and show them in relation to sex-specific lung cancer trends in Figure 3 to illustrate this concordance between causation at the individual and population levels between smoking and lung cancer. A similar argument for consistency between individual- and population-level causes might be made for *H. pylori* infection and peptic ulcer and stomach cancer (184, 185), for HPV infection and cervical cancer, for alcohol and liver cirrhosis (151), and for hepatitis C infection and liver cancer (172). However, such examples will be most pertinent in situations where the bulk of cases arise from a small number of sufficient causes with relatively few component causes (168).

Outcomes that have more diverse pathways and more complicated interactions of risk factors make it more difficult to map trends in a single exposure across different birth cohorts onto trends in disease. However, if we had integrated measures based on knowledge of the major risk factors for outcomes such as CHD and how they interacted, then it is likely that a large part of the population-level

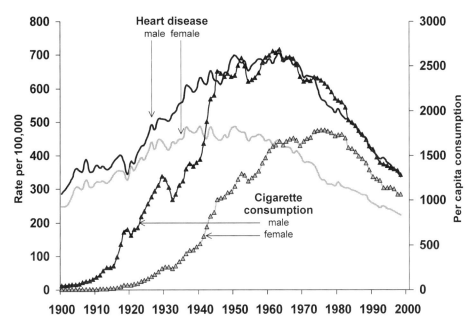

Figure 4   Age-adjusted heart disease mortality and estimated annual adult per capita cigarette consumption, males and females 1900–1998.

trend is explicable in terms of trends in combinations of major risk factors: lipids, hypertension, and smoking (12, 83, 133). Indeed, as we understand more about disease etiology, and about how many conditions that at first sight appear unitary— such as lymphoma—are in fact made up of many constituent diseases of distinct etiological processes and pathophysiology, we may discover that more diseases have a limited number of important sufficient causes. The clear multifactorial nature of CHD may, in fact, be an exception rather than the rule in this respect.

Figure 4 shows male and female heart disease in the United States from 1900–1998, demonstrating the twentieth-century epidemic pattern dominated by male heart disease mortality. An important limitation is that the category of "heart disease" used here is composed of a diverse set of pathological entities with potentially disparate causal mechanisms (131). The generic category of heart disease, which we are forced to use for temporal comparability, includes not only CHD but also congestive heart failure, rheumatic heart disease, arrhythmia, hypertensive heart disease, and others. In addition, the relative contributions of these subcomponents of the generic category of heart disease have changed over time. Nevertheless, it is reasonable to propose that the largest contributor to the rise and subsequent fall in the twentieth-century epidemic of heart disease was CHD.

For males, these patterns suggest that at the population level, the effect of smoking on heart disease is rather immediate. However, the apparent simultaneity of the rise and fall of smoking with heart disease in U.S. men has not been evident in all countries. For example, in the United Kingdom the zenith of smoking was about 10 years prior to the peak of the heart disease epidemic (25). In the United States there seems little or no time lag between the rapid rise of smoking in the population and the equally steep increase and decline in smoking and heart disease. This is not the case for women, where the peak in heart disease occurs 25–30 years before the zenith of smoking. There is clearly a need to examine these sex-specific links between smoking and CHD in more detail—especially concerning the age of initiation in various birth cohorts (78), age at smoking cessation, and their total exposure to smoking. The apparent sex difference in the causal immediacy between smoking and heart disease is not evident for lung cancer (Figure 3), where there is little sex difference in the time lag between the exposure of different birth cohorts to high rates of smoking and the subsequent population yield in lung cancer mortality.

There are three main processes implicated in CHD—development of atheroma, thrombo-embolic processes, and arrhythmia. Smoking may not only affect development of atheroma, but also operate through the thrombo-embolic and/or arrhythmic pathways, thus plausibly being able to influence, almost instantaneously, heart disease. This would be contingent on an underlying susceptibility owing to the development of vulnerable atherosclerotic plaque—itself associated with diet, blood lipids, and blood pressure. Data on blood pressure trends in the United States show strong birth cohort shifts in the whole distribution of blood pressure from the 1950s onward (79). This suggests that each successive generation born after the last decades of the nineteenth century carried with it a more favorable distribution of blood pressure. The U.S. epidemic of heart disease peaked in the 1960s for men— among cohorts born around the turn of the twentieth century. The rapid declines in heart disease after the 1960s are thus compatible with both period declines in smoking and cohort declines in blood pressure in the population. This implies different influences across successive birth cohorts in how both early- and later-life experiences of the conditions predisposing those particular cohorts to adverse risks for adopting (and maintaining) smoking and developing hypertension. With this complex mixture of cohort effects in the increases (and decreases) for some risk factors (hypertension), but period effects in others (smoking), combined with the generally multiplicative nature of the combined influence of CHD risk factors, (177) it is difficult to predict whether cohort or period effects in CHD should be seen. However, a reanalysis of U.K. data suggested that both were evident, but period effects were stronger (24).

The examples offered here of adopting a life course approach at the population level may be even more difficult to apply to other etiologically complex diseases. First, in some instances we have less knowledge of the main individual-level risk factors, so population-level trends in the known risk factors or their combinations do not map easily onto disease trends within and among populations (114); that said, some of the population trend is likely to be explained, even for breast cancer, by complicated interactions and trends in known risk factors. Nevertheless, complex diseases like breast cancer do present something of a paradox in this regard, which awaits greater biological insights into their etiology (124).

Importantly, from a life course perspective, even if we can explain the bulk of the twentieth-century epidemic of chronic diseases like CHD, with the traditional risk factors, we still do not understand the socio-environmental determinants of the changing distributions of these risk factors across the life course of different birth cohorts and social groups over time (45, 110). One important implication for adopting a life course approach would be that apparently novel life course risk factors—such as poor in utero growth, early-life deprivation, or psychosocial factors in adulthood—are most likely to increase CHD risk through their links with conventional risk factors, both at the individual and population level (35). Thus, life course processes are likely to work mainly through the established major proximal adult risk factors (smoking, lipids, hypertension, diabetes). Connections between early- and later-life exposures might occur in several ways. Early-life expsoures could modify the effects of adult exposures—as in lower birth weight, combined with higher adult BMI, and increased risk of diabetes and CHD (a critical period with later effect modification model according to the terminology in Table 1). Alternatively, early-life exposures may act as precursors—as in the tracking of blood pressure and obesity from childhood through adolescence (chain of risk model), or via the timing of exposure—where the amount of pre-pubertal weight gain and age at menarche affect health in adulthood (pathways model); or by accumulating negative exposure over time—as in the amount of smoking and COPD, or cholesterol and CHD.

METHODOLOGICAL CHALLENGES

Adopting a life course approach to chronic disease epidemiology presents multiple methodological and analytic challenges concerning study design, data collection, and interpretation. Fundamentally, investigating life course processes for chronic diseases requires measuring data at multiple time points from birth (or before) to middle and older ages (56, 182) and potentially across generations. Ideally, the timing of these data collections is informed by some knowledge of the relevant latency periods between particular life course exposures and outcomes. For some life course research questions, there are time lags of 50 or more years between exposures and outcomes of interest (e.g., *H. Pylori* infection and stomach cancer). That is why much of the current knowledge in the life course epidemiology of chronic diseases has been derived from reconstructed cohorts where information about early-life conditions and events was gathered from cohorts born in the late nineteenth and early twentieth centuries. One of the limitations of these data is that the life course processes studied in these cohorts are reflections of the past and may not in some cases be as applicable to current generations. Reconstructing early-life exposures from adult recall is limited because it introduces possibilities of bias and measurement error, so objective data collected at the relevant life course stage are most desirable. Innovative designs that combine individual and routinely collected register information for exposures, confounders, and outcomes will be important in this regard. Future life course studies that attempt to collect a diverse array of information about early- and later-life exposures will have high respondent burden, so recruitment and retention over long periods of time will be a major challenge.

Life course exposures may operate through the timing of their action and/or through their accumulation. Testing critical and sensitive-period exposures requires that the exposure is measured at multiple points spanning the hypothesized time period. Such repeatedly measured exposure data are rare and expensive to collect. Similarly, if the exposure is thought to affect the outcome through accumulation, then the exposure needs to be measured at multiple time points. Multiple measures present analytic challenges in how best to represent the accumulation of exposure. Exposure can be averaged across time points, but it is conceptually inadequate to capture accumulation, especially when differences in the tempo or pattern of accumulation are thought to confer differential disease risk. It makes little sense to consider a measure of average growth rate from infancy to adolescence, and innovative methods are beginning to be applied to capture the dynamic trajectories of exposure accumulation (50).

Finally, long-term life course studies of chronic disease will make the problems of missing data even more acute than they are currently, and so advances in multiple imputation techniques are likely to be important (157). Additionally, innovative design through replenishment samples and analytic methods will need to be applied to avoid making inferences from overly selected study samples.

CONCLUSIONS

We have provided a necessarily selective overview of life course approaches to chronic disease epidemiology, in terms of its background, theories, and empirical evidence. Additionally, we have underscored that a life course approach offers a way to conceptualize how underlying socio-environmental determinants of health, experienced at different life course stages, can differentially influence the development of chronic diseases, as mediated through proximal specific biological processes. The life course perspective has a long history in sociological and psychological sciences (57), but it is still in its relative infancy within epidemiology. We are certain that the contents of this review will seem simplistic and naive within a relatively short time period, thus demonstrating the vitality that a life course approach can bring to epidemiology.

ACKNOWLEDGMENTS

John Lynch and George Davey Smith were supported in part by the Robert Wood Johnson Foundation, Investigator Awards in Health Policy Research Program.

The *Annual Review of Public Health* is online at
http://publhealth.annualreviews.org

LITERATURE CITED

1. 2001. Gastric cancer and Helicobacter pylori: a combined analysis of 12 case control studies nested within prospective cohorts. *Gut* 49:347–53
2. Aboderin I, Kalache A, Ben-Shlomo Y, Lynch J, Yajnik C, Kuh D, eds. 2002. *Life Course Perspectives on Coronary Heart Disease, Stroke and Diabetes: Key Issues and Implications for Policy and Research.* Geneva: WHO
3. Ahlgren M, Sorensen T, Wohlfahrt J, Haflidadottir A, Holst C, Melbye M. 2003. Birth weight and risk of breast cancer in a cohort of 106,504 women. *Int. J. Cancer* 107:997–1000
4. Akerblom HK, Viikari J, Raitakari OT, Uhari M. 1999. Cardiovascular risk in young Finns Study: general outline and recent developments. *Ann. Med.* 31(Suppl. 1):45–54
5. Bao W, Threefoot SA, Srinivasan SR, Berenson GS. 1995. Essential hypertension predicted by tracking of elevated blood pressure from childhood to adulthood: the Bogalusa Heart Study. *Am. J. Hypertens.* 8:657–65
6. Barker DJ, Godfrey KM, Fall C, Osmond C, Winter PD, Shaheen SO. 1991. Relation of birth weight and childhood respiratory infection to adult lung function and death from chronic obstructive airways disease. *Br. Med. J.* 303(6804):671–75
7. Barker DJ, Osmond C. 1986. Infant mortality, childhood nutrition, and ischaemic heart disease in England and Wales. *Lancet* 1:1077–81
8. Barker DJ, Winter PD, Osmond C, Margetts B, Simmonds SJ. 1989. Weight in infancy and death from ischaemic heart disease. *Lancet* 2:577–80
9. Barker DJP, Forsén T, Uutela A, Os-

mond C, Eriksson JG. 2001. Size at birth and resilience to effects of poor living conditions in adult life: longitudinal study. *Br. Med. J.* 323:1273–76
10. Barker DJP, Osmond C. 1987. Death rates from stroke in England and Wales predicted from past maternal mortality. *Br. Med. J.* 295:83–86
11. Batty D, Leon D. 2003. Socioeconomic position and coronary heart disease risk factors in children and young people. See Ref. 77, pp. 79–118
12. Beaglehole R, Magnus P. 2002. The search for new risk factors for coronary heart disease: occupational therapy for epidemiologists? *Int. J. Epidemiol.* 31(6):1117–22
13. Beebe-Dimmer J, Lynch JW, Turrell G, Lustgarten S, Raghunathan T, Kaplan GA. 2004. Childhood and adult socioeconomic conditions and 31-year mortality risk in women. *Am. J. Epidemiol.* 159(5):481–90
14. Ben-Shlomo Y, Davey Smith G. 1991. Deprivation in infancy or in adult life: Which is more important for mortality risk? *Lancet* 337:530–34
15. Ben-Shlomo Y, Holly J, McCarthy A, Savage P, Davies D, et al. 2003. An investigation of fetal, postnatal and childhood growth with insulin-like growth factor I and binding protein 3 in adulthood. *Clin. Endocrinol.* 59(3):366–73
16. Ben-Shlomo Y, Kuh D. 2002. A life course approach to chronic disease epidemiology: conceptual models, empirical challenges and interdisciplinary perspectives. *Int. J. Epidemiol.* 31:285–93
17. Berenson GS, Srinivasan SR, Bao W, Newman WP, Tracy RE, Wattigney WA. 1998. Association between multiple cardiovascular risk factors and

atherosclerosis in children and young adults. *N. Engl. J. Med.* 338:1650–56

18. Berenson GS, Srinivasan SR, Freedman DS, Radhakrishnamurthy B, Dakferes ERJ. 1987. Atherosclerosis and its evolution in childhood. *Am. J. Med. Sci.* 294:429–40

19. Bhargava SK, Sachdev HS, Fall CH, Osmond C, Lakshmy R, et al. 2004. Relation of serial changes in childhood body-mass index to impaired glucose tolerance in young adulthood. *N. Engl. J. Med.* 350:865–75

20. Brenner H, Arndt V, Stegmaier C, Ziegler H, Rothenbacher D. 2004. Is helicobacter pylori infection a necessary condition for noncardia gastric cancer? *Am. J. Epidemiol.* 159(3):252–58

21. Burns DM, Lee L, Shen LZ, Gilpin E, Tolley HD, et al. 1997. Cigarette smoking behavior in the United States. In *Smoking and Tobacco Control Monograph 8: Changes in Cigarette-Related Disease Risks and Their Implications for Prevention and Control*, ed. DM Burns, L Garfinkel, JM Samet, pp. 13–42. Bethesda, MD: US Dept. HHS, Natl. Cancer Inst.

22. Burrows B, Bloom JW, Traver GA, Cline MG. 1987. The course and prognosis of different forms of chronic airways obstruction in a sample from the general population. *N. Engl. J. Med.* 317(21):1309–14

23. Cavill N, Biddle S. 2003. The determinants of young people's participation in physical activity, and investigation of tracking of physical activity from youth to adulthood. See Ref. 77, pp. 179–98

24. Charlton J, Murphy M, eds. 1994. *The Health of Adult Britain 1841–1994.* London: The Station. Off.

25. Charlton J, Murphy M, Khaw KT, Ebrahim S, Davey Smith G. 1997. Cardiovascular diseases. See Ref. 24, pp. 60–80

26. Ciocco A, Klein H, Palmer CE. 1941. Child health and the selective service physical standards. *Public Health Rep.* 56:2365–75

27. Claussen B, Davey Smith G, Thelle D. 2003. Impact of childhood and adulthood socioeconomic position on cause specific mortality: the Oslo Mortality Study. *J. Epidemiol. Community Health* 57(1):40–45

28. Colditz GA. 1993. Epidemiology of breast cancer. Findings from the nurses' health study. *Cancer* 71:1480–89

29. Correa P, Fontham ET, Bravo JC, Bravo LE, Ruiz B, et al. 2000. Chemoprevention of gastric dysplasia: randomized trial of antioxidant supplements and antihelicobacter pylori therapy. *J. Natl. Cancer Inst.* 92:1881–88

30. Coultas DB. 1998. Health effects of passive smoking. 8. Passive smoking and risk of adult asthma and COPD: an update. *Thorax* 53(5):381–87

31. Cremonini F, Gabrielli M, Gasbarrini G, Pola P, Gasbarrini A. 2004. The relationship between chronic H. pylori infection, CagA seropositivity and stroke: meta-analysis. *Atherosclerosis* 173(2):253–59

32. Davey Smith G. 1997. Socioeconomic differentials. See Ref. 111, pp. 242–73

33. Davey Smith G. 2001. Genetic risk factors in mothers and offspring. *Lancet* 358:1268

34. Davey Smith G. 2003. Lifecourse approaches to health inequalities. In *Health Inequalities: Lifecourse Approaches*, ed. G Davey Smith, pp. xii–lix. Bristol: Policy Press

35. Davey Smith G. 2004. The biopsychosocial approach: a note of caution. In *Understanding Illness: The Biopsychosocial Approach*, ed. PD White. Oxford: Oxford Univ. Press. In press

36. Davey Smith G, Ebrahim S. 2003. 'Mendelian randomization': Can genetic epidemiology contribute to understanding environmental determinants of disease? *Int. J. Epidemiol.* 32(1):1–22

37. Davey Smith G, Greenwood R, Gunnell D, Sweetnam P, Yarnell J, Elwood P.

2001. Leg length, insulin resistance, and coronary heart disease risk: The Caerphilly Study. *J. Epidemiol. Community Health* 55:867–72

38. Davey Smith G, Gunnell D, Ben Shlomo Y. 2000. Life-course approaches to socioeconomic differentials in cause-specific mortality. In *Poverty, Inequality and Health*, ed. D Leon, G Walt, pp. 88–124. London: Oxford Univ. Press

39. Davey Smith G, Gunnell D, Holly J. 2000. Cancer and insulin-like growth factor-I: a potential mechanism linking the environment with cancer risk. *Br. Med. J.* 321:847–48

40. Davey Smith G, Hart C, Blane D, Gillis C, Hawthorne V. 1997. Lifetime socioeconomic position and mortality: prospective observational study. *Br. Med. J.* 314(7080):547–52

41. Davey Smith G, Hart C, Blane D, Hole D. 1998. Adverse socioeconomic conditions in childhood and cause specific adult mortality: prospective observational study. *Br. Med. J.* 316(7145): 1631–35

42. Davey Smith G, Hart C, Ferrell C, Upton M, Hole D, et al. 1997. Birth weight of offspring and mortality in the Renfrew and Paisley study: prospective observational study. *Br. Med. J.* 315:1189–93

43. Davey Smith G, Hart C, Upton M, Hole D, Gillis C, et al. 2000. Height and risk of death among men and women: aetiological implications of associations with cardiorespiratory disease and cancer mortality. *J. Epidemiol. Community Health* 54:97–103

44. Davey Smith G, Kuh D. 2001. Commentary: William Ogilvy Kermack and the childhood origins of adult health and disease. *Int. J. Epidemiol.* 30:696–703

45. Davey Smith G, Lynch J. 2005. Life course influences on coronary heart disease. In *Coronary Heart Disease Epidemiology*, ed. M Marmot, P Elliot. London: Oxford Univ. Press. In press

46. Davey Smith G, Lynch JW. 2004. So-cioeconomic differentials. See Ref. 112, pp. 77–115. In press

47. Davey Smith G, Sterne JAC, Tynelius P, Rasmussen F. 2004. Birth characteristics of offspring and parental diabetes: evidence for the fetal insulin hypothesis. *J. Epidemiol. Community Health* 58(2):126–28

48. Davey Smith G, Whitley E, Gissler M, Hemminki E. 2000. Birth dimensions of offspring, premature birth, and the mortality of mothers. *Lancet* 256:2066–67

49. Davis PH, Dawson JD, Riley WA, Lauer RM. 2001. Carotid intimal-medial thickness is related to cardiovascular risk factors measured from childhood through middle age: the Muscatine study. *Circulation* 104:2815

50. De Stavola BL, dos Santos Silva I, McCormack V, Hardy RJ, Kuh DJ, Wadsworth MEJ. 2004. Childhood growth and breast cancer. *Am. J. Epidemiol.* 159(7):671–82

51. Doll R, Peto R, Boreham J, Sutherland I. 2004. Mortality in relation to smoking: 50 years' observations on male British doctors. *Br. Med. J.* 328(7455):1519–28

52. dos Santos Silva I, De Stavola B. 2002. Breast cancer etiology: Where do we go from here? See Ref. 115, pp. 44–63

53. Drake AJ, Walker BR. 2004. The intergenerational effects of fetal programming: non-genomic mechanisms for the inheritance of low birth weight and cardiovascular risk. *J. Endocrinol.* 180(1):1–16

54. Dubos R, Savage D, Schaedler R. 1966. Biological freudianism: lasting effects of early environment influences. *Pediatrics* 38:789–800

55. Duncan GJ, Yeung WJ, Brooks-Gunn J, Smith JR. 1998. How much does childhood poverty affect the life chances of children? *Am. Sociol. Rev.* 63:406–23

56. Eaton WW. 2002. The logic for a conception-to-death cohort study. *Ann. Epidemiol.* 12:445–51

57. Elder GH. 1994. Time, human agency,

and social change: perspectives on the life course. *Soc. Psychol. Q.* 57:4–14

58. Enos MW, Holmes LCR, Beyer CJ. 1953. Coronary disease among United States soldiers killed in action in Korea. *JAMA* 31:1117–22

59. Eriksson JG, Forsen T, Tuomilehto J, Osmond C, Barker DJ. 2001. Early growth and coronary heart disease in later life: longitudinal study. *Br. Med. J.* 322:949–53

60. Eriksson JG, Forsen T, Tuomilehto J, Osmond C, Barker DJ. 2003. Early adiposity rebound in childhood and risk of Type 2 diabetes in adult life. *Diabetologia* 46:190–94

61. Eriksson JG, Forsen T, Tuomilehto J, Winter PD, Osmond C, Barker DJ. 1999. Catch-up growth in childhood and death from coronary heart disease: longitudinal study. *Br. Med. J.* 318:427–31

62. Escobedo L, Peddicord J. 1996. Smoking prevalence in US birth cohorts: the influence of gender and education. *Am. J. Public Health* 86(2):231–36

63. Fang J, Madhavan S, Alderman MH. 1996. The association between birthplace and mortality from cardiovascular causes among black and white residents of New York City. *N. Engl. J. Med.* 335:1545–51

64. Felitti VJ, Anda RF, Nordenberg D, Williamson DF, Spitz AM, et al. 1998. Relationship of childhood abuse and household dysfunction to many of the leading causes of death in adults. The Adverse Childhood Experiences (ACE) Study. *Am. J. Prev. Med.* 14:245–58

65. Forouhi N, Hall E, McKeigue P. 2004. A life course approach to diabetes. See Ref. 112, pp. 166–99. In press

66. Forsdahl A. 1977. Are poor living conditions in childhood and adolescence an important risk factor for arteriosclerotic heart disease? *Br. J. Prev. Soc. Med.* 31: 91–95

67. Forsdahl A. 1978. Living conditions in childhood and subsequent development of risk factors for arteriosclerotic heart disease. The cardiovascular survey in Finnmark 1974–75. *J. Epidemiol. Community Health* 32:34–37

68. Forsdahl A. 2002. Observations throwing light on the high mortality in the county of Finnmark: Is the high mortality today a late effect of very poor living conditions in childhood and adolescence? *Int. J. Epidemiol.* 31(2): 302–8

69. Forsen T, Eriksson J, Tuomilehto J, Reunanen A, Osmond C, Barker D. 2000. The fetal and childhood growth of persons who develop type 2 diabetes. *Ann. Intern. Med.* 133:176–82

70. Frankel S, Davey Smith G, Gunnell D. 1999. Childhood socioeconomic position and adult cardiovascular mortality: the Boyd Orr cohort. *Am. J. Epidemiol.* 150:1081–84

71. Frankel S, Elwood P, Sweetnam P, Yarnell J, Davey Smith G. 1996. Birthweight, body-mass index in middle age, and incident coronary heart disease. *Lancet* 348:1478–80

72. Frankel S, Gunnell DJ, Peters TJ, Maynard M, Davey Smith G. 1998. Childhood energy intake and adult mortality from cancer: the Boyd Orr Cohort Study. *Br. Med. J.* 316:499–504

73. Freedman DS, Dietz WH, Srinivasan SR, Berenson GS. 1999. The relation of overweight to cardiovascular risk factors among children and adolescents: the Bogalusa Heart Study. *Pediatrics* 103(6):1175–82

74. Galobardes B, Lynch JW, Davey Smith G. 2004. Childhood socioeconomic circumstances and cause-specific mortality in adulthood: systematic review and interpretation. *Epidemiol. Rev.* 26:7–21. In press

75. Geleijnse JM, Hofman A, Witteman JC, Hazebroek AA, Valkenburg HA, Grobbee DE. 1997. Long-term effects of neonatal sodium restriction on blood pressure. *Hypertension* 29:913–17

76. Gerver WJM, Bruin RD. 1995. Relationship between height, sitting height and subischial leg length in Dutch children: presentation of normal values. *Acta Pediatr.* 84:532–35

77. Giles A, ed. 2003. *A Lifecourse Approach to Coronary Heart Disease Prevention.* London: Natl. Heart Forum/The Station. Off.

78. Glied S. 2003. Is smoking delayed smoking averted? *Am. J. Public Health* 93:412–16

79. Goff DC, Howard G, Russell GB, Labarthe DR. 2001. Birth cohort evidence of population influences on blood pressure in the United States, 1887–1994. *Ann. Epidemiol.* 11:271–79

80. Gold DR, Wang X, Wypij D, Speizer FE, Ware JH, Dockery DW. 1996. Effects of cigarette smoking on lung function in adolescent boys and girls. *N. Engl. J. Med.* 335(13):931–37

81. Goodman KJ, Correa P. 2000. Transmission of *Helicobacter pylori* among siblings. *Lancet* 355:358–62

82. Greenland P, Gidding SS, Tracy RP. 2002. Commentary: Lifelong prevention of atherosclerosis: the critical importance of major risk factor exposures. *Int. J. Epidemiol.* 31(6):1129–34

83. Greenland P, Knoll MD, Stamler J, Neaton JD, Dyer AR, et al. 2003. Major risk factors as antecedents of fatal and nonfatal coronary heart disease events. *JAMA* 290(7):891–97

84. Greer JR, Abbey DE, Burchette RJ. 1993. Asthma related to occupational and ambient air pollutants in nonsmokers. *J. Occup. Med.* 35(9):909–15

85. Gunnell D, Okasha M, Davey Smith G, Oliver SE, Sandhu J, Holly JMP. 2001. Height, leg length, and cancer risk: a systematic review. *Epidemiol. Rev.* 23:313–42

86. Hales CN, Barker DJ. 1992. Type 2 (non-insulin-dependent) diabetes mellitus: the thrifty phenotype hypothesis. *Diabetologia* 35:595–601

87. Halfon N, Hochstein M. 2002. Life course health development: an integrated framework for developing health, policy, and research. *Milbank Q.* 80(3):433–79

88. Hallqvist J, Lynch JW, Blane D, Bartley M, Lange T. 2004. Critical period, accumulation and social trajectory: Can we empirically distinguish lifecourse processes? *Soc. Sci. Med.* 58:1555–62

89. Harding JE. 2001. The nutritional basis of the fetal origins of adult disease. *Int. J. Epidemiol.* 30:15–23

90. Hart CL, Davey Smith G. 2003. Relation between number of siblings and adult mortality and stroke risk: 25 year follow up of men in the Collaborative study. *J. Epidemiol. Community Health* 57(5):385–91

91. Hart CL, Hole DJ, Davey Smith G. 2000. The relation between cholesterol and haemorrhagic or ischaemic stroke in the Renfrew/Paisley study. *J. Epidemiol. Community Health* 54(11):874–75

92. Hattersley AT, Tooke JE. 1999. The fetal insulin hypothesis: an alternative explanation of the association of low birthweight with diabetes and vascular disease. *Lancet* 353:1789–92

93. Heart Protection Study Collaborative Group. 2002. MRC/BHF Heart Protection Study of cholesterol lowering with simvastatin in 20,536 high-risk individuals: a randomised placebo-controlled trial. *Lancet* 360(9326):7–22

94. Hemminki K, Li X, Czene K. 2002. Cancer risks in first-generation immigrants to Sweden. *Int. J. Cancer* 99:218–28

95. Hofman A, Hazebroek A, Valkenburg HA. 1983. A randomized trial of sodium intake and blood pressure in newborn infants. *JAMA* 250(3):370–73

96. Holman RL. 1961. Atherosclerosis: a pediatric nutrition problem. *Am. J. Clin. Nutr.* 9:565–69

97. Hu G, Cassano PA. 2000. Antioxidant nutrients and pulmonary function: the Third National Health and Nutrition

Examination Survey (NHANES III). *Am. J. Epidemiol.* 151(10):975–81

98. Huxley RR, Neil HA. 2004. Does maternal nutrition in pregnancy and birth weight influence levels of CHD risk factors in adult life? *Br. J. Nutr.* 91(3):459–68

99. Hyppönen E, Leon DA, Kenward MG, Lithell H. 2001. Prenatal growth and risk of occlusive and haemorrhagic stroke in Swedish men and women born 1915–29: historical cohort study. *Br. Med. J.* 323:1033

100. Innes KE, Byers TE, Marshall JA, Baron A, Orleans M, Hamman RF. 2002. Association of a woman's own birth weight with subsequent risk for gestational diabetes. *JAMA* 287:2534–41

101. Jackson B, Kubzansky LD, Cohen S, Weiss S, Wright RJ. 2004. A matter of life and breath: childhood socioeconomic status is related to young adult pulmonary function in the CARDIA study. *Int. J. Epidemiol.* 33(2):271–78

102. Joseph KS, Kramer MS. 1996. Review of the evidence on fetal and early childhood antecedents of adults chronic disease. *Epidemiol. Rev.* 18:158–74

103. Juul A, Holm K, Kastrup KW, Pedersen SA, Michaelsen KF, et al. 1997. Free insulin-like growth factor I serum levels in 1430 healthy children and adults, and its diagnostic value in patients suspected of growth hormone deficiency. *J. Clin. Endocrinol. Metab.* 82:2497–502

104. Kannel WB, Dawber TR. 1972. Atherosclerosis as a pediatric problem. *J. Pediatr.* 80(4):544–54

105. Kawachi I, Colditz GA, Stampfer MJ, Willett WC, Manson JE, et al. 1994. Smoking cessation and time course of decreased risks of coronary heart disease in middle-aged women. *Arch. Intern. Med.* 154(2):169–75

106. Kermack WO, McKendrick AG, McKinlay PL. 2001. Death-rates in Great Britain and Sweden. Some general regu-

larities and their significance. *Int. J. Epidemiol.* 30:678–83

107. Kermack WO, McKendrick AG, McKinlay PL. 1934. Death-rates in Great Britain and Sweden. Some general regularities and their signifcance. *Lancet* 31:698–703 [Reprinted in 2001. *Int. J. Epidemiol.* 30:678–83]

108. King H, Aubert RE, Herman WH. 1998. Global burden of diabetes, 1995–2025: prevalence, numerical estimates, and projections. *Diabetes Care* 21:1414–31

109. Klag MJ, Ford DE, Mead LA, He J, Whelton PK, et al. 1993. Serum cholesterol in young men and subsequent cardiovascular disease. *N. Engl. J. Med.* 328:313–18

110. Krieger N, Davey Smith G. 2004. "Bodies count," and body counts: social epidemiology and embodying inquality. *Epidemiol. Rev.* 26:92–103

111. Kuh D, Ben-Shlomo Y. 1997. *A Life Course Approach to Chronic Disease Epidemiology.* New York: Oxford Univ. Press

112. Kuh D, Ben-Shlomo Y. 2004. *A Life Course Approach to Chronic Disease Epidemiology.* New York: Oxford Univ. Press. 2nd ed.

113. Kuh D, Ben-Shlomo Y, Lynch J, Hallqvist J, Power C. 2003. Life course epidemiology. *J. Epidemiol. Community Health* 57(10):778–83

114. Kuh D, dos Santos Silva I, Barrett-Connor E. 2002. Disease trends in women living in established market economies: evidence of cohort effects during the epidemiological transition. See Ref. 115, pp. 347–73

115. Kuh D, Hardy R, eds. 2002. *Life Course Approach to Women's Health.* Oxford: Oxford Univ. Press

116. Kuh DL, Power C, Rodgers B. 1991. Secular trends in social class and sex differences in adult height. *Int. J. Epidemiol.* 20:1001–9

117. Kvaavik E, Tell GS, Klepp KI. 2003. Predictors and tracking of body mass

index from adolescence into adulthood: follow-up of 18 to 20 years in the Oslo Youth Study. *Arch. Pediatr. Adolesc. Med.* 157(12):1212–18

118. Lampl M, Jeanty P. 2003. Timing is everything: a reconsideration of fetal growth velocity patterns identifies the importance of individual and sex differences. *Am. J. Hum. Biol.* 15:667–80

119. Lauer RM, Clarke WR. 1990. Use of cholesterol measurements in childhood for the prediction of adult hypercholesterolemia. The Muscatine Study. *JAMA* 264(23):3034–38

120. Lawlor D, Ben-Shlomo Y, Leon D. 2004. Pre-adult influences on cardiovascular disease. See Ref. 112, pp. 41–76

121. Lawlor DA, Davey Smith G, Leon D, Sterne J, Ebrahim S. 2002. Secular trends in mortality by stroke subtype over the twentieth century: resolution of the stroke-coronary heart disease paradox? *Lancet* 360:1818–23

122. Lawlor DA, Ebrahim S, Davey Smith G. 2002. The association between components of adult height and type II diabetes and insulin resistance: British Women's Heart Health Study. *Diabetologia* 45:1097–106

123. Lawlor DA, Ebrahim S, Davey Smith G. 2004. Association between self-reported childhood socioeconomic position and adult lung function: findings from the British Women's Heart and Health Study. *Thorax* 59:199–203

124. Leon D. 2002. Commentary on "Disease trends in women living in established market economies: evidence of cohort effects during the epidemiological transition." See Ref. 115, pp. 366–73

125. Leon DA. 2001. Common threads: underlying components of inequalities in mortality between and within countries. In *Poverty, Inequality and Health*, ed. DA Leon, G Walt, pp. 58–87. Oxford: Oxford Univ. Press

126. Leon DA, Davey Smith G. 2000. Infant mortality, stomach cancer, stroke, and

coronary heart disease: ecological analysis. *Br. Med. J.* 320:1705–6

127. Leon DA, Lithell HO, Vågerö D, Koupilová I, Mohsen R, et al. 1998. Reduced fetal growth rate and increased risk of death from ischaemic heart disease: cohort study of 15000 Swedish men and women born 1915–29. *Br. Med. J.* 317:241–45

128. Li S, Chen W, Srinivasan SR, Bond MG, Tang R, et al. 2003. Childhood cardiovascular risk factors and carotid vascular changes in adulthood: the Bogalusa Heart Study. *JAMA* 290(17):2271–76

129. Lopez AD. 1995. The lung cancer epidemic in developed countries. In *Adult Mortality in Developed Countries: From Description to Explanation*, ed. AD Lopez, G Caselli, T Valkonen, pp. 111–34. New York: Oxford Univ. Press

130. Lucas A, Fewtrell MS, Cole TJ. 1999. Fetal origins of adult disease: the hypothesis revisited. *Br. Med. J.* 319:245–49

131. Lynch J, Davey Smith G, Harper S, Hillemeier M. 2004. Is income inequality a determinant of population health? Part 2. U.S. national and regional trends in income inequality and age- and cause-specific mortality. *Milbank Q.* 82:355–400

132. Lynch JW, Kaplan GA, Shema SJ. 1997. Cumulative impact of sustained economic hardship on physical, cognitive, psychological, and social functioning. *N. Engl. J. Med.* 337(26):1889–95

133. Magnus P, Beaglehole R. 2001. The real contribution of the major risk factors to the coronary epidemics—time to end the 'only-50%' myth. *Arch. Intern. Med.* 161:2657–60

134. Mahoney LT, Lauer RM, Lee J, Clarke WR. 1991. Factors affecting tracking of coronary heart disease risk factors in children. The Muscatine Study. *Ann. NY Acad. Sci.* 623:120–32

135. Mann SL, Wadsworth ME, Colley JR. 1992. Accumulation of factors influencing respiratory illness in members of

a national birth cohort and their offspring. *J. Epidemiol. Community Health* 46(3):286–92

136. Martin RM, Ness AR, Gunnell D, Emmett P, Davey Smith G. 2004. Does breast-feeding in infancy lower blood pressure in childhood? The Avon Longitudinal Study of Parents and Children (ALSPAC). *Circulation* 109(10):1259–66

137. McCarron P, Davey Smith G. 2003. Physiological measurements in children and young people, and risk of coronary heart disease in adults. See Ref. 77, pp. 49–78

138. McCarron P, Davey Smith G, Okasha M, McEwen J. 2000. Blood pressure in young adulthood and mortality from cadiovascular disease. *Lancet* 355:1430–31

139. McCarron P, Hart CL, Hole D, Davey Smith G. 2001. The relation between adult height and haemorrhagic and ischaemic stroke in the Renfrew/Paisley study. *J. Epidemiol. Community Health* 55:404–5

140. McCarron P, Okasha M, McEwen J, Davey Smith G. 2001. Changes in blood pressure among students attending Glasgow University between 1948 and 1968: analyses of cross sectional surveys. *Br. Med. J.* 322:885–89

141. McCarron P, Davey Smith G, Okasha M, McEwen J. 2000. Blood pressure in young adulthood and mortality from cardiovascular disease. *Lancet* 355:1430–31

142. McCarron P, Davey Smith G, Okasha M, McEwen J. 2001. Smoking in adolescence and young adulthood and mortality in later life: prospective observational study. *J. Epidemiol. Community Health* 55:334–35

143. McNamara JJ, Molot MA, Stremple JF, Cutting RT. 1971. Coronary artery disease in combat casualties in Vietnam. *JAMA* 216:1185–87

144. Michels KB, Ekbom A. 2004. Caloric restriction and incidence of breast cancer. *JAMA* 291:1226–30

144a. Milton J. 1667. *Paradise Lost*. London: Peter Parker

145. Miura K, Daviglus ML, Dyer AR, Liu K, Garside DB, et al. 2001. Relationship of blood pressure to 25-year mortality due to coronary heart disease, cardiovascular diseases, and all causes in young adult men: the Chicago Heart Association Detection Project in Industry. *Arch. Intern. Med.* 161:1501–8

146. Moceri VM, Kukull WA, Emanual I, van Belle G, Starr JR, et al. 2001. Using census data and birth certificates to reconstruct the early-life socioeconomic environment and the relation to the development of Alzheimer's disease. *Epidemiology* 12:383–89

147. Mokdad AH, Ford ES, Bowman BA, Dietz WH, Vinicor F, et al. 2003. Prevalence of obesity, diabetes, and obesity-related health risk factors, 2001. *JAMA* 289(1):76–79

148. Munoz N, Bosch FX, de Sanjose S, Herrero R, Castellsague X, et al. 2003. Epidemiologic classification of human papillomavirus types associated with cervical cancer. *N. Engl. J. Med.* 348(6):518–27

149. Myers L, Coughlin SS, Webber LS, Srinivasan SR, Berenson GS. 1995. Prediction of adult cardiovascular multifactorial risk status from childhood risk factor levels. The Bogalusa Heart Study. *Am. J. Epidemiol.* 142:918–24

150. Newsome CA, Shiell AW, Fall CHD, Phillips DIW, Shier R, Law CM. 2003. Is birth weight related to later glucose and insulin metabolism?—a systematic review. *Diabet. Med.* 20:339–48

151. Norstrom T, Skog OJ. 2001. Alcohol and mortality: methodological and analytical issues in aggregate analyses. *Addiction* 96:S5–17

152. Okasha M, McCarron P, Gunnell D, Davey Smith G. 2003. Exposures in childhood, adolescence and early

adulthood and breast cancer risk: a systematic review of the literature. *Breast Cancer Res. Treat.* 78:223–76

153. Osmond C, Barker DJP, Winter PD, Fall CHD, Simmonds SJ. 1993. Early growth and death from cardiovascular disease in women. *Br. Med. J.* 307:1519–24

154. Peto R, Darby S, Deo H, Silcocks P, Whitley E, Doll R. 2000. Smoking, smoking cessation, and lung cancer in the UK since 1950: combination of national statistics with two case-control studies. *Br. Med. J.* 321(7257):323–29

155. Pollak MN, Schernhammer ES, Hankinson SE. 2004. Insulin-like growth factors and neoplasia. *Nat. Rev. Cancer* 4(7):505–18

156. Prescott SL. 2003. Allergy: the price we pay for cleaner living? *Ann. Allergy Asthma Immunol.* 90(Suppl. 3):64–70

157. Raghunathan TE. 2004. What do we do with missing data? Some options for analysis of incomplete data. *Annu. Rev. Public Health* 25(1):99–117

158. Raitakari OT, Juonala M, Kahonen M, Taittonen L, Laitinen T, et al. 2003. Cardiovascular risk factors in childhood and carotid artery intima-media thickness in adulthood: the Cardiovascular Risk in Young Finns Study. *JAMA* 290:2277–83

159. Rao A, Avni O. 2000. Molecular aspects of T-cell differentiation. *Br. Med. Bull.* 56(4):969–84

160. Rasmussen F, Davey Smith G, Sterne J, Tynelius P, Leon DA. 2001. Birth characteristics of offspring and parental diabetes. *Am. J. Epidemiol.* 153:S47

161. Rasmussen F, Sterne J, Davey Smith G, Tynelius P, Leon DA. 2001. Fetal growth is associated with parents' cardiovascular mortality. *Am. J. Epidemiol.* 153(Suppl.):S98

162. Reaven GM. 1988. Banting lecture 1988. Role of insulin resistance in human disease. *Diabetes* 37:1595–607

163. Renehan AG, Zwahlen M, Nimder C, O'Dwyer S, Shalet SM, Egger M. 2004. Insulin-like growth factor (IGF-1), IGF

binding protein-3, and cancer risk: systematic review and meta-regression analysis. *Lancet* 363:1346–53

164. Rich-Edwards JW, Colditz GA, Stampfer MJ, Willett WC, Gillman MW, et al. 1999. Birthweight and the risk for type 2 diabetes mellitus in adult women. *Ann. Intern. Med.* 130:278–84

165. Rich-Edwards JW, Manson JE, Stampfer MJ, Colditz GA, Willett WC, et al. 1995. Height and the risk of cardiovascular disease in women. *Am. J. Epidemiol.* 142:909–17

166. Rose G. 1982. Incubation period of coronary heart disease. *Br. Med. J. Clin. Res. Ed.* 284:1600–1

167. Roseboom TJ, van der Meulen JHP, Osmond C, Barker DJP, Ravelli ACJ, et al. 2000. Coronary heart disease after prenatal exposure to the Dutch famine, 1944–45. *Heart* 84:595–98

168. Rothman KJ. 1976. Causes. *Am. J. Epidemiol.* 104:587–92

169. Schiffman MH, Brinton LA. 1995. The epidemiology of cervical carcinogenesis. *Cancer* 76:1888–901

170. Scholl TO, Sowers M, Chen X, Lenders C. 2001. Maternal glucose concentration influences fetal growth, gestation, and pregnancy complications. *Am. J. Epidemiol.* 154:514–20

171. Shaheen SO, Barker DJ, Shiell AW, Crocker FJ, Wield GA, Holgate ST. 1994. The relationship between pneumonia in early childhood and impaired lung function in late adult life. *Am. J. Respir. Crit. Care Med.* 149(3):616–19

172. Shibuya K, Yano E. 2004. Regression analysis of trends in mortality from hepatocellular carcinoma in Japan, 1972–2001. *Int. J. Epidemiol.* In press

173. Song Y-M, Davey Smith G, Sung J. 2003. Adult height and cause-specific mortality: a large prospective study of South Korean men. *Am. J. Epidemiol.* 158(5):479–85

174. Deleted in proof

175. Song Y-M, Sung J, Davey Smith G,

Ebrahim S. 2004. Body mass index and ischemic and hemorrhagic stroke: a prospective study in Korean men. *Stroke* 35(4):831–36

176. Song Y-M, Sung J, Lawlor DA, Davey Smith G, Shin Y, Ebrahim S. 2004. Blood pressure, haemorrhagic stroke, and ischaemic stroke: the Korean national prospective occupational cohort study. *Br. Med. J.* 328(7435):324–25

177. Stamler J. 1992. Established major risk factors. In *Coronary Heart Disease Epidemiology: From Aetiology to Public Health*, ed. M Marmot, P Elliot, pp. 35–66. Oxford: Oxford Univ. Press

178. Stanner SA, Bulmer K, Andres C, Lantseva OE, Borodina V, et al. 1997. Does malnutrition in utero determine diabetes and coronary heart disease in adulthood? Results from the Leningrad siege study, a cross sectional study. *Br. Med. J.* 315:1342–48

179. Stein CE, Kumaran K, Fall CH, Shaheen SO, Osmond C, Barker DJ. 1997. Relation of fetal growth to adult lung function in south India. *Thorax* 52(10):895–99

180. Strachan DP. 1997. Respiratory and allergic diseases. See Ref. 111, pp. 101–20

181. Strachan DP, Sheikh A. 2004. A life course appraoch to respiratory and allergic diseases. See Ref. 112, pp. 240–59

182. Susser E, Terry MB. 2003. A conception-to-death cohort. *Lancet* 361:797–98

183. Deleted in proof

184. Susser M, Stein Z. 2002. Civilization and peptic ulcer. *Int. J. Epidemiol.* 31:13–17 [Reprint of 1962. *Lancet* 1:115–19]

185. Susser M, Stein Z. 2002. Commentary: civilization and peptic ulcer 40 years on. *Int. J. Epidemiol.* 31:18–21

186. Tammelin T, Nayha S, Laitinen J, Rintamaki H, Jarvelin MR. 2003. Physical activity and social status in adolescence as predictors of physical inactivity in adulthood. *Prev. Med.* 37(4):375–81

187. Uemura N, Okamoto S, Yamamoto S, Matsumura N, Yamaguchi S, et al. 2001. Helicobacter pylori infection and the development of gastric cancer. *N. Engl. J. Med.* 345:784–89

188. Upton MN, McConnachie A, McSharry C, Hart CL, Davey Smith G, et al. 2000. Intergenerational 20 year trends in the prevalence of asthma and hay fever in adults: the Midspan family study surveys of parents and offspring. *Br. Med. J.* 321(7253):88–92

189. Upton MN, Davey Smith G, McConnachie A, Hart CL, Watt GC. 2004. Maternal and personal cigarette smoking synergize to increase airflow limitation in adults. *Am. J. Respir. Crit. Care Med.* 169(4):479–87

190. Upton MN, Watt GCM, Davey Smith G, McConnachie A, Hart CL. 1998. Permanent effects of maternal smoking on offsprings' lung function. *Lancet* 352: 453

191. Wadsworth MEJ, Hardy RJ, Paul AA, Marshall SF, Cole TJ. 2002. Leg and trunk length at 43 years in relation to childhood health, diet, and family circumstances; evidence from the 1946 national birth cohort. *Int. J. Epidemiol.* 31: 383–90

192. Wannamethee SG, Lawlor DA, Whincup PH, Walker M, Ebrahim S, Davey Smith G. 2004. Birthweight of offspring and paternal insulin resistance and paternal diabetes in late adulthood: cross sectional survey. *Diabetologia* 47(1):12–18

193. Wannamethee SG, Shaper AG, Whincup PH, Walker M. 1995. Smoking cessation and the risk of stroke in middle-aged men. *JAMA* 274(2):155–60

194. Wannamethee SG, Shaper AG, Whincup PH, Walker M. 1998. Adult height, stroke, and coronary heart disease. *Am. J. Epidemiol.* 148:1069–76

195. Weitzman M, Gortmaker SL, Sobol AM, Perrin JM. 1992. Recent trends in the prevalence and severity of childhood asthma. *JAMA* 268(19):2673–77

196. Wise PH. 2003. Framework as metaphor: the promise and perils of MCH life-course perspectives. *Matern. Child Health* 7:151–56

197. Yusuf S, Reddy S, Ounpuu S, Anand S. 2001. Global burden of cardiovascular diseases: Part 1: general considerations, the epidemiologic transition, risk factors, and impact of urbanization. *Circulation* 104(22):2746–53

198. Yusuf S, Reddy S, Ounpuu S, Anand S. 2001. Global burden of cardiovascular diseases: Part 2: variations in cardiovascular disease by specific ethnic groups and geographic regions and prevention strategies. *Circulation* 104(23):2855–64

Annu. Rev. Public Health 2005. 26:37–60
doi: 10.1146/annurev.publhealth.26.021304.144402
First published online as a Review in Advance on October 25, 2004

ADVANCES IN CANCER EPIDEMIOLOGY: Understanding Causal Mechanisms and the Evidence for Implementing Interventions

David Schottenfeld[1,2] and Jennifer L. Beebe-Dimmer[1,3]

Departments of Epidemiology,[1] Internal Medicine,[2] and Urology,[3] School of Public Health, University of Michigan, Ann Arbor, Michigan 48109-2029; email: daschott@umich.edu, jbeebe@umich.edu

Key Words   chronic inflammation, obesity, tobacco carcinogenesis, gene-environment interactions, cancer control

■ **Abstract**   In a worldwide population of 6 billion, in the year 2000, approximately 10 million cancers were diagnosed, and there were an estimated 6.2 million cancer deaths. Whereas the universality of cancer incidence and mortality is established, the burden of cancer by type or organ site is distributed unequally between developing and industrialized nations. Populations in developing countries are disproportionately affected by cancers in which infectious agents are causal. Our review of advances in cancer epidemiology underscores the complexity of pathogenic mechanisms mediated by chronic inflammation, obesity, and gene-environment interactions as in tobacco and alcohol carcinogenesis. Ultimately, the implementation of effective cancer control interventions that will serve to alleviate the cancer burden must integrate basic and applied research in the behavioral, social, biomedical, and population sciences.

INTRODUCTION

Cancer is a global public health burden, but the summary of cancer incidence and mortality patterns in the relative rankings by cancer site reveal differences between industrialized and developing nations. Among U.S. men, cancers of the prostate, lung and bronchus, and colon and rectum account for an estimated 57% of all newly diagnosed invasive cancers. Among U.S. women, cancers of the breast, lung and bronchus, and colon and rectum account for an estimated 55% of invasive cancers. For the year 2003, there were an estimated 1.3 million invasive cancer cases, 556,000 cancer deaths, and 9.6 million surviving cancer patients. Proportionate mortality by cause was 29% for heart disease, 22.9% for cancer, and 6.8% for cerebrovascular disease. Cancer is the leading cause of death among women aged 40 to 79 years and among men aged 60 to 79 years (62).

In a worldwide population of 6 billion, in the year 2000, approximately 10 million cancers were diagnosed, 5.3 million in men and 4.7 million in women.

0163-7525/05/0421-0037$20.00

Concurrently, there were 6.2 million cancer deaths, for a deaths-to-cases ratio of 0.62, and an estimated 22.4 million persons surviving from cancer diagnosed in the previous 5 years. When rates of incidence and mortality are relatively stable, the ratio of mortality-to-incidence rates approximates case fatality rates or prognosis for individual cancer sites. The most common incident cancers proportionately, excluding the keratinocyte carcinomas of the skin, were lung (12.3%), breast (10.4%), and colorectum (9.4%). The three cancer sites contributing to the highest proportions of cancer deaths were lung (17.8%), stomach (10.4%), and liver (8.8%). Cancer mortality as a proportionate cause of all global deaths was 12% (42, 90, 94, 95).

Whereas the universality of cancer incidence and mortality is established, the burden of cancer by type or organ site is distributed unequally between developing countries in Africa, Asia, and Latin America and more-industrialized countries in North America, Europe, Australia, and New Zealand. The patterns observed in individual countries may also be quite heterogeneous, as in urban compared with rural regions or in relationship to racial, cultural, ethnic, and socioeconomic characteristics. For example, in the United States, the incidence rates of cancers of the uterine cervix, stomach, and liver are generally higher in the minority racial/ethnic groups than in the non-Hispanic white population, whereas breast, endometrium, ovary, and melanoma incidence rates are higher in the white population.

Populations in developing countries are disproportionately susceptible to cancers in which infectious agents are causal. These organ sites include uterine cervix (human papillomavirus), liver (hepatitis viruses B and C), stomach (*Helicobacter* pylori), endemic Burkitt's lymphoma (Epstein-Barr virus and a cofactor of recurring falciparum malaria), nasopharynx (Epstein-Barr virus), urinary bladder (schistosoma haematobium), and biliary tract (opisthorchis viverrini, clonorchis sinensis). The public health impact of these infections is substantial. The proportion of cancer deaths attributable to infectious agents is about 20%–25% in developing countries and 7%–10% in more industrialized countries (96). Approximately 35% of patients with human immunodeficiency virus (HIV) infection are likely to develop a neoplasm of lymphatic tissue (B- and T-cell lymphomas), Kaposi's sarcoma (human herpes virus −8), or a neoplasm of the anogenital tract (human papillomaviruses).

The Pace of New Discoveries

By the early 1980s, cancer epidemiologic studies had underscored the significance of exposures to tobacco smoke, ethyl alcohol, workplace chemicals, ionizing radiation, UV radiation, exogenous hormones, and other pharmaceuticals and the importance of macronutrient excesses and micronutrient deficiencies. Investigators hypothesized that uterine cervix cancer was caused by a sexually transmitted infectious agent, and the endocrinology of reproduction and menstruation was a major focus of research in distinguishing persons at risk for cancers of the breast, endometrium, and ovary.

In a review of salient developments in cancer epidemiology, Linet (73) commented on the "expanding purview of cancer epidemiology" and the profound influence of methodological and conceptual advances in molecular biology, immunology and virology, pathology, toxicology, and biostatistics. Examples described in detail included (*a*) the identification of oncogenic types of human papillomavirus in the pathogenesis of uterine cervical cancer, and (*b*) the etiology of malignant melanoma in relation to patterns of exposure to UV radiation and interactions with host susceptibility factors that influence skin pigmentation, immunologic responses, and DNA replication and repair (73).

Adami et al. (10) in their epilogue to the *Textbook of Cancer Epidemiology* commented, "If the past is prologue to the future, then the pace of new discoveries in the past decade suggest that we are in a golden age of epidemiologic inquiry into the causes of cancer."

They provided an illustrative listing of risk factors revealed in the past 20 years, which included microbial agents, smoking tobacco and environmental tobacco smoke, hormone replacement therapy, obesity, and level of physical activity. This listing of selected discoveries provides the context for the presentation that follows (10).

CHRONIC INFLAMMATION: A UNIFYING CONCEPT IN PATHOGENESIS

A causal link between chronic inflammation and cancer has been suspected for many years. The complex cascade of cellular and cytokine components of the inflammatory response are potentially interactive in stimulating clonally expansive tumor growth and progression. Cytokines are produced by lymphocytes, macrophages, epithelial cells, and mesenchymal cells. Under chronic inflammatory conditions, the upregulation of matrix metalloproteinases by the signaling of macrophages and fibroblasts results in the overproduction of tumor growth factors, new blood vessel formation (neoangiogenesis), and disruption of the normal architecture of the connective tissue compartment. Chronic inflammation is often accompanied by the formation of reactive oxygen and nitrogen species that are potentially damaging to DNA, lipoproteins, and cell membranes (15, 22, 29, 59, 61).

Obstructive Airway Disease and Lung Cancer

In the early 1960s, Passey (93) hypothesized that it was the irritating properties of tobacco smoke, resulting in chronic bronchitis and inflammatory destruction of lung tissue, that was of pathogenic significance in the causal pathway of lung cancer, rather than any direct action by volatile and particulate carcinogens in tobacco smoke. The experiments of Kuschner (65), however, suggested that bronchial and bronchiolar inflammation, accompanied by reactive proliferation, squamous metaplasia, and dysplasia in basal epithelial cells, provided a cocarcinogenic mechanism for neoplastic cell transformation upon exposure to polycyclic aromatic hydrocarbons. Continued smoking in association with chronic obstructive pulmonary disease (COPD), when accompanied by moderate or marked cytological atypia in exfoliated cells in the sputum, was significantly predictive of lung cancer in the Colorado Cancer Center Sputum Screening Cohort Study (100).

Although cigarette smoking is the predominant cause of COPD, with an estimated attributable (etiologic) risk fraction exceeding 80% in smoking-affected individuals, perhaps only 10%–15% of current smokers will eventually develop clinically significant sequellae of productive cough, exertional dyspnea, and cardiovascular disease (1). At least ten cohort studies indicate that chronic obstructive airway disease is an independent predictor of lung cancer risk, and numerous studies report an increased risk of lung cancer among adults with asthma, tuberculosis, or interstitial fibrosis in patients with systemic sclerosis (57, 58, 60, 64, 69, 106, 118, 127).

Chronic cigarette smoking retards mucociliary clearance of foreign particulates and respiratory tract secretions, evokes an inflammatory response accompanied by fibrosis and thickening in the membranous and respiratory bronchioles, and causes mucus gland hypertrophy, hyperplasia, and dysplasia in the proximal airways (122). The manifestations of COPD signal the extent of bronchopulmonary structural and functional damage arising from the interaction of sustained exposure to toxic products of tobacco combustion and host susceptibility. In this context, COPD is a biomarker of cumulative exposure dose level and tissue susceptibility. A conceptual model may be structured that incorporates the tumorigenic effects of chronic obstructive inflammatory disease in the causal pathway of cigarette smoke and lung cancer. The molecular events in the natural history of lung cancer comprise multiple genetic mutations that are determinants of neoplastic transformation and tumor progression and elaboration of autocrine growth factors that influence the clonal behavior and morphologic features of neoplastic cells (12, 26, 79, 107). Chronic inflammation in the proximal and distal bronchial airways is an important cause of obstructive symptoms and provides the dynamic setting for oxidative stress and the formation of free radicals that accompany the reparative proliferative response (102). Increased proliferation kinetics and the interaction of hydroxyl radicals with DNA augment the likelihood of DNA structural and transcriptional errors.

Microbial Agents, Chronic Infections, and Human Carcinogenesis

The oncogenic actions of viral, bacterial, and parasitic agents are mediated through mechanisms associated with chronic inflammation or by host somatic cell events associated with molecular controlling actions of the microbial genome. Each infectious agent has the capacity to persist in the host if not cleared by an effective immune response (Table 1).

TABLE 1 Chronic inflammation and human cancer

Causal mechanisms	Types of cancer
Helicobacter pylori and chronic gastritis	Adenocarcinoma of stomach B-cell lymphoma
Epstein-Barr	Non-Hodgkin's lymphoma Hodgkin's disease Nasopharyngeal carcinoma
Human papillomavirus	Anogenital carcinoma Oropharyngeal carcinoma
Hepatitis B or C	Hepatocellular carcinoma
HIV/AIDS	Non-Hodgkin's lymphoma Kaposi's sarcoma
Liver flukes (e.g., *Clonorchis sinensis*)	Cholangiocarcinoma
Schistosoma haematobium	Squamous carcinoma of urinary bladder
Gastroesophageal reflux	Adenocarcinoma of the distal esophagus and gastric cardia
Ulcerative colitis	Adenocarcinoma of the large intestine
Crohn's granulomatous colitis	Adenocarcinoma of the large intestine
Chronic obstructive lung disease	Carcinoma of the lung
Chronic lung infections	Carcinoma of the lung
Chronic cholecystitis	Gallbladder carcinoma
Inflammatory atrophy of prostate	Prostate carcinoma

Hepatitis C virus (HCV) is an RNA virus (family: Flaviviridae) transmitted predominantly by the parenteral route. More than 60% of cases in the United States occur in drug users from contaminated needles and syringes, 15%–20% through multiple sexual contacts, and 5% from infected mothers to their infants. Population-based studies reported from the Centers for Disease Control and Prevention (CDC) indicated that 40% of chronic liver disease incidences in the United States are due to persistent HCV infection, resulting in 8000 to 10,000 deaths per year. Hepatitis C virus chronic infection occurs in 55%–85% of cases after the acute infection and is prevalent in an estimated 1.8% of the U.S. population; among these cases, 30%–50% develop cirrhosis or fibrosis of the hepatic parenchyma resulting in nodule formation. Hepatic cellular proliferation is induced by cytokines, notably platelet-derived growth factor, whereas fibrogenesis is stimulated by transforming growth factor beta. After a period of 20–30 years from onset of infection, 2%–4% of those with chronic liver disease develop hepatocellular carcinoma. The rate of progression of chronic liver disease among HCV-infected individuals is increased in males, older age at initial infection (in contrast to hepatitis B viral infection), coinfections with hepatitis B and HIV, immunosuppression, and regular use of ethyl alcohol (39, 116).

Of the estimated 50 million new cases of hepatitis B virus (HBV) infection diagnosed globally per year, 5%–10% of adults and up to 90% of infants born to infected mothers will become chronically infected; 75% of chronically infected cases are prevalent in China and southeast Asian countries, where HBV is the leading cause of chronic hepatitis, cirrhosis, and hepatocellular carcinoma. HBV, a double-shelled enveloped DNA virus belonging to the family Hepadnaviridae, is transmitted by sexual contact, percutaneously or parenterally as in intravenous drug use, or perinatally from the infected mother to the infant. An estimated 0.33% of the U.S. population are HBV chronic carriers, as evidenced by antigenemia, HBsAg, for more than six months. High rates of hepatocellular carcinoma (HCC) are prevalent in southeast Asia and sub-Saharan Africa, and low rates are prevalent in the United States and Europe. The estimated population attributable risk percent of the burden of HBV-associated liver cancer varies in China and Africa (65%–70%) and in North America and Australia (<10%). The cumulative lifetime risk of HCC in those who are chronically infected is estimated to be 10%–25% (35, 37, 80, 115).

The latent period from the onset of infection to the diagnosis of HCC may range from 20 to 50 years. The enhancement of risk of neoplasia or liver degeneration will be influenced by onset of persistent infection in infancy or early childhood, immune suppression, coinfection with hepatitis C virus (HCV) or HIV, chronic ethyl alcohol exposure, exposure to the aflatoxin of the *Aspergillus* fungus, acquired or inherited iron storage disease, and possibly exposure to tobacco smoke (114). Cytotoxic T-lymphocytes and cytokines interact with infected hepatocytes, generating recurring cycles of cellular injury, apoptosis, necrosis, and regeneration. In addition, the HBV DNA integrates randomly into the host cell genome, which may provide an important promotional role in HBV-induced hepatocarcinogenesis. We assume that the resulting augmented proliferation of infected hepatocytes triggers genetic instability. The inflammatory process is associated with oxidative stress, which also may cause structural damage to DNA or impede DNA repair processes.

Another important example of an oncogenic viral agent is the group of human papillomaviruses (HPV). Of the ~90 HPV types that have been classified and numbered, the oncogenic types include HPV 16, 18, 31, 33, 35, 39, 45, 51, 52, 56, 58, 59, and 68. HPV infections are transmitted by sexual intercourse or by intimate interpersonal contact. HPV 16 is associated with ~50% of uterine cervical cancer incidences prevalent worldwide (120). In addition, HPV infects and is potentially oncogenic in the basal layers of the stratified epithelium or the mucous epithelium of the vagina, vulva, anus, penile urethral meatus, glans and shaft, and the oropharynx (55, 81). The persistence of infection, genotype, and viral load are predictive of the risk of neoplasia. In addition, other sexually transmitted infectious agents (e.g., chlamydia, herpes simplex), tobacco smoking, multiparity, sustained use of contraceptive steroids, nutritional deficiencies in antioxidant micronutrients, and immune dysfunction all enhance susceptibility for clonal expansion and progression.

The molecular mechanisms in HPV-associated carcinogenesis are of interest. The HPV genome codes for eight proteins. The L1 and L2 genes code for viral capsid proteins, and E1 and E2 code for viral replication and transcription. HPVs also encode E6 and E7 proteins that interfere with the p53 and the retinoblastoma (RB) cell cycle–regulating proteins of the host. The E5 protein complexes with host cell growth factor receptors, stimulating cell growth and proliferation and neoplastic transformation. Genotyping of HPV is based on DNA sequences of the L1, E6, and E7 genes.

Helicobacter pylori (H. pylori) is a gram-negative, multiflagellate, spiral bacterium that colonizes the luminal surface of the gastric epithelium. Its ability to survive in the acidic environment of the stomach is due to its capacity to penetrate the viscous mucous layer, to adhere to epithelial cells, and to increase the pH in the local gastric niche by secreting urease. H. pylori is genetically diverse with strains subdivided by their expression of the cytotoxin-associated gene A (Cag A) and vacuolating cytotoxin A (Vac A). H. pylori has been identified as the major cause of chronic gastritis, peptic ulcer, and adenocarcinoma of the gastric body and antrum. Chronic inflammation, destruction of mucosal epithelium with replacement of normal cells with intestinal metaplastic cells, and augmented cell proliferation appear to be critical events in the evolution of gastric adenocarcinoma. The marked geographical variations in gastric cancer incidence can be explained in part by differences in prevalence of H. pylori infection. H. pylori is acquired early in life, enters the environment in feces, saliva, or vomitus, and is observed most commonly in populations of low socioeconomic status that live in crowded households. Persons with chronic inflammation due to Cag A–positive H. pylori are at increased risk of both diffuse and intestinal types of gastric cancer. The intestinal pattern predominates in men and in high-risk populations and has declined most dramatically in recent decades. Morphologic features include large irregular nuclei, large cells arranged in a columnar pattern, inflammatory cell infiltration, and sparse connective tissue. Commonly, there is the association of intestinal metaplasia or atrophic gastritis. The diffuse pattern is characterized by clusters of small cells and morphologic patterns of scirrhous carcinoma. In low-risk areas, the diffuse type affects younger individuals, and the male:female incidence ratio is close to unity (13, 40, 87, 97).

The gastric mucosa is normally devoid of organized mucosa-associated lymphoid tissue (MALT), in contrast to Peyer's patches in the ileum. The immune response to H. pylori is manifested by the accumulation of organized lymphoid tissue comprising B-cell follicles and surrounding lymphoplasmacytic infiltrate in the gastric mucosa. In a nested case-control study, investigators observed that patients with gastric lymphoma were six times more likely (odds ratio 6.3; 95% confidence interval, 2.0 to 19.9) to have been infected with H. pylori than were matched controls (92). Gastric MALT-low-grade B-cell lymphomas are indolent neoplasms diagnosed most commonly in the antrum or distal corpus of the stomach, which reflects the sites of concentration of H. pylori organisms and acquired lymphoid tissue. Low-grade MALT lymphomas originate from a marginal-zone B-cell population and are genetically different from other low-grade B-cell lymphomas, such as those of follicle center cell and mantle cell origin. The low-grade MALT lymphomas have been associated cytogenetically with trisomy 3 or translocations [e.g., t (11:18) and t (1:14)]. Low-grade mucosa-associated lymphoid tissue lymphomas can be induced in mice after chronic infection with H. felis, H. heilmannii, or H. pylori. The low-grade superficial neoplastic lesions regress or can be eradicated after antimicrobial therapy.

Gastroesophageal Reflux and Esophagogastric Carcinoma

One of the most intriguing features of esophageal cancer is its geographic variability. The pattern around the world resembles a mosaic of contrasting incidence rates and incidence sex ratios that reflect a complex of environmental factors intimately correlated with sociocultural factors and ethnic characteristics. In most parts of the world, incidence rates per 100,000 are around 2.5–5.0 for males and 1.5–2.5 for females, but they may exceed 100.0 in areas of Asia to the north and east of the Caspian Sea. In high-incidence areas such as India, the Transkei (southern Africa), and the Gonbad region in northern Iran, the incidence in females approaches or exceeds that in males (77, 103). More than 60% of the annual esophageal cancer deaths in the world are reported in China, where it is the second most common cancer after stomach cancer.

The highest age-adjusted incidence rates in the United States have been registered in African Americans, Hawaiians, and Alaskan natives. Epidemiologic studies have implicated a variety of risk factors, including tobacco, alcohol, low consumption of fresh fruits and vegetables, deficiencies of specific antioxidant micronutrients, and consumption of foods contaminated by mycotoxins or containing nitrosamine precursors.

Previously, at least 90% of esophageal cancer incidences were classified as squamous cell carcinomas. During the past 20 years, particularly in U.S. white males, the incidence of adenocarcinoma of the esophagus has increased more rapidly than has the incidence of any other upper digestive or gastrointestinal cancer. Whereas the reported incidence of squamous cell carcinoma of the esophagus among U.S. white and black men and women was relatively stable during 1975–1995, incidences of adenocarcinoma of the esophagus increased by more than 100% among white men and by about 50% among white women. The black-white age-adjusted incidence-rate ratio or estimated relative risk was 5.6 for squamous cell carcinoma and 0.3 for adenocarcinoma of the esophagus (121).

Esophageal adenocarcinomas are generally located in the lower third of the esophagus, in association with Barrett's intestinal metaplasia, a condition wherein the squamous epithelium of the distal esophagus is replaced by columnar epithelium and mucus-secreting goblet cells. The diagnosis is made by endoscopy and biopsy. The histogenesis of Barrett's columnar epithelial metaplasia is attributable to chronic inflammatory injury as a result of protracted gastroesophageal reflux. Normally, gastroesophageal junctional structures, swallowing-induced primary peristalsis, and the upper esophageal sphincter serve as protective barriers against the retrograde escape of gastric refluxate.

The reported incidence of adenocarcinoma in Barrett's esophagus with dysplasia, 0.5% per year, is ~30–125 times that of the general population (110, 125). The probable morphologic sequence of events consists of chronic esophagitis,

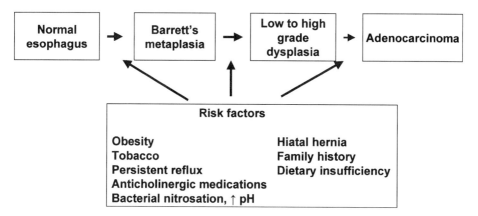

Figure 1 Epidemiology and pathogenesis of adenocarcinoma of the esophagus and gastric cardia.

mucosal ulcerations accompanied by partial epithelial regeneration and repair, Barrett's esophagus (metaplasia), high-grade dysplasia, and neoplasia (Figure 1). Biomarkers of neoplastic progression of Barrett's mucosa include loss of heterozygosity at chromosomes 9p and 17p, aneuploidy and polyploidy (16). Nitrosamines, nitrosamides, and N-nitroso compounds are potent experimental carcinogens for the esophagus. The nitrosamines that affect the esophagus are metabolized in the target organ and result in the formation of genotoxic compounds, which alkylate DNA at the 0^6 position of guanine. Humans may be exposed to nitrosamines and nitrosamine precursors through ingested foods, drinking water, the volatile fraction of tobacco smoke, industrial air emissions, and medications (17). Studies of lifestyle risk factors associated with adenocarcinoma of the esophagus have underscored current cigarette smoking, obesity, a history of hiatal hernia, and medications that relax or alter the gastroesophageal fibromuscular junctional structures (66–68).

In sharp contrast to the trend of declining incidence of gastric cancer located in the antrum or corpus, investigators in various countries of North America and Europe have reported rising incidence rates for adenocarcinoma of the gastric cardia in parallel with increases in esophageal adenocarcinoma. In the United States, on the basis of data from the Surveillance, Epidemiology, and End Results (SEER) program, the incidence of gastric cardia adenocarcinoma among white males has nearly equaled the rate for gastric cancers in other anatomic locations. In Sweden, the incidence of gastric cardia carcinoma has exhibited an average annual increase of 2.5% since 1970. Interpretation of the magnitude of the increasing trends for gastric cardia cancer may be biased by the extent of misclassification of esophageal adenocarcinoma and noncardia stomach cancer. However, the temporal and racial patterns by pathologic cell type and anatomic location, and the commonality of risk factors associated with gastroesophageal reflux disease, suggest that the classification of gastric cardia adenocarcinoma and esophageal adenocarcinoma represents a singular pathophysiologic and epidemiologic entity (30, 36).

Immune Dysfunction and Inflammatory Bowel Disease

In inflammatory bowel disease (IBD), the inflammatory response in ulcerative colitis (UC) is generally confined to the mucosa and submucosa, whereas in Crohn's disease (CD) the inflammation extends from the mucosa to serosa of the large intestine, ileum of the small intestine, or other segments of the intestinal tract. Analysis of inflamed tissues from UC and CD patients has revealed increased expression of proinflammatory cytokines such as the interleukins (IL) and tumor necrosis factor alpha (TNF-α) (89, 108). The pathogenesis of IBD assumes that there is a failure to suppress the inflammatory response in a genetically susceptible host or an inability to sustain mucosal immune tolerance of a luminal foreign antigen. Patients with extensive UC or pancolitis, associated with epithelial dysplasia, after an interval of 10–15 years, demonstrate increasing risk of colon cancer. The cumulative risk of colon cancer, after the latency interval, is an annual increment of about 1%. The neoplastic risk in patients with Crohn's granulomatous colitis will vary as in UC, with the extent and duration of disease.

Inflammatory Atrophy and Prostate Cancer

A suggestive association of prostatic inflammation and carcinogenesis has been described but investigators have not identified a causal infectious agent. In the prostate, a pathologic entity of chronic inflammation is associated with focal hyperplasia and inflammatory atrophy. Such lesions occur most frequently in the peripheral zone of the prostate, wherein most lesions (>70%) of intraepithelial neoplasia and invasive adenocarcinoma are observed. Merging or morphologic transition of proliferative inflammatory atrophy, intraepithelial neoplasia, and invasive adenocarcinoma has been reported by some but not all pathologists (21, 33, 34, 101).

The focal areas of inflammatory cell infiltration appear to exist in response to the extravasation of prostatic secretions in areas of eroded epithelium. The cyclooxygenase-2 (COX-2) enzyme is overexpressed in the macrophages and epithelial cells in lesions of proliferative inflammatory atrophy. COX-2 is the inducible isoform of COX that converts arachidonic acid to proinflammatory prostaglandins (e.g., PGE2) (43). Multiple examples of solid tumors, as in the colon, esophagus, pancreas, lung, urinary bladder, breast, and uterine cervix, have demonstrated overexpression of COX-2. COX-2 is induced by mediators of oxidative stress and environmental mitogenic agents.

OBESITY

"Banish plump Jack and banish all the world."

King Henry IV, Part I
Shakespeare (108a)

By the year 2000, 35% of the U.S. adult population was considered overweight, and 26%–30% obese. If current trends are extrapolated, then by the year 2010, more than 40% of the population will be classified as obese (i.e., Body Mass Index at 30 kg/m^2 or greater) (5). The World Health Organization has estimated that more than one billion adults are overweight and that more than 300 million are obese (6). The average population weight gain in U.S. adults varies between 0.5 to 2.0 pounds per year (56). In a 30-year survey from 1971 to 2000, the caloric intake in women increased on average each day by 22% and in men by less than 10%. Of particular note was the increasing percentage of calories derived from carbohydrates: in women from 45% to ~52%, and for men, from 42% to 49% (8).

An estimated mortality burden of at least 300,000 deaths (all causes) per year and $90 billion in direct health care costs have been attributed to excess weight and relatively sedentary lifestyle (27, 78). Data from the National Health and Nutrition Examination Survey (NHANES) indicated that severe obesity (BMI >45 kg/m^2) was associated with a 17% reduction, or the equivalent of 13 years, in life expectancy in white males and a 10% reduction (8 years) in white females (45). In a prospective study of 900,053 volunteers participating in the American Cancer Society (ACS) Cancer Prevention Study II, excess risk of cancer mortality was estimated in relationship to self-reported weight and height at baseline. The attributable risk of the cancer mortality burden to excess body weight was influenced by the estimated relative risks for various cancer sites, after controlling for history of cigarette smoking, and the prevalence of increased BMI in the study population. On the basis of the estimated population attributable risk proportions in the ACS cohort, the preventive impact of maintaining a recommended BMI below the category of overweight (BMI <25) was 15%–20% of cancer deaths in women and 10%–14% in men, or a total of 90,000 cancer deaths per year (25). Cancer sites associated with the metabolic sequelae of obesity included esophagus (adenocarcinoma), gastric cardia, pancreas, colon, liver, gallbladder, biliary duct and ampulla of Vater, kidney (adenocarcinoma), endometrium and breast (postmenopausal women), thyroid, and multiple myeloma. These associations with obesity have been reported in most studies (20, 88, 98, 99, 104).

The pathophysiology of obesity may be viewed as a dysfunctional disparity between energy intake (kilocalories), mechanisms controlling appetite, and energy expenditure (metabolic equivalents of physical activity or METS) or thermogenesis. The genetic and hormonal mechanisms controlling appetite and the optimal mass of fat cells more efficiently protect humans from the evolutionary effects of food deprivation than do the mechanisms for maintaining optimal body mass standardized for height. The metabolic consequences of central abdominal obesity include insulin resistance, hyperinsulinemia, glucose intolerance, or Type II diabetes; increased triglyceride levels; altered bile acid metabolism as evidenced by cholesterol cholelithiasis; increased production of proinflammatory cytokines and elevated C-reactive protein; and increased endogenous production of bioavailable sex-steroid hormones. The increased levels of insulin are positively correlated with increased production of bioavailable insulin-like growth factor I (IGF-I) in the liver, fat cells, and other organs. IGF-I exhibits mitogenic and antiapoptotic actions that have been associated with risk of solid organ cancers (31, 50, 63, 76, 105).

TOBACCO CARCINOGENESIS: THE SEARCH FOR GENETIC INTERACTIONS

The complexity of tobacco smoke, namely that it contains more than 4000 chemicals, has made it difficult to identify the contribution of more than 50 specific putative carcinogenic agents. The contributions in tobacco smoke include the polynuclear aromatic hydrocarbons or PAHs (benz[a]anthracene, benzo[a]pyrene), N-nitrosamines (N-nitrosodimethylamine, N-nitrosonornicotine), aromatic amines or arylamines (2-naphthylamine, 4-aminobiphenyl), aldehydes (formaldehyde, acetaldehyde), other organic (benzene, acrylonitrile) and inorganic (arsenic, chromium) compounds, and polonium 210 (41, 48, 52–54). The composition of the smoke depends on the ambient conditions of smoking, the blend of tobacco leaf, filtration, additives, paper wrapping, and other factors. Most of the components are produced in an oxygen-deficient, hydrogen-rich environment and arise from pyrolysis and distillation in the region immediately behind the burning tip of the cigarette. The chemical analysis of tobacco smoke is separated into particulate or tar and gaseous phases (113, 124). The curing, fermentation, and aging of smokeless tobacco products favor the formation of various N-nitrosamines from tobacco alkaloids. Among the nitrosamines in smokeless tobacco, N-nitrosonornicotine and 4(methyl, nitrosamino)-1-(3-pyridyl)-1-butanone are carcinogenic in various tested rodents. During chewing or snuff dipping, additional amounts of carcinogenic tobacco-specific N-nitrosamines are formed endogenously in the oral cavity.

Epidemiologic studies conducted in many countries have established that the risks of oral cavity, pharyngeal, laryngeal, lung, esophageal, stomach, pancreatic, liver, colorectal, anal, kidney and urinary bladder, and uterine cervical carcinomas are increased among cigarette smokers (2, 109). In countries such as India, Pakistan, Thailand, Sri Lanka, and Afghanistan, where the use of snuff and chewing tobacco is quite common, oral and pharyngeal cancer mortality rates are among the highest in the world (91).

In the United States, on average, men and women who smoke experience a reduction in life expectancy of 13 and 14–15 years, respectively (9). Tobacco use in the United States is estimated to contribute directly to 30% of total cancer mortality; the corresponding attributable proportion of all cancer deaths in men is estimated to be 40%–45% and 20%–25% in women (Figure 2). Tobacco control in the United States has evolved since the publication in 1964 of the Surgeon General's report on the health consequences of smoking. In 2002, the National Health Interview Survey estimated that 22.5% or about 45.8 million adults were current smokers and that 46 million adults were former smokers. Current smoking prevalence was highest among persons aged 18–24 years (28.5%) and 25–44 years (25.7%) and was lowest among those aged 65+ years (9.3%). A variety of interventions have

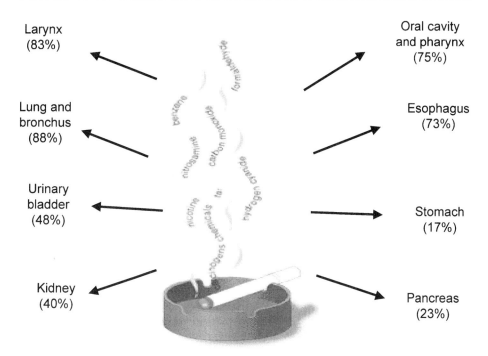

Figure 2 Population attributable risk percentage for tobacco and cancer deaths: United States, 1995–1999, men (117).

been advocated to influence smoking cessation and smoking initiation: school-based health education programs; reducing minors' access to tobacco products; developing and enacting clean indoor air policies and legislation; restricting or eliminating advertising directed toward persons aged <18 years; and increasing tobacco excise taxes. A 10% increase in the price of cigarettes has resulted in a 4% decrease in adult consumption and a 14% decrease in teenage consumption (7).

Public Health officials are concerned that the cancer incidence and mortality rates due to smoking will shift in relative magnitude after the year 2000 from the industrialized nations to developing nations. Whereas tobacco smoking prevalence proportions have been gradually declining by about 1% per year in men and women in North America and Western Europe, they have been rising at ~2% per year in Eastern European and Asian countries. In the early 1970s the average annual per capita consumption of cigarettes in North America and Western Europe was 3.3 times the level in Asian countries; by the early 1990s, this ratio decreased to 1.8. In a prospective study conducted in Shanghai, 61% of men described themselves as current cigarette smokers. Among the Chinese men, about 20% of all deaths were attributed to cigarette smoking; of these deaths, one third were due to lung cancer, and in the smoking men the relative risks were increased for lung, esophageal and liver cancers, coronary heart disease, and chronic obstructive pulmonary disease.

The 1990 report of the Surgeon General, *The Health Benefits of Smoking Cessation*, comprehensively reviewed the epidemiologic evidence for the long-term benefits of cessation of tobacco use. The patterns of changing risk after cessation may be illustrated with an analysis of respiratory cancers. The risk of lung cancer incidence increases with the number of cigarettes smoked daily and with the total number of years smoked (38). Former smokers experience a 20%–90% reduction in risk of lung cancer when compared with current smokers. The rate of decline in former smokers is influenced by health status at the time of quitting and previous patterns of smoking duration, age at initiation, and average daily intensity of exposure. The magnitude of risk reduction is considerably greater among light smokers (<20 cigarettes/day), smokers of short duration, or those who quit at younger ages, and among smokers who inhaled less often or less deeply (4, 49).

Interaction of Tobacco and Ethyl Alcohol

Alcoholic beverages interact commonly with tobacco smoking in the natural history of cancers of the upper respiratory and gastrointestinal tracts. In addition, regular alcohol consumption in excess of three drinks per day (40–45 ml or 32–36 grams of ethyl alcohol) is associated with an increased risk of mortality due to liver cancer and cirrhosis, breast cancer, colorectal cancer, cardiomyopathy, and hemorrhagic stroke (3). Exposure to ethyl alcohol and tobacco combined in the United States accounts for 75%–85% of cancers of the oral cavity, pharynx, larynx, and esophagus (23). Of public health significance is the demonstration of synergy by the interaction of increasing levels of exposure to tobacco and ethyl alcohol. For oral and pharyngeal cancer, joint exposure to tobacco and ethyl alcohol results in odds ratios 2–2.5 times those expected if the effects of alcohol and tobacco were only additive (32). For laryngeal cancer, the interaction of ethyl alcohol and tobacco increases the risk by ~50% more than the increase predicted if the effects were only additive (44). Other subsites within the upper aerodigestive tract exhibiting interaction with previous tobacco and ethyl alcohol exposures are the hypopharynx, supraglottis, and esophagus (3).

Possible carcinogenic mechanisms postulated for ethanol include congeners, derivatives, or contaminants present in alcoholic beverages; induction of cytochrome P450 microsomal activating enzymes; solvent action with increased penetration or absorption of concurrent exposure to a genotoxic agent as in tobacco smoke; cytoxic damage with increased reparative proliferation; exacerbation of deficiencies in antioxidant micronutrients; and perturbation in cell-mediated immune responses or in DNA repair mechanisms. The oxidative metabolism of ethyl alcohol results in the production of acetaldehyde. Acetaldehyde is a reactive compound that forms adducts with various proteins, interferes with DNA repair, induces sister chromatid exchanges, and promotes depletion of glutathione. Minute amounts of acetaldehyde inactivate O^6-methylguanine transferase, the enzyme responsible for repairing adducts resulting from alkylation at the O^6 position of guanine (47, 71, 72). Individual susceptibility may be influenced by genetically determined variations in the activity of metabolic enzymes such as alcohol dehydrogenase, cytochrome P-450 and the microsomal ethanol-oxidizing system, and DNA repair enzymes that influence the rate of removal of damaged DNA as a result of formation of toxic electrophilic metabolites and free-radical reactive intermediates (47).

Genetic Interactions

The search for genetic interactions with environmental risk factors in epidemiologic studies of lung, laryngeal, kidney, and urinary bladder cancer has focused on genes that activate or eliminate tobacco carcinogens. The molecular pathophysiology of gene-environment interactions is complex and varies for specific types of cancer (85). The genes influencing cancer susceptibility may consist of polymorphic alleles at one locus or a combination of alleles at multiple loci (84). Mechanistic interactions of genes and exogenous agents may result from (*a*) environmental agents altering the expression of genes involved in the regulation of the cell cycle, intercellular signaling, and cell-cycle arrest and apoptosis; (*b*) inheritance of susceptibility genes concerned with the fidelity of DNA repair, DNA replication, genomic stability, and the integrity of immune function; or (*c*) metabolic polymorphisms or pharmacogenetic mechanisms that affect the ability to detoxify mutagenic or electrophilic agents (111, 123).

Aromatic amines or arylamines from cigarette smoke are classified as bladder and kidney carcinogens in animals and humans. Arylamines are metabolically activated to electrophilic compounds in the liver through N-hydroxylation by cytochrome P4501A2. If metabolites such as N-hydroxyarylamines are not detoxified by N-acetyltransferases (NAT), they can react with urothelial DNA. The human NAT gene family is located on the short arm of chromosome 8 and is comprised of polymorphic NAT-1 and NAT-2 functional loci. The acetylator phenotype rapid/intermediate or slow influences the rate of metabolism and excretion. Cigarette smokers and slow acetylators are at increased relative risk, with positive interaction or synergy, for urothelial cancers and renal cell adenocarcinoma. Smokers who are slow acetylators exhibit a higher mean level of the hemoglobin adduct of 4-aminobiphenyl than do smokers who are rapid acetylators. The ranking of urinary bladder cancer incidence rates in U.S. whites, blacks, and Asians parallels the proportion of slow acetylators in these three racial groups.

The cytochrome P450 enzymes (CYPs) are a multigene superfamily of mixed-function monooxygenases that are responsible for phase I metabolic activation of structurally diverse substrates. CYP1A1 metabolizes polycyclic aromatic hydrocarbons (PAHs) in tobacco smoke (18, 70). CYP1A2 is expressed in the metabolism of nitrosamines, heterocyclic arylamines, and aflatoxin B1 (46). Epidemiologic analysis of the role of a single polymorphism may reveal inconsistent, false-negative or false-positive results, perhaps because of methodologic limitations in study design. The expression of any single enzyme system must be viewed in relation to the totality of activation and detoxification enzyme systems and the extent of interindividual variability in the metabolic disposition of any potential carcinogenic agent (82).

Various phase II detoxification systems serve to modulate risk in relation to cumulative levels of exposure to chemical metabolites and dietary constituents. These include the glutathione S-transferase (GST) superfamily, N-acetyltransferases (NATs), and genetic mechanisms controlling DNA repair capacity. Glutathione S-transferase genes (GSTs) encode a family of phase II cytosolic enzymes that catalyze the conjugation of electrophilic substrates formed during phase I metabolism (83, 86, 119). There are at least four classes of GSTs: alpha(GSTA), mu(GSTM), pi(GSTP), and theta(GSTT). In addition to their primary function in the detoxification of reactive electrophilic metabolites, the GST enzymes in conjunction with selenium and via glutathione peroxidase have an important function in scavenging free radicals and protecting cells from the metabolic products of oxidative stress. The incorporation of glutathione enhances the molecule's water solubility and excretability. Metabolites of cigarette smoke constituents, including polycyclic aromatic hydrocarbons, arylamines, and nitrosamines, are potential substrates for GSTM1. GSTM1 is polymorphic in humans; inherited homozygous deficiency $(-/-)$, the null genotype, is associated with no measurable enzymatic activity. About 50%–60% of American whites, 20%–25% of American blacks, and 35%–50% of Asian Americans possess the homozygous null genotype. Epidemiologic studies have suggested that the homozygous null GSTM1 genotype potentiates the toxic effects of cigarette smoking in lung, urinary bladder, and aerodigestive tract cancers (75, 126). Studies in Japan report that subjects with the combined GSTM1 null genotype and CYP1A1 polymorphisms were at increased risk (51). The risk is greater than additive in cigarette smokers with homozygous deletions of GSTM1 and CYP1A1 polymorphisms. Alexandrov et al. (11) noted that with both variant genes, the concentration levels of benzo(a)pyrene diol epoxide adducts of DNA were increased in lung parenchyma.

Inherited genetic traits can influence an individual's addictive smoking behavior. The candidate genes affecting smoking behavior include the dopamine receptors, dopamine and serotonin transporter alleles, and the cytochrome P450 alleles (e.g., CYP2A6). These genetic factors collectively influence binding and metabolism of nicotine and other neurotransmitters (14).

ALLEVIATING THE CANCER BURDEN

In 1996, the American Cancer Society (ACS) projected a cancer control objective of a 25% reduction in cancer incidence and a 50% reduction in cancer mortality by 2015. Byers et al. (24) examined the feasibility of achieving the targeted goals by exploring the impact of varying rates of reduction on the prevalence of behavioral risk factors. The risk factors included currently smoking tobacco, dietary patterns of high fat or low fruit and vegetable consumption, frequent or heavy use of alcohol, nonuse of antagonists of endogenous estrogens (e.g., tamoxifen), failure to have screening with sigmoidoscopy or mammography, or failure to receive optimal treatment for cancer. Under various assumptions and the application of population attributable risk estimates, if current trends in the prevalence of cancer risk factors continue, by the year 2015, the projection would be a 13% decline in cancer incidence and a 21% decline in cancer mortality, compared with the rates in 1990. This analysis—on the basis of the synthesis of epidemiologic, clinical oncologic, and behavioral risk factor surveillance data—underscores the strategic significance of the interdisciplinary research required to assign priorities in planning cancer control interventions.

National cancer control priorities include (*a*) eliminating use of tobacco; (*b*) limiting consumption of alcohol; (*c*) avoiding overexposure to sunlight; (*d*) controlling exposures to microbial agents that may be sexually transmitted or transmitted by sharing contaminated needles or personal articles, or prevented by immunization; and (*e*) consuming a prudent diet that includes an abundant distribution of fruits and vegetables and achieves a balance between energy intake and regular physical activity (28). We estimate that for industrialized countries, on the basis of epidemiologic studies, effective interventions to eliminate tobacco smoking and environmental tobacco smoke, to moderate alcohol consumption, and to reverse the rising prevalence of obesity would result in a 50% reduction in cancer mortality. Whereas 30% of cancer deaths in the United States may be attributed to tobacco, the current estimate for global cancer deaths is 16% (117). In contrast,

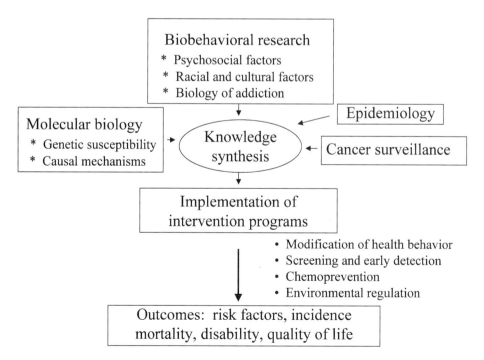

Figure 3 Strategy for population-based cancer control.

the proportion of cancer deaths attributable to infectious agents is ∼20%–25% in developing countries and 7%–10% in industrialized countries.

Cancer control research integrates basic and applied research in the behavioral, social, biomedical, and population sciences. The goals include identifying, quantifying, and ultimately reducing prevalences of cancer risk factors and cancer incidence, morbidity (disability), and mortality (Figure 3) (19). Current and future challenges in cancer epidemiology and cancer control research will include the effective integration of genetic and biochemical biomarkers that measure cancer susceptibility, effects of exposure on target organs and tissues to genotoxic agents, and predictive intermediate endpoints in a pathway of tumorigenesis (74, 112).

**The *Annual Review of Public Health* is online at
http://publhealth.annualreviews.org**

LITERATURE CITED

1. 1984. U.S. Dep. Health Hum. Serv. *The Health Consequences of Smoking: Chronic Obstructive Lung Diseaset. A Report of the Surgeon General.* Rockville, MD: Off. Smok. Health. DHHS Publ. No. 84-50205

2. 2004. Int. Agency Res. Cancer (IARC). *Tobacco Smoking and Involuntary Smoking. IARC Monogr. Evaluation of Carcinogenic Risks to Humans.* Lyon, Fr.: IARC. Vol. 83

3. 1988. Int. Agency Res. Cancer (IARC). *Alcohol Drinking*, Vol. 44. Lyon, Fr.: IARC

4. 1990. U.S. Dep. Health Hum. Serv. *A Report of the Surgeon General: The Health Benefits of Smoking Cessation.* Public Health Serv., Cent. Chronic Dis. Prev. Health Promot. Off. Smok. Health. DHSS Publ. No. (CDC) 90-8416

5. 1999. Natl. Cent. Health Stat. http://www.cdc.gov/nchs/products/pubs/pubd/hestats/obese/obse99.htm

6. 2004. WHO. http://www.who.int/nut/obs.htm

7. 2004. *MMWR* 53:427–36

8. 2004. *JAMA*. Trends in intake of energy and macronutrients–United States, 1971–2000 MMWR. *JAMA* 291:1193–94

9. 2004. U.S. Dep. Health Hum. Serv. *The Health Consequences of Smoking: A Report of the Surgeon General, 1964–2004.* Atlanta, GA: Cent. Dis. Control Prev., Off. Smok. Health

10. Adami HO, Hunter D, Trichopoulos D, eds. 2002. *Textbook of Cancer Epidemiology*, pp. 573–75. New York: Oxford Univ.

11. Alexandrov K, Cascorbi I, Rojas M, Bouvier G, Kriek E, Bartsch H. 2002. CYP1A1 and GSTM1 genotypes affect benzo[a]pyrene DNA adducts in smokers' lung: comparison with aromatic/hydrophobic adduct formation. *Carcinogenesis* 23:1969–77

12. Aoyagi Y, Yokose T, Minami Y, Ochiai A, Iijima T, et al. 2001. Accumulation of losses of heterozygosity and multistep carcinogenesis in pulmonary adenocarcinoma. *Cancer Res.* 61:7950–54

13. Aragones N, Pollan M, Rodero I, Lopez-Abente G. 1997. Gastric cancer in the European Union (1968–1992): mortality trends and cohort effect. *Ann. Epidemiol.* 7:294–303

14. Arinami T, Ishiguro H, Onaivi ES. 2000. Polymorphisms in genes involved in neurotransmission in relation to smoking. *Eur. J. Pharmacol.* 410:215–26

15. Balkwill F, Mantovani A. 2001. Inflammation and cancer: back to Virchow? *Lancet* 357:539–45

16. Bani-Hani K, Martin IG, Hardie LJ, Mapstone N, Briggs JA, et al. 2000. Prospective study of cyclin D1 overexpression in Barrett's esophagus: association with increased risk of adenocarcinoma. *J. Natl. Cancer Inst.* 92:1316–21

17. Bartsch H. 1991. N-nitroso compounds and human cancer: Where do we stand? *IARC Sci. Publ.* 105:1–10

18. Bartsch H, Nair U, Risch A, Rojas M, Wikman H, Alexandrov K. 2000. Genetic polymorphism of CYP genes, alone or in combination, as a risk modifier of tobacco-related cancers. *Cancer Epidemiol. Biomark. Prev.* 9:3–28

19. Best A, Hiatt RA, Cameron R, Rimer BK, Abrams DB. 2003. The evolution of cancer control research: an international perspective from Canada and the United States. *Cancer Epidemiol. Biomark. Prev.* 12:705–12

20. Bianchini F, Kaaks R, Vainio H. 2002. Overweight, obesity, and cancer risk. *Lancet Oncol.* 3:565–74

21. Billis A, Magna LA. 2003. Inflammatory atrophy of the prostate. Prevalence and significance. *Arch. Pathol. Lab. Med.* 127:840–44

22. Block G, Dietrich M, Norkus EP, Morrow JD, Hudes M, et al. 2002. Factors associated with oxidative stress in human populations. *Am. J. Epidemiol.* 156:274–85

23. Blot WJ, McLaughlin JK, Winn DM, Austin DF, Greenberg RS, et al. 1988. Smoking and drinking in relation to oral and pharyngeal cancer. *Cancer Res.* 48:3282–87

24. Byers T, Mouchawar J, Marks J, Cady B, Lins N, et al. 1999. The American Cancer Society challenge goals. How far can cancer rates decline in the U.S. by the year 2015? *Cancer* 86:715–27

25. Calle EE, Rodriguez C, Walker-Thurmond K, Thun MJ. 2003. Overweight, obesity, and mortality from cancer in a prospectively studied cohort of U.S. adults. *N. Engl. J. Med.* 348:1625–38

26. Carbone DP, Minna JD. 1992. The molecular genetics of lung cancer. *Adv. Intern. Med.* 37:153–71

27. Colditz GA. 1999. Economic costs of obesity and inactivity. *Med. Sci. Sports. Exerc.* 31:S663–67

28. Colditz GA, Samplin-Salgado M, Ryan CT, Dart H, Fisher L, et al. 2002. Harvard Report on Cancer Prevention. Volume 5: Fulfilling the potential for cancer prevention: policy approaches. *Cancer Causes Control* 13:199–212

29. Coussens LM, Werb Z. 2002. Inflammation and cancer. *Nature* 420:860–67

30. Craanen ME, Dekker W, Blok P, Ferwerda J, Tytgat GN. 1992. Time trends in gastric carcinoma: changing patterns of type and location. *Am. J. Gastroenterol.* 87:572–79

31. Davi G, Guagnano MT, Ciabattoni G, Basili S, Falco A, et al. 2002. Platelet activation in obese women: role of inflammation and oxidant stress. *JAMA* 288:2008–14

32. Day GL, Blot WJ, Shore RE, McLaughlin JK, Austin DF, et al. 1994. Second cancers following oral and pharyngeal cancers: role of tobacco and alcohol. *J. Natl. Cancer Inst.* 86:131–37

33. De Marzo AM, Marchi VL, Epstein JI, Nelson WG. 1999. Proliferative inflammatory atrophy of the prostate: implications for prostatic carcinogenesis. *Am. J. Pathol.* 155:1985–92

34. De Marzo AM, Meeker AK, Zha S, Luo J, Nakayama M, et al. 2003. Human prostate cancer precursors and pathobiology. *Urology* 62:55–62

35. Deuffic S, Poynard T, Buffat L, Valleron AJ. 1998. Trends in primary liver cancer. *Lancet* 351:214–15

36. Devesa SS, Blot WJ, Fraumeni JF Jr. 1998. Changing patterns in the incidence of esophageal and gastric carcinoma in the United States. *Cancer* 83:2049–53

37. De Vos, Irvine H, Goldberg D, Hole DJ, McMenamin J. 1998. Trends in primary liver cancer. *Lancet* 351:215–16

38. Doll R, Peto R. 1978. Cigarette smoking and bronchial carcinoma: dose and time relationships among regular smokers and lifelong non-smokers. *J. Epidemiol. Community Health* 32:303–13

39. El Serag HB, Mason AC. 1999. Rising incidence of hepatocellular carcinoma in the United States. *N. Engl. J. Med.* 340:745–50

40. Enroth H, Kraaz W, Engstrand L, Nyren O, Rohan T. 2000. Helicobacter pylori strain types and risk of gastric cancer: a case-control study. *Cancer Epidemiol. Biomark. Prev.* 9:981–85

41. Fearon ER. 1997. The smoking gun and the damage done: genetic alterations in the lungs of smokers. *J. Natl. Cancer Inst.* 89:834–36

42. Ferlay J, Bray F, Pisani P, Parkin DM, Ferlay J. 2001. *GLOBOCAN 2000: Cancer Incidence, Mortality and Prevalence Worldwide. IARC CancerBase No. 5.* Lyon, Fr.: IARC

43. FitzGerald GA, Patrono C. 2001. The coxibs, selective inhibitors of cyclooxygenase-2. *N. Engl. J. Med.* 345:433–42

44. Flanders WD, Rothman KJ. 1982. Interaction of alcohol and tobacco in laryngeal cancer. *Am. J. Epidemiol.* 115:371–79

45. Fontaine KR, Redden DT, Wang C, Westfall AO, Allison DB. 2003. Years of life lost due to obesity. *JAMA* 289:187–93

46. Garcia-Closas M, Kelsey KT, Wiencke JK, Xu X, Wain JC, Christiani DC. 1997. A case-control study of cytochrome P450 1A1, glutathione S-transferase M1, cigarette smoking and lung cancer susceptibility (Massachusetts, United States). *Cancer Causes Control* 8:544–53

47. Garro AJ, Lieber CS. 1990. Alcohol and cancer. *Annu. Rev. Pharmacol. Toxicol.* 30:219–49

48. Goldman R, Enewold L, Pellizzari E, Beach JB, Bowman ED, et al. 2001. Smoking increases carcinogenic polycyclic aromatic hydrocarbons in human lung tissue. *Cancer Res.* 61:6367–71

49. Halpern MT, Gillespie BW, Warner KE. 1993. Patterns of absolute risk of lung cancer mortality in former smokers. *J. Natl. Cancer Inst.* 85:457–64

50. Harvie M, Hooper L, Howell AH. 2003. Central obesity and breast cancer risk: a systematic review. *Obesity Rev.* 4:157–73

51. Hayashi S, Watanabe J, Kawajiri K. 1992. High susceptibility to lung cancer analyzed in terms of combined genotypes of P450IA1 and Mu-class glutathione S-transferase genes. *Jpn. J. Cancer Res.* 83:866–70

52. Hecht SS. 1999. Tobacco smoke carcinogens and lung cancer. *J. Natl. Cancer Inst.* 91:1194–210

53. Hecht SS. 2002. Cigarette smoking and lung cancer: chemical mechanisms and approaches to prevention. *Lancet Oncol.* 3:461–69

54. Hecht SS. 2003. Tobacco carcinogens, their biomarkers and tobacco-induced cancer. *Nat. Rev. Cancer* 3:733–44

55. Herrero R, Castellsague X, Pawlita M, Lissowska J, Kee F, et al. 2003. Human papillomavirus and oral cancer: the International Agency for Research on Cancer multicenter study. *J. Natl. Cancer Inst.* 95:1772–83

56. Hill JO, Wyatt HR, Reed GW, Peters JC. 2003. Obesity and the environment: Where do we go from here? *Science* 299:853–55

57. Hinds MW, Cohen HI, Kolonel LN. 1982. Tuberculosis and lung cancer risk in nonsmoking women. *Am. Rev. Respir. Dis.* 125:776–78

58. Hole DJ, Watt GC, Davey-Smith G, Hart CL, Gillis CR, Hawthorne VM. 1996. Impaired lung function and mortality risk in men and women: findings from the Renfrew and Paisley prospective

population study. *Br. Med. J.* 313:711–15

59. Hussain SP, Hofseth LJ, Harris CC. 2003. Radical causes of cancer. *Nat. Rev. Cancer* 3:276–85

60. Islam SS, Schottenfeld D. 1994. Declining FEV1 and chronic productive cough in cigarette smokers: a 25-year prospective study of lung cancer incidence in Tecumseh, Michigan. *Cancer Epidemiol. Biomark. Prev.* 3:289–98

61. Jaiswal M, LaRusso NF, Gores GJ. 2001. Nitric oxide in gastrointestinal epithelial cell carcinogenesis: linking inflammation to oncogenesis. *Am. J. Physiol. Gastrointest. Liver Physiol.* 281:G626–34

62. Jemal A, Murray T, Samuels A, Ghafoor A, Ward E, Thun MJ. 2003. Cancer statistics, 2003. *CA Cancer J. Clin.* 53:5–26

63. Kaaks R, Lukanova A, Kurzer MS. 2002. Obesity, endogenous hormones, and endometrial cancer risk: a synthetic review. *Cancer Epidemiol. Biomark. Prev.* 11:1531–43

64. Kuller LH, Ockene J, Meilahn E, Svendsen KH. 1990. Relation of forced expiratory volume in one second (FEV1) to lung cancer mortality in the Multiple Risk Factor Intervention Trial (MRFIT). *Am. J. Epidemiol.* 132:265–74

65. Kuschner M. 1968. The causes of lung cancer. *Am. Rev. Respir. Dis.* 98:573–90

66. Lagergren J, Bergstrom R, Adami HO, Nyren O. 2000. Association between medications that relax the lower esophageal sphincter and risk for esophageal adenocarcinoma. *Ann. Intern. Med.* 133:165–75

67. Lagergren J, Bergstrom R, Nyren O. 1999. Association between body mass and adenocarcinoma of the esophagus and gastric cardia. *Ann. Intern. Med.* 130:883–90

68. Laheij RJ, Straatman H, Verbeek AL, Jansen JB. 1999. Mortality trend from cancer of the gastric cardia in The Netherlands, 1969–1994. *Int. J. Epidemiol.* 28:391–95

69. Lange P, Nyboe J, Appleyard M, Jensen G, Schnohr P. 1990. Ventilatory function and chronic mucus hypersecretion as predictors of death from lung cancer. *Am. Rev. Respir. Dis.* 141:613–17

70. Le Marchand L, Guo C, Benhamou S, Bouchardy C, Cascorbi I, et al. 2003. Pooled analysis of the CYP1A1 exon 7 polymorphism and lung cancer (United States). *Cancer Causes Control* 14:339–46

71. Lieber CS. 1988. Biochemical and molecular basis of alcohol-induced injury to liver and other tissues. *N. Engl. J. Med.* 319:1639–50

72. Lieber CS. 1995. Medical disorders of alcoholism. *N. Engl. J. Med.* 333:1058–65

73. Linet MS. 2000. Evolution of cancer epidemiology. *Epidemiol. Rev.* 22:35–56

74. Lippman SM, Hong WK. 2002. Cancer prevention science and practice. *Cancer Res.* 62:5119–25

75. London SJ, Daly AK, Cooper J, Navidi WC, Carpenter CL, Idle JR. 1995. Polymorphism of glutathione S-transferase M1 and lung cancer risk among African-Americans and Caucasians in Los Angeles County, California. *J. Natl. Cancer Inst.* 87:1246–53

76. Lukanova A, Lundin E, Zeleniuch-Jacquotte A, Muti P, Mure A, et al. 2004. Body mass index, circulating levels of sex-steroid hormones, IGF-I and IGF-binding protein-3: a cross-sectional study in healthy women. *Eur. J. Endocrinol.* 150:161–71

77. Mahboubi E, Kmet J, Cook PJ, Day NE, Ghadirian P, Salmasizadeh S. 1973. Oesophageal cancer studies in the Caspian Littoral of Iran: the Caspian cancer registry. *Br. J. Cancer* 28:197–214

78. Manson JE, Skerrett PJ, Greenland P, VanItallie TB. 2004. The escalating pandemics of obesity and sedentary lifestyle.

A call to action for clinicians. *Arch. Intern. Med.* 164:249–58

79. Mao L, Lee JS, Kurie JM, Fan YH, Lippman SM, et al. 1997. Clonal genetic alterations in the lungs of current and former smokers. *J. Natl. Cancer Inst.* 89:857–62

80. McGlynn KA, Tsao L, Hsing AW, Devesa SS, Fraumeni JF Jr. 2001. International trends and patterns of primary liver cancer. *Int. J. Cancer* 94:290–96

81. Melbye M, Frisch M. 1998. The role of human papillomaviruses in anogenital cancers. *Semin. Cancer Biol.* 8:307–13

82. Miller DP, Liu G, de Vivo I, Lynch TJ, Wain JC, et al. 2002. Combinations of the variant genotypes of GSTP1, GSTM1, and p53 are associated with an increased lung cancer risk. *Cancer Res.* 62:2819–23

83. Miller DP, Neuberg D, de Vivo I, Wain JC, Lynch TJ, et al. 2003. Smoking and the risk of lung cancer: susceptibility with GSTP1 polymorphisms. *Epidemiology* 14:545–51

84. Mucci LA, Wedren S, Tamimi RM, Trichopoulos D, Adami HO. 2001. The role of gene-environment interaction in the aetiology of human cancer: examples from cancers of the large bowel, lung and breast. *J. Intern. Med.* 249:477–93

85. Nakachi K, Imai K, Hayashi S, Watanabe J, Kawajiri K. 1991. Genetic susceptibility to squamous cell carcinoma of the lung in relation to cigarette smoking dose. *Cancer Res.* 51:5177–80

86. Nazar-Stewart V, Motulsky AG, Eaton DL, White E, Hornung SK, et al. 1993. The glutathione S-transferase mu polymorphism as a marker for susceptibility to lung carcinoma. *Cancer Res.* 53:2313–18

87. Nyren O. 1998. Is Helicobacter pylori really the cause of gastric cancer? *Semin. Cancer Biol.* 8:275–83

88. Pan SY, Johnson KC, Ugnat AM, Wen SW, Mao Y. 2004. Association of obesity and cancer risk in Canada. *Am. J. Epidemiol.* 159:259–68

89. Papadakis KA, Targan SR. 2000. Role of cytokines in the pathogenesis of inflammatory bowel disease. *Annu. Rev. Med.* 51:289–98

90. Parkin DM. 2001. Global cancer statistics in the year 2000. *Lancet Oncol.* 2:533–43

91. Parkin DM, Pisani P, Lopez AD, Masuyer E. 1994. At least one in seven cases of cancer is caused by smoking. Global estimates for 1985. *Int. J. Cancer* 59:494–504

92. Parsonnet J, Hansen S, Rodriguez L, Gelb AB, Warnke RA, et al. 1994. Helicobacter pylori infection and gastric lymphoma. *N. Engl. J. Med.* 330:1267–71

93. Passey RD. 1962. Some problems of lung cancer. *Lancet* 2:107–12

94. Pisani P, Bray F, Parkin DM. 2002. Estimates of the world-wide prevalence of cancer for 25 sites in the adult population. *Int. J. Cancer* 97:72–81

95. Pisani P, Parkin DM, Bray F, Ferlay J. 1999. Estimates of the worldwide mortality from 25 cancers in 1990. *Int. J. Cancer* 83:18–29

96. Pisani P, Parkin DM, Munoz N, Ferlay J. 1997. Cancer and infection: estimates of the attributable fraction in 1990. *Cancer Epidemiol. Biomark. Prev.* 6:387–400

97. Plummer M, Vivas J, Fauchere JL, Del Giudice G, Pena AS, et al. 2000. Helicobacter pylori and stomach cancer: a case-control study in Venezuela. *Cancer Epidemiol. Biomark. Prev.* 9:961–65

98. Polednak AP. 2003. Trends in incidence rates for obesity-associated cancers in the US. *Cancer Detect. Prev.* 27:415–21

99. Pomerleau J, McKee M, Lobstein T, Knai C. 2003. The burden of disease attributable to nutrition in Europe. *Public Health Nutr.* 6:453–61

100. Prindiville SA, Byers T, Hirsch FR, Franklin WA, Miller YE, et al. 2003. Sputum cytological atypia as a predictor of incident lung cancer in a cohort

of heavy smokers with airflow obstruction. *Cancer Epidemiol. Biomark. Prev.* 12:987–93

101. Putzi MJ, De Marzo AM. 2000. Morphologic transitions between proliferative inflammatory atrophy and high-grade prostatic intraepithelial neoplasia. *Urology* 56:828–32

102. Ryrfeldt A, Bannenberg G, Moldeus P. 1993. Free radicals and lung disease. *Br. Med. Bull.* 49:588–603

103. Saidi F, Sepehr A, Fahimi S, Farahvash MJ, Salehian P, et al. 2000. Oesophageal cancer among the Turkomans of northeast Iran. *Br. J. Cancer* 83:1249–54

104. Samanic C, Gridley G, Chow WH, Lubin J, Hoover RN, Fraumeni JF Jr. 2004. Obesity and cancer risk among white and black United States veterans. *Cancer Causes Control* 15:35–44

105. Sandhu MS, Gibson JM, Heald AH, Dunger DB, Wareham NJ. 2004. Association between insulin-like growth factor-I: insulin-like growth factor-binding protein-1 ratio and metabolic and anthropometric factors in men and women. *Cancer Epidemiol. Biomark. Prev.* 13: 166–70

106. Santillan AA, Camargo CA Jr, Colditz GA. 2003. A meta-analysis of asthma and risk of lung cancer (United States). *Cancer Causes Control* 14:327–34

107. Sekido Y, Fong KM, Minna JD. 2003. Molecular genetics of lung cancer. *Annu. Rev. Med.* 54:73–87

108. Seril DN, Liao J, Yang GY, Yang CS. 2003. Oxidative stress and ulcerative colitis-associated carcinogenesis: studies in humans and animal models. *Carcinogenesis* 24:353–62

108a. Shakespeare W. *King Henry IV, Part I.*

109. Shopland DR, Eyre HJ, Pechacek TF. 1991. Smoking-attributable cancer mortality in 1991: Is lung cancer now the leading cause of death among smokers in the United States? *J. Natl. Cancer Inst.* 83:1142–48

110. Spechler SJ. 2002. Clinical practice. Barrett's Esophagus. *N. Engl. J. Med.* 346:836–42

111. Spitz MR, Wei Q, Dong Q, Amos CI, Wu X. 2003. Genetic susceptibility to lung cancer: the role of DNA damage and repair. *Cancer Epidemiol. Biomark. Prev.* 12:689–98

112. Steinberg K, Beck J, Nickerson D, Garcia-Closas M, Gallagher M, et al. 2002. DNA banking for epidemiologic studies: a review of current practices. *Epidemiology* 13:246–54

113. Stellman SD, Garfinkel L. 1989. Lung cancer risk is proportional to cigarette tar yield: evidence from a prospective study. *Prev. Med.* 18:518–25

114. Stern MC, Umbach DM, Yu MC, London SJ, Zhang ZQ, Taylor JA. 2001. Hepatitis B, aflatoxin B(1), and p53 codon 249 mutation in hepatocellular carcinomas from Guangxi, People's Republic of China, and a meta-analysis of existing studies. *Cancer Epidemiol. Biomark. Prev.* 10:617–25

115. Stuver SO. 1998. Towards global control of liver cancer? *Semin. Cancer Biol.* 8:299–306

116. Tanaka K, Hirohata T, Koga S, Sugimachi K, Kanematsu T, et al. 1991. Hepatitis C and hepatitis B in the etiology of hepatocellular carcinoma in the Japanese population. *Cancer Res.* 51:2842–47

117. Thune MJ, Henley SJ. 2005. Tobacco. In *Cancer Epidemiology and Prevention*, ed. D Schottenfeld, JF Fraumeni Jr. New York: Oxford Univ. Press

118. Tockman MS, Anthonisen NR, Wright EC, Donithan MG. 1987. Airways obstruction and the risk for lung cancer. *Ann. Intern. Med.* 106:512–18

119. To-Figueras J, Gene M, Gomez-Catalan J, Pique E, Borrego N, et al. 1999. Genetic polymorphism of glutathione S-transferase P1 gene and lung cancer risk. *Cancer Causes Control* 10:65–70

120. Villa LL. 1997. Human papillomaviruses

and cervical cancer. *Adv. Cancer Res.* 71:321–41

121. Vizcaino AP, Moreno V, Lambert R, Parkin DM. 2002. Time trends incidence of both major histologic types of esophageal carcinomas in selected countries, 1973–1995. *Int. J. Cancer* 99:860–68

122. Wanner A, Salathe M, O'Riordan TG. 1996. Mucociliary clearance in the airways. *Am. J. Respir. Crit. Care Med.* 154:1868–902

123. Wei Q, Cheng L, Hong WK, Spitz MR. 1996. Reduced DNA repair capacity in lung cancer patients. *Cancer Res.* 56:4103–7

124. Wilcox HB, Schoenberg JB, Mason TJ, Bill JS, Stemhagen A. 1988. Smoking and lung cancer: risk as a function of cigarette tar content. *Prev. Med.* 17:263–72

125. Wild CP, Hardie LJ. 2003. Reflux, Barrett's oesophagus and adenocarcinoma: burning questions. *Nat. Rev. Cancer* 3:676–84

126. Yu MC, Ross RK, Chan KK, Henderson BE, Skipper PL, et al. 1995. Glutathione S-transferase M1 genotype affects aminobiphenyl-hemoglobin adduct levels in white, black and Asian smokers and nonsmokers. *Cancer Epidemiol. Biomark. Prev.* 4:861–64

127. Zheng W, Blot WJ, Liao ML, Wang ZX, Levin LI, et al. 1987. Lung cancer and prior tuberculosis infection in Shanghai. *Br. J. Cancer* 56:501–4

Annu. Rev. Public Health 2005. 26:61–88
doi: 10.1146/annurev.publhealth.26.021304.144415
First published online as a Review in Advance on August 20, 2004

COMPETING DIETARY CLAIMS FOR WEIGHT LOSS: Finding the Forest Through Truculent Trees

David L. Katz

Yale Prevention Research Center, Derby, Connecticut 06418; email: katzdl@pol.net

Key Words   obesity, overweight, BMI, pandemic, diet, carbohydrate

■ **Abstract**   In response to an accelerating obesity pandemic, competing weight-loss diets have propagated; those touting carbohydrate restriction are currently most in vogue. Evidence that sustainable weight loss is enhanced by means other than caloric restriction, however, is lacking. Whereas short-term weight loss is consistently achieved by any dietary approach to the restriction of choice and thereby calories, lasting weight control is not. Competing dietary claims imply that fundamental knowledge of dietary pattern and human health is lacking; an extensive literature belies this notion. The same dietary and lifestyle pattern conducive to health promotion is consistently associated with weight control. A bird's eye view of the literature on diet and weight reveals a forest otherwise difficult to discern through the trees. Competing diet claims are diverting attention and resources from what is actually and urgently needed: a dedicated and concerted effort to make the basic dietary pattern known to support both health and weight control more accessible to all.

INTRODUCTION

In the United States, obesity is not only epidemic, but arguably the gravest and most poorly controlled public health threat of our time (62, 93, 151). Some 65%–80% of adults in the United States are overweight or obese, defined as a body mass index (BMI) at or above 25kg/m^2 (100). The rate of childhood obesity has tripled in the past two decades and appears to be worsening at an accelerating rate (109). Despite a conservative definition of overweight in children based on the 95th percentile for age- and sex-adjusted BMI, intended to be more specific than sensitive (http://www.cdc.gov/nccdphp/dnpa/bmi/bmi-for-age.htm), at least 15% of children in the population are considered overweight. In some ethnic minority groups, this figure rises to 50% (36, 110, 153).

The increasingly global economy has rendered obesity an increasingly global problem; the United States is the putative epicenter of an obesity pandemic (32, 35, 77). Rates of obesity are already high and rising in most developed countries and are lower but rising faster in countries undergoing a cultural transition (38). In China, India, and Russia, the constellation of enormous population, inadequate

0163-7525/05/0421-0061$20.00

control of historical public health threats such as infectious disease, and the advent of epidemic obesity and attendant chronic disease represent an unprecedented challenge (61, 98, 139).

The health consequences of obesity are well characterized, as is the economic toll (148, 149). In the United States, some 300,000–400,000 premature deaths each year are thought to result from direct and indirect effects of the obesity epidemic (101). A linear relationship exists between the BMI and all-cause mortality (27); obesity contributes substantially to cardiovascular risk (91, 126, 142); and excess body weight is a potent risk factor for most prevalent cancers (26). The toll of the epidemic is most starkly conveyed by the impact on children. In the past two decades, due to childhood obesity, type 2 diabetes has been transformed from a condition occurring almost exclusively at or after middle age into a pediatric epidemic affecting children as young as six (16).

The strong link between diabetes and cardiovascular disease suggests that on the current trajectory, cardiovascular events in adolescence will become routine in the near future. Data from the *National Center for Health Statistics* indicate that children growing up in the United States today will ultimately suffer more chronic disease and premature death from poor dietary habits and lack of physical activity than from exposure to tobacco, drugs, and alcohol combined (http://www.cdc.gov/nchs/data/series/sr_10/sr10_216.pdf). These data also suggest that current U.S. trends will translate into a shorter life expectancy for children than for their parents.

Against the backdrop of this increasingly acute need, the identification of practical and generalizable solutions to the obesity crisis has proved elusive. From research interventions, to commercial weight-loss programs, to supplements, potions, and devices, innumerable approaches to weight loss have been devised. That none of these has yet met the need of the population is clearly reflected in the worsening epidemiology of obesity.

Obesity is as relevant to prevailing views on beauty, fashion, and body image as it is to public health and thus engenders unique preoccupations (2, 6, 25, 104, 115, 144, 150). Individuals reluctant to take antihypertensive or lipid-lowering medication for fear of side effects may aggressively pursue pharmacotherapy, or even surgery, for weight control (7, 90, 99). The visibility of obesity, the stigma associated with it (89, 121, 122) (it is often said that antiobesity sentiment is the last bastion of socially acceptable prejudice), and the difficulty most people experience in their efforts to resist it contribute to its novel influences on attitude and behavior. This widespread state of volatile frustration renders the public susceptible to almost any persuasive sales pitch for a weight-loss lotion, potion, or program.

The natural consequence of acute and substantially unmet need is frustration. This public frustration has created a seemingly limitless market for weight-loss approaches. This same frustration has engendered a prevailing gullibility so that virtually any weight-loss claim is accepted at face value. Dual aphorisms might be considered for characterizing the obesity epidemic. Until recently, organized responses to this degenerating crisis have been tepid at best, suggesting that among public health professionals, familiarity breeds if not outright contempt then at least complacency. Among members of the general public, desperation breeds gullibility.

It is thus a sellers market for weight-loss wares. The ensuing litany of competing claims for effective weight loss is producing increasing confusion among both the public at large and health care professionals (67). In the mix is everything from science to snake oil, with no assurances that science is the more popular choice. Sorting among the competing claims—and finding a forest through the trees—is the goal of this review and synthesis. This chapter endeavors to provide a comprehensive overview and objective assessment of competing claims for weight loss and an examination of the implications within the context of what is known about dietary pattern and human health and within the bounds of reason.

METHODS

This report reviews and synthesizes the available evidence related to dietary approaches to weight loss and control. An examination of other approaches to weight loss—such as physical activity alone, pharmacotherapy, liquid diets, and surgery—is excluded unless relevant to the consideration of competing dietary claims. Eight principal areas within the expansive literature addressing diet and weight regulation are examined, as shown in Table 1.

The overall assessment method utilized was strictly qualitative and, while intended to be thorough, nonsystematic. However, subsumed within the overview, and informing it, is a Center for Disease Control (CDC)-funded systematic review of the obesity prevention and control literature conducted at the Yale Prevention Research Center (PRC) (170). This project involved the detailed abstraction of

TABLE 1   Eight principal domains within the literature covering diet, health, and weight control reviewed/considered for this report

1	Dietary interventions studied for weight loss
2	Diets in wide use by the general public; popular diet books
3	Reports related to the long-term sustainability of weight loss or long-term prevention of weight gain
4	Studies characterizing the effects of various weight-loss diets on body composition
5	Anthropology literature characterizing the "native" human diet and its health implications
6	Reports of associations between dietary pattern and health outcomes for diverse populations, healthy or otherwise
7	Reported hazards of specific weight-loss diets
8	Reviews, position statements, and dietary guidelines addressing weight control, health promotion, or both

roughly 350 intervention studies spanning four decades and was recently completed with manuscript preparation ongoing. The results of this systematic review will provide the content for the chapter on obesity prevention and control in *The Guide to Community Preventive Services* (24, 146).

Methods for the systematic review, in brief, were as follows. The literature search spanned November 2000–February 2001 using Medical Subject Headings (MeSH) terms agreed on by the Prevention Research Center core investigative team and members of a collaborating expert panel, including content experts at the CDC. Four databases were searched (using identical MeSH terms), including

1. PubMed,
2. HealthStar,
3. Embase, and
4. Cochrane Library.

All related articles published in peer-reviewed journals from 1966 to the present were considered. Manual reference searches (using meta-analyses, review articles, and some articles written by prominent authors in this area) were also performed, resulting in the identification of several studies not catalogued in the above-mentioned databases. Many of these studies were identified as being published in behavioral science/psychology journals; therefore, the *Psych Info* database was also searched. However, using the entire list of MeSH terms was not necessary because only a small number of articles were found using very general terms such as "obesity and control." Additional MeSH terms were added at the end of the searching phase (February 2001) to allow consideration of other physical outcomes (such as improved body composition) resulting from diet and exercise interventions regardless of whether weight was lost. Articles describing weight-loss interventions used as treatment for other medical conditions, such as cardiovascular disease, hypertension, and sleep apnea, were also included at this stage.

Eligibility criteria were applied to the studies before retrieval on the basis of information provided in abstracts. Full articles were retrieved for studies meeting criteria; articles that did not provide an abstract; or when abstracts did not include all required pertinent information.

Studies included in the systematic review met the following criteria:

■ Papers must report a community/population-based intervention in school, clinical, workplace, general community, or family settings; interventions (diet, physical activity, combinations) must be clearly defined;

■ outcomes must be clearly defined and commonly used (e.g., BMI, body weight, skin fold);

■ a control measurement must be made (either with baseline and follow-up measurements or using a control group(s);

■ and subjects must be followed for at least six months from the beginning of the intervention.

Meta analyses and systematic reviews were also retrieved. Articles were excluded that met the above criteria but focused only on inpatients; used pharmacotherapy, surgery, or very-low calorie liquid diets (VLCDs); intervened with individual patients only; or tested commercial weight loss diets (unless at the community level).

Citations were downloaded into Endnote libraries and sorted for duplicates. A research assistant retrieved the majority of articles at the Yale Medical Library; the remainder were ordered through interlibrary loan via the Griffin Hospital (Derby, Connecticut) Resource Center.

Articles ($n = 343$) were retrieved and catalogued by research assistants who identified the settings, intervention methods, population targeted, sample size, and mode of intervention-prevention/control or treatment. Several articles that did not meet the inclusion criteria were identified by reviewing full text (this could not be determined on the basis of abstracts alone). More than 550 articles were retrieved initially, with approximately 200 being discarded (saved for later reference/further bibliography search). The primary reasons for article disqualification were (*a*) insufficient length of follow-up with subjects and (*b*) studies that did not describe an intervention or were only descriptive. The core study team reviewed any articles that were difficult to categorize. The fate of all papers initially retrieved is shown in Figure 1.

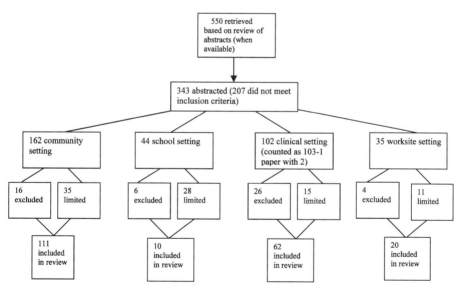

Figure 1   Fate of papers diagram from OOPS literature "flow" diagram. Excluded papers were found to not meet inclusion criteria during/after data abstraction. Reasons for exclusion include the following: <6-month follow-up, no weight-related outcomes, uninterpretable data/lack of useful data, review articles, commercial program, population was not generalizable. Limited studies were found to have poor methodology.

Each article was abstracted using a standardized data abstraction form developed by the CDC Community Guide branch. Articles were abstracted by two independent reviewers and audited by a third party when necessary to reconcile discrepant interpretations. The final versions of the forms were entered into an Access database. Evidence tables (a one-page summary of the evidence from each article) were created for all studies with adequate methodological quality (208 of the initial 343 studies) and used to summarize evidence across studies by setting, target group, type of intervention, etc. Meta-analytic methods were applied as indicated.

Other than the systematic review, the pertinent literature was accessed using online search engines, principally PubMed (http://www.pubmed.gov), in a manner intended to be balanced, representative, and as objective as possible, but not systematic (20). Searches were based on a wide array of pertinent search terms and strings, using key words and/or MeSH terms, as well as explode functions as indicated. Given the expansiveness of pertinent literature, searches were restricted to studies in humans and published in English.

In addition to these sources of information, this overview was informed by considering the anthropology literature addressing human dietary intake patterns over time, as well as an even more extensive assessment of the nutrition literature undertaken during the recent preparation of a nutrition textbook (76).

RESULTS

The CDC-funded systematic review of obesity prevention and control, on which this report is partially based, retrieved 343 studies; the complete bibliography is available at http://www.yalegriffinprc.org/obesityreviewcitations. The full systematic review will be published separately. Relevant to the current review are those studies that used various diets in an effort to produce weight loss or prevent weight gain. Interventions conducted in school, work site, community, and clinical settings were examined; the inclusion and exclusion criteria for the review are available at http://www.yalegriffinprc.org/obesityreviewcitations.

In all settings studied, diets that restricted calories by any means produced weight loss in the short term. The search was terminated in 2001, thus some currently popular diets were not represented. Caloric restriction was achieved by various means, ranging from direct provision of food (168); systems of incentive/disincentive (63); cognitive behavioral therapy (125); fat restriction (54); and the color-coding of food choices based on nutrient density (46). In general, those interventions achieving the most extreme degrees of caloric restriction also produced the greatest initial weight loss (152, 160). However, a rebound weight gain was observed; the more rapid the initial weight loss, in general the greater and more rapid the subsequent weight gain (152, 160). This observation appears to be of generalizable significance, likely owing to the fact that the extreme caloric restriction necessary for very rapid weight loss is intrinsically unsustainable. When the means used to achieve initial weight loss are unsustainable, weight regain is consistently observed.

Dietary Interventions for Weight Loss

The current popularity of carbohydrate-restricted diets for weight loss (1) is little less than a national phenomenon and is literally reshaping the American food supply. An assessment of diet and weight loss thus requires particular consideration of entries in this category. The one published review (21) of low-carbohydrate diets to date suggests that short-term weight loss is consistently achieved but that neither weight loss sustainability nor effects on overall health have been determined yet.

Two studies of low-carbohydrate diets that received widespread attention are those by Samaha et al. (132) and Foster et al. (49), published in the same issue of the *New England Journal of Medicine* in 2003. Samaha and colleagues compared a very low carbohydrate diet (<30 g carbohydrate per day) to a fat- and calorie-restricted diet in 132 adults with a BMI of ≥35 over a 6-month period. The carbohydrate-restricted diet resulted in greater weight loss at 6 months than did the low-fat diet but was also associated with a far greater reduction in daily calorie intake (a mean reduction of 271 kcal per day for the low-fat diet and 460 kcal for the low-carbohydrate diet). Foster et al. compared the Atkins diet as described in *Dr. Atkins' New Diet Revolution* (14) to a fat- and calorie-restricted diet in 63 obese adults followed for 12 months. The low-carbohydrate diet produced significantly greater weight loss at 6 months but not at 12 months. Calorie intake was not reported. In both studies, attrition and recidivism were high; Samaha and colleagues noted that their trial was unblinded, whereas Foster et al. made no mention of blinding.

Brehm and colleagues (23) examined weight loss, cardiac risk factors, and body composition in 53 obese women randomly assigned to a very low carbohydrate diet, or a calorie-restricted, balanced diet with 30% of calories from fat. Subjects assigned to the very low carbohydrate diet group lost more weight (8.5 +/− 1.0 versus 3.9 +/− 1.0 kg; P < 0.001) and more body fat (4.8 +/− 0.67 versus 2.0 +/− 0.75 kg; P < 0.01) than those assigned to the low-fat diet group; cardiac risk measures improved comparably in both groups.

Sondike et al. (141a) ran a 12-week weight-loss trial comparing low-carbohydrate to moderately fat-restricted diets in 30 overweight adolescents. There was significantly greater weight loss with the low-carbohydrate assignment. LDL cholesterol levels improved with fat restriction, but not with carbohydrate restriction.

In 2000, Spieth and colleagues (143) reported the results of a retrospective cohort study comparing a low glycemic index (GI) to a low-fat diet for weight loss in 107 obese children. Greater reduction in the BMI was observed at approximately 4 months in the low GI group (−1.53 kg/m(2) [95% confidence interval, −1.94 to −1.12]) as compared to the low-fat diet group (−0.06 kg/m(2) [−0.56 to +0. 44], P < .001).

Interest in carbohydrate restriction for weight loss is not new; Atkins' *Diet Revolution* was first published in 1972 (13). In 1978, Rabast and colleagues used isocaloric formula diets to compare fat- and carbohydrate-restricted approaches to weight loss in 45 obese adults (123). Carbohydrate restriction resulted in greater weight loss (14 +/− 7.2 kg versus 9.8 +/− 4.5 kg) at 30 days.

Such results are not seen universally, however. Golay and colleagues (52) assigned 68 overweight adults to approximately isocaloric low- (25% of calories) and moderate- (45% of calories) carbohydrate diets for 12 weeks and observed comparable losses of weight, waist circumference, and body fat in both groups. For the most part, metabolic indices were favorably, and comparably, influenced by both diets as well. The matching of calorie levels is noteworthy.

Poppitt and colleagues (120) achieved significant weight loss among 46 adult subjects with metabolic syndrome followed for 6 months by substituting carbohydrate for fat. Complex carbohydrate substitution for fat was associated with both weigh loss and amelioration of the lipid profile; the substitution of simple carbohydrate for fat did not result in weight gain.

In 1999, Skov et al. (141) reported an interesting variation on the low-carbohydrate diet theme by comparing two fat-restricted (30% of calories) diets, one high in carbohydrate (58% of calories) and the other high in protein (25% of calories). Subjects were 65 overweight adults followed for 6 months and were provided diets strictly controlled with regard to nutritional composition but unrestricted in calories. More weight was lost with high protein (8.9 kg) intake than with high carbohydrate (5.1 kg) intake; no weight loss occurred in a control group.

Golay and colleagues assessed the relative effects of carbohydrate versus calorie restriction on weight loss by keeping 43 obese adults in the hospital for 6 weeks (51). Subjects were assigned isoenergetic diets that differed in macronutrient distribution; one diet provided 15% of calories from carbohydrate, the other, 45%. At 6 weeks, weight loss, body-fat loss, and anthropometric changes were comparable between groups. The authors concluded that energy intake rather than macronutrient distribution determined weight loss over the short term. The implication is that in many other weight-loss studies, reductions in the former are masquerading as adjustments of the latter.

Finally, a recent trial by Ebbeling et al. (44) reveals some of the potential distortions introduced when means of improving dietary intake pattern are considered as mutually exclusive of one another. This group of investigators compared a diet reduced in glycemic load, with 30%–35% of calories from fat, with a diet termed conventional in which fat was restricted to 25%–30% of calories, but the quality of the carbohydrate choices was not addressed. The reduced glycemic load diet resulted in slightly greater weight loss and control of insulin resistance than did the control diet in the 16 obese adolescents followed. What seems most noteworthy, however, is that the range of fat intake for the low-fat and low-glycemic load diets are contiguous. Thus, this study actually compared two diets that differed little with regard to fat content, one in which glycemic load was controlled and the other in which it was not. This is very much like comparing complex to simple carbohydrates and finding that complex carbohydrates have preferable health effects. Regrettably, in the rush to defend competing dietary claims, this simple message is obscured.

The current preoccupation with carbohydrate restriction appears to be reactionary to the recent era during which fat restriction was prioritized. The popular press and media reports suggest that the public feels misled by promises that fat restriction would lead to weight loss. In particular, the widely known United States Department of Agriculture (USDA) food guide pyramid has come under attack as a contributor to worsening obesity rates (164). The adulteration of messages in the pyramid under the influence of special interest groups is the subject of a recent book (106). The CDC has recently released data indicating that over the past several decades, weight has gone up as carbohydrate consumption has risen (169).

An impassive examination of these trends and related scientific evidence paints a rather different picture, however. Dietary guidelines have long emphasized consumption of specific low-fat foods, namely whole grains, vegetables, and fruits. In response to the public's interest in fat restriction, the food industry generated a vast array of low-fat, but not necessarily low-calorie, foods over the past two decades, prototypical of which is Snackwell® cookies. On close inspection, the CDC data reveal that total fat intake never meaningfully declined; rather, fat as a proportion of total calories was diluted somewhat by an increase in total calorie intake (30, 56, 169). The increase in calories was driven by increased consumption of calorie-dense, nutrient-dilute, fat-restricted foods, contemporaneous with a trend toward increasing portion sizes in general (8, 53, 96, 107, 130).

The competition between low-fat and low-carbohydrate diets for weight loss has in some ways polarized debate beyond the point of reason or utility. Lowering the fat content of processed foods while increasing consumption of simple sugars and starch is not consistent with the long-standing recommendations of nutrition authorities to moderate intake of dietary fat. Yet it is this distorted approach to dietary fat "restriction" that best characterizes secular trends in dietary intake at the population level and that subtends the contention that dietary fat is unrelated to obesity.

An extensive literature belies this claim. Dietary fat is the most energy dense and least satiating of the macronutrient classes (57, 116, 134). When fat restriction is in accord with prevailing views on nutrition— i.e., achieved by shifting from foods high in fat to naturally low-fat foods such as vegetables, whole grains, and fruits— the results are consistently favorable with regard to energy balance and body weight (22). High dietary fat intake is a powerful predictor of weight gain (133).

Transcultural comparisons dating back at least to the work of Ancel Keys consistently indicate that higher intake of dietary fat is associated with higher rates of obesity and chronic disease (80–82). Most authorities concur that high intake of dietary fat contributes to obesity at the individual and population levels (116), and studies suggesting facilitation of weight loss by dietary fat restriction are numerous (66). The theoretical basis for weight loss through dietary fat restriction is strong, given the widely acknowledged primacy of calories in weight governance and the energy density of fat (72). Also noteworthy are data from the *National Weight Control Registry*, which indicate that lasting weight loss is consistently attributable to relatively fat-restricted, balanced diets in conjunction with regular physical activity (167). The weight-loss benefit of advice to follow fat-restricted diets is, however, no more enduring than that of advice to restrict calories by any other means (117).

Despite the extensive literature supporting dietary fat restriction for weight loss and control, there are dissenting voices (165). For the most part, dissent is predicated on the failure of dietary fat restriction to achieve population-level weight control in the United States and on the good health of Mediterranean populations with fat intake as high as 40% of calories (86). In addition, the evidence is clear that when energy restriction can be achieved on a diet relatively high in fat content, weight loss is achieved (136), suggesting the primacy of energy intake over macronutrient intake in weight regulation.

Recent U.S. trends suggest that fat intake over recent decades was held constant, not reduced, and that intake of total calories has risen to dilute the percent of food energy derived from fat; increased consumption of highly processed, fat-reduced foods is the principal basis for these trends (169). Thus, the failure of dietary fat restriction to facilitate weight control is more a problem of adherence than effectiveness (65). The Mediterranean diet differs from the typical American diet not only in the quantity of fat but in the type of fat and the quantity of unrefined grains, vegetables, fruit, and lean protein sources (140). Further, many of the Mediterranean populations enjoying good health have traditionally high rates of physical activity compared to Western societies; the effects of physical inactivity and high dietary fat intake may be synergistic with regard to weight gain (10).

Some evidence suggests that dietary protein may preserve resting energy expenditure following weight loss (163). This finding, together with protein's high satiety index, suggests a benefit of protein intake at the high end of the range advisable for overall health as an aid to weight loss and control efforts (69, 141).

Reports Related to the Long-Term Sustainability of Weight Loss or Long-Term Prevention of Weight Gain

As opposed to most people who commit a lifetime to sequential dieting, the literature on long-term weight loss success is thin; frequency of dieting is a negative predictor of lasting weight control (114). The best available data are from observational studies (95), trans-cultural comparison, and the National Weight Control Registry (167). The Registry was established to characterize the behavioral patterns of individuals successful at long-term maintenance of considerable weight loss (an average loss of 30 kg maintained for more than 5 years). Registry data indicate that a relatively low-fat, and therefore energy-dilute, diet is a mainstay of successful weight maintenance, as is regular physical activity (84, 97, 137).

Studies Characterizing the Effects of Various Weight-Loss Diets on Body Composition

One of the most tantalizing claims of popular weight-loss diets is that weight loss can be achieved or facilitated by means other than energy restriction. De-emphasizing calories is, in fact, quite characteristic of popular weight-loss approaches. Proponents of carbohydrate restriction contend that limiting intake of carbohydrate allows for weight loss regardless of calorie intake (15). At least one study reported at the 2003 meeting of the North American Association for the Study of Obesity (NAASO; http://www.naaso.org) suggested greater weight loss over a 12-week period among subjects on a low-carbohydrate diet than among those on a low-fat diet, despite consuming 300 more calories per day on the carbohydrate-restricted assignment.

However, only limited data are available to date on the effects of carbohydrate restriction on body composition. There is clear evidence of a dehydrating effect of very low carbohydrate diets and of ketosis in the short term (77); thus, some of the early weight loss on low-carbohydrate diets is almost certainly water. An association between increasing dietary fat and increasing body fat has been noted (88). Nelson and colleagues reported a positive association between dietary fat and body fat and negative associations with body fat for both total and complex carbohydrate (105).

Hays and colleagues recently reported that a diet rich in complex carbohydrate resulted in an increase in lean body mass and a decrease in body fat among 34 subjects with impaired glucose tolerance (55). Similar results have been observed by other groups (138). Volek and colleagues, however, reported a loss of body fat and an increase in lean body mass with carbohydrate restriction in 12 volunteers followed for 6 weeks (159). Thus, the independent effects of redistributing macronutrients on body composition remain the subject of controversy; more science is clearly required for closure. The effects of physical activity on body composition are, of course, clear and noncontroversial; increased activity leads to relative increases in lean body mass at the expense of body fat (83, 124).

Overall, little evidence supports a claim that loss of body fat is achieved preferentially by redistributing macronutrients at isoenergetic levels. Worth noting is that a pound of body fat represents an energy reserve of over 4000 kcal; a pound of muscle, a reserve of roughly 1800 kcal; and a pound of water, no latent energy whatsoever. Although each weighs a pound, each requires a markedly different energy deficit to be lost; water can be lost with no energy deficit. Thus until proved otherwise, the most plausible explanation for enhanced weight loss at any given level of energy intake is the loss of body compartments that represent lesser energy reserves. Such losses of water and muscle protein are undesirable.

Diets in Wide Use by the General Public; Popular Diet Books

A search on Amazon.com using the terms "diet," "weight loss," and "weight control," yields bibliographies of 85,645; 96,722; and 101,099, respectively (http://www.amazon.com, as of April 30, 2004). The same terms entered into a web search on Google yield 25,900,000, 8620,000, and 7770,000 sites, respectively (http://www.google.com, as of April 30, 2004). Thus, it is far beyond the scope of this or any review, or even plausibility, to characterize even a representative sample of weight-loss diets, programs, or products being promoted to the general public.

The best that can be done to characterize these myriad claims on the basis of evidence is to apply a process of exclusion. In a systematic review of the obesity prevention and control literature (170), strategies that emerge as most promising with regard to lasting weight control involve achieving an energy-controlled and balanced diet along with regular physical activity. Fundamentally, claims for virtually any other approach to sustainable weight loss are unsubstantiated. There is little or no scientific evidence to support the contentions of the most popular diets, including those based on carbohydrate restriction (e.g., the Atkins' diet), those based on food combination or food proportioning (e.g., the Zone diet), or those based on the glycemic index (e.g., the South Beach Diet, the GI Diet). There is, of course, no shortage of anecdotal support and testimonials for virtually all of the popular diets.

Worth noting is that a modest proportion of the books on the subject of diet address not so much the "what" of weight loss but the "how," describing strategies for achieving a diet and lifestyle the evidence indicates to be associated with both lasting weight control and good health. Among the offerings in this category are approaches based on energy density (111, 157); water and fiber content (128); and the array of skills and strategies needed to navigate through the modern, "toxic" nutritional environment (78). Related to these are books dedicated to the same goal for children and/or families (e.g., 135).

Potential Hazards of Popular Weight-Loss Diets

Little evidence suggests that dietary fat restriction as a weight loss method is harmful. To the contrary, a rich and varied literature argues that restriction of dietary fat is both conducive to weight loss and is health-promoting (11, 33). Many cultures recognized for good health and longevity have native diets very low in fat (40); few free-living societies adhere to dietary patterns low in carbohydrate. The worst that can be said of fat restriction for weight loss is that if extreme it may not be optimal for health (68). Even critics of dietary fat restriction appear to agree that low-fat diets offer health benefits relative to the typical American diet, which is high in saturated and trans fat.

Carbohydrate restriction, in contrast, is actually or potentially linked to an array of adverse health effects (77). Evidence indicates that weight loss attributable to carbohydrate restriction is in part body water loss. Gluconeogenesis consumes water along with glycogen, and ketone bodies cause increased renal excretion of sodium and water (37). Studies suggest dizziness, fatigue, and headache are common side effects (145) of ketosis.

Ketosis is potentially harmful, with possible long-term sequelae including hyperlipidemia, impaired neutrophil function, optic neuropathy, osteoporosis, and protein deficiency as well as alterations in cognitive function (37). Children on ketogenic diets as part of an antiseizure regimen have developed dehydration, constipation, and kidney stones. In response to ketosis, renal calcium excretion increases. To make up for the loss of calcium in urine, it is mobilized from bone to circulation (37). One study of adolescents on a ketogenic diet showed decreased bone mineral density after just three months, despite vitamin D and calcium supplementation (145). Sustained ketosis causes bone resorption, suggesting a risk for osteoporosis (45).

Comparison of eight high-protein, low-carbohydrate diets indicates that the Atkins diet advises the highest level of total fat, saturated fat, and cholesterol (145). Consuming a diet high in saturated fat may raise total and low-density lipoprotein cholesterol levels, both of which contribute to cardiovascular disease. A significant increase in LDL has been reported among subjects on the Atkins diet (37), although this finding is inconsistent. An increase in C-reactive protein (CRP) on the Atkins diet has been observed as well (145), suggesting an inflammatory response. A high intake of saturated fat increases the risk of insulin resistance (145), contradicting the contention of low-carbohydrate diet proponents that carbohydrates are to blame for insulin resistance (15). High-fat diets may also predispose to cancer (71).

High-protein intake may negatively affect renal function in healthy individuals and certainly accelerates renal disease in diabetes. In patients with renal dysfunction on a high-protein diet, there is glomerular damage causing spillage of plasma proteins and resultant tubular injury and fibrosis (145). As noted, urinary calcium excretion is also increased and hypercalciuria may ensue, predisposing to calcium stone formation (37). High-protein intake imposes a metabolic burden on both the liver and kidneys, requiring additional excretion of urea and ammonia (64).

Extreme carbohydrate restriction is potentially associated with increased risk of dysthymia, if not depression, through a serotonergic mechanism (73). The production of serotonin in the brain requires delivery and uptake of tryptophan, which is influenced by both the availability of tryptophan and the actions of insulin. With very low carbohydrate intake and blunted insulin release, tryptophan delivery to the brain is impaired, serotonin production is limited, and mood instability has been reported to ensue (19); the public health significance of this mechanism remains uncertain.

Finally, high-protein, low-carbohydrate diets simply do not allow for adequate intake of fruits and vegetables, restricting nutrient and fiber-rich foods shown to protect against cancer, cardiovascular disease, diabetes, diverticular disease, as well as constipation (112, 147, 156, 162). Fiber lowers cholesterol, reducing the risk for cardiovascular disease, and lowers insulin secretion after meals by slowing nutrient absorption (29, 145).

The known and potential hazards of carbohydrate restriction are summarized in Table 2.

Reports of Associations Between Dietary Pattern and Health Outcomes for Diverse Populations, Healthy and Otherwise

In the Diabetes Prevention Program, a low-calorie, low-fat diet coupled with moderately intense physical activity for at least 150 min per week reduced the incidence of type 2 diabetes by 58% (85). Similarly, the DASH Collaborative Research Group

TABLE 2   Known and potential adverse effects of extreme restriction of dietary intake of carbohydrate. Derived from Reference 113a

Adverse effect	Mechanism
Constipation	An established effect attributable to low intake of dietary fiber.
Dehydration	Gluconeogenesis consumes water along with glycogen, and ketone bodies cause increased renal excretion of sodium and water.
Depression/dysthymia	A theoretical risk due to impaired delivery of tryptophan to the brain and impaired serotonin production.
Halitosis	An established effect of ketosis.
Hepatic injury	A potential sequela of high protein intake over time.
Increased cancer risk	A potential sequela of increased consumption of animal products and decreased consumption of grains and fruit.
Increased cardiovascular disease risk	A potential sequela of increased consumption of animal products and decreased consumption of grains and fruit.
Nausea	An established side effect of ketosis.
Nephropathy	A potential consequence of high intake of protein over time.
Osteopenia	An established effect of ketosis. Hypercalciuria is induced by high intake of dietary protein.
Renal calculi	A known sequela of ketosis. Risk is increased by dehydration.

has shown that hypertension can be prevented and treated by reducing intake of saturated and total fat and adopting a diet rich in fruits, vegetables, grains, and low-fat dairy (131). Cardiovascular disease prevention has been demonstrated with both low-fat (113) and Mediterranean dietary patterns (92). Weight loss is a common element in all of these successful interventions.

Reviews of diet for optimal health do not necessarily demonstrate complete accord on all points but are nonetheless substantially confluent with regard to fundamentals. Diets rich in fruits, vegetables, and whole grains; restricted in animal fats and trans fat from processed foods; limited in refined starches and sugar; providing protein principally from lean sources; and offering fat principally in the form of monounsaturated and polyunsaturated oils are linked to good health (58–60, 74, 79, 94, 127, 164). With regard to diet and optimal health, debate is substantially limited to variations on this basic theme, rather than any fundamental departures from it.

Anthropology Literature Characterizing the Native Human Diet and Its Health Implications

A final contribution is made by the anthropology literature to considerations of dietary pattern and human health. Quite distinct from biomedical research, a fairly

TABLE 3   A comparison of the energy density and satiety indices of the macronutrient classes. The satiety index is a measure of how filling a food is based on comparison of isoenergetic servings (70)

Macronutrient class	Energy density	Satiety index	Comments
Fat	Highest; 9 kcal/g	Lowest	The notion seems to prevail that fat is filling; but on a calorie-for-calorie basis, it is the least satiating of the macronutrient classes.
Carbohydrate; simple	4 kcal/g	Intermediate; lower than for complex carbohydrate	The satiety threshold for sugar is higher than that for other nutrients, thus making sugar an important contributor to caloric excess in most people.
Carbohydrate; complex	<4 kcal/g	Intermediate; higher than for simple carbohydrate	Sources of complex carbohydrate—whole grains, fruits, and vegetables—are rich in water and fiber, both of which increase food volume and contribute to satiety, yet provide no calories.
Protein	3–4 kcal/g	Highest	Protein is generally more filling, calorie-for-calorie, than other food classes, although this finding may not be true when compared with complex carbohydrates very high in fiber and/or water content.

extensive body of work characterizes what is and is not known about the native nutritional habitat of our species. Although researchers debate many details, there is general consensus that humanity adapted over eons to an environment in which calories were relatively scarce and physical activity demands were high (43). Saturated and trans fat intake were low and negligible, respectively; micronutrient intake was high; and protein intake was from lean sources (17, 41). The traditional human diet was, of course, low in both starch and sugar but rich in complex carbohydrate from a variety of plant foods (41). Many, but not all, anthropologists suggest we were more gatherers than hunters and that meat likely contributed less to our subsistence than did the gathering of diverse plant foods (42, 75). That this should be relevant to human health requires nothing more than acknowledging that human beings are creatures. For all other species under our care, epitomized by zoological parks, the diet we provide is an adaptation of the diet consumed in the wild. The native human diet appears to have provided roughly 25% of calories from fat, 20%–25% of calories from protein, and the remainder from complex carbohydrate (41); this pattern is remarkably confluent with that demonstrating compelling health benefits in clinical trials (85, 131).

Reviews, Position Statements, and Dietary Guidelines Addressing Weight Control, Health Promotion, or Both

On the basis of its review of evidence linking dietary pattern to health outcomes, *The United States Preventive Services Task Force* advises clinicians to endorse to all patients over the age of two a diet restricted in fat, particularly saturated fat, and abundant in fruits, vegetables, and grains (155a). These recommendations are highly concordant with those of the National Heart Lung and Blood Institute at the National Institutes of Health (http://www.nhlbi.nih.gov/guidelines/obesity/prctgd_b.pdf). The United States Department of Agriculture recommendations (155), depicted in the USDA food guide pyramid (154), emphasize abundant intake of grains, vegetables, and fruits, with restricted intake of both simple sugars and total fat. The National Cancer Institute sponsors the 5-a-day program encouraging fruit and vegetable intake and endorses dietary guidelines that include 20–35 g of fiber per day, with 30% or less of calories from fat (103). The American Heart Association offers dietary guidelines that call for 55% or more of calories from carbohydrate, 30% or less from fat (7%–10% saturated/trans fat, 10% polyunsaturated, and 15% monounsaturated fats), and 15%–20% from protein (5). The American Dietetic Association supports the USDA Dietary Guidelines and recommends intake of a variety of grains and at least five servings of fruits and vegetables daily, restriction of saturated fat and cholesterol, and limited sugar and sweet consumption (4). The American Diabetes Association advocates 55% of calories from carbohydrate, up to 30% from fat (10% saturated/trans fat, 10% polyunsaturated fat), and 15%–20% from protein (50). Differing only in detail, all of these recommendations are substantially congruent.

In 2002, The National Academies of Science's Institute of Medicine (IOM) released dietary guidelines calling for 45%–65% of calories from carbohydrate, 20%–35% from fat, and 10%–35% from protein, in conjunction with 60 min each day of moderately intense physical activity (47). The IOM guidelines further emphasize the restriction of saturated and trans fat and their replacement with monounsaturated and polyunsaturated fat. Also in 2002, on the basis of consensus opinion, the American College of Preventive Medicine formally adopted a position supporting dietary recommendations within the IOM ranges and in opposition to carbohydrate restriction for purposes of weight control (3).

There are numerous reviews on the subject of diet for weight loss (9, 12, 18, 31, 39, 66, 102, 118, 119, 129, 158, 161, 166). In the aggregate, this literature lends strongest support to diets abundant in fruits, vegetables, and whole grains and restricted in total fat (see Table 3).

DISCUSSION

A comprehensive examination of the weight control literature and assessment of competing dietary claims for weight loss pose some unique challenges. At a time of rapidly worsening epidemic obesity, it is self-evident that no generally effective approach to reliable weight control has been established and applied. This at once belies the exaggerated claims of most popular diets but also, to some degree, legitimizes them all. If nothing works to stem the rising tides of our dietary tribulations, then no one claim rings substantially less true than any other.

Thus, a proximal examination of the weight control evidence base leads to uncertainty and confusion. Short-term weight loss is achieved by virtually any means conducive to the restriction of choice and calories. Various amounts of weight have been lost with varying alacrity on diets restricting fat, diets restricting carbohydrate, diets requiring specific combinations of foods or macronutrient classes, diets based on rice, diets based on grapefruit, low and very low calorie liquid diets, meal replacement systems, calorie-counting systems, programs based on incentives and disincentives, programs based on emotional troubleshooting, programs based on the energy-density of foods, and virtually every conceivable combination of and variation on these themes. Yet sustainability of weight loss in the aftermath of almost any short-term approach has been elusive. The relative effectiveness of various dietary approaches to weight loss and weight control involving food exclusions, food combinations, and the redistribution of macronutrient classes is substantially unclear.

But this proximal view is rather like looking at a mosaic from several inches away or inspecting a dense forest from within. The former results in perception of a blur of random color, an apparently haphazard placement of tiles, and the latter, proverbially, in a failure to see the forest through the trees. The weight-control literature is like this, too.

A step back from specific dietary contentions and contradictions so that the whole lay of the land may be viewed lends clarity. Although we have little definitive evidence regarding dietary interventions effective at achieving sustainable weight loss and control for an increasingly overweight public, we have substantial and compelling evidence regarding the basic dietary pattern conducive to human health. There is, as well, considerable evidence from multiple sources to suggest an association between a health-promoting diet and lifestyle and lasting weight control. From a prudent distance, sorting among competing diet claims ceases to be daunting, because—by and large—it ceases to be relevant.

Multiple sources of evidence point to a dietary pattern, or relatively narrow range of patterns, conducive to the long-term health promotion, and weight control, of *Homo sapiens*. These sources—trial data, observational studies, trans-cultural comparisons, and paleo-anthropology—together comprise a triangulation method of considerable robustness. The common ground is characterized in Table 4.

Popular diets tend to emphasize weight loss while ignoring the importance of dietary pattern to overall health. The responsible practitioner should do just the opposite, encouraging healthful dietary and physical activity practices, with a secondary emphasis on weight control. This approach, coupled with guidance toward the skills and strategies for eating well in a challenging environment, should serve to blunt the public's appetite for fad diets and thereby safeguard health.

Perennially reinventing our destination for weight control in the form of the hot diet du jour is a discredit to our common sense, a digression from our cultural

TABLE 4   Dietary pattern recommended for health promotion. Adapted from Reference 78

Nutrient class/nutrient		Recommended intake
Carbohydrate, predominately complex		Approximately 55%–60% of total calories
Fiber, both soluble and insoluble		At least 25 g per day, with additional potential benefit from up to 50 g per day
Protein, predominantly plant-based sources		Up to 20% of total calories
Total Fat	**Types of Fat**	Not more than 30%, and preferably 20%–25% of total calories
	Monounsaturated fat	10%–15% of total calories
	Polyunsaturated fat Omega-3 and Omega-6 fat	10% of total calories between 1:1 to 1:4 ratio
	Saturated fat and trans fat (partially hydrogenated fat)	Less than 5% of total calories
Sugar		Less than 10% of total calories
Sodium		Up to 2400 mg per day
Cholesterol		Up to 300 mg per day
Water		Approximately 64 oz per day
Alcohol		Up to one drink per day for women Up to two drinks per day for men
Calorie level		Adequate to achieve and maintain a healthy weight
Physical activity/exercise		Daily moderate activity for 30 min Strength training twice weekly

imperatives about confronting challenges, an indictment of our collective judgment, and a neglect of a robust base of evidence characterizing the effects of dietary pattern on the health of human beings across the life span. But it is something far worse. It is a bona fide public health threat in and of itself. As long as we remain distracted by competing dietary claims and beguiled by the prospect of weight-loss magic, we will fail to take the requisite steps or mobilize the requisite political will to make healthful eating more accessible to all. In other words, the more resources we devote to questioning where we ought to go, the longer it will be before we get anywhere.

Ongoing examination of competing diets appears to apply a very different standard of evidence than that applied in other cases. The most plausible rationale for genuine uncertainty about the basic dietary pattern conducive to long-term human health and weight control is the lack of definitive trial evidence. In response to this, it is instructive to consider what such trials would look like. It may be that dietary exposures at different times in the life cycle have differential effects on weight management; obesigenic exposures in early childhood and at puberty, for example, contribute disproportionately to hyperplasia of adipose tissue (108). Thus, a definitive trial of alternative diets for lifelong weight control should begin in early childhood at worst and preferably at or even before birth; it is well established that exposures in utero influence susceptibility to obesity (28, 34, 159a). To examine the outcome of interest—lifelong health and weight control—would require following subjects across the entire life span. Thus, what we need to answer the question, what diet is best for lasting weight control?, is a randomized controlled trial of every diet we deem worthy of evaluation, with subjects enrolled as fetuses and followed through senescence. Anything other than strict adherence to the assigned diet over the length of the trial would compromise the results.

This ridiculously implausible trial highlights how easy it is to allow notions of evidence to become tyrannical and counterproductive and how readily "perfect" can be made the enemy of "good." Somehow, we seem willing to do this for diet, and yet we apply more reasonable standards of evidence elsewhere.

Consider the state of both knowledge and public health practice with regard to physical activity. It is widely, perhaps even universally, accepted that a lifetime of regular physical activity promotes health. On this basis, current pertinent effort is directed toward identifying practical means of raising the ambient level of daily activity. In other words, "what" is established, so we are wrestling collectively with "how," from encouraging use of stairs, to making sure neighborhoods have sidewalks, to reestablishing physical education in our schools.

But do we, in fact, actually know that there is no alternative to regular physical activity? Have we systematically examined every conceivable means of being sedentary—different postures, different positions, different couches on which to perch—and proved that none is as good as being regularly active? Of course we have not. Yet it seems if we were to apply the standard we are using for diet, this is exactly what we would do. Rather than work to promote the activity pattern abundant but not truly definitive evidence indicates promotes health, we would devote our resources to studying every conceivable alternative to that pattern.

We have, in the aggregate, as much evidence regarding the association between diet and health as we do regarding physical activity and health. Diet may be a more complex variable, but the parallel is still strong. The evidence we have in support of a particular dietary pattern for health suggests that our resources should be devoted to getting us there, not looking for alternatives. If we are committed to looking for alternatives, we should apply a single standard in our commitment to evidence, abandon efforts to promote physical activity, and start studying the myriad ways of being sedentary until we have disproved the benefits of each.

One is tempted to wonder why such dichotomous standards of evidence have developed in the first place. The fact that there would be financial liability for some powerful special interests were consensus regarding diet to emerge and none such for physical activity is irrefutable. That we are all somehow influenced by this circumstance is a prospect at once both tantalizing and appalling.

We cannot afford to delay a dedicated effort to establish consensus regarding a health-promoting dietary pattern conducive to sustainable weight control. Already, some 65%–80% of us are overweight or obese, and most of the rest of us are slowly succumbing. Already, we are raising children subject to epidemic type 2 diabetes, a disease accurately referred to as "adult onset" a mere two decades ago. Already, we are raising children on a trajectory toward cardiovascular disease in adolescence. Already, we are raising children more subject to chronic disease and premature death from a lifetime of bad eating habits than from exposure to tobacco, illicit drugs, and alcohol combined. Already, we are raising a generation of children so threatened by epidemic obesity that they are projected to have a shorter life span than their parents, an unprecedented travesty in our modern history.

Popular diets generally appeal to the public because they offer clear and simple guidelines that people can follow. In contrast, most people struggle to adopt prevailing guidelines for healthful eating. There is reason to hope that if the public were better instructed in how to overcome the obstacles to healthful eating so abundant in the modern world, they would be less vulnerable to fad diets. Further, fad diets promise, and deliver, rapid weight loss. They do not seem to deliver sustainable weight loss, however. Sustainable weight loss is most consistently achieved with diets corresponding to prevailing nutrition guidelines. Finally, fad diets imply a solution to weight-control problems that is independent of calories. This is simply a false allure; fad diets produce weight loss by restricting calories.

One cannot offer ironclad evidence that fad diets are harmful in the long term simply because such long-term studies have not been conducted. They may never be conducted. The onus of proof lies with those suggesting radical departures from patterns of behavior known to support human health; the community of nutrition experts is not obligated to prove the harmfulness of every new diet proposed.

Health promotion is the forest through the truculent trees of competing dietary claims. We have a long way to go to achieve population-wide weight control in a toxic nutritional environment. But that is not because we are clueless about the basic care and feeding of *Homo sapiens*. We are not! (See Table 4.) The challenge before us is determining how best to get where we need to go, not deciding where that is. The sooner we accept that we know where we should be going, the sooner we may actually hope to advance toward that destination. Stated differently, we will need to espouse a common vision of the forest through the trees before we can hope to get out of the woods.

ACKNOWLEDGMENTS

The assistance of Meghan O'Connell, MPH, and Ather Ali, ND, is gratefully acknowledged, as is the technical support of Michelle Larovera.

This work was partially supported by grants U48-CCU115802 and U48-CCU115802 from the Centers for Disease Control and Prevention.

The *Annual Review of Public Health* is online at
http://publhealth.annualreviews.org

LITERATURE CITED

1. 2004. Low carb nation. *Time Mag.* May, Vol. 163
2. Akan GE, Grilo CM. 1995. Sociocultural influences on eating attitudes and behaviors, body image, and psychological functioning: a comparison of African-American, Asian-American, and Caucasian college women. *Int. J. Eat Disord.* 18:181–87
3. Am. Coll. Prev. Med. Position Statement. 2002. *Diet in the prevention and control of obesity, insulin resistance, and type II diabetes.* http://www.acpm.org/2002–057(F).htm
4. Am. Diet. Assoc. 2002. Weight management—position of ADA. *J. Am. Diet. Assoc.* 102:1145–55
5. Am. Heart Assoc. 2001. *Step I and step II diets.* http://www.americanheart.org/presenter.jhtml?identifier=4764
6. Anderson LA, Eyler AA, Galuska DA, Brown DR, Brownson RC. 2002. Relationship of satisfaction with body size and trying to lose weight in a national survey of overweight and obese women aged 40 and older, United States. *Prev. Med.* 35:390–96
7. Ashworth M, Clement S, Wright M. 2002. Demand, appropriateness and prescribing of 'lifestyle drugs', a consultation survey in general practice. *Fam. Pract.* 19:236–41
8. Astrup A. 1998. The American paradox: the role of energy-dense fat-reduced food in the increasing prevalence of obesity. *Curr. Opin. Clin. Nutr. Metab. Care* 1:573–77
9. Astrup A. 1999. Dietary approaches to reducing body weight. *Baillieres Best Pract. Res. Clin. Endocrinol. Metab.* 13:109–20
10. Astrup A. 1999. Macronutrient balances and obesity: the role of diet and physical activity. *Public Health Nutr.* 2:341–47
11. Astrup A. 2001. The role of dietary fat in the prevention and treatment of obesity. Efficacy and safety of low-fat diets. *Int. J. Obes. Relat. Metab. Disord.* 25:S46–50
12. Astrup A, Ryan L, Grunwald GK, Storgaard M, Saris W, et al. 2000. The role of dietary fat in body fatness: evidence from a preliminary meta-analysis of ad libitum low-fat dietary intervention studies. *Br. J. Nutr.* 83:S25–32
13. Atkins RC. 1972. *Dr. Atkins' Diet Revolution.* New York: Bantam
14. Atkins RC. 1999. *Atkins' New Diet Revolution.* New York: Evans
15. Atkins RC. 2002. *Dr. Atkins' New Diet Revolution.* New York: HarperCollins
16. Aye T, Levitsky LL. 2003. Type 2 diabetes: an epidemic disease in childhood. *Curr. Opin. Pediatr.* 15:411–15
17. Baschetti R. 1997. Paleolithic nutrition. *Eur. J. Clin. Nutr.* 51:715–16
18. Bedno SA. 2003. Weight loss in diabetes management. *Nutr. Clin. Care* 6:62–72
19. Benton D. 2002. Carbohydrate ingestion, blood glucose and mood. *Neurosci. Biobehav. Rev.* 26:293–308
20. Bramwell VH, Williams CJ. 1997. Do authors of review articles use systematic methods to identify, assess and synthesize information? *Ann. Oncol.* 8:1185–95
21. Bravata DM, Sanders L, Huang J, Krumholz HM, Olkin I, et al. 2003. Efficacy and safety of low-carbohydrate diets: a systematic review. *JAMA* 289:1837–50
22. Bray G, Popkin B. 1998. Dietary fat intake does affect obesity! *Am. J. Clin. Nutr.* 68:1157–73
23. Brehm BJ, Seeley RJ, Daniels SR,

D'Alessio DA. 2003. A randomized trial comparing a very low carbohydrate diet and a calorie-restricted low fat diet on body weight and cardiovascular risk factors in healthy women. *J. Clin. Endocrinol. Metab.* 88:1617–23

24. Briss P, Zaza S, Pappaioanou M, Fielding J, Aguero LW-D, et al. 2000. Developing an evidence-based guide to community preventive services—methods. The task force on community preventive services. *Am. J. Prev. Med.* 18:35–43

25. Caldwell MB, Brownell KD, Wilfley DE. 1997. Relationship of weight, body dissatisfaction, and self-esteem in African American and white female dieters. *Int. J. Eat Disord.* 22:127–30

26. Calle EE, Rodriguez C, Walker-Thurmond K, Thun MJ. 2003. Overweight, obesity, and mortality from cancer in a prospectively studied cohort of U.S. adults. *N. Engl. J. Med.* 348:1625–38

27. Calle EE, Thun MJ, Petrelli JM, Rodriguez C, Heath CW Jr. 1999. Body-mass index and mortality in a prospective cohort of U.S. adults. *N. Engl. J. Med.* 341:1097–105

28. Catalano PM, Thomas A, Huston-Presley L, Amini SB. 2003. Increased fetal adiposity: a very sensitive marker of abnormal in utero development. *Am. J. Obstet. Gynecol.* 189:1698–704

29. Chandalia M, Garg A, Lutjohann D, von Bergmann K, Grundy SM, Brinkley LJ. 2000. Beneficial effects of high dietary fiber intake in patients with type 2 diabetes mellitus. *N. Engl. J. Med.* 342:1392–98

30. Chanmugam P, Guthrie JF, Cecilio S, Morton JF, Basiotis PP, Anand R. 2003. Did fat intake in the United States really decline between 1989–1991 and 1994–1996? *J. Am. Diet. Assoc.* 103:867–72

31. Cheuvront SN. 2003. The Zone Diet phenomenon: a closer look at the science behind the claims. *J. Am. Coll. Nutr.* 22:9–17

32. Chopra M, Galbraith S, Darnton-Hill I. 2002. A global response to a global problem: the epidemic of overnutrition. *Bull. World Health Organ.* 80:952–58

33. Connor W, Connor S. 1997. Should a low-fat, high-carbohydrate diet be recommended for everyone? The case for a low-fat, high-carbohydrate diet. *N. Engl. J. Med.* 337:562–63

34. Dabelea D, Hanson RL, Lindsay RS, Pettitt DJ, Imperatore G, et al. 2000. Intrauterine exposure to diabetes conveys risks for type 2 diabetes and obesity: a study of discordant sibships. *Diabetes* 49:2208–11

35. Damcott CM, Sack P, Shuldiner AR. 2003. The genetics of obesity. *Endocrinol. Metab. Clin. North Am.* 32:761–86

36. Davis SP, Northington L, Kolar K. 2000. Cultural considerations for treatment of childhood obesity. *J. Cult. Divers.* 7:128–32

37. Denke M. 2001. Metabolic effects of high-protein, low-carbohydrate diets. *Am. J. Cardiol.* 88:59–61

38. Drewnowski A. 2000. Nutrition transition and global dietary trends. *Nutrition* 16:486–87

39. Drewnowski A. 2003. The role of energy density. *Lipids* 38:109–15

40. Drewnowski A, Popkin BM. 1997. The nutrition transition: new trends in the global diet. *Nutr. Rev.* 55:31–43

41. Eaton SB, Eaton SB III, Konner M. 1997. Paleolithic nutrition revisited: a twelve-year retrospective on its nature and implications. *Eur. J. Clin. Nutr.* 51:207–16

42. Eaton SB, Eaton SB III, Konner M, Shostak M. 1996. An evolutionary perspective enhances understanding of human nutritional requirements. *J. Nutr.* 126:1732–40

43. Eaton SB, Strassman BI, Nesse RM, Neel JV, Ewald PW, et al. 2002. Evolutionary health promotion. *Prev. Med.* 34:109–18

44. Ebbeling CB, Leidig MM, Sinclair

KB, Hangen JP, Ludwig DS. 2003. A reduced-glycemic load diet in the treatment of adolescent obesity. *Arch. Pediatr. Adolesc. Med.* 157:773–79

45. Eisenstein J, Roberts SB, Dallal G, Saltzman E. 2002. High-protein weight-loss diets: Are they safe and do they work? A review of the experimental and epidemiologic data. *Nutr. Rev.* 60:189–200

46. Epstein LH. 1996. Family-based behavioural intervention for obese children. *Int. J. Obes. Relat. Metab. Disord.* 20:S14–21

47. Food Nutr. Board, Inst. Med., Natl. Acad. Sci. 2002. *Dietary Reference Intakes for Energy, Carbohydrate, Fiber, Fat, Fatty Acids, Cholesterol, Protein, and Amino Acids* (*Macronutrients*). Washington, DC: Natl. Acad. Press

48. Deleted in proof

49. Foster GD, Wyatt HR, Hill JO, McGuckin BG, Brill C, et al. 2003. A randomized trial of a low-carbohydrate diet for obesity. *N. Engl. J. Med.* 348:2082–90

50. Franz MJ, Bantle JP, Beebe CA, Brunzell JD, Chiasson J, et al. 2002. Evidence-based nutrition. Principles and recommendations for the treatment and prevention of diabetes and related complications. *Diabetes Care* 25:148–98

51. Golay A, Allaz A, Morel Y, de Tonnac N, Tankova S, Reaven G. 1996. Similar weight loss with low- and high-carbohydrate diets. *Am. J. Clin. Nutr.* 63:174–78

52. Golay A, Eigenheer C, Morel Y, Kujawski P, Lehmann T, deTonnac N. 1996. Weight-loss with low or high carbohydrate diet? *Int. J. Obes. Relat. Metab. Disord.* 20:1067–72

53. Harnack LJ, Jeffery RW, Boutelle KN. 2000. Temporal trends in energy intake in the United States: an ecologic perspective. *Am. J. Clin. Nutr.* 71:1478–84

54. Harvey-Berino J. 1998. The efficacy of dietary fat vs. total energy restriction for weight loss. *Obes. Res.* 6:202–7

55. Hays NP, Starling RD, Liu X, Sullivan DH, Trappe TA, et al. 2004. Effects of an ad libitum low-fat, high-carbohydrate diet on body weight, body composition, and fat distribution in older men and women—a randomized controlled trial. *Arch. Intern. Med.* 164:210–17

56. Heitmann BL, Lissner L, Osler M. 2000. Do we eat less fat, or just report so? *Int. J. Obes. Relat. Metab. Disord.* 24:435–42

57. Hill JO, Melanson EL, Wyatt HT. 2000. Dietary fat intake and regulation of energy balance: implications for obesity. *J. Nutr.* 130:284S–88

58. Hu FB. 2003. Plant-based foods and prevention of cardiovascular disease: an overview. *Am. J. Clin. Nutr.* 78:544S–51

59. Hu FB, Manson JE, Willett WC. 2001. Types of dietary fat and risk of coronary heart disease: a critical review. *J. Am. Coll. Nutr.* 20:5–19

60. Hu FB, Willett WC. 2002. Optimal diets for prevention of coronary heart disease. *JAMA* 288:2569–78

61. Jahns L, Baturin A, Popkin BM. 2003. Obesity, diet, and poverty: trends in the Russian transition to market economy. *Eur. J. Clin. Nutr.* 57:1295–302

62. Jeffery RW, Utter J. 2003. The changing environment and population obesity in the United States. *Obes. Res.* 11:12S–22

63. Jeffery RW, Wing RR. 1995. Long-term effects of interventions for weight loss using food provision and monetary incentives. *J. Consult. Clin. Psychol.* 63:793–96

64. Jeor SS, Howard B, Prewitt E, Bovee V, Bazzarre T, Eckel R. 2001. Dietary protein and weight reduction: a statement for healthcare professionals from the Nutrition Committee of the Council on Nutrition, Physical Activity, and Metabolism of the American Heart Association. *Circulation* 104:1869–74

65. Jequier E. 2002. Pathways to obesity. *Int. J. Obes. Relat. Metab. Disord.* 26:S12–17

66. Jequier E, Bray GA. 2002. Low-fat diets are preferred. *Am. J. Med.* 113:41S–46

67. Kappagoda CT, Hyson DA, Amsterdam EA. 2004. Low-carbohydrate-high-protein diets: Is there a place for them in clinical cardiology? *J. Am. Coll. Cardiol.* 43:725–30

68. Katan M, Grundy S, Willett W. 1997. Should a low-fat, high-carbohydrate diet be recommended for everyone? Beyond low-fat diets. *N. Engl. J. Med.* 337:563–66

69. Katz D. 2001. Diet, obesity, and weight regulation. See Ref. 76, pp. 37–62

70. Katz D. 2001. Hunger, appetite, taste, and satiety. See Ref. 76, pp. 260–67

71. Katz DL. 2001. Diet and cancer. See Ref. 76, pp. 114–26

72. Katz DL. 2001. Clinically relevant fat metabolism. See Ref. 76, pp. 9–15

73. Katz DL. 2001. Diet, sleep-wake cycles, and mood. See Ref. 76, pp. 243–47

74. Katz DL. 2001. Dietary recommendations for health promotion and disease prevention. See Ref. 76, pp. 291–98

75. Katz DL. 2001. Evolutionary biology, culture, and determinants of dietary behavior. See Ref. 76, pp. 279–90

76. Katz DL. 2001. *Nutrition in Clinical Practice*. Philadelphia, PA: Lippincott Williams & Wilkins

77. Katz DL. 2003. Pandemic obesity and the contagion of nutritional nonsense. *Public Health Rev.* 31:33–44

78. Katz DL, Gonzalez MH. 2002. *The Way to Eat*. Naperville, Ill.: Sourcebooks

79. Key TJ, Schatzkin A, Willett WC, Allen NE, Spencer EA, Travis RC. 2004. Diet, nutrition and the prevention of cancer. *Public Health Nutr.* 7:187–200

80. Keys A. 1955. Relative obesity and its health significance. *Diabetes* 4:447–55

81. Keys A, Aravanis C, Blackburn H, Buchem FSV, Buzina R, et al. 1972. Coronary heart disease: overweight and obesity as risk factors. *Ann. Intern. Med.* 77:15–27

82. Keys A, Menotti A, Aravanis C, Black-burn H, Djordevic BS, et al. 1984. The seven countries study: 2,289 deaths in 15 years. *Prev. Med.* 13:141–54

83. Kirk EP, Jacobsen DJ, Gibson C, Hill JO, Donnelly JE. 2003. Time course for changes in aerobic capacity and body composition in overweight men and women in response to long-term exercise: the Midwest Exercise Trial (MET). *Int. J. Obes. Relat. Metab. Disord.* 27:912–19

84. Klem ML, Wing RR, McGuire MT, Seagle HM, Hill JO. 1997. A descriptive study of individuals successful at long-term maintenance of substantial weight loss. *Am. J. Clin. Nutr.* 66:239–46

85. Knowler WC, Barrett-Connor E, Fowler SE, Hamman RF, Lachin JM, et al. 2002. Reduction in the incidence of type 2 diabetes with lifestyle intervention or metformin. *N. Engl. J. Med.* 346:393–403

86. Kok FJ, Kromhout D. 2004. Epidemiological studies on the health effects of a Mediterranean diet. *Eur. J. Nutr.* 43:I2–5

87. Deleted in proof

88. Larson D, Tataranni P, Ferraro RT, Ravussin E. 1995. Ad libitum food intake on a "cafeteria diet" in Native American women: relations with body composition and 24-h energy expenditure. *Am. J. Clin. Nutr.* 62:911–17

89. Latner JD, Stunkard AJ. 2003. Getting worse: the stigmatization of obese children. *Obes. Res.* 11:452–56

90. Lexchin J. 2001. Lifestyle drugs: issues for debate. *CMAJ* 164:1449–51

91. Lindsay RS, Howard BV. 2004. Cardiovascular risk associated with the metabolic syndrome. *Curr. Diab. Rep.* 4:63–68

92. deLorgeril M, Salen P, Martin JL, Monjaud I, Delaye J, Mamelle N. 1999. Mediterranean diet, traditional risk factors, and the rate of cardiovascular complications after myocardial infarction: final report of the Lyon Diet Heart Study. *Circulation* 99:779–85

93. Mascie-Taylor CG, Karim E. 2003.

The burden of chronic disease. *Science* 302:1921–22

94. Mathers JC. 2003. Nutrition and cancer prevention: diet-gene interactions. *Proc. Nutr. Soc.* 62:605–10

95. Mattes RD. 2002. Feeding behaviors and weight loss outcomes over 64 months. *Eat Behav.* 3:191–204

96. McCrory MA, Fuss PJ, Saltzman E, Roberts SB. 2000. Dietary determinants of energy intake and weight regulation in healthy adults. *J. Nutr.* 130:276S–79

97. McGuire MT, Wing RR, Klem ML, Seagle HM, Hill JO. 1998. Long-term maintenance of weight loss: Do people who lose weight through various weight loss methods use different behaviors to maintain their weight? *Int. J. Obes. Relat. Metab. Disord.* 22:572–77

98. Misra A, Vikram NK. 2004. Insulin resistance syndrome (metabolic syndrome) and obesity in Asian Indians: evidence and implications. *Nutrition* 20:482–91

99. Mitka M. 2003. Surgery for obesity: demand soars amid scientific, ethical questions. *JAMA* 289:1761–62

100. Mokdad AH, Ford ES, Bowman BA, Dietz WH, Vinicor F, et al. 2003. Prevalence of obesity, diabetes, and obesity-related health risk factors, 2001. *JAMA* 289:76–79

101. Mokdad AH, Marks JS, Stroup DF, Gerberding JL. 2004. Actual causes of death in the United States, 2000. *JAMA* 291:1238–45

102. Moloney M. 2000. Dietary treatments of obesity. *Proc. Nutr. Soc.* 59:601–8

103. Natl. Cancer Inst. 2004. *National Cancer Institute dietary guidelines.* http://www.pueblo.gsa.gov/cic_text/food/guideeat/guidelns.html

104. Neff LJ, Sargent RG, McKeown RE, Jackson KL, Valois RF. 1997. Black-white differences in body size perceptions and weight management practices among adolescent females. *J. Adolesc. Health* 20:459–65

105. Nelson LH, Tucker LA. 1996. Diet composition related to body fat in a multivariate study of 203 men. *J. Am. Diet. Assoc.* 96:771–77

106. Nestle M. 2002. *Food Politics.* Berkeley: Univ. Calif. Press

107. Nestle M. 2003. Increasing portion sizes in American diets: more calories, more obesity. *J. Am. Diet. Assoc.* 103:39–40

108. Noppa H, Bengtsson C, Isaksson B, Smith U. 1980. Adipose tissue cellularity in adulthood and its relation to childhood obesity. *Int. J. Obes.* 4:253–63

109. Ogden CL, Carroll MD, Flegal KM. 2003. Epidemiologic trends in overweight and obesity. *Endocrinol. Metab. Clin. North Am.* 32:741–60

110. Ogden CL, Flegal KM, Carroll MD, Johnson CL. 2002. Prevalence and trends in overweight among US children and adolescents, 1999–2000. *JAMA* 288:1728–32

111. Ornish D. 2000. *Eat More, Weigh Less: Dr. Dean Ornish's Life Choice Program for Losing Weight Safely While Eating Abundantly.* New York: Quill

112. Ornish D. 2004. Was Dr. Atkins right? *Am. J. Diet. Assoc.* 104:537–42

113. Ornish D, Scherwitz LW, Billings JH, Brown SE, Gould KL, et al. 1998. Intensive lifestyle changes for reversal of coronary heart disease. *JAMA* 280:2001–7

113a. Pagano-Therrien J, Katz DL. 2003. The low-down on low-carbohydrate diets: responding to your patients' enthusiasm. *Nurse Pract.* 28(3):5, 14

114. Pasman W, Saris W, Westerterp-Plantenga M. 1999. Predictors of weight maintenance. *Obes. Res.* 7:43–50

115. Perez M, Joiner TE Jr. 2003. Body image dissatisfaction and disordered eating in black and white women. *Int. J. Eat Disord.* 33:342–50

116. Peters JC. 2003. Dietary fat and body weight control. *Lipids* 38:123–27

117. Pirozzo S, Summerbell C, Cameron C, Glasziou P. 2002. Advice on low-fat

diets for obesity. *Cochrane Database Syst. Rev.* CD003640

118. Pirozzo S, Summerbell C, Cameron C, Glasziou P. 2003. Should we recommend low-fat diets for obesity? *Obes. Rev.* 4:83–90

119. Plodkowski RA, St. Jeor S. 2003. Medical nutrition therapy for the treatment of obesity. *Endocrinol. Metab. Clin. North Am.* 32:935–65

120. Poppitt SD, Keogh GF, Prentice AM, Williams DE, Sonnemans HM, et al. 2002. Long-term effects of ad libitum low-fat, high-carbohydrate diets on body weight and serum lipids in overweight subjects with metabolic syndrome. *Am. J. Clin. Nutr.* 75:11–20

121. Puhl R, Brownell KD. 2003. Ways of coping with obesity stigma: review and conceptual analysis. *Eat Behav.* 4:53–78

122. Puhl RM, Brownell KD. 2003. Psychosocial origins of obesity stigma: toward changing a powerful and pervasive bias. *Obes. Rev.* 4:213–27

123. Rabast U, Kasper H, Schonborn J. 1978. Comparative studies in obese subjects fed carbohydrate-restricted and high carbohydrate 1,000-calorie formula diets. *Nutr. Metab.* 22:269–77

124. Racette SB, Schoeller DA, Kushner RF, Neil KM, Herling-Iaffaldano K. 1995. Effects of aerobic exercise and dietary carbohydrate on energy expenditure and body composition during weight reduction in obese women. *Am. J. Clin. Nutr.* 61:486–94

125. Rapoport L, Clark M, Wardle J. 2000. Evaluation of a modified cognitive-behavioural programme for weight management. *Int. J. Obes. Relat. Metab. Disord.* 24:1726–37

126. Reaven G, Abbasi F, McLaughlin T. 2004. Obesity, insulin resistance, and cardiovascular disease. *Recent. Prog. Horm. Res.* 59:207–23

127. Reddy KS, Katan MB. 2004. Diet, nutrition and the prevention of hypertension and cardiovascular diseases. *Public Health Nutr.* 7:167–86

128. Rolls BJ, Barnett RA. 2000. *The Volumetrics Weight-Control Plan: Feel Full on Fewer Calories.* New York: Quill

129. Rolls BJ, Ello-Martin JA, Tohill BC. 2004. What can intervention studies tell us about the relationship between fruit and vegetable consumption and weight management? *Nutr. Rev.* 62:1–17

130. Rolls BJ, Miller DL. 1997. Is the low-fat message giving people a license to eat more? *J. Am. Coll. Nutr.* 16:535–43

131. Sacks FM, Svetkey LP, Vollmer WM, Appel LJ, Bray GA, et al. 2001. Effects on blood pressure of reduced dietary sodium and the Dietary Approaches to Stop Hypertension (DASH) diet. DASH-Sodium Collaborative Research Group. *N. Engl. J. Med.* 344:3–10

132. Samaha FF, Iqbal N, Seshadri P, Chicano KL, Daily DA, et al. 2003. A low-carbohydrate as compared with a low-fat diet in severe obesity. *N. Engl. J. Med.* 348:2074–81

133. Schrauwen P, Westerterp KR. 2000. The role of high-fat diets and physical activity in the regulation of body weight. *Br. J. Nutr.* 84:417–27

134. Schutz Y. 1995. Macronutrients and energy balance in obesity. *Metabolism* 44:7–11

135. Sears W. 1999. *The Family Nutrition Book: Everything You Need to Know About Feeding Your Children—From Birth to Age Two.* New York: Little Brown

136. Shah M, Garg A. 1996. High-fat and high-carbohydrate diets and energy balance. *Diabetes Care* 19:1142–52

137. Shick SM, Wing RR, Klem ML, McGuire MT, Hill JO, Seagle H. 1998. Persons successful at long-term weight loss and maintenance continue to consume a low-energy, low-fat diet. *J. Am. Diet. Assoc.* 98:408–13

138. Siggaard R, Raben A, Astrup A. 1996. Weight loss during 12 weeks ad libitum

carbohydrate-rich diet in overweight and normal weight subjects at a Danish work site. *Obes. Res.* 4:347–56

139. Silventoinen K, Sans S, Tolonen H, Monterde D, Kuulasmaa K, et al. 2004. WHO MONICA Project. Trends in obesity and energy supply in the WHO MONICA Project. *Int. J. Obes. Relat. Metab. Disord.* 28:710–18

140. Simopoulos AP. 2001. The Mediterranean diets: What is so special about the diet of Greece? The scientific evidence. *J. Nutr.* 131:3065S–73

141. Skov A, Toubro S, Ronn B, Holm L, Astrup A. 1999. Randomized trial on protein vs. carbohydrate in ad libitum fat reduced diet for the treatment of obesity. *Int. J. Obes. Relat. Metab. Disord.* 23:528–36

141a. Sondike SB, Copperman N, Jacobson MS. 2003. Effects of a low-carbohydrate diet on weight loss and cardiovascular risk factor in overweight adolescents. *J. Pediatr.* 142:253–58

142. Sowers JR, Frohlich ED. 2004. Insulin and insulin resistance: impact on blood pressure and cardiovascular disease. *Med. Clin. North Am.* 88:63–82

143. Spieth LE, Harnish JD, Lenders CM, Raezer LB, Pereira MA, et al. 2000. A low-glycemic index diet in the treatment of pediatric obesity. *Arch. Pediatr. Adolesc. Med.* 154:947–51

144. Stevens J, Kumanyika SK, Keil JE. 1994. Attitudes toward body size and dieting: differences between elderly black and white women. *Am. J. Public Health* 84:1322–25

145. Tapper-Gardzina Y, Cotugna N, Vickery C. 2002. Should you recommend a low-carb, high-protein diet? *Nurse Pract.* 27:52–57

146. Task Force Community Prev. Serv. 2004. *Guide to community preventive services.* http://www.thecommunityguide.org

147. Terry P, Terry JB, Wolk A. 2001. Fruit and vegetable consumption in the prevention of cancer: an update. *J. Intern. Med.* 250:280–90

148. Thompson D, Edelsberg J, Colditz GA, Bird AP, Oster G. 1999. Lifetime health and economic consequences of obesity. *Arch. Intern. Med.* 159:2177–83

149. Thompson D, Wolf AM. 2001. The medical-care cost burden of obesity. *Obes. Rev.* 2:189–97

150. Thompson SH, Sargent RG. 2000. Black and White women's weight-related attitudes and parental criticism of their childhood appearance. *Women Health* 30:77–92

151. Tillotson JE. 2004. Pandemic obesity: What is the solution? *Nutr. Today* 39:6–9

152. Torgerson JS, Lissner L, Lindroos AK, Kruijer H, Sjostrom L. 1997. VLCD plus dietary and behavioural support versus support alone in the treatment of severe obesity. A randomised two-year clinical trial. *Int. J. Obes. Relat. Metab. Disord.* 21:987–94

153. Troiano RP, Flegal KM. 1998. Overweight children and adolescents: description, epidemiology, and demographics. *Pediatrics* 101:497–504

154. U.S. Dep. Agric. 1992. *The Food Guide Pyramid.* Washington, DC: http://www.nal.usda.gov:8001/py/pmap.htm

155. U.S. Dep. Agric. 2000. *Dietary guidelines for Americans 2000.* http://www.health.gov/dietaryguidelines/dga2000/document/contents.htm

155a. U.S. Prev. Serv. Task Force. 1996. *Guide to Clinical Preventive Services.* Baltimore, MD: Williams and Wilkins

156. Van Duyn MA, Pivonka E. 2000. Overview of the health benefits of fruit and vegetable consumption for the dietetics professional: selected literature. *J. Am. Diet. Assoc.* 100:1511–21

157. Vartabedian RE, Matthews K. 1994. *Nutripoints: The Breakthrough Point System for Optimal Health.* New York: Harper Collins

158. Vermunt SH, Pasman WJ, Schaafsma G,

Kardinaal AF. 2003. Effects of sugar intake on body weight: a review. *Obes. Rev.* 4:91–99

159. Volek JS, Sharman MJ, Love DM, Avery NG, Gomez AL, et al. 2002. Body composition and hormonal responses to a carbohydrate-restricted diet. *Metabolism* 51:864–70

159a. von Kries R, Toschke AM, Koletzko B, Slikker W Jr. 2002. Maternal smoking during pregnancy and childhood obesity. *Am. J. Epidemiol.* 156:954–61

160. Wadden T, Foster G, Letizia K. 1994. One-year behavioral treatment of obesity: comparison of moderate and severe caloric restriction and the effects of weight maintenance therapy. *J. Consult. Clin. Psychol.* 62:165–71

161. Wadden TA, Butryn ML. 2003. Behavioral treatment of obesity. *Endocrinol. Metab. Clin. North Am.* 32:981–1003

162. Weisburger JH. 2000. Eat to live, not live to eat. *Nutrition* 16:767–73

163. Westerterp-Plantenga MS, Lejeune MP, Nijs I, van Ooijen M, Kovacs EM. 2004. High protein intake sustains weight maintenance after body weight loss in humans. *Int. J. Obes. Relat. Metab. Disord.* 28:57–64

164. Willett WC. 2001. *Eat, Drink, and Be Healthy*. New York: Simon & Schuster Source

165. Willett WC, Leibel RL. 2002. Dietary fat is not a major determinant of body fat. *Am. J. Med.* 113:47S–59

166. Wing RR, Gorin AA. 2003. Behavioral techniques for treating the obese patient. *Prim. Care* 30:375–91

167. Wing RR, Hill JO. 2001. Successful weight loss maintenance. *Annu. Rev. Nutr.* 21:323–41

168. Wing RR, Jeffery RW. 2001. Food provision as a strategy to promote weight loss. *Obes. Res.* 9:271S–75

169. Wright JD, Kennedy-Stephenson J, Wang CY, McDowell MA, Johnson CL, et al. 2004. Trends in Intake of Energy and Macronutrients—United States, 1971–2000. *MMWR* 53:80–82

170. Yale-Griffin Prev. Res. Cent. 2000–2003. *Obesity Systematic Review*. Derby, CT: Cent. Dis. Control, Grant #U48-CCU115802

Annu. Rev. Public Health 2005. 26:89–113
doi: 10.1146/annurev.publhealth.26.021304.144528

POPULATION DISPARITIES IN ASTHMA

Diane R. Gold and Rosalind Wright

*Harvard Medical School, Channing Laboratory, Brigham and Women's Hospital,
Boston, Massachusetts 02467; email: diane.gold@channing.harvard.edu,
rosalind.wright@channing.harvard.edu*

Key Words   children, hygiene hypothesis, smoking, allergens, traffic pollution,
obesity

■ **Abstract**   The prevalence of asthma in the United States is higher than in many
other countries in the world. Asthma, the most common chronic disease of childhood in
the United States, disproportionately burdens many socioeconomically disadvantaged
urban communities. In this review we discuss hypotheses for between-country disparities in asthma prevalence, including differences in "hygiene" (e.g., family size, use of
day care, early-life respiratory infection exposures, endotoxin and other farm-related
exposures, microbial colonization of the infant bowel, exposure to parasites, and exposure to large domestic animal sources of allergen), diet, traffic pollution, and cigarette
smoking. We present data on socioeconomic and ethnic disparities in asthma prevalence
and morbidity in the United States and discuss environmental factors contributing to
asthma disparities (e.g., housing conditions, indoor environmental exposures including
allergens, traffic air pollution, disparities in treatment and access to care, and cigarette
smoking). We discuss environmental influences on somatic growth (low birth weight,
prematurity, and obesity) and their relevance to asthma disparities. The relevance of
the hygiene hypothesis to the U.S. urban situation is reviewed. Finally, we discuss
community-level factors contributing to asthma disparities.

INTRODUCTION

Asthma, the most common chronic disease of childhood in the United States,
disproportionately burdens many socioeconomically disadvantaged urban communities (61, 142, 143). The Centers for Disease Control and Prevention (CDC)
has estimated that there are ~17.3 million people in the United States with the
illness (107). Approximately one third of these asthmatics are children (12). The
social and economic costs of asthma are considerable. In the United States in 1996,
there were 474,000 asthma hospitalizations and 11.9 million medical visits for the
disease (48).

DEFINITIONS OF ASTHMA

The estimated prevalence of asthma can vary widely according to the epidemiologic or clinical definition utilized; nevertheless, certain between-country and within-U.S. disparities in asthma prevalence and morbidity have been well documented and are not likely to be a function of definition. In the U.S. National Institutes of Health Guidelines for Management and Diagnosis of Asthma (61, 92), asthma is defined as

> a chronic inflammatory disorder of the airways in which many cells and cellular elements play a role, in particular, mast cells, eosinophils, T lymphocytes, macrophages, neutrophils, and epithelial cells. In susceptible individuals, this inflammation causes recurrent episodes of wheezing, breathlessness, chest tightness, and coughing. . ... These episodes are usually associated with widespread but variable airflow obstruction that is often reversible either spontaneously or with treatment. The inflammation also causes an associated increase in the existing bronchial hyper-responsiveness to a variety of stimuli. (p. 8)

In large-scale epidemiologic studies, the diagnosis of asthma has generally been elicited by a series of questions related to wheeze (doctor-diagnosed or parentally/self-observed) and its persistence or chronicity (5), often with evaluation of secondary phenotypes including allergic sensitization and airway hyperreactivity (138). In the United States, the majority of those with asthma have allergy or elevated IgE, but a minority of asthmatics have symptoms, airway inflammation, and airway hyperreactivity without identifiable allergy (41).

BETWEEN-COUNTRY DISPARITIES IN ASTHMA PREVALENCE

The prevalence of asthma in the United States is higher than in many other countries in the world (Figure 1). Using standardized questionnaires, the International Study of Asthma and Allergy in Childhood (ISAAC) (158) has shown an almost thirty-fold between-country variation in asthma prevalence rates (62). Urbanized, more "Westernized" countries tend to have higher asthma rates than do less developed countries, though exposures related to urbanization and Westernization do not explain all the between-country differences noted in this international effort to understand the patterns of asthma and allergy in children. A number of hypotheses have been proposed as potential partial explanations for between-country and within-country disparities in asthma prevalence, including differences in (*a*) "hygiene," (*b*) diet, (*c*) cigarette smoking, (*d*) traffic pollution, (*e*) antenatal exposures, and (*f*) physical activity/obesity. Despite a growing body of worldwide literature reporting studies testing these hypotheses, the significance of most of these factors in the development of asthma has yet to be fully understood,

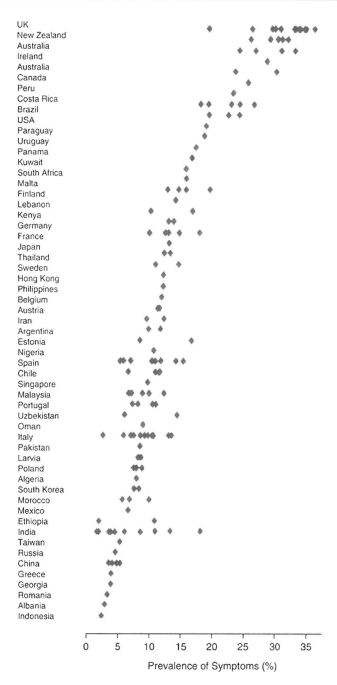

Figure 1   Prevalence of asthma symptoms (percentage) from a questionnaire in the ISAAC database. Source: ISAAC Steer. Comm. (62).

and their significance for explaining between-region or -country disparities in asthma prevalence is uncertain (61). One exception is in utero/early infancy exposure to cigarette smoking, which is consistently found to be an important risk factor for development of wheeze and early asthma. However, its relationship to development of allergy and allergic inflammation is uncertain (61). Environmental factors contributing to increased asthma morbidity are far better understood and are reviewed here only in relation to asthma disparities in the United States (61). But first we present theories potentially explaining worldwide asthma disparities, with a focus on the hygiene and diet hypotheses.

THE HYGIENE HYPOTHESES

The hygiene hypothesis is actually a series of hypotheses that have expanded since the original English and Swiss observations in the late nineteenth and early twentieth centuries that hay fever and wheeze appeared to be diseases of more affluent urban areas, compared with rural farming areas (128, 157). The hypotheses have evolved to include (*a*) small families, earlier birth order, and less use of day care (8, 23, 128); (*b*) less exposure to respiratory infection in early childhood (128); (*c*) a reduction in endotoxin or other farm-related exposures (15); (*d*) a change in microbial colonization of the infant's large bowel through diet or antibiotics (86); (*e*) reduced exposure to parasites (17); or (*f*) reduced exposure to large domestic animal sources of allergens (102) as potential explanations for increases in asthma prevalence in more Westernized urban communities compared with more rural communities.

Family Size, Day Care, and Viral Exposure

In longitudinal U.S. studies, having siblings (8) and early life exposure to day care (8, 23) have been associated with more wheeze in early childhood but with decreased risk of persistent childhood wheeze and with lower IgE levels in later childhood. Later birth order is also associated with reduced allergic disease risk (129). The very early-life increase in wheeze associated with increased exposure to siblings/day care has been attributed to the proinflammatory effects of increased viral infection exposure on small airways and not to allergic responses. The later childhood reduction in wheeze associated with early-life exposure to siblings/day care has been attributed to possible downregulation of chronic allergic immune inflammatory responses by early-life infections. Some investigators hypothesized that early-life respiratory viral or mycobacterial exposure may modify T-regulatory lymphocyte cell behavior and may downregulate T helper 1 (Th1) and Th2 lymphocyte secretion of proinflammatory cytokines (57, 144). The potential of early day care/viral exposure to be protective against later allergic asthmatic responses is likely to vary by familial inheritance. Celedon et al. (26) found that for children of mothers without asthma, day care was protective; for children of mothers with asthma, day care was a risk factor for wheeze. The associations of day care, siblings, or birth order with later protection against wheeze may well represent effects of exposures other than viral illness. In a review of the literature, the Institute of Medicine (61) report "Clearing the Air" concluded that association with allergy of infant viral exposure to later childhood asthma is uncertain; conflicting results have come from the few prospective studies that directly measure the number and type of viral illnesses encountered in infancy (61).

Endotoxin

Endotoxin is a biologically active lipopolysaccharide, a primary component of the outer cell membrane of gram-negative bacteria (110). The endotoxin hypothesis has come from reproducible observations in Swiss, German, and Austrian individual and combined studies, demonstrating lower rates of allergy-associated wheeze/asthma and allergic sensitization in children of farming families, compared with children from nonfarming families in the same region (15, 112, 139). In a recent West European multi-country cross-sectional study of school-aged rural children, endotoxin in the bed mattress was associated with lower rates of asthma with allergy and atopic sensitization but not with asthma/wheeze without allergy (15). On the basis of animal and human studies, investigators have hypothesized that at certain doses, with the right timing in the life cycle, endotoxin may downregulate allergic airway inflammation, perhaps by increasing Th1-type lymphocytes through increasing macrophage interleukin-12 secretion, (110) or by alteration of T regulatory cell behavior early in life (144). The effect of endotoxin may depend on the timing of exposure and dose, as well as genotype (7, 42); endotoxin is well known to have an irritant effect causing wheeze symptoms in adults in the occupational setting (110). Endotoxin exposure may reduce the risk of allergy or asthma if encountered in infancy, yet it may increase wheeze risk once individuals have established asthma (89).

Microbial Colonization of the Infant's Large Bowel

The European farm studies have also found that taking children into the barn in infancy and feeding young children raw milk may be protective of wheeze and allergy (112). If farm exposures are protective, then it is possible that bacterial exposures encountered in raw milk, fermented foods (86), and additional farm-associated exposures other than endotoxin may be protective (65, 66). Some researchers have suggested that antibiotic use has increased risk of allergy and asthma by altering bowel flora and intestinal immune mechanisms, but recent prospective articles on antibiotic use in infancy that adjust for infection do not support that hypothesis.

Domestic Allergen Exposure

There is no question that asthmatic individuals who are sensitized to animals such as cats, and who have higher exposure to these animals, have an increase in allergic symptoms compared with sensitized asthmatic individuals with lower exposure (82). However, multiple studies also suggest an association between early-life exposure to dog or cat in the home and reduced risk of asthma or allergic sensitization (96, 100). The data on cat and protection against asthma are not as consistent as those related to dog. Dogs are associated with endotoxin (97), but domestic dogs kept in the home are also associated with the presence of large quantities of aerosolized dog allergen. Similarly, homes with cats have very high levels of aerosolized cat allergen (104), though there is not a clear-cut correlation between cat allergen levels and measurable dust or air endotoxin in the home. Platts-Mills (102) has hypothesized that for some children, high allergen exposure may result in a "modified Th2 response," leading to increased interleukin 10 antiinflammatory cytokine production, increased IgG4 production, and reduced proinflammatory interleukin 4 production. Yet the data on cat in the home and allergy or asthma are contradictory, perhaps because of both the unmeasured exposures to cat outside the home (depending on the prevalence of cat in the community) and on familial factors. There is likely familial or genetic variation in response to high levels of allergen exposure—not all people will respond in a similar fashion. For example, in a Boston longitudinal study, early exposure to cat in the home appeared protective for children of mothers without asthma, yet it was a risk factor for wheeze for children with asthma (22). In a Wisconson longitudinal study, the relation of dog in the home to atopic dermatitis was modified by the CD14 genotype (42).

DIET

Differences in dietary intake also may contribute to disparities in allergy and asthma. Particularly in the Westernized English-speaking countries such as the United States, the United Kingdom, Australia, and New Zealand, dietary intake of fresh fruits and vegetables containing antioxidants has decreased (135). Asthma was negatively associated with consumption of foods containing Vitamin E in the prospective U.S. Nurses' Health Study of 77,866 female nurses (54). Increases in allergy and asthma may be related also to decreases in dietary intake of n-3 polyunsaturated fatty acids (PUFA), such as eicosapentaenoic acid (EPA) and docosahexaenoic acid (DHA) found in oily fish (tuna, salmon, mackerel, and herring) and leafy green vegetables, and to increases in n-6 polyunsaturated fatty acids, such as linoleic acid (LA) and arachidonic acid (AA) found in vegetable oils (13, 54, 106, 125). Investigators have noted a very low prevalence of asthma among Greenland Eskimos, who have a high intake of n-3 fatty acid EPA (59). Peat found an 8% versus 16% prevalence of asthma in regular fish eaters versus nonfish eaters (98). In a more recent Australian dietary intervention trial, children whose mothers were randomized to supplementation with omega-3 fatty acids during pregnancy had less wheeze in the first 18 months of life than did controls (90). Early-life exposure to N-3 PUFA may decrease asthma or allergy risk through decreasing chronic allergic inflammation, including airway inflammation.

Differences in breast-feeding practices also have been suggested as a factor influencing asthma risk but are not reviewed here in depth. Breast-feeding is complex, as a source of bonding between mother and infant, and a source of small amounts of antigen, antibodies, and protection against potentially diluted formula or bacterial contamination introduced by bottle-feeding using dirty water. The association between breast-feeding and protection (or risk) of allergy and asthma in the child will likely vary depending on other environmental as well as genetic factors (151).

SOCIOECONOMIC AND ETHNIC DISPARITIES IN ASTHMA PREVALENCE, MORBIDITY, AND MORTALITY IN THE UNITED STATES

For almost two decades, socioeconomic and racial/ethnic disparities in asthma prevalence and asthma morbidity in the United States have been well documented (41, 46, 124, 143, 146), though the environmental exposures contributing to these disparities are only partially understood. What is the nature of the disparities in asthma in the United States, and what factors have been considered potential partial explanations for those disparities?

Asthma Disparities: Black/African American versus White/Non-Hispanic Ethnicity in the United States

In the United States, asthma prevalence, hospitalization, and mortality are higher for Black/African American compared to Caucasian (White) children and adults (61). In a Southfield, Michigan, cross-sectional study of childhood asthma in an integrated middle class population (93), the lifetime prevalence of asthma was twice as high for Black compared with White children; this finding suggests that even in middle class communities unmeasured socioeconomic factors (e.g., racial discrimination, differential access to medical care, differential access to housing, differential patterns of medical care use), and perhaps biologic factors [e.g., genetic variation in vulnerability to effects of exposures (81)], may contribute to these disparities.

The disparity in asthma morbidity is greater than the disparity in asthma prevalence, which suggests that once asthma is established, many factors converge to make asthma worse for children and adults who are Black (46, 114, 124, 146). In New York City, asthma hospitalization and death rates among Blacks and Hispanics were 3–5 times those of Whites, in a study of data from all hospital discharges obtained from the New York State Department of Health (19). Asthma hospitalization and mortality were highly correlated with living in the city's poorest neighborhoods, making it impossible to separate ethnicity/race from poverty. Similarly, in a Boston study, asthma hospitalization was positively correlated with the poverty rate of the neighborhood within Boston and also with the proportion of non-White residents (47).

Asthma Disparities in the U.S. Hispanic/Latino Communities

Hispanic or Latino peoples are of many racial, ethnic, cultural, and national origins. A 1999 survey in North Brooklyn, New York, found that the reported asthma prevalence was 5.3% among Dominican Latinos, compared with 13.2% among Puerto Rican Latinos. These differences could not be explained by location, household size, use of home remedies, educational attainment, or country where education was completed (80). Asthma mortality is rare, but in the United States, Puerto Ricans had the highest asthma mortality rates among Hispanics, followed by Cuban Americans and Mexican Americans. Mortality rates for Hispanics were higher in the Northeast than in any other region (58). A 1993–1994 multiethnic study of asthma rates among children in Connecticut found significantly higher asthma rates among Puerto Rican Hispanics, compared with non-Hispanic Whites, and these differences could not be explained by active smoking in the home or various measures of socioeconomic status (SES) (9). In Hartford, Connecticut, Puerto Rican ethnicity was associated with an increased risk of sensitization to indoor and outdoor allergens among children with asthma (25).

ENVIRONMENTAL FACTORS CONTRIBUTING TO ASTHMA DISPARITIES IN THE U.S.

In trying to define and explain ethnic/racial disparities in asthma prevalence or morbidity in the United States, a number of investigators have analyzed national data from the National Health and Nutrition and Examination Surveys I, II, (124) and III (114); the National Health Interview Surveys (3, 146); and the Six Cities Study of air pollution and respiratory health (46). These data have advantages, in that they survey large populations from many regions of the United States, but they also have disadvantages, in that they often offer relatively sparse or specifically selective environmental exposure data on individuals within specific communities. Most investigators have evaluated whether it is possible to explain ethnic/racial disparities in asthma by urban living or by indices of disadvantage. Using data from four U.S. cities, Black children still had 1.6 times the odds of asthma diagnosis compared with White children, after taking into account exposures including cigarette smoke, body-mass index, air-conditioning use, city of residence, parental respiratory illness, parental education, only-child status, and single-parent household (46). Similarly, in the Second National Health Interview Survey, younger maternal age, residence in the central city, family income, low birth weight, and measures of overweight or obesity partially, but not fully, explain the increased prevalence of asthma among Black compared with White children (124). More recently, investigators analyzing data from the 1988 National Health Interview Survey reported that after controlling for multiple factors, Black children did not have higher rates of asthma, but living in an urban setting, regardless of race or income, increased the risk of asthma (3). Using Maryland hospital discharge data for the period 1979–1982, investigators found that Black children had higher rates of hospitalization for asthma than did White children, but these racial/ethnic differences could be explained by indices of poverty (149). More detailed small-area analyses suggest that this finding may not be the case. Small-area ecologic analyses of Los Angeles and New York City suggested that Black race/ethnicity and poverty were each associated with increased asthma hospitalization, and that Black race/ethnicity remained a strong predictor of hospitalization after controlling for the available socioeconomic variables (109). Blacks in Los Angeles and New York City had similar rates of hospitalization, but Mexican Hispanics in Los Angeles had far lower rates than did Puerto Rican Hispanics in New York City. Not all poverty and socioeconomic disadvantages are associated with higher rates of asthma, or worse asthma morbidity, as demonstrated in the ISAAC surveys (62). Studies within communities have enabled investigators to dig layers deeper to understand the exposures connected with poverty and disadvantage in U.S. urban life that increase the risk of significant asthma morbidity, particularly in children.

The Hygiene Hypothesis—Is it Relevant?

The hygiene hypotheses has been challenged as being irrelevant to the U.S. setting for explained disparities in asthma prevalence or asthma morbidity. If anything, some investigators have argued, endotoxin and early-life infectious exposures must be higher, yet asthma rates are not lower but higher in U.S. cities. They argue that home endotoxin levels in U.S. urban regions must be higher because of the higher levels of dirt and garbage present in the city, but it is not known whether this is the case. Two important sources of endotoxin—dog and dampness (97)—are often lower in overheated urban apartments where dogs may not be kept for cultural reasons or because the landlord does not allow pets. Similarly, it has been hypothesized that in the United States urban infants have higher exposure to other siblings and to children in day care than do more affluent suburban children, resulting in more exposure to early-life infections, but this hypothesis has not been systematically tested.

Housing Conditions and Indoor Environmental Exposures Including Allergens

Independent of income and ethnicity, the degree of housing disrepair has been associated with increased cockroach allergen levels (108), which has been demonstrated to increase childhood asthma morbidity in sensitized children (117). The associations of indoor environmental exposures with asthma morbidity have been well summarized and are not reviewed here (61). The type of allergens differ by building status and by socioeconomic status, but it is not certain whether, regardless of type of indoor allergen, the total amount of allergen exposure (the allergen burden) differs by socioeconomic status or by ethnicity (28, 75). Certain allergens, such as cockroach, mouse, or rat, may be more potent sources of allergic or nonallergic airway inflammation, or environmental cofactors such as community stress may increase vulnerability to the effects of these exposures in sensitized individuals.

The multicenter National Cooperative Inner City Asthma Study demonstrated an increase in asthma morbidity in children both sensitized and exposed to cockroach (117). In studies in metropolitan Boston, Massachusetts, and Connecticut, cockroach allergen levels were higher in households of Black and Hispanic families compared with White non-Hispanic families, but dust mite levels were lower (28, 75, 79). In a one-year multicity U.S. environmental intervention trial among urban children with asthma, education and remediation for exposure to both allergens and environmental tobacco smoke resulted in fewer days with asthma symptoms during the intervention, compared with the control group (91). Allergen levels in the home were significantly reduced during the year of intervention. Allergen reduction trials have not been uniformly successful in reducing asthma morbidity in allergic asthmatic adults (150), either because of the more fixed nature of long-established asthma or because these trials have not been as comprehensive as the Inner-City Asthma Study trial.

Traffic Air Pollution

Environmental cofactors may also increase vulnerability to adverse effects of air pollution on asthma morbidity (94). Direct exposure to traffic and industrial pollutants is often high in socioeconomically disadvantaged urban neighborhoods (94), though many secondary pollutants (e.g., ozone) can form some distance from their sources of emission. Increased levels of air pollution from both traffic and industrial sources have been reproducibly demonstrated to be associated with increased asthma morbidity in children, whether measured as increased airway obstruction, increased symptoms, or increased hospitalizations for asthma (123). The relation of air pollution to asthma development is less certain. In the United States and Europe, pollution from industrial sources has often been associated with lower levels of lung function and higher rates of cough and bronchitis but not with higher rates of asthma or allergy (123, 139). In contrast, accumulating evidence suggests a possible association between living near traffic pollution and wheeze or asthma (55, 123); diesel exhaust has been proposed as a potential adjuvant that might increase vulnerability to development of allergy (32). Additional research is needed to ascertain whether these associations represent a relation between traffic pollution and the development of allergic asthma.

Disparities in Treatment for Asthma and Access to Care

Asthma is one of many chronic diseases in the United States in which disparities in treatment and access to care have been documented (29). Even those with apparently equal access to the same health care system may experience disparities in care, and communication with the medical system is far more subtle than expressions of overt racism. In one study, the asthma hospitalization rate was inversely correlated with the ratio of inhaled anti-inflammatory to beta agonist medication use, which suggests that asthmatics in poor neighborhoods were undertreated for their asthma (47). The National Cooperative Inner-City Asthma Study (NCICAS) found that lack of access to care and adherence to treatment (as well as environmental factors including smoking) were potential contributors to increased asthma morbidity among inner-city children (68), and it demonstrated the efficacy and cost-effectiveness of a comprehensive social worker–based education program and environmental control in the reduction of asthma morbidity (132). Individual-level solutions to disparities in treatment and access to care have severe limitations; community-level approaches to reducing disparities are discussed in subsequent sections of this review.

Maternal Cigarette Smoking

The respiratory health effects of smoking have been well documented. Maternal cigarette smoking is associated with high risk of asthma prevalence in early childhood (130, 131) and with high risk of asthma morbidity, wheeze, and respiratory infection in children (61). Smoke exposure in-utero is associated with increased airway resistance/obstruction in infancy and childhood, but its influence on allergic, as opposed to irritant, airway inflammation is uncertain (53, 61). Cigarette smoking varies by ethnicity and by national origin, and cigarette companies have targeted minorities in an attempt to increase smoking where rates have traditionally been low. In a national survey of U.S. Latino individuals, smoking rates were higher among Puerto Rican women than among other women. Central American men and women had the lowest smoking rates (99). Whereas the overall prevalence of cigarette smoking in the United States declined from 40% in 1965 to 29% in 1987, the decline has been marginal among individuals with low education aspirations (61, 136). More worrisome is the fact that after several years of substantial decline among adolescents in four ethnic minority groups, in the 1990s smoking prevalence increased among African American and Hispanic youth (21). Successful smoking cessation is more difficult among pregnant women and mothers dealing with the circumstances surrounding socioeconomic disadvantage. Moreover environmental tobacco smoke (ETS) exposure of children at greatest risk of adverse asthma outcomes (e.g., children of low-income families) may come from caregivers other than the mother or father (e.g., grandparents, day care), and successful interventions must consider all early childhood sources of ETS (61).

Disparities in Asthma and Somatic Growth (Low Birth Weight, Prematurity, and Obesity)

Smoking and other environmental factors influencing both fetal growth and asthma are more prevalent in many (but not all) socioeconomically disadvantaged populations in the United States (133). Prematurity and low birth weight adjusted for gestational age can be influenced not only by maternal smoking, but also by placental insufficiency, maternal:fetal nutrition, infection, and maternal psychologic as well as physical stress (11, 35). The risk of all these environmental influences on adverse fetal growth may be higher in many socioeconomically disadvantaged U.S. groups, increasing the risk of prematurity and low birth weight (50, 118, 137). Prematurity and low birth weight are risk factors for early life wheeze (43), but their relationship to allergic airway inflammation in asthma that persists into the school-aged years and adolescence is less certain.

Underweight and obesity may both be risk factors for wheeze or asthma (24, 45), and paradoxically, they may even have similar origins in fetal life or early childhood. Overweight has increased markedly in the United States over the past decade, for all Americans (77). The relation of obesity to respiratory disease has been reviewed recently (145). Accumulating evidence suggests that obesity may be not only a result of asthma symptoms, but also a factor contributing to asthma development and the persistence of wheeze (20, 45). The circumstances of urban living and socioeconomic disadvantage, as well as cultural factors, may contribute to obesity (40, 84). Obesity may be a primary contributor to asthma risk; additionally the circumstances leading to obesity may influence risk. The need to keep children indoors because of community violence (decreasing activity, increasing indoor allergen exposures) and the lack of access to playgrounds or healthy foods during school and after-school periods are all factors leading to obesity and may explain some of the association of obesity with asthma (77).

COMMUNITY-LEVEL FACTORS CONTRIBUTING TO ASTHMA DISPARITIES

The etiology of health problems is increasingly recognized as a result of the complex interplay of influences operating at several levels, including the individual, the family, and the community levels (140). Evidence points to the potential influence on health of diverse community (or group-level) characteristics in addition to the economic and individual-level characteristics and exposures (71). The observed wide geographic and sociodemographic variation in asthma expression has led to reconsideration of the interplay among biological and social determinants in understanding such disparities in the asthma burden (153, 155). The balance of this chapter emphasizes how this variation in asthma burden may be explained by community-level factors, including both physical environmental determinants of asthma and the potential influence of social, cultural, and institutional structures.

Neighborhood Contextual Factors

Community-level social variables are receiving increased attention for their potential role in determining inequalities across several health outcomes (33, 51, 72, 78, 113, 115, 147). Few studies have directly examined the influence of such contextual factors on asthma. Two recent studies have shown significant associations between greater neighborhood income inequality and higher childhood asthma hospitalization rates (60, 141). In New Zealand, Salmond and colleagues

(119) used small-area analysis to find a linear increase in a 12-month period prevalence of asthma with increasing area deprivation. In addition, they demonstrated a persistent independent effect for ethnicity.

Given the range of variables that may be considered, identifying pathways that may link community influences, which are supported in existing research, to asthma morbidity may be most informative. Plausible pathways include (*a*) differential environmental exposures, (*b*) stress, and (*c*) impact on health behaviors.

Differential Environmental Exposures

To date, much of the literature has focused on the potential importance of physical environmental characteristics on asthma morbidity: outdoor air pollution (101); crowding, as it may predispose to viral respiratory illness (122); and changing housing stock, which may increase exposure to indoor allergens (31, 103). Future research may need to pay increased attention to social, political, and economic forces that result in marginalization of certain populations in disadvantaged neighborhoods, which may increase exposure to these known environmental risk factors (49, 95). We also need to understand better how the physical and psychological demands of living in a relatively deprived environment may potentiate an individual's susceptibility to such exposures.

Stress

There is a renewed interest in the influence of psychological stress on asthma (18, 37, 155). This is a useful way to conceptualize community-level (or group-level) influences on health, whether one operationalizes the environment as a social or a physical construct. Both physical and social factors can be a source of environmental demands that contribute to stress experienced by populations living in a particular area (37). Differential exposure to and perception of stress may, in part. explain the associations between SES and health (2). Various sociodemographic characteristics (e.g., lower social class, ethnic minority status, gender) may predispose individuals to particular pervasive forms of chronic life stress (34, 88, 105), which may, in turn, be significantly influenced by the characteristics of the communities in which they live (134). Growing evidence in prospective population-based and laboratory studies support the role of differential life stress experiences and asthma expression. In a prospective birth-cohort study, our laboratory demonstrated that greater levels of caregiver-perceived stress was independently associated with subsequent risk of recurrent wheeze (2 or more) episodes in early childhood (152), controlling for variables that may have been related to stress (i.e., birth weight, parental asthma, race/ethnicity, and socioeconomic status). Moreover, high levels of caregiver stress predicted an increased risk of wheeze in the index children even after adjusting for potential mediators (i.e., maternal smoking, lower respiratory illness, allergen levels, and breast feeding), which suggests that the relation between stress and early childhood repeated wheeze may not be primarily mediated through these caregiver behaviors or through susceptibility to lower respiratory infections. A plausible alternative hypothesis may be that there is a more direct effect on airway inflammation through influences on the immune system, which may promote airway obstruction and wheeze. In this same Boston-based cohort study, we have examined the influence of chronic caregiver stress in early childhood on the expression of intermediate phenotypes potentially related to the development of atopy (156a). Increased stress in the home predicted higher levels of IgE expression, enhanced allergen-specific lymphocyte proliferation, and differential cytokine expression in the index children. Sandberg and colleagues (121) found an increased risk of asthma exacerbations among children aged 6–13 years to be associated with acute severe life events. This effect was enhanced in the context of chronic ongoing stress. Two prospective studies of preschool-aged children attending day care in California found that children with high autonomic and immune reactivity to stress had higher subsequent rates of respiratory infections during high environmental stress experienced during follow-up (14). Lower respiratory infections, particularly during childhood, play a role in asthma exacerbations (44).

Recent evidence links stress and differential immunological responses among asthmatic adolescents. Chen and colleagues (27) recently reported differential neuroendocrine and immune reactivity in a group of adolescent asthmatics relative to SES. Adolescents in the low-SES group had significantly higher levels of a mitogen-stimulated cytokine associated with a Th-2 immune response (IL-5), higher levels of a stimulated cytokine associated with a Th-1 immune response (IFN-γ), and marginally lower morning cortisol values compared with the high-SES group. Low SES adolescents also had greater stress experiences and lower beliefs about control over their health, which partially explained the relationship between SES and IL-5/IFN-γ.

One type of chronic stress that has been investigated in relation to the well-being of U.S. urban populations is neighborhood disadvantage (ND), characterized by the presence of a number of community-level stressors including poverty, unemployment, substandard housing, and high crime/violence rates (6). Some data suggest that the health implications of low income are significantly different for individuals living in areas with high ND (52). In the United States, trends in social environmental factors over the past few decades have resulted in many urban communities characterized by high ND (148). Changes have occurred in the residential distribution of the U.S. population and have resulted in the disproportionate concentration of minority groups in areas of concentrated poverty (74). Similar to ND are the constructs of social organization, social capital, or community assets (83). Closely related to these are physical features of the environment such as crowding and noise. Research has linked these to stress, but few studies have evaluated their relationship to asthma outcomes (37).

The broad constructs of ND or low levels of community assets subsume key exposures such as living in the presence of pervasive violence and crime. Violent crime undermines social cohesion (70, 73, 120) and is associated with the erosion of social capital and community resilience. Crime is most prevalent in societies with large disparities in the material standards of living (70). Thus, in addition to direct impacts on community residents, crime and violence (or the lack thereof) can be used as indicators of collective well-being, social relations, or social cohesion within a community and society. Furthermore, the conditions known to be associated with violence exposure are related to experienced stress (16), and chronic violence exposure has been conceptualized as a pervasive environmental stressor imposed on already vulnerable populations (63).

Violence exposure has been associated with asthma in both the clinical (156) and research settings. We examined the association between exposure to community violence and caretaker-reported asthma symptoms and behaviors in the Inner-City Asthma Study (ICAS) (154). We hypothesized that those families and children living with high levels of violence would have increased asthma morbidity. Greater community violence exposure was independently associated with asthma morbidity after simultaneous adjustment for income, employment status, caretaker education, a number of housing problems, and other adverse life events, which suggests that violence was not merely a marker for these other factors. Psychological stress and caretaker behaviors (keeping children indoors, smoking, and skipping medications) partially explained the association between higher violence and increased asthma morbidity.

Minority group status may predispose individuals to pervasive chronic stressors (e.g., discrimination, racism) and societal factors that link minorities and ND. For example, the broader political and economic forces that result in marginalization of minority populations in disadvantaged inner-city neighborhoods may lead to increased stress experienced by these populations and thus greater disease morbidity (70). Future studies need to examine the links among ND, minority group status, low levels of social capital, violence exposure, and other social influences (and the heightened stress that they may elicit) as risk factors for childhood asthma analogous to physical environmental exposures (e.g., allergens, tobacco smoke, air pollution). Such studies are likely to further our understanding of the increased asthma burden on populations of children living in poverty in urban areas or other disadvantaged communities.

Health Behaviors and Other Psychological Factors

Smoking can be viewed as a strategy to cope with negative affect or stress (1, 4, 10). This relationship among stress and smoking may be considered from a neighborhood perspective as well. Studies have demonstrated effects of neighborhood social factors on smoking behavior (67, 76, 111). Neighborhood SES may be related to increased social tolerance and norms supporting behavioral risk factors such as smoking (30).

In adult African American populations, prevalence of smoking is higher relative to Whites. Evidence from the 1987 General Social Survey suggests that stress may be one factor promoting increased prevalence of smoking in African American communities (38). Romano and colleagues (116) surveyed adults from 1137 African American households and found that the strongest predictor of smoking was household report of high-level stress, represented by an abbreviated hassles index. The hassles index was a ten-item scale based on items chosen to represent a dimension that community residents perceived to be especially relevant. Among the items were neighborhood-level factors including concern about living in an unsafe area. Community violence exposure has been linked to smoking rates in Harlem (39).

In addition to community-level stress influences on health behaviors such as smoking, evidence has linked community-level variables to key individual characteristics such as perceived control. A large body of research indicates the importance of constructs such as perceived control (global feeling of the ability to deal with an event) over health as, for example, they mediate the relationship between illness experience, understanding, and compliance (126). Perceived control has been found to correlate with many aspects of disease burden (56, 127).

Evidence indicates that exposure to indicators of neighborhood disadvantage including violence reduces perceived control. DuRant and colleagues (36) examined the relationships between exposure to community violence and depression, hopelessness, and purpose in life among Black urban youth. These authors found that higher current depression and hopelessness and lower purpose in life were significantly associated with the reported higher frequency of exposure to, or victimization by, violence in a youth's lifetime. Thus, tying together several of the findings discussed here, exposure to violence or living in a community with high ND may lead to reduced perceived control, which may, in turn, be associated with poorer asthma management and outcomes. An important methodological issue should be raised here. If increased exposure to tobacco smoke or reduced perceived control is a result of increased stress caused by the physical or social environment, then they should be considered as mediators rather than confounders of the relationships between community-level variables and asthma outcomes. Inappropriate adjustment for such factors may result in the attenuation of a true effect (37, 69).

Populations in communities that experience environmental inequities may also be characterized by high levels of poverty, low social capital, lack of opportunity and employment, high violence or crime rates, lack of perceived control, and hopelessness. The health problems of these disadvantaged populations are not likely to be solved without understanding the potential role of such social determinants of health.

CONCLUSION

Community-level and individual-level factors both contribute to disparities in asthma morbidity and the incidence/prevalence of asthma. We understand more about factors that influence asthma morbidity (the worsening of asthma in allergic asthmatic individuals) than we do about factors that influence the development of allergy and asthma. Our understanding of asthma morbidity comes from both observational studies and intervention trials. Recent evidence suggests that in the United States, among socioeconomically disadvantaged children with asthma and allergy, asthma morbidity can be improved with targeted interventions (91).

The effects of individual environmental factors on asthma morbidity and asthma development are likely to be modified by other environmental factors and by genes. With the exception of cigarette smoking cessation, policy makers should be cautious when recommending global solutions for protection against development of early-life asthma, given the lack of certainty regarding factors influencing asthma development and the likelihood that individual responses to environmental interventions will be significantly modified by genetic and other environmental factors. It is not trite to say that "more research is needed" to improve our understanding of factors responsible for disparities in asthma prevalence. However, where community-level or individual-level interventions have been demonstrated to decrease asthma morbidity with reasonable certainty (85, 91), policy makers should develop the means to apply the lessons learned through changes in governmental and social policy as well as through recommendations to individuals (64). Subsequently, the outcome of changes in policy should be systematically evaluated. In the United States, effective reduction in disparities in asthma morbidity will be dependent only in part on specific measures like establishment of smoking cessation programs, home allergen reduction in sensitized asthmatic children, physician feedback, and/or health education. The long-term success of any of these specific measures is likely to depend, in great part, on more general improvements in living conditions and life opportunities (64, 87).

ACKNOWLEDGMENTS

Many thanks are given to Dr. Dominic Hodgkin for reviewing this manuscript, to Dr. Juan Celedón for sharing information on asthma disparities in the U.S. Hispanic/Latino communities and to Ms. Marisa Barr and Ms. Nancy Beattie for their secretarial assistance. These analyses were supported by NIH R01 #AI/EHS 35786 (DRG), K08 HL04187 (RW), ES10932 (RW), and U01 HL72494 (RW).

**The *Annual Review of Public Health* is online at
http://publhealth.annualreviews.org**

LITERATURE CITED

1. Acierno R, Kilpatrick DG, Rsesnick HS, Saund CL. 1996. Violent assault, post-traumatic stress disorder, and depression: risk factors for cigarette use among adult women. *Behav. Modif.* 20:363–84
2. Adler NE, Boyce T, Chesney MA, Cohen S, Folkman S, et al. 1994. Socioeco-

nomic status and health: the challenge of the gradient. *Am. Psychol.* 49:15–24
3. Aligne CA, Auinger P, Byrd RS, Weitzman M. 2000. Risk factors for pediatric asthma. Contributions of poverty, race, and urban residence. *Am. J. Respir. Crit. Care Med.* 162:873–77
4. Anda RF, Williamson DF, Escobedo LG,

Mast EE, Giovino GA, Remington PL. 1990. Depression and the dynamics of smoking: a national perspective. *JAMA* 264:1541–45

5. Asher MI, Keil U, Anderson HR. 1995. International study of asthma and allergies in childhood (ISAAC): rational and methods. *Eur. Respir. J.* 8:483–91

6. Attar BK, Guerra NG, Tolan PH. 1994. Neighborhood disadvantage, stressful life events and adjustment in urban elementary-school children. *J. Clin. Child Psychol.* 23:391–40

7. Baldini M, Lohman IC, Halonen M, Erickson RP, Holt PG, Martinez FD. 1999. A polymorphism in the 5′ flanking region of the CD14 gene is associated with circulating soluble CD14 levels and with total serum immunoglobulin E. *Am. J. Respir. Cell Mol. Biol.* 20:976–83

8. Ball TM, Castro-Rodriguez JA, Griffith KA, Holberg CJ, Martinez F, Wright AL. 2000. Siblings, day-care attendance, and the risk of asthma and wheezing during childhood. *N. Engl. J. Med.* 343:538–43

9. Beckett WS, Belanger K, Gent JF, Holford TR, Leaderer BP. 1996. Asthma among Puerto Rican Hispanics: a multiethnic comparison study of risk factors. *Am. J. Respir. Crit. Care Med.* 154:894–99

10. Beckham J, Roodman A, Shipley R, Hetzberg M, Cunha G, et al. 1995. Smoking in Vietnam combat veterans with posttraumatic stress disorder. *J. Trauma Stress* 8:461–72

11. Benson CB, Doubilet PM. 1998. Fetal measurements: normal and abnormal fetal growth. In *Diagnostic Ultrasound*, ed. CM Rumack, SR Wilson, JW Charboneau, pp. 1013–31. St. Louis: Mosby-Year Book

12. Benson V, Marano M. 1998. Current estimates from the National Health Interview Survey, 1995. Vital Health Stat. 10 (199). Hyattsville, MD: Natl. Cent. Health Stat.

13. Black PN, Sharpe S. 1997. Dietary fat and asthma: Is there a connection? *Eur. Respir. J.* 10:6–12

14. Boyce TW, Chesney M, Alkon A, Tschann JM, Adams S, et al. 1995. Psychobiologic reactivity to stress and childhood respiratory illnesses: results of two prospective studies. *Psychosom. Med.* 57:411–22

15. Braun-Fahrlander C, Riedler J, Herz U, Eder W, Waser M, et al. 2002. Environmental exposure to endotoxin and its relation to asthma in school-age children. *N. Engl. J. Med.* 347:869–77

16. Breslau N, Davis G, Andreski P, Petersen E. 1991. Traumatic events and posttraumatic stress disorder in an urban population of young adults. *Arch. Gen. Psychiatry* 48:216–22

17. Britton J. 2003. Parasites, allergy, and asthma. *Am. J. Respir. Crit. Care Med.* 168:266–67

18. Busse W, Kiecolt-Glaser J, Coe C, Martin R, Weiss S, Parker S. 1994. Stress and asthma: NHLBI Workshop Summary. *Am. J. Respir. Crit. Care Med.* 151:249–52

19. Carr W, Zeitel L, Weiss K. 1992. Variations in asthma hospitalizations and deaths in New York City. *Am. J. Public Health* 82:59–65

20. Castro-Rodriguez JA, Holberg CJ, Morgan WJ, Wright AL, Martinez FD. 2001. Increased incidence of asthmalike symptoms in girls who become overweight or obese during the school years. *Am. J. Respir. Crit. Care Med.* 163:1344–49

21. CDC. 1998. *Tobacco Use Among U.S. Racial/Ethnic Minority Groups-African American, America Indians and Alaska Natives, Asian American and Pacific Islanders, and Hispanics: A Report of the Surgeon General.* Atlanta, GA: US Dep. Health Hum. Serv., Natl. Cent. Chronic Dis. Prev. Health Promot. Off. Smok. Health

22. Celedon JC, Litonjua AA, Ryan L, Platts-Mills T, Weiss ST, Gold DR. 2002. Exposure to cat allergen, maternal

history of asthma, and wheezing in first 5 years of life. *Lancet* 360:781–82

23. Celedon JC, Litonjua AA, Ryan L, Weiss ST, Gold DR. 2002. Day care attendance, respiratory tract illnesses, wheezing, asthma, and total serum IgE level in early childhood. *Arch. Pediatr. Adolesc. Med.* 156:241–45

24. Celedon JC, Palmer LJ, Litonjua AA, Weiss ST, Wang B, et al. 2001. Body mass index and asthma in adults in families of subjects with asthma in Anqing, China. *Am. J. Respir. Crit. Care Med.* 164:1835–40

25. Celedon JC, Sredl D, Weiss ST, Pisarski M, Wakefield D, Cloutier M. 2004. Ethnicity and skin test reactivity to aeroallergens among asthmatic children in Connecticut. *Chest* 125:85–92

26. Celedon JC, Wright RJ, Litonjua AA, Sredl D, Ryan L, et al. 2003. Day care attendance in early life, maternal history of asthma, and asthma at the age of 6 years. *Am. J. Respir. Crit. Care Med.* 167:1239–43

27. Chen E, Fisher EB, Bacharier LB, Strunk RC. 2003. Socioeconomic status, stress, and immune markers in adolescents with asthma. *Psychosom. Med.* 65:984–92

28. Chew GL, Burge HA, Dockery DW, Muilenberg ML, Weiss ST, Gold DR. 1998. Limitations of a home characteristics questionnaire as a predictor of indoor allergen levels. *Am. J. Respir. Crit. Care Med.* 157:1536–41

29. Comm. Underst. Elimin. Racial Ethn. Disparities Health Care, Board Health Sci. Policy, Inst. Med. 2002. *Unequal Treatment Confronting Racial and Ethnic Disparities in Health Care.* Washington, DC: Natl. Acad. Press

30. Curry SJ, Wagner EH, Cheadle A, Diehr P, Koepsell T, et al. 1993. Assessment of community-level influences on individual's attitudes about cigarette smoking, alcohol use, and consumption of dietary fat. *Am. J. Prev. Med.* 9:78–84

31. Dekker C, Dales R, Bartlett S, Brunekree B, Zwanenburg H. 1991. Childhood asthma and the indoor environment. *Chest* 100:922–26

32. Diaz-Sanchez D, Dotson AR, Takenaka H, Saxon A. 1994. Diesel exhaust particles induce local IgE production in vivo and alter the pattern of IgE messenger RNA isoforms. *J. Clin. Invest.* 94:1417–25

33. Diez-Roux AV, Nieto FJ, Muntaner C, Tyroler HA, Comstock GW, et al. 1997. Neighborhood environments and coronary heart disease: a multilevel analyses. *Am. J. Epidemiol.* 146:48–63

34. Dohrenwend BP, Dohrenwend BS. 1969. *Social Status and Psychological Disorder.* New York: Wiley

35. Doubilet PM, Benson CB, Callen PW. 2000. Ultrasound evaluation of fetal growth. In *Ultrasonography in Obstetrics and Gynecology*, ed. PW Callen, pp. 206–20. Philadelphia: Saunders

36. DuRant R, Getts A, Cadenhead C, Emans S, Woods E. 1995. Exposure to violence and victimization and depression, hopelessness, and purpose in life among adolescents living in and around public housing. *Dev. Behav. Pediatr.* 16:233–37

37. Evans G. 2001. Environmental stress and health. In *Handbook of Health Psychology*, ed. A Baum, T Revenson, J Singer, pp. 365–85. Mahwah, NJ: Erlbaum

38. Feigelman W, Gorman B. 1989. Toward explaining the higher incidence of cigarette smoking among Black Americans. *J. Psychoactive Drugs* 21:299–305

39. Ganz ML. 2000. The relationship between external threats and smoking in central Harlem. *Am. J. Public Health* 90:367–71

40. Gennuso J, Epstein LH, Paluch RA, Cerny F. 1998. The relationship between asthma and obesity in urban minority children and adolescents. *Arch. Pediatr. Adolesc. Med.* 152:1197–200

41. Gergen PJ, Mullally DI, Evans R. 1988. National survey of prevalence of asthma

among children in the United States. *Pediatrics* 81:1–7

42. Gern JE, Reardon CL, Hoffjan S, Nicolae D, Li Z, et al. 2004. Effects of dog ownership and genotype on immune development and atopy in infancy. *J. Allergy Clin. Immunol.* 113:307–14

43. Gold DR, Burge HA, Carey V, Milton DK, Platts-Mills T, Weiss ST. 1999. Predictors of repeated wheeze in the first year of life: the relative roles of cockroach, birth weight, acute lower respiratory illness, and maternal smoking. *Am. J. Resp. Crit. Care Med.* 160:227–36

44. Deleted in proof

45. Gold DR, Damokosh AI, Dockery DW, Berkey CS. 2003. Body-mass index as a predictor of incident asthma in a prospective cohort of children. *Pediatr. Pulmonol.* 36:514–21

46. Gold DR, Rotnitzky A, Damokosh AI, Ware JH, Speizer FE, et al. 1993. Race and gender differences in respiratory illness prevalence and their relationship to environmental exposures in children 7 to 14 years of age. *Am. Rev. Resp. Dis.* 148:10–18

47. Gottlieb DJ, Beiser AS, O'Connor GT. 1995. Poverty, race, and medication use are correlates of asthma hospitalization rates. A small area analysis in Boston. *Chest* 108:28–35

48. Graves E, Kozak L. 1998. *Detailed diagnoses and procedures. National Hospital Discharge Survey, 1996.* Natl. Cent. Health Stat. Vital Health Stat. Ser. 13: Data from the National Health Survey (138):i–iii

49. Green RS, Smorodinsky S, Kim JJ, McLaughlin R, Ostro B. 2003. Proximity of California public schools to busy roads. *Environ. Health Perspect.* 112: 61–66

50. Grischkan J, Storfer-Isser A, Rosen CL, Larkin EK, Kirchner HL, et al. 2004. Variation in childhood asthma among former preterm infants. *J. Pediatr.* 144:321–26

51. Haan M, Kaplan G, Camacho T. 1987. Poverty and health: prospective evidence from the Alameda County Study. *Am. J. Epidemiol.* 125:989–98

52. Haan M, Kaplan N, Syme S. 1989. Socioeconomic status and health: old observations and new thoughts. In *Pathways in Health*, ed. J Bunder, D Gomby, B Kehrer, pp. 76–135. Menlo Park, CA: Henry J. Kaiser Family Found.

53. Hanrahan JP, Tager IB, Segal MR, Tosteson TD, Castile RG, et al. 1992. The effect of maternal smoking during pregnancy on early infant lung function. *Am. Rev. Respir. Dis.* 145:1129–35

54. Hodge L, Salome CM, Peat JK, Haby MM, Xuan W, Woolcock AJ. 1996. Consumption of oily fish and childhood asthma risk. *Med. J. Aust.* 164:137–40

55. Hoek G, Brunekreef B, Goldbohm S, Fischer P, van den Brandt PA. 2002. Association between mortality and indicators of traffic-related air pollution in the Netherlands: a cohort study. *Lancet* 360:1203–9

56. Holden G. 1991. The relationship of self-efficacy appraisals to subsequent health related outcomes: a meta-analysis. *Soc. Work Health Care* 16:53–93

57. Holt PG, O'Keeffe P, Holt BJ, Upham JW, Baron-Hay MJ, et al. 1995. T-cell "priming" against environmental allergens in human neonates: sequential deletion of food antigen reactivity during infancy with concomitant expansion of responses to ubiquitous inhalant allergens. *Pediatr. Allergy Immunol.* 6:85–90

58. Homa DM, Mannino DM, Lara M. 2000. Asthma mortality in U.S. Hispanics of Mexican, Puerto Rican, and Cuban heritage, 1990–1995. *Am. J. Respir. Crit. Care Med.* 161:504–9

59. Horrobin DF. 1987. Low prevalences of coronary heart disease (CHD), psoriasis, asthma and rheumatoid arthritis in Eskimos: Are they caused by high dietary intake of eicosapentaenoic acid (EPA), a genetic variation of essential fatty acid

(EFA) metabolism or a combination of both? *Med. Hypotheses* 22:421–28

60. Howard DE, Cross SI, Li X, Huang W. 1999. Parent-youth concordance regarding violence exposure: relationship to youth psychosocial functioning. *J. Adolesc. Health* 25:396–406

61. Inst. Med. Comm. Assess. Asthma Indoor Air. 2000. *Clearing the Air: Asthma and Indoor Air Exposures.* Washington, DC: IOM

62. Int. Study Asthma Allerg. Childhood (ISAAC) Steer. Comm. 1998. Worldwide variation in prevalence of symptoms of asthma, allergic rhinoconjunctivitis, and atopic eczema: ISAAC. *Lancet* 351:1225–32

63. Isaacs M. 1992. *Violence: The Impact of Community Violence on African American Children and Families.* Arlington, VA: Natl. Cent. Educ. Matern. Child Health

64. Isaacs SL, Schroeder SA. 2004. Class—the ignored determinant of the nation's health. *N. Engl. J. Med.* 351:1137–42

65. Kalliomaki M, Kirjavainen P, Eerola E, Kero P, Salminen S, Isolauri E. 2001. Distinct patterns of neonatal gut microflora in infants in whom atopy was and was not developing. *J. Allergy Clin. Immunol.* 107:129–34

66. Kalliomaki M, Salminen S, Arvilommi H, Kero P, Koskinen P, Isolauri E. 2001. Probiotics in primary prevention of atopic disease: a randomized placebo-controlled trial. *Lancet* 357:1076–79

67. Karvaonen S, Rimpela A. 1996. Socio-regional context as a determinant of adolescents' health in Finland. *Soc. Sci. Med.* 43:1467–74

68. Kattan M, Mitchell H, Eggleston P, Gergen P, Crain E, et al. 1997. Characteristics of inner-city children with asthma: the National Cooperative Inner-City Asthma Study. *Pediatr. Pulmonol.* 24:253–62

69. Kaufman J, Kaufman S. 2001. Assess-

ment of structured socioeconomic effects on health. *Epidemiology* 12:157–67

70. Kawachi I. 1999. Social capital and community effects on population and individual health. *Ann. NY Acad. Sci.* 896:120–30

71. Kawachi I, Berkman LF, eds. 2003. *Neighborhoods and Health.* New York: Oxford Univ. Press

72. Kennedy B, Kawachi I, Prothrow-Smith D. 1996. Income distribution and mortality: test of the Robin Hoos Index in the United States. *Br. Med. J.* 312:1004–7

73. Kennedy B, Kawachi I, Prothrow-Smith D, Lochner K, Gupta V. 1998. Social capital, income inequality, and firearm violent crime. *Soc. Sci. Med.* 47:7–17

74. Kilpatrick KL, Williams LM. 1998. Potential mediators of post-traumatic stress disorder in child witnesses to domestic violence. *Child Abuse Negl.* 22:319–30

75. Kitch BT, Chew G, Burge HA, Muilenberg ML, Weiss ST, et al. 2000. Socioeconomic predictors of high allergen levels in homes in the greater Boston area. *Environ. Health Perspect.* 108:301–7

76. Kleinschmidt I, Hills M, Elliott P. 1997. Smoking behavior can be predicated by neighborhood deprivation measures. *J. Epidemiol. Community Health* 87:1113–18

77. Krebs NF, Jacobson MS. 2003. Prevention of pediatric overweight and obesity. *Pediatrics* 112:424–30

78. La Veist T. 1993. Segregation, poverty, and empowerment: health consequence for African Americans. *Milbank Q.* 71:41–64

79. Leaderer BP, Belanger K, Triche E, Holford T, Gold DR, et al. 2002. Dust mite, cockroach, cat, and dog allergen concentrations in homes of asthmatic children in the northeastern United States: impact of socioeconomic factors and population density. *Environ. Health Perspect.* 110:419–25

80. Ledogar RJ, Penchaszadeh A, Garden CC, Iglesias G. 2000. Asthma and Latino

cultures: different prevalence reported among groups sharing the same environment. *Am. J. Public Health* 90:929–35

81. Lester LA, Rich SS, Blumenthal MN, Togias A, Murphy S, et al. 2001. Ethnic differences in asthma and associated phenotypes: collaborative study on the genetics of asthma. *J. Allergy Clin. Immunol.* 108:357–62

82. Lewis SA, Weiss ST, Platts-Mills TA, Burge H, Gold DR. 2002. The role of indoor allergen sensitization and exposure in causing morbidity in women with asthma. *Am. J. Respir. Crit. Care Med.* 165:961–66

83. Lochner K, Kawachi I, Kennedy B. 1999. Social capital: a guide to its measurement. *Health Place* 5:259–70

84. Luder E, Melnick TA, DiMaio M. 1998. Association of being overweight with greater asthma symptoms in inner city black and Hispanic children. *J. Pediatrics* 132:699–703

85. Martinez FD, Wright AL, Taussig LM, Holberg CJ, Halonen M, Morgan WJ. 1995. Asthma and wheezing in the first six years of life. The Group Health Medical Associates. *N. Engl. J. Med.* 332:133–38

86. Matricardi PM, Rosmini F, Rapicetta M, Gasbarrini G, Stroffolini T. 1999. Atopy, hygiene, and anthroposophic lifestyle. San Marino Study Group. *Lancet* 354:430

87. McKinlay J. 1975. The help-seeking behavior of the poor. In *Poverty and Health: A Sociological Analysis*, ed. J Kosa, A Antonovsky, I Zoal, pp. 224–73. Cambridge, MA: Harvard Univ. Press

88. McLean D, Hatfield-Timajchy K, Wingo P, Floyd R. 1993. Psychosocial measurement: implications for the study of preterm delivery in black women. *Am. J. Prev. Med.* 9(Suppl. 6):39–81

89. Michel O, Kips J, Duchateau J, Vertongen F, Robert L, et al. 1996. Severity of asthma is related to endotoxin in house dust. *Am. J. Respir. Crit. Care Med.* 154:1641–46

90. Mihrshahi S, Peat JK, Marks GB, Mellis CM, Tovey ER, et al. 2003. Eighteen-month outcomes of house dust mite avoidance and dietary fatty acid modification in the Childhood Asthma Prevention Study (CAPS). *J. Allergy Clin. Immunol.* 111:162–68

91. Morgan WJ, Crain EF, Gruchalla RS, O'Connor GT, Kattan M, et al. 2004. Results of a home-based environmental intervention among urban children with asthma. *N. Engl. J. Med.* 351:1068–80

92. Murphy S. 1997. *Expert Panel Report 2: Guidelines for the Diagnosis and Management of Asthma. Rep. 97–4051.* Bethesda, MD: Natl. Inst. Health, Natl. Heart, Lung, Blood Inst.

93. Nelson DA, Johnson CC, Divine GW, Strauchman C, Joseph CL, Ownby DR. 1997. Ethnic differences in the prevalence of asthma in middle class children. *Ann. Allergy Asthma Immunol.* 78:21–26

94. O'Neill MS, Jerrett M, Kawachi I, Levy JI, Cohen AJ, et al. 2003. Health, wealth, and air pollution: advancing theory and methods. *Environ. Health Perspect.* 111:1861–70

95. Deleted in proof

96. Ownby DR, Johnson CC, Peterson EL. 2002. Exposure to dogs and cats in the first year of life and risk of allergic sensitization at 6 to 7 years of age. *JAMA* 288:963–72

97. Park JH, Spiegelman DL, Gold DR, Burge HA, Milton DK. 2001. Predictors of airborne endotoxin in the home. *Environ. Health Perspect.* 109:859–64

98. Peat JK, Salome CM, Woolcock AJ. 1992. Factors associated with bronchial hyperresponsiveness in Australian adults and children. *Eur. Respir. J.* 5:921–29

99. Perez-Stable EJ, Ramirez A, Villareal R, Talavera GA, Trapido E, et al. 2001. Cigarette smoking behavior among US Latino men and women from different

countries of origin. *Am. J. Public Health* 91:1424–30

100. Perzanowski MS, Ronmark E, Platts-Mills TA, Lundback B. 2002. Effect of cat and dog ownership on sensitization and development of asthma among pre-teenage children. *Am. J. Respir. Crit. Care Med.* 166:696–702

101. Pierson WE, Koenig JQ. 1992. Respiratory effects of air pollution on allergic disease. *J. Allergy Clin. Immunol.* 90: 557–66

102. Platts-Mills T, Vaughan J, Squillace S, Woodfolk J, Sporik R. 2001. Sensitisation, asthma, and a modified Th2 response in children exposed to cat allergen: a population-based cross-sectional study. *Lancet* 357:752–56

103. Platts-Mills TA, Ward GW Jr, Sporik R, Gelber LE, Chapman MD, Heymann PW. 1991. Epidemiology of the relationship between exposure to indoor allergens and asthma. *Int. Arch. Allergy Appl. Immunol.* 94:339–45

104. Platts-Mills TAE, Erwin EA, Allison AB, Blumenthal K, Barr M, et al. 2003. The relevance of maternal immune responses to inhalant allergens to maternal symptoms, passive transfer to the infant, and development of antibodies in the first 2 years of life. *J. Allergy Clin. Immunol.* 111:123–30

105. Rabkin J, Struening E. 1976. Life events, stress and illness. *Science* 194:1013–20

106. Raper NR, Cronin FJ, Exler J. 1992. Omega-3 fatty acid content of the US food supply. *J. Am. Coll. Nutr.* 11:304–8

107. Rappaport S, Boodram B. 1998. Forecasted state-specific estimates of self-reported asthma prevalence–United States, 1998. *MMWR* 47:1022–25

108. Rauh VA, Chew GR, Garfinkel RS. 2002. Deteriorated housing contributes to high cockroach allergen levels in inner-city households. *Environ. Health Perspect.* 110(Suppl. 2):323–27

109. Ray NF, Thamer M, Fadillioglu B, Gergen PJ. 1998. Race, income, urbanicity, and asthma hospitalization in California: a small area analysis. *Chest* 113:1277–84

110. Reed CE, Milton DK. 2001. Endotoxin-stimulated innate immunity: a contributing factor for asthma. *J. Allergy Clin. Immunol.* 108:157–66

111. Reijneveld S. 1998. The impact of individual and area characteristics on urban socioeconomic differences in health and smoking. *Int. J. Epidemiol.* 27:33–40

112. Riedler J, Braun-Fahrlander C, Eder W, Schreuer M, Waser M, et al. 2001. Exposure to farming in early life and development of asthma and allergy: a cross-sectional survey. *Lancet* 358:1129–33

113. Roberts EM. 1997. Neighborhood social environments and the distribution of low birth weight in Chicago. *Am. J. Public Health* 87:597–603

114. Roberts EM. 2002. Racial and ethnic disparities in childhood asthma diagnosis: the role of clinical findings. *J. Natl. Med. Assoc.* 94:215–23

115. Roberts S. 1998. Community-level socioeconomic status effects on adult health. *J. Health Soc. Behav.* 39:18–37

116. Romano P, Bloom J, Syme S. 1991. Smoking, social support, and hassles in an urban African-American Community. *Am. J. Public Health* 81:1415–22

117. Rosenstreich DL, Eggleston P, Kattan M, Baker D, Slavin RG, et al. 1997. The role of cockroach allergy and exposure to cockroach allergen in causing morbidity among inner-city children with asthma. *N. Engl. J. Med.* 336:1356–63

118. Rowley DL. 2001. Closing the gap, opening the process: why study social contributors to preterm delivery among black women. *Matern. Child Health J.* 5: 71–74

119. Salmond C, Crampton P, Hales S, Lewis S, Pearce N. 1999. Asthma prevalence and deprivation: a small area analysis. *J. Epidemiol. Community Health* 53:476–80

120. Sampson R, Raudenbush S, Earls F. 1997. Neighborhoods and violent crime:

a multilevel study of collective efficacy. *Science* 277:918–24

121. Sandberg S, Paton JY, McCann DC, McGuiness D, Hillary CR, Oja H. 2000. The role of acute and chronic stress in asthma attacks in children. *Lancet* 356: 982–87

122. Schenker M, Samet J, Speizer F. 1983. Risk factors for childhood respiratory disease. *Am. Rev. Respir. Dis.* 128:1038–43

123. Schwartz J. 2004. Air pollution and children's health. *Pediatrics* 113:1037–43

124. Schwartz J, Gold DR, Dockery DW, Weiss ST, Speizer FE. 1990. Predictors of asthma and persistent wheeze in a national sample of children in the United States. Association with social class, perinatal events and race. *Am. Rev. Respir. Dis.* 142:555–62

125. Seaton A, Godden DJ, Brown K. 1994. Increase in asthma: a more toxic environment or a more susceptible population? *Thorax* 49:171–74

126. Shagena M, Sandler H, Perrin E. 1988. Concepts of illness and perception of control in healthy children and in children with chronic illnesses. *J. Dev. Behav. Pediatr.* 9:252–56

127. Stein M, Wallston K, Nicassio P, Castner N. 1988. Correlates of a clinical classification schema for the Arthritis Helplessness Index. *Arthritis Rheum.* 31:876–81

128. Strachan DP. 1989. Hay fever, hygiene, and household size. *Br. Med. J.* 299: 1259–60

129. Strachan DP. 2000. Family size, infection and atopy: the first decade of the "hygiene hypothesis." *Thorax* 55(Suppl. 1):S2–10

130. Strachan DP, Cook DG. 1997. Health effects of passive smoking. 1. Parental smoking and lower respiratory illness in infancy and early childhood. *Thorax* 52:905–14

131. Strachan DP, Cook DG. 1998. Health effects of passive smoking. 6. Parental smoking and childhood asthma: longitudinal and case-control studies. *Thorax* 53:204–12

132. Sullivan SD, Weiss KB, Lynn H, Mitchell H, Kattan M, et al. 2002. The cost-effectiveness of an inner-city asthma intervention for children. *J. Allergy Clin. Immunol.* 110:576–81

133. Tager IB. 1998. Smoking and childhood asthma—Where do we stand? *Am. J. Respir. Crit. Care Med.* 158:349–51

134. Taylor SE, Repetti RL, Seeman T. 1997. Health psychology: What is an unhealthy environment and how does it get under the skin? *Annu. Rev. Psychol.* 48:411–47

135. Troisi RJ, Willett WC, Weiss ST, Trichopoulos D, Rosner B, Speizer FE. 1995. A prospective study of diet and adult-onset asthma. *Am. J. Respir. Crit. Care Med.* 151:1401–8

136. U.S. Dep. Health Hum. Serv. 1991. *Healthy People 2000: National Health Promotion and Disease Prevention Objectives. DHHS Publ. No. (PHS) 91–50212.* Washington, DC: Off. Assist. Secretary Health

137. Vintzileos AM, Ananth CV, Smulian JC, Scorza WE, Knuppel RA. 2002. The impact of prenatal care in the United States on preterm births in the presence and absence of antenatal high-risk conditions. *Am. J. Obstet. Gynecol.* 187:1254–57

138. von Mutius E, Illi S, Hirsch T, Leupold W, Keil U, Weiland SK. 1999. Frequency of infections and risk of asthma, atopy and airway hyperresponsiveness in children. *Eur. Respir. J.* 14:4–11

139. von Mutius E, Martinez FD, Fritzsch C, Nicolai T, Roell G, Thiemann HH. 1994. Prevalence of asthma and atopy in two areas of West and East Germany. *Am. J. Respir. Crit. Care Med.* 149:358–64

140. Wagener D, Williams D, Wilson P. 1993. Equity and environmental health: data collection and interpretation issues. *Toxicol. Ind. Health* 9:775–95

141. Watson J, Cowen P, Lewis R. 1996. The relationship between asthma admission rates, routes of admission, and

socioeconomic deprivation. *Eur. Respir. J.* 9:2087–83

142. Weiss KB, Gergen PJ, Hodgson TA. 1992. An economic evaluation of asthma in the United States. *N. Engl. J. Med.* 326:862–66

143. Weiss KB, Gergen PJ, Wagener DK. 1993. Breathing better or wheezing worse? The changing epidemiology of asthma morbidity and mortality. *Annu. Rev. Public Health* 14:491–513

144. Weiss ST. 2002. Eat dirt—the hygiene hypothesis and allergic diseases. *N. Engl. J. Med.* 347:930–31

145. Weiss ST, Shore S. 2004. Obesity and Asthma: Directions for Research NHLBI Workshop, Bethesda, MD, July 15, 2002. *Am. J. Respir. Crit. Care Med.* 169:963–68

146. Weitzman M, Gortmaker S, Sobol A. 1990. Racial, social, and environmental risks for childhood asthma. *Am. J. Dis. Child.* 144:1189–94

147. Wilkinson R. 1996. *Unhealthy Societies. The Afflictions of Inequality.* London: Routledge

148. Wilson WJ. 1987. *The Truly Disadvantaged: The Inner-City, the Underclass, and Public Policy.* Chicago: Univ. Chicago Press

149. Wissow LS, Gittelsohn AM, Szklo M, Starfield B, Mussman M. 1988. Poverty, race, and hospitalization for childhood asthma. *Am. J. Public Health* 78:777–82

150. Woodcock A, Forster L, Matthews E, Martin J, Letley L, et al. 2003. Control of exposure to mite allergen and allergen-impermeable bed covers for adults with asthma. *N. Engl. J. Med.* 349:225–36

151. Wright AL, Sherrill D, Holberg CJ, Halonen M, Martinez FD. 1999. Breastfeeding, maternal IgE, and total serum IgE in childhood. *J. Allergy Clin. Immunol.* 104:589–94

152. Wright RJ, Cohen S, Carey V, Weiss ST, Gold DR. 2002. Parental stress as a predictor of wheezing in infancy: a prospective birth-cohort study. *Am. J. Respir. Crit. Care Med.* 165:358–65

153. Wright RJ, Fisher EB. 2003. Putting asthma into context: influences on risk, behavior, and intervention. In *Neighborhoods and Health*, ed. I Kawachi, LF Berkman, pp. 233–62. New York: Oxford Univ. Press

154. Wright RJ, Mitchell H, Visness CM, Cohen S, Stout J, et al. 2004. Community violence and asthma morbidity in the Inner-City Asthma Study. *Am. J. Public Health* 94:625–32

155. Wright RJ, Rodriguez M, Cohen S. 1998. Review of psychosocial stress and asthma: an integrated biopsychosocial approach. *Thorax* 53:1066–74

156. Wright RJ, Steinbach SF. 2001. Violence: an unrecognized environmental exposure that may contribute to greater asthma morbidity in high risk inner-city populations. *Environ. Health Perspect.* 109:1085–89

156a. Wright RJ, Wright RO, Finn P, Staudenmayer J, Contreras JP, et al. 2004. Chronic caregiver stress and IgE expression, allergen-induced proliferation, and cytokine profiles in a birth cohort predisposed to atopy. *J. Allergy Clin. Immunol.* 113:1051–57

157. Wuthrich B. 1989. Epidemiology of the allergic diseases: Are they really on the increase? *Int. Arch. Allergy Appl. Immunol.* 90(Suppl. 1):3–10

158. Yamada E, Vanna AT, Naspitz CK, Sole D. 2002. International Study of Asthma and Allergies in Childhood (ISAAC): validation of the written questionnaire (eczema component) and prevalence of atopic eczema among Brazilian children. *J. Investig. Allergol. Clin. Immunol.* 12:34–41

Annu. Rev. Public Health 2005. 26:115–40
doi: 10.1146/annurev.publhealth.26.021304.144637

THE RISE AND FALL OF MENOPAUSAL HORMONE THERAPY

Elizabeth Barrett-Connor,[1] Deborah Grady,[2] and Marcia L. Stefanick[3]

[1]*Division of Epidemiology, Department of Family and Preventive Medicine, University of California, San Diego, La Jolla, California 92093-0607; email: ebarrettconnor@ucsd.edu*
[2]*Department of Epidemiology and Biostatistics, University of California, San Francisco, California 94105; email: dgrady@itsa.ucsf.edu*
[3]*Stanford Prevention Research Center, School of Medicine, Stanford University, Stanford, California 94305; email: stefanick@stanford.edu*

Key Words   estrogen therapy, menopause, heart disease, stroke, breast cancer

■ **Abstract**   Clinical trials show that hormone therapy (HT) is an effective treatment for vasomotor symptoms and vaginal dryness. HT improves other symptoms including sleep and quality of life in women who have menopause symptoms. In the Women's Health Initiative controlled clinical trials, both estrogen therapy (ET) and estrogen plus progestin therapy (EPT) reduced fracture risk, neither reduced the risk of heart disease, and both increased the risk of stroke, deep vein thrombosis, and dementia. EPT, but not ET, increased breast cancer risk and reduced colon cancer risk. Differences between EPT and ET may reflect chance, baseline differences between the EPT and ET cohorts, or a progestin effect. Studies of younger women and lower HT doses with intermediate endpoints are beginning.

INTRODUCTION

The prescription of estrogens to relieve menopause-related symptoms was approved by the Food and Drug Administration (FDA) more than 60 years ago. Over the years, enthusiasm for hormone therapy (HT) has fluctuated dramatically. As expectations of benefit increased in the 1960s, widespread estrogen use was advocated to prevent postmenopausal estrogen deficiency and the "tragedy of the menopause" (99). In the 1970s prescriptions decreased, reflecting public awareness of an increase in endometrial cancer in hormone users (84, 100) and subsequently increased again with evidence that the addition of a progestin could prevent estrogen-induced endometrial changes. In the 1980s there was a renewed emphasis on potential long-term benefits, as epidemiological evidence mounted for a reduced risk of osteoporotic fractures (66, 96) and an equally dramatic reduction in coronary heart disease (18, 88).

In 1992, a landmark systematic review and meta-analysis of the results of observational studies of postmenopausal HT described four outcomes plausibly related to HT: heart disease, hip fracture, breast cancer, and uterine cancer (32). On the basis of summary odds ratios from the observational studies and life-table models, the authors concluded that the reduced risk of heart disease and hip fracture would outweigh the cancer risks. This favorable risk benefit ratio, based on observational evidence and driven largely by the apparent cardiovascular benefit, increased the recognition that coronary heart disease was the main killer of women, and led to the recommendation that "hormone replacement therapy" be considered for all women. In the United States, by the mid-1990s, recommendation of HT was counted as a criterion for good medical practice in managed care organizations, the annual number of HT prescriptions filled increased from 58 million in 1995 to 90 million in 1999 (43), and estrogen became the biggest selling prescription drug.

By 2002, however, results from two large, randomized, placebo-controlled clinical trials, Heart and Estrogen/Progestin Replacement Study (HERS) and the Women's Health Initiative estrogen plus progestin trial (WHI-EPT), both comparing conjugated equine estrogen (CEE) plus daily medroxyprogesterone acetate (MPA) with placebo, did not show the expected coronary benefit (49, 75). Postmenopausal estrogen prescriptions decreased by 33% and combined estrogen/progestin therapy prescriptions decreased by 66%, with total hormone prescriptions dropping by 50% as shown in Figure 1 (43). In April of 2004, the main results from the Women's Health Initiative trial of unopposed estrogen (WHI-ET), which compared unopposed CEE with placebo, also reported no reduction in risk of coronary events, with as yet unknown effects on future hormone use (6).

This chapter reviews the major randomized, placebo-controlled clinical trials of hormone therapy published in the past 10 years, first in a section most relevant to the management of menopause-related symptoms, and second in a section related to common chronic diseases possibly related to estrogen use. We also briefly describe large cohort studies and meta-analyses of observational data because volunteers in trials may differ from women in the community, outcome collection methods differ, and larger and longer observational studies provide information about rare events and about the risks and benefits of extended use. Because of space limitations, we do not discuss laboratory evidence for favorable or unfavorable outcomes.

Finally, because postmenopausal hormone therapy is pharmacologic not physiologic, we do not use the term hormone replacement therapy. Instead we use hormone therapy (HT) as a comprehensive term for postmenopausal estrogen with or without a progestin, estrogen therapy (ET) to describe unopposed estrogen, and estrogen plus progestin therapy (EPT) to describe continuous or cyclic combined therapy.

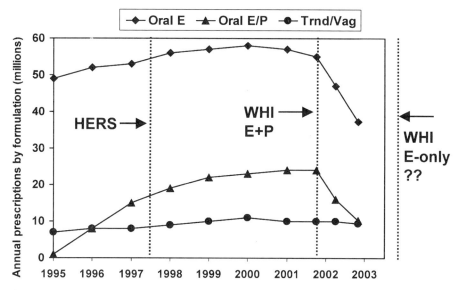

Figure 1   Annual number of U.S. prescriptions for hormone therapy by formulation, 1995 to July 2003. Data taken from the National Prescription Audit Plus, IMS HEALTH. Abbreviations: HERS, Heart and Estrogen/Progestin Replacement Study; WHI, Women's Health Initiative. Permission to reprint from Hersch AL, Stefanick ML, Stafford RS. 2004. National use of postmenopausal hormone therapy. *JAMA* 291:47–53 (43, figure 3, p. 50). Copyright © 2004 American Medical Association. All rights reserved.

HORMONE THERAPY FOR MENOPAUSE-RELATED SYMPTOMS

Vasomotor and genital symptoms are the symptoms most unequivocally associated with menopause and are consistently shown in clinical trials to respond better to estrogen than to placebo (58). As described below, other common complaints often attributed to menopause, such as mood swings, depression, disturbed sleep, and "fuzzy thinking," are either unchanged by HT in controlled trials or are improved primarily or exclusively in women who have severe vasomotor symptoms.

Vasomotor Symptoms

Hot flashes, sudden waves of heat sensation typically spreading over the upper body and face, are experienced by about 75% of U.S. and European women at some point in the menopause transition (52, 91). Hot flashes tend to decrease in severity and frequency over a few months to a few years (53) but sometimes persist into old age. Severe hot flashes may compromise quality of life by causing discomfort, as well as embarrassing visible changes in skin color and sweating; severe night sweats may require change of bedding and interfere with sleep.

Clinical Trials of HT for Vasomotor Symptoms

Estrogen is the most effective treatment for troublesome vasomotor symptoms. The first systematic review of randomized controlled clinical trials found 40 trials showing that HT reduces the severity of vasomotor symptoms, often with improvement beginning within the first week of treatment (76). Summary estimates of hot-flash frequency and severity from another meta-analysis of the results of 21 trials of 3 months–3 years duration reported that standard doses of estrogen (equivalent to about 0.625 mg of conjugated estrogen) reduced weekly hot-flash frequency by 77%, compared with placebo (58). Unopposed estrogen and estrogen plus progestin regimens were equally effective in relieving hot flashes in peri- and postmenopausal women, as were various types of estrogen, both oral and transdermal (58). Lower-than-standard doses of estrogen, such as 0.3 mg/day oral conjugated estrogen (93) and 0.02 to 0.025 mg/day transdermal 17-beta estradiol (87, 92), are also effective for treatment of hot flashes. Many of these trials included only women who were compliant with HT in the analysis. Studies limited to compliant women tend to overestimate benefit and underestimate side effects.

Estrogen therapy also appears to be effective in older women who have had hot flashes for many years. The 3-year Postmenopausal Estrogen/Progestin Intervention (PEPI) trial, which included 875 women who were within 10 years of menopause (average age 56), showed a 58% reduction in vasomotor symptoms in women receiving ET (alone or combined with a progestin) compared with placebo (35). In the Heart and Estrogen/Progestin Replacement Study (HERS), 85% of the 434 women (average age 67) who reported hot flashes at baseline improved after 1 year of hormone therapy, compared with 48% of women assigned to placebo (44). In the WHI-EPT trial, a subset of 1072 women in the EPT group and 974 women in the placebo group reported moderate-to-severe vasomotor symptoms at baseline. After 1 year, 77% in the hormone group had reduced severity of hot flashes, compared with 52% in the placebo group (40); more women assigned to active treatment also showed improvement in the severity of night sweats (71% compared with 53% in women assigned to placebo) (40).

Quality of Life, Sleep, Mood, and Depression

Results from randomized placebo-controlled trials suggest ET improves quality of life, as estimated by standard quantitative tests (76). This improvement in general quality of life is likely due to improvement in vasomotor symptoms (44). For example, in the HERS trial, improved quality of life related to EPT was limited to women who had vasomotor symptoms; women who reported no vasomotor symptoms at baseline also reported no improvement in quality of life on EPT and, in fact, reported less vigor and well-being than did women assigned to placebo (44).

Among HERS women who reported trouble sleeping before treatment, a slightly higher proportion on EPT (39%) than on placebo (33%) reported improvement after 1 year (44). In WHI-EPT, EPT was associated with a statistically significant small benefit in terms of sleep disturbance, physical functioning, and bodily pain at one year; however, these differences were not clinically meaningful (the mean benefit of sleep disturbance was 0.4 point on a 20-point scale, physical functioning was 0.8 point on a 100-point scale, and pain was 1.9 points on a 100-point scale). No differences were seen at three years between the women assigned to EPT versus placebo with regard to any quality-of-life outcome (40). In a subset analysis, 574 women aged 50–54 who reported moderate-to-severe vasomotor symptoms at baseline showed a significant improvement in sleep disturbance on EPT versus placebo, with no difference in other quality-of-life outcomes (40).

Feeling depressed is a common complaint during the menopause transition. Evidence that HT improves depressed mood is mixed. A 1997 review of 14 clinical trials (101) concluded that estrogen therapy improved depressed mood during the menopause transition or after oophorectomy, but the review included several clinical trials without placebo controls. In another review, significant improvement in mood was reported in the majority of 13 observational studies of nondepressed women, but half of the 14 clinical trials found no significant improvement in mood (62). The most recent review included 9 trials of ET for diverse depressive disorders among women in the menopause transition; 6 of these were placebo controlled, and 4 suggested that ET was superior to placebo (86). The most impressive results were reported from two trials of transdermal estrogen in the treatment of severe clinical depression (78, 85).

In the HERS trial, emotional health was improved by ET only in women with vasomotor symptoms at baseline. In this trial of 2763 older women, 3 years of EPT had no significant effect on depressive symptoms overall; but women with flushing who were assigned to EPT experienced significantly fewer depressive symptoms and reported improved mental health compared with women with flushing in the placebo group (44). In contrast, the same combined-hormone treatment had no effect on an 8-item depression score in the overall WHI-EPT cohort or in the subset of 574 women aged 50–54 who reported moderate-to-severe vasomotor symptoms at baseline (40).

Weight Gain

One clinical trial has demonstrated that weight gain during the menopause transition can be prevented by diet and exercise (54). In that trial, premenopausal women ages 44–50 were randomly assigned to a lifestyle intervention of reduced calories and saturated fat plus increased physical activity or to assessment only. Although the proportion of women who became menopausal over the 5-year period is not reported, 55% of the lifestyle intervention participants were at or below baseline weight compared with 26% of controls after 4.5 years, and the mean weight in the intervention group was 0.1 kg below baseline compared with an average gain of 2.4 kg in the control group; waist circumference decreased 2.9 cm in the intervention group compared with a decrease of 0.5 cm in the control group.

A quantitative review (68) of 22 randomized controlled trials found no consistent evidence that postmenopausal estrogen alone or in combination with a progestin promotes or prevents weight gain. These results contrast with the 3-year PEPI trial results, where women within 10 years of menopause who were assigned to HT (estrogen with or without one of three progestational agents) had, on average, 1.0-kg less weight gain and 1.2-cm less increase in waist girth than women assigned to placebo (24). Similarly, WHI women assigned to EPT reduced weight by 0.4% and waist circumference by 0.9% from baseline to year 1, compared with placebo (59).

Urogenital Symptoms and Sexual Function

GENITAL COMPLAINTS   After menopause, the urogenital mucosa becomes thinner, less elastic, and less vascular. The vagina shortens and narrows, developing a thin, friable surface, generally called vaginal atrophy. Vulvovaginal symptoms, which do not necessarily parallel clinical findings, include dryness, pruritis, discharge, dyspareunia, and postcoital bleeding. Nevertheless, older women often report a satisfactory sex life without HT. In the Massachusetts Women's Health Study (8), factors such as marital status and sexual dysfunction of partner, physical and mental health, and cigarette smoking had a greater impact on sexual functioning than menopause status. Studies of symptomatic women generally suggest that HT improves genital symptoms and sexuality, but there are no quantitative reviews and diverse definitions of sexual function impede synthesis (9). In WHI-EPT, active treatment of older women had no effect on sexual satisfaction as assessed by a 4-point response scale (40).

VAGINAL DRYNESS   A meta-analysis of 10 randomized, controlled clinical trials showed that oral, transdermal, and intravaginal ET (cream, tablet, or vaginal ring) reduced vaginal symptoms among women with vaginal dryness or dyspareunia (19). In HERS, 61% of women assigned to oral EPT and 47% assigned to placebo reported improvement in genital dryness (11). Although there are few head-to-head comparisons, vaginal application seems to provide superior relief compared with systemic ET and raises circulating estrogen concentrations less than oral ET, which may improve the safety profile.

LIBIDO   There is no evidence that reduced sexual desire beginning during the menopause transition is caused by estrogen deficiency or improved by ET. The reverse is plausible because oral estrogen increases sex hormone-binding globulin, which reduces bioavailable testosterone and estradiol (83). This effect on sex hormone–binding globulin may explain why estrogen plus testosterone improved sexual enjoyment, desire, and arousal more than estrogen alone in two clinical trials (57, 76).

URINARY COMPLAINTS   Urinary tract symptoms previously attributed to estrogen deficiency include dysuria, frequency, nocturia, urinary incontinence, and urinary tract infection. Of these, only the frequency of recurrent urinary tract infection has been shown in clinical trials to be reduced by estrogen treatment (23, 71). However, HT did not prevent urinary tract infections in HERS women without prior urinary tract infections (17).

No good evidence supports the notion that HT improves or protects against stress or urge incontinence. In the HERS trial, women with incontinence at baseline who were treated with EPT reported worsened incontinence compared with those treated with placebo; similarly, women without incontinence at baseline were more likely to develop incontinence when assigned to EPT (29).

HORMONE THERAPY TO PREVENT CHRONIC DISEASE

The potential of ET to prevent diverse conditions that are common in later life was a major impetus for long-term HT. Observational studies reported that women using HT had fewer fractures, less heart disease, less colon cancer, and less dementia, but a healthy-user bias could explain some or all of these putative benefits. For example, women physicians in Britain who continued HT were more likely than non-hormone-using physicians to report a healthy diet and vigorous physical activity (51). In a U.S. prospective study, women who elected to use HT after menopause were healthier before menopause than those who did not choose to use HT (60).

Only randomized, placebo-controlled clinical trials, the basis of evidence-based medicine, can control for the effects of known and unknown differences between postmenopausal women who do or do not take hormones. Nowhere has the importance of clinical trials been so evident as in the past five years, when the results of HT trials have contradicted several of the findings of earlier observational studies of HT.

Table 1 shows characteristics of the participants, the intervention, and the duration for the three large chronic disease–outcome trials: HERS and the two WHI hormone trials. Table 2 summarizes the results from these trials with regard to major clinical outcomes. Figure 2 shows the absolute risks in rates per 10,000 women per year from WHI-EPT and WHI-ET. When comparing and contrasting WHI-EPT and WHI-ET results, it is important to understand that these are two different trials, not only with regard to treatment, size, and duration (See Table 1), but also because the trial cohorts are quite different. To be eligible for WHI-ET, women were required to have had a hysterectomy, and more than 40% reported a bilateral oophorectomy. In addition, a substantially greater percentage of WHI-ET women had used HT in the past, and on average they had first births at younger ages and had had more live births than had WHI-EPT participants. WHI-ET women were also more overweight and had more hypertension and diabetes at baseline than did women in WHI-EPT. Furthermore, the percentage of minority women was

TABLE 1   Characteristics of three hormone therapy outcome trials

Trial	N	Study drug (mg/d)	Eligibility criteria	Primary outcomes	Duration (years)
HERS	2763	CEE 0.625 MPA 2.5	Heart disease No hysterectomy	Heart disease	4.1
WHI-EPT	16,608	CEE 0.625 MPA 2.5	No hysterectomy	Heart disease Breast cancer Global index	5.2
WHI-ET	10,739	CEE 0.625	Hysterectomy	Heart disease Breast cancer Global index	6.8

substantially greater in the WHI-ET, particularly for African American women (89).

WHI-EPT results were first published in 2002. More detailed subsequent reports from WHI-EPT have been published for most of the major outcomes, which include somewhat longer follow-up (5.6 vs. 5.2 years), additional cases, and central adjudication of outcomes that was not available at the time of the first publication. This has not materially changed the results, but small differences may confuse the

TABLE 2   Hazard ratios from three hormone therapy trials

Clinical event	Hazard ratio (95% confidence interval)*		
	HERS (estrogen + progestin) (49, 82)	WHI (estrogen + progestin) (75)	WHI (estrogen) (6)
CHD events	0.99 (0.80–1.22)	1.29 (1.02–1.63)	0.91 (0.75–1.12)
Stroke	1.23 (0.89–1.70)	1.41 (1.07–1.85)	1.39 (1.10–1.77)
Pulmonary embolism	2.79 (0.89–8.75)	2.13 (1.39–3.25)	1.34 (0.87–2.06)
Breast cancer	1.30 (0.77–2.19)	1.26 (1.00–1.59)	0.77 (0.59–1.01)
Colon cancer	0.69 (0.32–1.49)	0.63 (0.43–0.92)	1.08 (0.75–1.55)
Hip fracture	1.10 (0.49–2.50)	0.66 (0.45–0.98)	0.61 (0.41–0.91)
Death	1.08 (0.84–1.38)	0.98 (0.82–1.18)	1.04 (0.88–1.22)
Global index[†]	—	1.15 (1.03–1.28)	1.01 (0.91–1.12)

Abbreviations: CHD, coronary heart disease; HERS, Heart and Estrogen/Progestin Replacement Study; WHI, Women's Health Initiative; —, not calculated.

*These data are from the initial WHI reports for EPT and CEE and differ slightly from subsequent updated reports presented in this review. Data are based on the intent-to-treat analyses. For the primary CHD events outcome (myocardial infarction plus CHD death), the three trials had similar numbers of events and thus similar power. For other outcomes the smaller HERS trial had fewer events and less-precise hazard ratios.

[†]The global index was composed of the first occurrence of any of the events listed in the table.

Permission to reprint from Hulley SB, Grady D. 2004. The WHI Estrogen-Alone Trial—Do things look any better? *JAMA* 291:1769–71 (48a, table 1, p. 1770). Copyright © 2004 American Medical Association. All rights reserved.

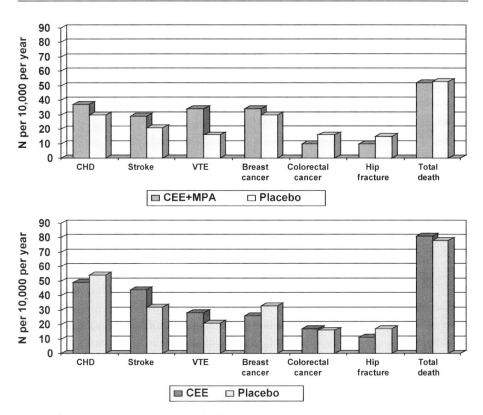

Figure 2   Clinical outcomes by randomization assignment (*N* per 10,000 per year) for the Women's Health Initiative Estrogen plus Progestin (*upper panel*) and Estrogen alone (*lower panel*) trials.

unwary reader. The second papers on each of the seven primary outcomes include stratified analyses and tests for interaction, seeking subgroups of women for whom HT might show particular risk or benefit.

Another cautionary note about the WHI trials is that both the percentage of women who stopped taking study pills ("drop-out") and the percentage who initiated active hormone therapy through their personal health care providers ("drop-in") exceeded design projections within the first year in both active and placebo arms and steadily increased over the course of the trials; in addition, although some women resumed study pills at some point, only cumulative drop-in and drop-out rates were reported. At the time the WHI-EPT trial was stopped, i.e., after an average of 5.2 years of follow-up, the cumulative drop-out rates were 42% for EPT and 38% for placebo, and the cumulative drop-in rates were 6.2% for EPT and 10.7% for placebo. At the time the WHI-ET trial was terminated, i.e., after an average of 6.8 years of follow-up, cumulative drop-out rates were 54% for both ET and placebo and drop-in rates were 5.7% for ET and 9.1% for placebo. Nonadherence can spuriously reduce the true benefit and the true harm of treatment.

Osteoporosis and Fractures

BONE DENSITY AND BONE LOSS   The balance between bone formation and bone resorption is disturbed during the menopause transition, before menses cease, when follicle-stimulating hormone (FSH) levels are high but estrogen levels are relatively normal. Bone loss is often, but not always, accelerated for several years after menopause, averaging 2% per year (range <1%–5%), after which there is a steady slow bone loss of about 0.5% per year. Some women show little change in bone mineral density after menopause (37). In very old age, bone loss may accelerate again, probably related to immobility, intercurrent illness, poor nutrition, or secondary hyperparathyroidism.

Fracture risk increases with age and is closely related to bone density, bone connectivity, body size, balance, strength, and the propensity to fall. In the United States, a 50-year-old white woman has a 15% lifetime risk of hip fracture, usually occurring after age 70, a 40% risk of at least one spine fracture, and a 15% risk of wrist fracture, the latter two generally occurring before age 60 (72). Long before the estrogen-prevents-heart-disease hypothesis prompted widespread use of HT, the prevention of osteoporosis and fractures was the main indication for HT in women not seeking therapy for menopause symptoms.

Many clinical trials have shown that estrogen therapy increases bone density in postmenopausal women, whether therapy began at menopause or in old age. A systematic review and meta-analysis that included results of 57 randomized, placebo-controlled clinical trials published between 1966 and 1999 reported a statistically significant increase in bone density in favor of HT (97). After one year, the change in bone density was 5.4% better at the lumbar spine, 3.0% better at the forearm, and 2.5% better at the femoral neck compared with placebo. After two years of treatment the percent change favoring HT increased further by about 1.5% at each site. At the end of two years, there was a significant dose-response effect with better bone density at the hip and spine in women taking higher doses of HT (0.9 mg) than lower doses (0.3 mg). HT also increased bone mineral density (BMD) at the hip and spine in the PEPI trial (37), with no significant differences between the bone effects of ET alone or given with any of three progestational regimens. Low doses may be adequate to maintain bone, however. In one small, randomized, placebo-controlled trial, an ultralow dose (0.25 mg/d) of oral micronized 17 beta-estradiol increased bone density at the hip and spine (69). In another larger randomized trial, 14 μg of transdermal estradiol per day increased bone density at the spine and hip compared with placebo (25).

HT must be continued to maintain the bone sparing effect (27). On the basis of data from the large National Osteoporosis Risk Assessment (NORA) observational study, women who used HT for 5–10 years after menopause and then quit had no better bone density at the radius or heel at age 70 than did women who had never used HT (14). Recency of use was much more important than duration of use, compatible with the observation that bone loss accelerates when HT is discontinued.

FRACTURE   In a large observational study of more than 138,737 postmenopausal English women followed for an average of 2.8 years, current HT was associated with a significantly reduced risk of fracture (RR 0.62, 95% CI 0.58–0.66), and the benefit was similar for ET and EPT (10). Fracture incidence rates returned to those of never-users about one year after discontinuing HT (10).

Until recently the best trial evidence that HT prevents fractures came from systematic reviews of small clinical trials. A review of 22 small trials reported a 27% summary relative risk reduction in nonvertebral fractures (90). A meta-analysis of the results of 7 clinical trials of HT with fracture outcomes (5 vertebral and 6 nonvertebral) found a 34% summary relative risk reduction for vertebral fractures and a 13% reduction for nonspine fractures; in neither case were the differences statistically significant (97).

WHI-EPT was the first trial large enough to unequivocally show that HT prevents fractures, even in women unselected for osteoporosis (75). Less than 6% of WHI-EPT women probably had osteoporosis, on the basis of BMD measured in 1024 women at 3 of the 40 WHI sites. About 5 years of combined continuous EPT reduced the risk of all fractures by 24% and the risk of hip fractures by 33% compared with placebo (see Table 2, Figure 2). Overall, 733 (8.6%) women in the EPT arm and 896 women (11.1%) in the placebo group had a fracture during the average 5.6-year follow-up (20). The effect of HT on fracture risk did not differ significantly by age, time since menopause, body mass index, smoking, personal or family history of fracture, past use of HT, or bone density. Even in the highest fracture risk group, the reduced hip fracture benefit did not exceed the other harms of HT (20). In subset analyses of WHI-EPT, there was only one statistically significant interaction: a 60% greater reduction in risk of hip fracture among women who reported a baseline dietary calcium intake of more than 1200 mg/day, compared with women who reported less calcium intake. This finding is compatible with the results of observational studies that consistently show better bone preservation in women who take both estrogen and calcium (65).

The unopposed estrogen arm of the WHI showed a similar statistically significant reduction in fracture risk with ET versus placebo in 10,739 women who were followed for an average of 6.8 years (6). In WHI-ET, the risk of hip fracture was reduced by 39% and the risk of clinical spine fracture was reduced by 38%.

Coronary Heart Disease

Coronary heart disease is the leading cause of death in women in most of the westernized world. Enthusiasm for nearly universal use of HT stemmed from observations that the risk might be reduced by as much as 50%, and this apparent protection would outweigh any other potential risks (32). Although a plethora of putative cardioprotective mechanisms were observed (including favorable changes in LDL and HDL cholesterol, Lp(a), vasoreactivity, fibrinogen, fasting blood glucose, homocysteine, and nitric oxide), the most persuasive evidence came from more than thirty epidemiologic studies that suggested a 30%–50% reduced risk of heart disease in women using estrogen compared with nonusers (13, 32). On the basis of this evidence, estrogen was promoted for the prevention of heart disease. A recent meta-analysis restricted to 18 "good quality" observational studies reported similar cardiac protection, but this apparent benefit disappeared when the analysis was restricted to the few observational studies that controlled for socioeconomic status, for alcohol consumption and physical activity, or both (50).

The first clinical trial evidence that HT might not prevent coronary heart disease in postmenopausal women came from a 1997 systematic review of 22 small, short, clinical trials performed to test the effect of HT on a variety of outcomes. Myocardial infarction and coronary death were not primary outcomes but were collected as adverse events or reasons for discontinuation. The summary results of these trials showed an increased cardiovascular risk in women assigned to HT (42).

Published in 1998, HERS was the first large, placebo-controlled clinical trial of EPT with coronary heart disease as the primary outcome (49). The 2763 HERS participants, all of whom had documented heart disease at baseline and an intact uterus (necessary for the test of efficacy of combined hormone therapy), experienced a 50% increased risk of coronary events during the first year and no overall reduction in the risk of fatal and nonfatal coronary disease or stroke after 4 years. A 3-year extension of HERS showed no evidence of later protection (relative hazard after 6.8 years of follow-up 1.00; 95% CI 0.77–1.29) (31). An extensive search for subgroups of women who might have been helped or harmed in HERS produced no convincing explanation for the early harm or overall absent benefit (26). Two of the most popular explanations for this unexpected result were that HT could not decrease the risk of cardiovascular events in women who already had coronary artery atherosclerosis or that the progestin offset the benefit of estrogen.

In July 2002, the 16,608 WHI-EPT participants were informed that the trial was being stopped 3.3 years early because an increased risk of breast cancer crossed a preestablished stopping boundary and was accompanied by an overall balance of harm greater than benefit with respect to 8 prespecified outcomes. As shown in Table 2, there was a 29% increased risk of coronary heart disease, a 41% increased stroke risk, and a 113% increased risk of pulmonary embolism (75). The increased risk of myocardial infarction and venous clotting in the hormone group was apparent in the first year of the trial, whereas the increased stroke risk was not seen until after the first year. Figure 2 shows that the number of additional cases of vascular disease attributed to EPT exposure (above rates in the placebo group) was small but greater than the number of other conditions prevented. In an updated report, the hazard ratio for CHD was 1.24 (CI 1.00–1.54) (59). There was a higher relative risk for coronary events associated with EPT among women with high LDL-cholesterol compared with those with low baseline LDL-cholesterol. However, this subgroup finding was one of more than 20 subgroup analyses performed and may have occurred by chance. There was no interaction of treatment effect with age, years since menopause, C-reactive protein, or other biomarkers. EPT had no effect on rates of revascularization procedures, confirmed angina, acute coronary syndrome, or congestive heart failure (59).

WHI-ET, the estrogen-only trial with 10,739 women enrolled, was stopped 2 years prematurely in 2004, after an average of 6.6 years (6). The main reason for stopping this trial early was a 39% increased incidence of stroke among ET users and a very low likelihood for future cardiac benefit. The fact that there was no overall benefit and the improbability of showing a more favorable balance of benefits and risks by continuing the trial were also considerations in stopping the trial (Table 2).

Women in WHI-ET assigned to unopposed estrogen, unlike women in HERS and WHI trials of combined therapy, experienced no early excess risk of coronary events. Similar to the previous trials, there was also no reduction in risk of coronary events during the trial (Table 2 and Figure 2). As shown in Figure 2, the risk of heart disease among women assigned to placebo was higher in WHI-ET than in WHI-EPT, possibly owing to greater baseline risk for heart disease [i.e., more obesity, hypertension, diabetes, or prior heart disease, which may be associated with hysterectomy or factors leading to the hysterectomy (59)]. Several other smaller randomized trials, some using unopposed oral or transdermal estradiol, also found no protection against coronary artery disease (12). Thus, there is no evidence that HT with or without a progestin prevents coronary heart disease.

The null results with unopposed ET should lay to rest the notion that the use of a progestin explains the lack of cardioprotection in HERS and WHI-EPT but leaves open the possibility that the early harm observed in HERS and WHI-EPT was related to daily use of medroxyprogesterone. However, women enrolled in WHI-EPT and -ET were sufficiently different that the small differences in early harm between the trials cannot be attributed necessarily to the presence or absence of a progestin.

Stroke

A meta-analysis of 9 observational studies among women with no history of stroke showed a small but significant increased risk of stroke associated with hormone use (relative risk 1.12; 95% CI 1.01–1.23) (4). The risk of stroke in the 2763 women in the HERS trial, who all had documented coronary artery disease, was increased but not significantly so (hazard ratio 1.23; 95% CI 0.80–1.22; Table 2) (82). In the Women's Estrogen for Stroke Trial (WEST) (94), 664 women who had a history of stroke or transient ischemic attack at enrollment were randomly assigned to unopposed 17 beta-estradiol or placebo and followed for an average of 2.8 years. Women assigned to ET experienced a nearly threefold increased risk of fatal stroke (RR 2.9; 95% CI 0.9–9.0). There was no excess risk of nonfatal stroke in the ET group, but the stroke survivors had slightly worse neurologic or functional deficits.

The first trial evidence of a statistically significant excess risk of stroke with HT came from the WHI trials (6, 75), with a hazard ratio of 1.41 for combined therapy in WHI-EPT and 1.39 for unopposed estrogen in WHI-ET (Table 2). In an updated report, the hazard ratio for total stroke was 1.31 (CI 1.02–1.68); the authors suggested that the risk was likely underestimated owing to the relatively low adherence rates in WHI: In an analysis restricted to women who were adherent to study medication, the hazard ratio increased to 1.50 (95% CI 1.08–2.08) (95). The increased risk with EPT was predominantly for ischemic stroke (HR 1.44; 95% CI 1.09–1.90) and was similar across all age groups, in all categories of baseline stroke risk, and in women with and without hypertension, prior history of cardiovascular disease, or use of statins or aspirin.

In WHI-ET, stroke was the only statistically significant adverse event attributable to unopposed estrogen. As shown in Figure 2, WHI-ET women assigned to ET experienced 12 additional stroke events per 10,000 treated women per year. In age-specific analyses, the hazard ratio was highest among women aged 60–69 (1.65; 95% CI 1.16–2.36). There were very few strokes in women younger than age 60.

Breast Cancer

Breast cancer accounts for 32% of new cancers diagnosed in women each year and is second only to lung cancer as the leading cause of cancer death in U.S. women (15% versus 25%). Breast cancer risk is related to endogenous estrogen, as shown in a pooled analysis of 9 prospective studies of postmenopausal women. in which a doubling of estradiol levels was associated with a 23%–35% increased risk of breast cancer with no evidence of a threshold effect (3).

The results of early observational studies of the association of HT and breast cancer were inconsistent, likely reflecting failure to consider duration of HT use and the role of obesity, reproductive history, and oophorectomy. A pooled reanalysis of data from 51 of 63 published observational studies of HT and breast cancer, which included 52,705 women with breast cancer and 108,411 without breast cancer, showed an increased risk of breast cancer that was clearly evident after 5 years of ET (2). Breast cancer risk increased 2.3% for each year of use beyond 5 years, the same as the increased risk for each year of delayed menopause, providing internal consistency to the thesis that estrogen promotes breast cancer. In women who used HT for more than 5 years, the increased risk of breast cancer was slightly but not significantly higher in women using EPT (OR = 1.53) than those using ET alone (OR 1.34); only 12% reported using EPT. Most of the observational studies included in this large pooling project were from the United States, where women who use HT are more likely than women who do not use HT to have frequent mammograms—making diagnostic detection bias a possible explanation for any observed excess breast cancer risk.

The Million Women Study, an observational study that included 828,923 postmenopausal British women who had breast cancer screening every third year, largely excludes diagnostic detection bias (15). After 2.6 years of follow-up, women who were current HT users at baseline were significantly more likely to develop breast cancer. The relative risk of breast cancer in women taking EPT (the predominant progestin was norgestrel or levonorgestrel) was higher than the relative risk in women taking unopposed ET (relative risk 2.0; 95% CI 1.88–2.12 vs. 1.30; 95% CI 1.21–1.40). Results were similar for oral, transdermal, or implanted estrogen, and varied little by specific estrogens or progestins or their doses. In an analysis combining women who were current users of ET or EPT, the HT treated women were more likely to have fatal breast cancer.

Despite the strong epidemiologic evidence that estrogen is a cause of breast cancer, WHI was the first clinical trial of sufficient size and duration to test this hypothesis. In WHI-EPT, a 26% increased risk of invasive breast cancer (95% CI 1.00–1.59) was first apparent after 4 years of combined HT, with a calculated absolute excess risk of 8 more invasive breast cancers per 10,000 persons per year attributable to estrogen plus progestin (Table 2 and Figure 2) (75). In an updated report, the hazard ratio was 1.24 (CI 1.01–1.54) (21). This increased relative risk is similar to the (nonsignificantly) increased risk observed in the smaller HERS study (hazard ratio 1.30; Table 2). Contrary to expectations, the invasive breast cancers observed in WHI-EPT women assigned to EPT were significantly larger and at a more advanced stage than breast cancers observed in women assigned to placebo (21).

In contrast, no significant increase in risk of breast cancer was found in women assigned to unopposed conjugated estrogen in WHI-ET (6). In fact, there was a trend to reduced breast cancer risk among women assigned to the estrogen group (relative risk 0.77; P = 0.06). This pattern of decreased risk of breast cancer differs from the findings of prior observational studies and clinical trials and could be due to chance. Despite previously described relevant differences in body mass index and parity between the WHI-ET and -EPT cohorts, the annualized rates for breast cancer were very similar in the placebo groups for the two trials. Future analyses from the WHI-ET, including information regarding the tumor characteristics, may clarify this situation. The higher risk of breast cancer observed in WHI-EPT but not in WHI-ET may be due to the progestin, concordant with the results in the Million Women Study (15).

Higher breast density is a strong risk factor for breast cancer in postmenopausal women (16). Evidence for a true difference between ET and EPT comes from the breast density changes observed in PEPI, showing that EPT increases breast density more than treatment with estrogen alone. In the PEPI trial of 875 relatively young postmenopausal women, no women taking placebo showed increased mammographic parenchymal density after one year while 16.4%–23.5% women taking an estrogen-plus-progestin regimen developed increased breast density, compared with only 3.5% of women taking unopposed estrogen (36). After one year in WHI-EPT, nearly twice as many women assigned to EPT had abnormal mammograms compared with placebo (21). Similar data are not yet available for WHI-ET.

Women with breast cancer who were surgically or chemically castrated before the age of natural menopause often experience severe menopause symptoms. The Hormonal Replacement Therapy after Breast Cancer (HABITS) trial was designed to determine whether ET is safe for the treatment of menopause symptoms in relatively young (mean age 55) breast cancer survivors (46). Eligible women had less than four positive lymph nodes and were free of breast cancer recurrence. The specific HT regimen used was chosen by the patient's physician. This trial was stopped early, after two years, because there was a significant excess of breast cancer in women assigned to HT compared with placebo (RH 3.5; 95% CI 1.5–8.1). The risk was highest in women who had used ET prior to the diagnosis of breast cancer and in women with estrogen-receptor-positive breast cancers (47). A concurrent trial in Stockholm that had previously planned to pool results with HABITS was also stopped early on the basis of recruiting difficulties and the HABITS results.

Endometrial Cancer

Endometrial cancer, the most common gynecological cancer in women, was the first cancer to be definitely associated with ET. In a 1995 meta-analysis of the results from 29 observational studies (30), 5 years of unopposed estrogen increased the endometrial cancer risk four- to fivefold, and 10 years of use increased risk approximately tenfold; overall there was a two- to threefold increased risk (95% CI 2.1–2.5) in women who used unopposed ET. The summary risk for fatal endometrial cancer after 5 or more years of ET in 4 observational studies was 2.7 (95% CI 0.9–8.0). A meta-analysis of 6 observational studies and 1 trial that evaluated EPT found no increased risk of endometrial cancer (RR 0.8; 95% CI 0.6–1.2) (30). In another review, EPT with continuous combined or cyclic progestin used for 10 or more days per cycle carried no increased risk (7). In a more recent prospective observational study, treatment with up to 5 years of continuous combined estradiol (2 mg) plus norethisterone (1 mg) daily was not associated with endometrial hyperplasia, and preexisting hyperplasia reverted to normal in HT-treated women (98).

Endometrial hyperplasia, particularly atypical hyperplasia, is a precursor for endometrial cancer, and prevention of hyperplasia prevents endometrial cancer (63). The best clinical trial evidence is from the PEPI trial, which found that using daily estrogen plus a progestin for 10–12 days each month or daily estrogen plus daily progestin prevents endometrial hyperplasia, and presumably endometrial cancer (1). In PEPI women, unopposed estrogen increased the risk of endometrial hyperplasia by 10% per year (1). These endometrial changes were not observed in women taking CEE plus continuous or cyclic MPA or cyclic micronized progesterone. Both HERS and WHI-EPT confirmed that the risk of endometrial cancer was not increased among women assigned to EPT compared with placebo (relative risk in HERS 0.25; 95% CI 0.05–1.18; relative risk in WHI-EPT 0.81; 95% CI 0.48–1.36) (5, 48). These results indicate that progestin prevents the increased risk of endometrial cancer associated with unopposed ET. More recent trials with low-dose unopposed ET show very low rates of endometrial hyperplasia, which suggests that a smaller dose of progestin (93), or perhaps no added progestin (25), will be required to prevent endometrial hyperplasia and cancer.

Colon Cancer

Colorectal cancer is the third most common cancer in women in the United States. In a systematic review of 21 published observational studies of HT and colorectal cancer, 9 reported a significant reduction in colorectal cancer, 9 reported no significant protective effect, and 3 reported a small nonsignificant increased risk (41). Another meta-analysis restricted to 18 studies that met specific inclusion criteria found a significantly reduced risk of colon cancer that was greater among current users (38).

WHI-EPT demonstrated a 44% reduced risk of invasive colon cancer in women assigned to EPT compared with placebo (0.56: 95% CI 0.38–0.81), with an absolute risk reduction of 6 fewer colorectal cancers per 10,000 women per year (22, 75). There was a similar reduced risk of colon and rectal cancer. More than 20 subgroups were tested for interactions with no significant differences found. Although there were fewer colorectal cancers, the authors reported that WHI women in the EPT group had a significantly greater number of positive lymph nodes and a more advanced stage at diagnosis (22).

In contrast with the reduced risk of colon cancer observed among women in WHI-EPT, colon cancer diagnoses were not reduced among women assigned to unopposed estrogen in WHI-ET (HR 1.08; 95% CI 0.75–1.55) (6). Although the numbers were too small for definitive interpretation, there was a suggestion of reduced colon cancer risk in HERS after 6.8 years of follow-up (RR 0.69; 95% CI 0.32–1.49) (48). Given the inconsistency of observational studies and the trial results, it is impossible at this point to conclude that EPT prevents colon cancer.

Ovarian Cancer

Ovarian cancer is the most lethal gynecologic cancer. It is relatively uncommon (4% of new cancers in women; 6% of annual cancer deaths) but not rare, diagnosed in 1 in every 57 U.S. women. Although some case-control studies reported an excess risk of ovarian cancer in women taking EPT or unopposed estrogen (55, 73, 74), most found no association. In a meta-analysis of ten observational studies, use of HT was associated with an increased risk of invasive epithelial ovarian cancer (OR 1.14; 95% CI 1.05–1.27); the risk was highest in women who had used HT for more than 10 years (28). In a more recently reported U.S. cohort study, estrogen alone, but not EPT, was associated with a significantly increased risk of ovarian cancer (55). A Swedish study reported an increased risk of ovarian cancer after ET and sequential EPT (OR 1.43; 95% CI 1.02–2.00, and OR 1.54; 95% CI 1.15–2.05, respectively) but found no increased risk after continuous combined EPT (73). Death rates in a very large U.S. prospective study found that women using HT at baseline (presumably primarily unopposed estrogen) had a significantly increased risk (RR 1.51; 95% CI 1.16–1.96) compared with nonusers, with a similar risk in former users of 10 or more years duration (74). Risk decreased with time since last use.

In the only published clinical trial, the WHI-EPT trial (5), women assigned to EPT had a 58% increased risk for ovarian cancer compared with placebo (1.58; 95%

CI 0.77–3.24), a difference that was not statistically significant. In WHI-EPT there were no differences in histological grade, state, or interactions by race/ethnicity, body mass index, family history of breast or ovarian cancer, or prior oral contraceptive or HT use.

Cognition and Dementia

Memory loss, cognitive dysfunction, and dementia are some of the most feared complications of aging. Many observational studies suggested that ET could improve postmenopausal memory loss or prevent dementia, and several short clinical trials in recently oophorectomized women showed improved verbal memory (79). A systematic review of the results of 12 clinical trials (56) found a significantly reduced relative risk of developing dementia in healthy women taking estrogen, but there was substantial heterogeneity in the results. A meta-analysis of 5 trials including 210 women with dementia found a clinically nonsignificant improvement in cognitive function scores among women treated with 0.625 mg of CEE (but not higher doses), and only for the first few months (45). After correcting for multiple testing, only a short-term improvement in memory remained among women treated with ET, compared with those treated with placebo.

Other clinical trials have not confirmed these benefits. No benefit of treatment with estrogen was shown in a one-year clinical trial in which 120 women with early Alzheimer's dementia were randomly assigned to placebo or unopposed CEE (either 0.625 mg or 1.25 mg) (64). In this trial, scores on the clinical dementia rating scale were actually significantly worse in women assigned to estrogen compared with the results in women assigned to placebo.

At the end of HERS, approximately 1000 older women with heart disease completed 6 standard cognitive function tests; women assigned to HT did not perform better on any test than did women assigned to placebo (34). In the Women's Health Initiative Memory Study (WHIMS), 7479 women aged 65 and older who were participating in the WHI-EPT ($N = 4532$) or -ET ($N = 2947$) trials (i.e., more than 92% of age-eligible WHI-HT participants) completed the Modified Mini-Mental State Examination (3MSE). When the WHI-EPT was stopped, after an average of 4.1 years of WHIMS EPT follow-up, more women in the EPT group had a substantial [≥ 2 standard deviations (SD)] decline in 3MSE total score than did women in the placebo group (6.7% vs. 4.8%, P $= 0.008$) (70). After an average of 5.2 years of WHIMS follow-up when the WHI-ET was stopped, 3MSE scores averaged 0.26 units lower among ET women compared with placebo (P $= 0.04$), and the odds of ≥ 2 SDs decline in 3MSE scores was increased by 50% (this was not significant) (70). For pooled EPT and ET, the mean decrement on the 3MSE was 0.21 among women treated with HT compared with placebo (P $= 0.005$). Findings were similar among subgroups classified by prior use of HT, age, and markers of socioeconomic status and health. The adverse impact of either HT regimen was more pronounced among women with lower cognitive function at baseline (70). The risk of probable dementia in WHI women assigned to EPT was increased twofold (HR 2.05; 95% CI 1.21–3.48) (81). In the 2947 WHIMS women from WHI-ET, the incidence of probable dementia following ET was increased by 49% (HR 1.49 95% CI 0.83–2.66) (80). This increased risk does not differ significantly from that observed with EPT; for pooled WHIMS data from WHI-EPT and WHI-ET the overall hazard ratio was 1.76 (95% CI 1.19–2.60) (80). The authors suggest that the higher risk of dementia in women assigned to ET or EPT could be due to micro infarcts or other vascular brain disease, consistent with the increased risk of stroke in both trials.

Venous Thromboembolic Disease

Oral contraceptives increase the risk of venous thromboembolic events (VTE) including deep vein thrombosis and pulmonary emboli, but the association of VTE with the lower-dose estrogen regimens used in postmenopausal women has been controversial. There is now little doubt that VTE is a complication of HT. A meta-analysis of 12 studies (including 3 trials) found a summary relative risk of 2.14 (95% CI 1.64–2.81) for VTE among HT users compared with nonusers, or 1.5 excess cases per 10,000 women per year of use (61). However, these studies included only idiopathic venous thromboembolic events, and excluded high-risk women. The excess rate of any VTE in unselected HT users is likely higher. On the basis of population rates of 34 per 10,000 in women more than 50 years old and 42 per 10,000 in women more than 60 years old (67), excess risk likely ranges from ~6–12 per 1000 HT users per year. In the older women in the HERS trial, the absolute risk was high, ~1 per 250 users per year (even though many HERS women were taking aspirin and statins, medications that may reduce the risk of venous thromboembolism) (33). Compatible with observational studies (39), the risk for VTE among HERS women assigned to EPT was highest in the first two years of treatment (three- to fourfold higher than placebo), decreased over the next three years, and was not different from placebo by the fifth year of follow-up (48).

Among the generally healthy women enrolled in WHI-EPT, EPT approximately doubled the risk of VTE (RH 2.11; CI: 1.58–2.82) (75). The relative risk was greatest in the first year but was still apparent after 4–5 years of treatment. In WHI-ET, women in the ET group had a smaller, nonsignificant increase in risk for VTE (relative risk 1.33; 95% CI 0.99–1.79) versus placebo. The apparent difference between EPT and ET in the WHI is not statistically significant. The mechanism whereby HT causes VTE is not clear, but it may be related to changes in coagulation factors that are the result of liver metabolism of oral estrogen. If this is true, transdermal estrogens, which avoid first-pass liver metabolism, might avoid the increase in risk of VTE associated with oral estrogens. Some observational data support this hypothesis (77), but there are no clinical trials large enough to provide definitive data.

Global Index

WHI investigators constructed a global index for eight clinically significant disease outcomes (coronary disease events, stroke, hip fracture, pulmonary embolism, breast, colon, and endometrial cancer, and death from other causes). Figure 2 shows the global index for the treatment groups in WHI-EPT and ET. In the WHI-EPT analysis, small risks exceeded the small benefits of combined therapy. In WHI-ET, the small benefits of unopposed estrogen equal the small risks. Other trials with other regimens, routes, and doses are beginning, although none apparently is large enough to examine clinical cardiovascular events or cancer. Such regimens may be safer or more dangerous.

CONCLUSIONS

Despite the apparent ubiquity of estrogen receptors in diverse human tissues, and estrogen's multiple biologic effects, clear randomized, clinical trial evidence of benefit for systemic HT is presently limited to relief of vasomotor and vaginal symptoms. For longer use, HT prevents bone loss and fractures but also increases the risk of other life-threatening events resulting in no overall benefit. On the basis of WHI-EPT and WHI-ET, the risks for combined or unopposed therapy are an increased risk of stroke that does not decrease with time, an increased risk of VTE that may wane over time, and, in older women, an increased risk of dementia.

None of these trials excludes the possibility that other doses, routes, or regimens would have a better risk-benefit ratio for the prevention of disease. The two areas of greatest current interest, with clinical trials in development, are the possibility that younger women may have a better risk-benefit ratio than older women and the possibility that the bone benefits of HT could be maintained at much lower doses, possibly below the threshold for causing stroke, breast cancer, and other untoward effects. These trials have mainly intermediate outcomes such as bone density and atherosclerosis but could serve as pilot tests for trials with clinical outcomes if the results suggest benefit greater than harm.

Meanwhile, it seems that the title of this chapter is also a work in progress. To quote from a financial forecasting document used by industry, a Women's Reproductive Health 2004 report received via email on April 7, 2004, "Negative press regarding the side-effects associated with hormone replacement therapy (HRT) has slowed this market down slightly, leaving a vacuum of market share for other osteoporosis therapies. HRT will, however, rebound during the forecast period and reachieve strong growth" (Y. Sule, personal communication). One hopes also for improved understanding.

The *Annual Review of Public Health* is online at
http://publhealth.annualreviews.org

LITERATURE CITED

1. 1996. Effects of hormone replacement therapy on endometrial histology in post-menopausal women. The Postmenopausal Estrogen/Progestin Interventions (PEPI) Trial. The Writing Group for the PEPI Trial. *JAMA* 275:370–75
2. 1997. Breast cancer and hormone replacement therapy: collaborative reanalysis of

data from 51 epidemiological studies of 52,705 women with breast cancer and 108,411 women without breast cancer. Collaborative Group on Hormonal Factors in Breast Cancer. *Lancet* 350:1047–59

3. 2002. Endogenous sex hormones and breast cancer in postmenopausal women: reanalysis of nine prospective studies. *J. Natl. Cancer Inst.* 94:606–16

4. 2002. Postmenopausal hormone replacement therapy for primary prevention of chronic conditions: recommendations and rationale. *Ann. Intern. Med.* 137:834–39

5. Anderson GL, Judd HL, Kaunitz AM, Barad DH, Beresford SA, et al. 2003. Effects of estrogen plus progestin on gynecologic cancers and associated diagnostic procedures: the Women's Health Initiative randomized trial. *JAMA* 290:1739–48

6. Anderson GL, Limacher M, Assaf AR, Bassford T, Beresford SA, et al. 2004. Effects of conjugated equine estrogen in postmenopausal women with hysterectomy: the Women's Health Initiative randomized controlled trial. *JAMA* 291:1701–12

7. Archer DF. 2001. The effect of the duration of progestin use on the occurrence of endometrial cancer in postmenopausal women. *Menopause* 8:245–51

8. Avis NE, Stellato R, Crawford S, Johannes C, Longcope C. 2000. Is there an association between menopause status and sexual functioning? *Menopause* 7:297–309

9. Bachmann GA, Leiblum SR. 2004. The impact of hormones on menopausal sexuality: a literature review. *Menopause* 11:120–30

10. Banks E, Beral V, Reeves G, Balkwill A, Barnes I. 2004. Fracture incidence in relation to the pattern of use of hormone therapy in postmenopausal women. *JAMA* 291:2212–20

11. Barnabei VM, Grady D, Stovall DW, Cauley JA, Lin F, et al. 2002. Menopausal symptoms in older women and the effects

of treatment with hormone therapy. *Obstet. Gynecol.* 100:1209–18

12. Barrett-Connor E. 2003. Clinical review 162: cardiovascular endocrinology 3: an epidemiologist looks at hormones and heart disease in women. *J. Clin. Endocrinol. Metab.* 88:4031–42

13. Barrett-Connor E, Grady D. 1998. Hormone replacement therapy, heart disease, and other considerations. *Annu. Rev. Public Health* 19:55–72

14. Barrett-Connor E, Wehren LE, Siris ES, Miller P, Chen YT, et al. 2003. Recency and duration of postmenopausal hormone therapy: effects on bone mineral density and fracture risk in the National Osteoporosis Risk Assessment (NORA) study. *Menopause* 10:412–19

15. Beral V. 2003. Breast cancer and hormone-replacement therapy in the Million Women Study. *Lancet* 362:419–27

16. Boyd NF, Byng JW, Jong RA, Fishell EK, Little LE, et al. 1995. Quantitative classification of mammographic densities and breast cancer risk: results from the Canadian National Breast Screening Study. *J. Natl. Cancer Inst.* 87:670–75

17. Brown JS, Vittinghoff E, Kanaya AM, Agarwal SK, Hulley S, Foxman B. 2001. Urinary tract infections in postmenopausal women: effect of hormone therapy and risk factors. *Obstet. Gynecol.* 98:1045–52

18. Bush TL, Barrett-Connor E, Cowan LD, Criqui MH, Wallace RB, et al. 1987. Cardiovascular mortality and noncontraceptive use of estrogen in women: results from the Lipid Research Clinics Program Follow-up Study. *Circulation* 75:1102–9

19. Cardozo L, Bachmann G, McClish D, Fonda D, Birgerson L. 1998. Meta-analysis of estrogen therapy in the management of urogenital atrophy in postmenopausal women: second report of the Hormones and Urogenital Therapy Committee. *Obstet. Gynecol.* 92:722–27

20. Cauley JA, Robbins J, Chen Z, Cummings SR, Jackson RD, et al. 2003. Effects of

estrogen plus progestin on risk of fracture and bone mineral density: the Women's Health Initiative randomized trial. *JAMA* 290:1729–38

21. Chlebowski RT, Hendrix SL, Langer RD, Stefanick ML, Gass M, et al. 2003. Influence of estrogen plus progestin on breast cancer and mammography in healthy postmenopausal women: the Women's Health Initiative Randomized Trial. *JAMA* 289:3243–53

22. Chlebowski RT, Wactawski-Wende J, Ritenbaugh C, Hubbell FA, Ascensao J, et al. 2004. Estrogen plus progestin and colorectal cancer in postmenopausal women. *N. Engl. J. Med.* 350:991–1004

23. Eriksen B. 1999. A randomized, open, parallel-group study on the preventive effect of an estradiol-releasing vaginal ring (Estring) on recurrent urinary tract infections in postmenopausal women. *Am. J. Obstet. Gynecol.* 180:1072–79

24. Espeland MA, Stefanick ML, Kritz-Silverstein D, Fineberg SE, Waclawiw MA, et al. 1997. Effect of postmenopausal hormone therapy on body weight and waist and hip girths. Postmenopausal Estrogen-Progestin Interventions Study Investigators. *J. Clin. Endocrinol. Metab.* 82:1549–56

25. Ettinger B, Ensrud KE, Wallace R, Johnson KC, Cummings SR, et al. 2004. Effects of ultralow-dose transdermal estradiol on bone mineral density: a randomized clinical trial. *Obstet. Gynecol.* 1104:443–51

26. Furberg CD, Vittinghoff E, Davidson M, Herrington DM, Simon JA, et al. 2002. Subgroup interactions in the Heart and Estrogen/Progestin Replacement Study: lessons learned. *Circulation* 105:917–22

27. Gallagher JC, Rapuri PB, Haynatzki G, Detter JR. 2002. Effect of discontinuation of estrogen, calcitriol, and the combination of both on bone density and bone markers. *J. Clin. Endocrinol. Metab.* 87:4914–23

28. Garg PP, Kerlikowske K, Subak L, Grady D. 1998. Hormone replacement therapy and the risk of epithelial ovarian carcinoma: a meta-analysis. *Obstet. Gynecol.* 92:472–79

29. Grady D, Brown JS, Vittinghoff E, Applegate W, Varner E, Snyder T. 2001. Postmenopausal hormones and incontinence: the Heart and Estrogen/Progestin Replacement Study. *Obstet. Gynecol.* 97: 116–20

30. Grady D, Gebretsadik T, Kerlikowske K, Ernster V, Petitti D. 1995. Hormone replacement therapy and endometrial cancer risk: a meta-analysis. *Obstet. Gynecol.* 85:304–13

31. Grady D, Herrington D, Bittner V, Blumenthal R, Davidson M, et al. 2002. Cardiovascular disease outcomes during 6.8 years of hormone therapy: Heart and Estrogen/Progestin Replacement Study follow-up (HERS II). *JAMA* 288:49–57

32. Grady D, Rubin SM, Petitti DB, Fox CS, Black D, et al. 1992. Hormone therapy to prevent disease and prolong life in postmenopausal women. *Ann. Intern. Med.* 117:1016–37

33. Grady D, Wenger NK, Herrington D, Khan S, Furberg C, et al. 2000. Postmenopausal hormone therapy increases risk for venous thromboembolic disease. The Heart and Estrogen/Progestin Replacement Study. *Ann. Intern. Med.* 132:689–96

34. Grady D, Yaffe K, Kristof M, Lin F, Richards C, Barrett-Connor E. 2002. Effect of postmenopausal hormone therapy on cognitive function: the Heart and Estrogen/Progestin Replacement Study. *Am. J. Med.* 113:543–48

35. Greendale GA, Reboussin BA, Hogan P, Barnabei VM, Shumaker S, et al. 1998. Symptom relief and side effects of postmenopausal hormones: results from the Postmenopausal Estrogen/Progestin Interventions Trial. *Obstet. Gynecol.* 92:982–88

36. Greendale GA, Reboussin BA, Sie A, Singh HR, Olson LK, et al. 1999.

Effects of estrogen and estrogen-progestin on mammographic parenchymal density. Postmenopausal Estrogen/Progestin Interventions (PEPI) Investigators. *Ann. Intern. Med.* 130:262–69

37. Greendale GA, Wells B, Marcus R, Barrett-Connor E. 2000. How many women lose bone mineral density while taking hormone replacement therapy? Results from the Postmenopausal Estrogen/Progestin Interventions Trial. *Arch. Intern. Med.* 160:3065–71

38. Grodstein F, Newcomb PA, Stampfer MJ. 1999. Postmenopausal hormone therapy and the risk of colorectal cancer: a review and meta-analysis. *Am. J. Med.* 106:574–82

39. Gutthann SP, Garcia Rodriguez LA, Raiford DS. 1997. Individual nonsteroidal antiinflammatory drugs and other risk factors for upper gastrointestinal bleeding and perforation. *Epidemiology* 8:18–24

40. Hays J, Ockene JK, Brunner RL, Kotchen JM, Manson JE, et al. 2003. Effects of estrogen plus progestin on health-related quality of life. *N. Engl. J. Med.* 348:1839–54

41. Hebert-Croteau N. 1998. A meta-analysis of hormone replacement therapy and colon cancer in women. *Cancer Epidemiol. Biomarkers Prev.* 7:653–59

42. Hemminki E, McPherson K. 1997. Impact of postmenopausal hormone therapy on cardiovascular events and cancer: pooled data from clinical trials. *BMJ* 315:149–53

43. Hersh AL, Stefanick ML, Stafford RS. 2004. National use of postmenopausal hormone therapy. *JAMA* 291:47–53

44. Hlatky MA, Boothroyd D, Vittinghoff E, Sharp PC, Whooley M. 2002. Quality-of-life and depressive symptoms in postmenopausal women after receiving hormone therapy: results from the Heart and Estrogen/Progestin Replacement Study (HERS) trial. *JAMA* 287:591–97

45. Hogervorst E, Yaffe K, Richards M, Huppert F. 2002. Hormone replacement therapy to maintain cognitive function in women with dementia. *Cochrane Database Syst. Rev.* CD003799

46. Holmberg L, Anderson H. 2004. HABITS (hormonal replacement therapy after breast cancer—Is it safe?), a randomised comparison: trial stopped. *Lancet* 363:453–55

47. Holmberg L, Anderson H. 2004. Stopping HABITS. *Lancet* 363:1477

48. Hulley S, Furberg C, Barrett-Connor E, Cauley J, Grady D, et al. 2002. Noncardiovascular disease outcomes during 6.8 years of hormone therapy: Heart and Estrogen/Progestin Replacement Study follow-up (HERS II). *JAMA* 288:58–66

48a. Hulley SB, Grady D. 2004. The WHI Estrogen-Alone Trial—Do things look any better? *JAMA* 291:1769–71

49. Hulley S, Grady D, Bush T, Furberg C, Herrington D, et al. 1998. Randomized trial of estrogen plus progestin for secondary prevention of coronary heart disease in postmenopausal women. Heart and Estrogen/Progestin Replacement Study (HERS) Research Group. *JAMA* 280:605–13

50. Humphrey LL, Chan BK, Sox HC. 2002. Postmenopausal hormone replacement therapy and the primary prevention of cardiovascular disease. *Ann. Intern. Med.* 137:273–84

51. Isaacs AJ, Britton AR, McPherson K. 1997. Why do women doctors in the UK take hormone replacement therapy? *J. Epidemiol. Community Health* 51:373–77

52. Kaufert P, Boggs PP, Ettinger B, Woods NF, Utian WH. 1998. Women and menopause: beliefs, attitudes, and behaviors. The North American Menopause Society 1997 Menopause Survey. *Menopause* 5:197–202

53. Kronenberg F. 1990. Hot flashes: epidemiology and physiology. *Ann. N.Y. Acad. Sci.* 592:52–86; discussion pp. 123–33

54. Kuller LH, Simkin-Silverman LR, Wing RR, Meilahn EN, Ives DG. 2001.

Women's Healthy Lifestyle Project: a randomized clinical trial: results at 54 months. *Circulation* 103:32–37

55. Lacey JV Jr, Mink PJ, Lubin JH, Sherman ME, Troisi R, et al. 2002. Menopausal hormone replacement therapy and risk of ovarian cancer. *JAMA* 288:334–41

56. LeBlanc ES, Janowsky J, Chan BK, Nelson HD. 2001. Hormone replacement therapy and cognition: systematic review and meta-analysis. *JAMA* 285:1489–99

57. Lobo RA, Rosen RC, Yang HM, Block B, Van Der Hoop RG. 2003. Comparative effects of oral esterified estrogens with and without methyltestosterone on endocrine profiles and dimensions of sexual function in postmenopausal women with hypoactive sexual desire. *Fertil. Steril.* 79:1341–52

58. MacLennan A, Lester S, Moore V. 2001. Oral estrogen replacement therapy versus placebo for hot flushes: a systematic review. *Climacteric* 4:58–74

59. Manson JE, Hsia J, Johnson KC, Rossouw JE, Assaf AR, et al. 2003. Estrogen plus progestin and the risk of coronary heart disease. *N. Engl. J. Med.* 349:523–34

60. Matthews KA, Kuller LH, Wing RR, Meilahn EN, Plantinga P. 1996. Prior to use of estrogen replacement therapy, are users healthier than nonusers? *Am. J. Epidemiol.* 143:971–78

61. Miller J, Chan BK, Nelson HD. 2002. Postmenopausal estrogen replacement and risk for venous thromboembolism: a systematic review and meta-analysis for the U.S. Preventive Services Task Force. *Ann. Intern. Med.* 136:680–90

62. Miller KJ. 2003. The other side of estrogen replacement therapy: outcome study results of mood improvement in estrogen users and nonusers. *Curr. Psychiatry Rep.* 5:439–44

63. Montgomery BE, Daum GS, Dunton CJ. 2004. Endometrial hyperplasia: a review. *Obstet. Gynecol. Surv.* 59:368–78

64. Mulnard RA, Cotman CW, Kawas C, van Dyck CH, Sano M, et al. 2000. Estrogen replacement therapy for treatment of mild to moderate Alzheimer disease: a randomized controlled trial. Alzheimer's Disease Cooperative Study. *JAMA* 283:1007–15

65. Nieves JW, Komar L, Cosman F, Lindsay R. 1998. Calcium potentiates the effect of estrogen and calcitonin on bone mass: review and analysis. *Am. J. Clin. Nutr.* 67:18–24

66. Nilas L, Christiansen C. 1987. Bone mass and its relationship to age and the menopause. *J. Clin. Endocrinol. Metab.* 65:697–702

67. Nordstrom M, Lindblad B, Bergqvist D, Kjellstrom T. 1992. A prospective study of the incidence of deep-vein thrombosis within a defined urban population. *J. Intern. Med.* 232:155–60

68. Norman RJ, Flight IH, Rees MC. 2000. Oestrogen and progestogen hormone replacement therapy for peri-menopausal and post-menopausal women: weight and body fat distribution. *Cochrane Database Syst. Rev.* CD001018

69. Prestwood KM, Kenny AM, Kleppinger A, Kulldorff M. 2003. Ultralow-dose micronized 17beta-estradiol and bone density and bone metabolism in older women: a randomized controlled trial. *JAMA* 290:1042–48

70. Rapp SR, Espeland MA, Shumaker SA, Henderson VW, Brunner RL, et al. 2003. Effect of estrogen plus progestin on global cognitive function in postmenopausal women: the Women's Health Initiative Memory Study: a randomized controlled trial. *JAMA* 289:2663–72

71. Raz R, Stamm WE. 1993. A controlled trial of intravaginal estriol in postmenopausal women with recurrent urinary tract infections. *N. Engl. J. Med.* 329:753–56

72. Riggs BL, Melton LJ 3rd. 1995. The worldwide problem of osteoporosis: insights afforded by epidemiology. *Bone* 17:505S–11

73. Riman T, Dickman PW, Nilsson S, Correia N, Nordlinder H, et al. 2002.

Hormone replacement therapy and the risk of invasive epithelial ovarian cancer in Swedish women. *J. Natl. Cancer Inst.* 94:497–504

74. Rodriguez C, Patel AV, Calle EE, Jacob EJ, Thun MJ. 2001. Estrogen replacement therapy and ovarian cancer mortality in a large prospective study of US women. *JAMA* 285:1460–65

75. Rossouw JE, Anderson GL, Prentice RL, LaCroix AZ, Kooperberg C, et al. 2002. Risks and benefits of estrogen plus progestin in healthy postmenopausal women: principal results from the Women's Health Initiative randomized controlled trial. *JAMA* 288:321–33

76. Rymer J, Morris EP. 2000. Extracts from "clinical evidence": menopausal symptoms. *BMJ* 321:1516–19

77. Scarabin PY, Oger E, Plu-Bureau G. 2003. Differential association of oral and transdermal oestrogen-replacement therapy with venous thromboembolism risk. *Lancet* 362:428–32

78. Schmidt PJ, Nieman L, Danaceau MA, Tobin MB, Roca CA, et al. 2000. Estrogen replacement in perimenopause-related depression: a preliminary report. *Am. J. Obstet. Gynecol.* 183:414–20

79. Sherwin BB. 1999. Can estrogen keep you smart? Evidence from clinical studies. *J. Psychiatry Neurosci.* 24:315–21

80. Shumaker SA, Legault C, Kuller L, Rapp SR, Thal L, et al. 2004. Conjugated equine estrogen alone and incidence of probable dementia and mild cognitive impairment in postmenopausal women: results from the Women's Health Initiative Memory Study. *JAMA* 291:2947–58

81. Shumaker SA, Legault C, Rapp SR, Thal L, Wallace RB, et al. 2003. Estrogen plus progestin and the incidence of dementia and mild cognitive impairment in postmenopausal women: the Women's Health Initiative Memory Study: a randomized controlled trial. *JAMA* 289:2651–62

82. Simon JA, Hsia J, Cauley JA, Richards C, Harris F, et al. 2001. Postmenopausal

hormone therapy and risk of stroke: the Heart and Estrogen-Progestin Replacement Study (HERS). *Circulation* 103: 638–42

83. Slater CC, Zhang C, Hodis HN, Mack WJ, Boostanfar R, et al. 2001. Comparison of estrogen and androgen levels after oral estrogen replacement therapy. *J. Reprod. Med.* 46:1052–56

84. Smith DC, Prentice R, Thompson DJ, Herrmann WL. 1975. Association of exogenous estrogen and endometrial carcinoma. *N. Engl. J. Med.* 293:1164–67

85. Soares CN, Almeida OP, Joffe H, Cohen LS. 2001. Efficacy of estradiol for the treatment of depressive disorders in perimenopausal women: a double-blind, randomized, placebo-controlled trial. *Arch. Gen. Psychiatry* 58:529–34

86. Soares CN, Poitras JR, Prouty J. 2003. Effect of reproductive hormones and selective estrogen receptor modulators on mood during menopause. *Drugs Aging* 20:85–100

87. Speroff L, Whitcomb RW, Kempfert NJ, Boyd RA, Paulissen JB, Rowan JP. 1996. Efficacy and local tolerance of a low-dose, 7-day matrix estradiol transdermal system in the treatment of menopausal vasomotor symptoms. *Obstet. Gynecol.* 88:587–92

88. Stampfer MJ, Willett WC, Colditz GA, Rosner B, Speizer FE, Hennekens CH. 1985. A prospective study of postmenopausal estrogen therapy and coronary heart disease. *N. Engl. J. Med.* 313:1044–49

89. Stefanick ML, Cochrane BB, Hsia J, Barad DH, Liu JH, Johnson SR. 2003. The Women's Health Initiative postmenopausal hormone trials: overview and baseline characteristics of participants. *Ann. Epidemiol.* 13:S78–86

90. Torgerson DJ, Bell-Syer SE. 2001. Hormone replacement therapy and prevention of nonvertebral fractures: a meta-analysis of randomized trials. *JAMA* 285:2891–97

91. Utian WH, Boggs PP. 1999. The North American Menopause Society

1998 Menopause Survey. Part I: Post-menopausal women's perceptions about menopause and midlife. *Menopause* 6: 122–28

92. Utian WH, Burry KA, Archer DF, Gallagher JC, Boyett RL, et al. 1999. Efficacy and safety of low, standard, and high dosages of an estradiol transdermal system (Esclim) compared with placebo on vasomotor symptoms in highly symptomatic menopausal patients. The Esclim Study Group. *Am. J. Obstet. Gynecol.* 181:71–79

93. Utian WH, Shoupe D, Bachmann G, Pinkerton JV, Pickar JH. 2001. Relief of vasomotor symptoms and vaginal atrophy with lower doses of conjugated equine estrogens and medroxyprogesterone acetate. *Fertil. Steril.* 75:1065–79

94. Viscoli CM, Brass LM, Kernan WN, Sarrel PM, Suissa S, Horwitz RI. 2001. A clinical trial of estrogen-replacement therapy after ischemic stroke. *N. Engl. J. Med.* 345:1243–49

95. Wassertheil-Smoller S, Hendrix SL, Limacher M, Heiss G, Kooperberg C, et al. 2003. Effect of estrogen plus progestin on stroke in postmenopausal women: the Women's Health Initiative: a randomized trial. *JAMA* 289:2673–84

96. Weiss NS, Ure CL, Ballard JH, Williams AR, Daling JR. 1980. Decreased risk of fractures of the hip and lower forearm with postmenopausal use of estrogen. *N. Engl. J. Med.* 303:1195–98

97. Wells G, Tugwell P, Shea B, Guyatt G, Peterson J, et al. 2002. Meta-analyses of therapies for postmenopausal osteoporosis. V. Meta-analysis of the efficacy of hormone replacement therapy in treating and preventing osteoporosis in postmenopausal women. *Endocr. Rev.* 23:529–39

98. Wells M, Sturdee DW, Barlow DH, Ulrich LG, O'Brien K, et al. 2002. Effect on endometrium of long term treatment with continuous combined oestrogen-progestogen replacement therapy: follow up study. *BMJ* 325:239–43

99. Wilson RA. 1966. *Feminine Forever.* New York: Evans (distributed by Lippincott)

100. Ziel HK, Finkle WD. 1975. Increased risk of endometrial carcinoma among users of conjugated estrogens. *N. Engl. J. Med.* 293:1167–70

101. Zweifel JE, O'Brien WH. 1997. A meta-analysis of the effect of hormone replacement therapy upon depressed mood. *Psychoneuroendocrinology* 22: 189–212

Annu. Rev. Public Health 2005. 26:141–63
doi: 10.1146/annurev.publhealth.26.021304.144410
Copyright © 2005 by Annual Reviews. All rights reserved
First published online as a Review in Advance on October 12, 2004

ADVANCES IN RISK ASSESSMENT AND COMMUNICATION

Bernard D. Goldstein

Graduate School of Public Health, Office of the Dean, University of Pittsburgh,
Pittsburgh, Pennsylvania 15261; email: bdgold@pitt.edu

Key Words   risk characterization, exposure assessment, dose-response analysis,
precautionary principle, environmental justice, long-term stewardship

■ **Abstract**   Risk analysis continues to evolve. There is increasing depth and breadth
to each component of the four-step risk-assessment paradigm of hazard identification,
dose-response analysis, exposure assessment, and risk characterization. Basic conceptual approaches to understanding how people perceive risk are being tested against a
growing body of empirical observations, many involving stakeholders. Emerging ideas
such as the precautionary principle have provided challenges that have led to a rethinking of the role of risk assessment in environmental health. Newer problems, such as
intergenerational issues posed by long-lasting radiation pollution, environmental justice, and the assessment and communication of risks related to terrorism, have spurred
innovative approaches to risk analysis.

INTRODUCTION

The field of risk analysis continues to grow. There has been an increase in the
breadth and depth of the scientific disciplines involved in assessing and managing
risk; an evolution of policies aimed at preventing and controlling risk; new threats
to be considered; and an expanding geographical base of risk analysts. This review
arbitrarily touches on some of the highlights. My focus is on those issues that have
developed out of the challenges posed by the science leading to the assessment
of human health risk and to its communication. The emphasis is on public health
rather than on ecological risk, and on risk assessment and communication rather
than risk management.

The four-step risk paradigm consists of hazard identification; exposure assessment; dose-response analysis, and risk characterization. The twentieth anniversary
of the 1983 National Research Council (NRC) report (90), known as the Red Book,
which led to the institutionalization of this paradigm, was marked in a variety of
ways, including a volume of articles that provide both a history of the events and
an expanded view of current areas of interest (70).

A myth about the early development of risk assessment was that it was believed
to be fully independent of risk management. The simple dichotomy between risk

assessment as science and risk management as policy has never really existed. From the very beginning, the Environmental Protection Agency (EPA) has recognized that there are at least three steps to the process. Before risk assessment begins there is a fundamental need to have guidelines in place, which delineate how to perform the four-step risk-assessment paradigm (42, 94, 106). These science policy guidelines establish uniform processes for default assumptions, extrapolation approaches, and other aspects of risk assessment that could greatly change the outcome and comparability of the risk assessment if left to a case-by-case basis. They also establish the criteria needed to replace a default assumption with actual data, thus leveling the playing field for stakeholders involved in the outcome of the risk assessment. The fourth and last step in risk assessment, risk characterization, also includes elements of risk communication and has long been recognized to overlap with risk management (45). A common theme by those involved in assessing and managing risk has been the need to integrate risk assessment and risk communication.

The NRC committee that produced the Red Book clearly recognized that risk assessment was only one part of the approach to making reasoned decisions concerning environmental and public health risks. A more formal approach to a framework for the overall management of risks was produced by the Presidential/Congressional Commission on Risk Assessment and Risk Management, which began meeting in 1994 (11, 96, 101, 102). The framework for environmental health risk management has six steps: formulation of the problem within the context of public or ecosystem health; analysis of the risks; determination of options for risk management; choice of an option; action on the decision; and evaluation of the outcome. Stakeholders are involved in every stage of the process; in fact, the first step, problem formulation, emphasizes stakeholder involvement. Their involvement is particularly needed as the lack of an appropriate context for the risk process often has led to paralysis rather than risk reduction.

HAZARD IDENTIFICATION

Hazard identification is based on the toxicological principle that assigns unique properties to the physicochemical structure of a molecule and to the specificity of the biological niche in which it reacts. The first recorded statement of this principle of specificity of chemical effects has been attributed to Paré who in the seventeenth century disappointed the King of France by demonstrating that the King's treasured alleged universal antidote could not possibly work for all poisons because "[p]oyson. . .kils by a certaine specifick antipathy contrary to our nature" (50).

Quantitative Structure Activity Relationships

Identifying the hazards of new chemicals has traditionally depended on costly and time-consuming animal studies, including thorough pathological and physiological evaluation. Toxicologists have long been interested in the prediction of chemical toxicity based on physical and chemical structure. Structure activity relationship (SAR) is heavily relied on in the evaluation of new chemicals submitted by industry for Environmental Protection Agency (EPA) review under the Toxic Substances Control Act. There are numerous examples in which SAR has served as a very powerful tool to predict chemical effects. There are other examples in which the effect of one chemical is not predictable from the effects of close structural analogs (e.g., the hematological effects of benzene but not toluene, or the neurotoxic effects of n-hexane but not n-heptane or n-pentane). In recent years investigators have developed newer approaches to SAR on the basis of the explosive growth of computing power and of informatics (107). This combinatorial toxicology is analogous to combinatorial pharmacology, which, in the search for new drugs, uses computer models to predict the potential pharmacological effects of minor variations in chemical structure. Although highly promising, a recent review of the use of quantitative SAR for developmental toxicants by the Risk Science Institute noted a variety of challenges, including the definition of the activity of a chemical or its score on any given characteristic; the incorporation of new data within a broader data set; the relative lack of chemical coverage and of data for validation; and the lack of transparency in the models regarding input and output criteria.

DOSE-RESPONSE ANALYSIS

Shape of the Lower End of the Dose-Response Curve

A continuing controversial issue in dose-response assessment is that of the shape of the dose-response curve at lower doses. Two types of dose-response curves have been considered to be central to risk assessment. The hallmark of one of these curves is a threshold, or better put, a no–observed-effect level, below which the compound is considered to be harmless. The second type of dose-response relationship, the nonthreshold relationship, has generally been reserved for mutagens. The belief that any one molecule of a mutagen has a risk of causing a major effect is based on the recognition that, theoretically, one molecule can cause a genetic change that is carried through progeny cells so that it then codes for cancer or, if in germ cells, for an inheritable mutation. Some known carcinogens act through apparent threshold mechanisms. For example, workplace exposure to sulfuric acid mist is causally related to cancer of the upper respiratory tract through a mechanism that appears to be related to inflammation, but one molecule of sulfuric acid would be readily buffered in the mucus layer of the airway and highly unlikely to be carcinogenic. Similarly, saccharine is now generally accepted to produce bladder cancer in rats through a threshold mechanism unrelated to human risk at usual saccharin doses. Public policy in the United States, sustained through many administrations, has put the burden of proof on industry to demonstrate that a chemical that is known or appears likely to cause cancer in humans occurs through a threshold mechanism. Attempts to prove a threshold have generally been unsuccessful. Cohen et al. (13) recently reviewed the issue of the human relevance of information on the mechanism of action of carcinogens (13), although not all researchers agree with their conclusion that evidence for carcinogenicity of chemicals has been overstated (85). A variant approach to addressing the lower end of the dose-response curve is provided by the concept of hormesis (10), in essence a biphasic response in low doses produces stimulation and high doses lead to inhibition. There is yet to be sufficient scientific evidence favoring hormesis for this concept to replace standard approaches to risk assessment.

Bench Mark Dose (BMD)

Expansion in the use of the BMD in risk assessment continues (15, 114, 127). Briefly, the BMD is an estimate of the lowest dose at which a prespecified effect occurs. It has the advantage of a greater degree of stability than the usual determination of the experimental no-observed-effect level (NOEL) to which safety factors are added (3). As the usual regulatory use of the BMD is based on the lower bound of its confidence interval, the method used to determine the confidence interval is particularly important, especially when the dose-response data are nonlinear. Moerbeek et al. (86) recently reviewed different statistical methods for calculating confidence intervals for the BMD and concluded that the likelihood-ratio method is more attractive for routine dose-response analysis but that the more time-consuming bootstrap method had the advantage of linking directly to Monte Carlo analysis in a probabilistic risk assessment. Dourson & Patterson (22) have provided an excellent overview of BMD as well as other noncancer-assessment methods.

Increasingly, attempts have been made to treat cancer and noncancer endpoints with similar risk models (16). The impetus for this approach has included advances in developing harmonized risk models, in part based on the BMD (7). The impetus also comes from findings, in essence, of no apparent threshold for the effects of particulates on mortality or the effects of ozone on symptoms, in at least some epidemiological studies. Although EPA has pursued approaches to similar dose-response analysis of cancer and noncancer endpoints, it has been difficult to obtain full agreement among the scientific community.

Multi-Step Carcinogenesis

For most known common human cancers, there is a multi-step process in which a series of mutational events occurs, leading to a progressively more neoplastic and invasive cancer (74). Risk analysts have considered this in a variety of multi-stage models of carcinogenesis (87). But a multi-hit model, in my view, should not be considered to be equivalent to a threshold model. For example, assume that the clinical manifestation of a common tumor requires five different mutations for it to occur. It is highly likely that many people develop four mutations but do not live long enough to develop the fifth before dying from other causes. For individuals with four mutations, presumably a significant subset of the population, an environmental agent causing that one additional mutation could result in a clinically detectable case of cancer. Accordingly, that there are multiple mutations often involved in carcinogenesis is not inconsistent with assuming a one-hit model for risk analysis.

The increasing emphasis on children's environmental health has led to efforts to understand the dose-response issues that are particularly pertinent to children (89). See below for exposure analysis in children. In many cases, the absorption, distribution, metabolism, or excretion of chemicals is different in children than in adults—often, but not always (21), putting children at greater risk. Using physiologically based pharmacokinetics (PBPK) to understand these differences is crucial to having the information needed to protect children or other high risk groups (76). For example, Ginsberg (40) has presented a method combining exposure and PBPK information to assess long-term cancer risks from short-term exposure periods in children.

Threats to the Use of Biomarkers to Link Low-Level Exposure with Effects

Extrapolation, whether from high to low dose, or from animal to human studies, is a central scientific challenge to risk assessment. The inherent methodological limitations of epidemiology and of animal toxicology make it exceptionally difficult to determine dose-response relationships at realistic levels of human environmental exposure, and particularly at the low-risk levels demanded by society. With rare exceptions, direct determination of a one-in-a-thousand risk level for an environmental effect, let alone a one-in-a-million risk, is beyond the capability of environmental health science without using extrapolation techniques. Biological markers capable of linking exposure with effect, particularly in the context of human susceptibility, provide a potential mechanism for linking dose with response.

Modern biological techniques, particularly advances in molecular biology and the new field of toxicogenomics, provide the basis for a better understanding of the role of toxic agents in human diseases (18, 128, 129) and the development of new biomarkers linking exposure and effect. The standard pathway for developing and validating such biomarkers begins with laboratory animal toxicology and progresses through controlled human exposure studies that explore the dose-response relationship of the biomarker at real-world exposure levels. Unfortunately, such studies are under unwarranted attack for allegedly being against ethical principles: laboratory animal studies by animal rights activists and controlled human exposure studies by "ethicists."

The arguments of animal rights activists are not new but are gathering force and require continued rebuttal. A particularly cogent rebuttal for the many pet owners who are frightened into being the chief financial supporters of organizations such as the so-called People for the Ethical Treatment of Animals (PETA) is the value of animal research to their own pets. Just consider the outdated numerical equation of a dog's age as 7 times that of a human: There are now many 15-year-old dogs but very few 105-year-old humans. Biomedical research advocates need to focus more on being responsive to the protective feelings of pet owners as we search for ways to protect the value of animal research.

Attacks on controlled human-exposure studies are partially fueled by scientific, legal, and political issues related to the additional tenfold protection factor required in the absence of definitive data to the contrary by the Food Quality Protection Act (93, 113). Controlled exposure of human volunteers should be subject to the highest standards. But there has been talk of banning such studies and a growing hesitation among agencies to support them. Discussion of the issues has generally lacked two major points. First, allowing a federal agency to subject the U.S. population to a given level of human exposure should ethically require it to accept the responsibility of learning how a human responds to such exposures. Second, there is a mistaken generalization from clinical research to controlled exposure to environmental agents. Controlled experimental exposures to agents at levels we would normally be subjected to in foods, or to levels of air pollutants to which we are routinely and involuntarily subjected to at a gasoline station, are surely different than a volunteer receiving an experimental treatment for a disease. Controlled human research is important not only because it provides a reasonable opportunity to understand the risk of low-level exposures, but also because it is pertinent to effective environmental protection through allowing attribution of effects to one or more of the usual components of mixtures of pollutants present in the real world.

EXPOSURE ASSESSMENT

In the past decade, exposure assessment has moved more rapidly than perhaps any other aspect of the four-step risk paradigm (99). Both theory and practice have progressed beyond the simplifying default assumptions of the past. Area measurements have been replaced by studies of microenvironments in which humans are likely to be exposed (12), and sophisticated theoretical approaches are being validated using data from direct exposure measurements such as the National Human Exposure Assessment Survey (NHEXAS) study (108). The concept of exposure efficiency, which relates exposure to source emissions by calculating the extent of eventual human uptake of material released from a source, has received additional emphasis (28). Further, there has been an expansion in the ability to utilize mundane exposure indicators, such as dust (78).

Among the many interesting advances has been the increasing availability of observational data to understand the extent and variability of human exposure and to test models (17, 88). Of particular value have been studies of exposure patterns that are responsible for greater risk among children. Videotapes of normal children's activities have clearly demonstrated the significant potential for exposure through ingestion and through the skin, concerns which have been validated in studies using blood lead levels or urinary pesticide markers (1, 34, 36). Of note were the findings of Freeman et al. (33), who demonstrated pesticide exposure in ten children following chlorpyrifos application on cracks and crevices. Despite the absence of aerosol application, exposure occurred owing to the pesticide vaporizing and redepositing, particularly on absorbent objects such as plush toys, and owing to the children's object-to-mouth behavior, which was confirmed by videotape. Freeman and her colleagues have also evaluated household exposure factors in relation to asthma and school absenteeism (35).

Recent review of the controversial issue of children's exposure to arsenic from playground wood treated with chromated copper arsenate as a preservative considered the different routes of exposure. As noted by the authors (62), the estimates are highly uncertain and need to be validated by studies of arsenic levels in children actually playing on such surfaces. This need for validation is often ignored in the rush to develop models. Such models are highly valuable for estimating exposure. But once exposure is occurring in the real world, and in the absence of overtly observable health effects, it should be mandatory for investigators to evaluate exposure rather than solely depending on mathematical models or laboratory animals. Once validated, simple models can be very useful in replacing the need for complex observational studies of human activity, as suggested by a model developed by Riley et al. (104) for intermittent dermal contact. Comparison of measured and modeled exposures in complex urban environments is particularly problematic.

Exposure Scenarios

The development and use of exposure scenarios to assess human risk have been particularly helpful. A theoretical basis for risk scenarios has been developed (71). Specific uses of exposure scenarios include the estimation that the greatest variability in transmission of tuberculosis in a hypothetical hospital was waiting time (75). Scenarios that included cultural factors such as hunting, fishing, and gathering patterns were of value in estimating the multipathway exposure of the Spokane tribal community to a superfund site (59). Life-cycle analysis of chemical solvents has been coupled with scenario-based risk assessment of solvent use (112).

Exposure Assessment as a Causal Link

Exposure assessment can also contribute to assessing hypothetical cause-and-effect relations. As one example, the finding by Opiekun et al. (97) that individuals who self-report symptoms from the gasoline fuel additive methyl tertiary-butyl ether (MTBE) have driving habits and automobiles likely to produce higher MTBE exposure levels is consistent with a cause-and-effect relationship and adds to the weight of the evidence. Similarly, accurate exposure evaluation is a necessary part of intervention studies aimed at decreasing adverse outcomes from hazardous chemicals.

Exposure Assessment in Relation to Genomics, Proteomics, and Other Advances in Molecular Biology

The promise of understanding gene-environment interactions is a significant part of the excitement about the potential value of recent advances in molecular biology. The enormous relevance of molecular biology to risk analysis includes the identification of susceptible populations and the provision of a biological basis for the individual variability observed in responses to environmental agents.

Perhaps most importantly, modern molecular biology presents the possibility of reversing the usual direction of environmental health science research. The standard approach, using increasingly complex systems, has been to begin with an isolated chemical or physical agent and ask what effect it has on human disease. Preferably, we want to begin with human diseases and work backward to understand cause—to understand which environmental condition(s) is responsible for an asthma attack or for chronic renal disease.

Exposure assessment is key to unraveling gene-environment interactions and to improving our ability to attribute disease to cause. Genetic propensities to environmental disease will often be manifest as the disease appearing at a lower dose, and through accurate exposure assessment, this dose-genetic relationship will be discovered and the pathway to disease will be interrupted.

RISK CHARACTERIZATION

The final step of the risk-assessment paradigm, risk characterization, clearly overlaps risk communication and management (45). The choice of how to depict a number can readily sway the response to the number: For example, consider the differing responses to a single situation characterized as being "99% free of any risk," or having "a 1% likelihood of serious side effects including death." A quantitative risk can be presented in various ways beyond just a bald statement of a risk number over time. Simply changing the characterization to how much time will lapse for each adverse effect will alter perception of the intensity of risk in a more understandable way (131). Risk can also be characterized as a change from background, rather than an absolute. Risk characterization should best use the same questions asked and answered by a journalist about an event: who, what, when, where, how many, etc.

Integrating risk perception into risk assessment occurs primarily at the risk characterization step (92, 117). This topic is discussed more fully below (see Risk Perception).

There are many uses for the number provided by a risk analysis, some of which go beyond the intent or the data-quality objective of the risk analyst. Critics of risk assessment often mistakenly base concerns on how risks are then managed. Tal (121) has encouraged environmental groups to become more engaged in risk assessment, pointing out the many proenvironmental decisions that have been based on risk assessment.

Specifying the risk to vulnerable populations is an important aspect of risk characterization. As briefly discussed above, the genomic revolution will lead to an identification of populations with relatively small degrees of susceptibility to environmental exposures. Inevitably, there will be a need to consider the implication of these newly discovered variations in human susceptibility to laws, such as portions of the United States Clean Air Act, that are specifically based on the protection of susceptible populations.

Uncertainty Analysis

Uncertainty is built into any analytic process. Quantitative risk analysis has aspects that foster uncertainty—particularly when extrapolation is used to estimate a risk at levels below which scientific validation is likely or even possible. Our society's public health and environmental protection goals are at risk levels below those which can usually be measured scientifically. For example, no current epidemiological or toxicological approaches can validate EPA's extrapolated risk potency factor for benzene-induced leukemia to the maximally exposed individual at the one-in-a-million risk objective of the 1990 Clean Air Act. Owing to the uncertainties inherent in risk assessment, and particularly in the extrapolation to low-level risk, there have been many calls for the routine characterization of uncertainty in any risk assessment. Much work has been done to develop and evaluate techniques, such as the Monte Carlo analysis, to measure and report uncertainty (53, 98, 105).

Understanding uncertainty can have practical application to analyses of risk issues. For example, Hattis et al. (60) have pointed out that the interindividual variability in human response to airborne particulates is sufficient to account for the small increases in daily mortality observed in epidemiological studies, and that this variability could account for the relative lack of toxicological evidence of an effect on the average individual at these low levels.

A continuing argument concerns whether a measure of uncertainty should always accompany a quantitative risk assessment. There is much to be said for such a requirement, including the often great uncertainty in a risk estimate and the overreliance of regulators and the public on a single number. The key elements of uncertainty should always be spelled out. But there are compelling arguments against the routine use of numerical uncertainty. These arguments include the difficulty in communicating uncertainty to nonscientists. I note that uncertainty is not specified with common metrics such as the gross domestic product or the unemployment rate. Should this be done for risk analysis it would be overstating its importance in the decision process. Most importantly, in the absence of agreement as to how to calculate or communicate uncertainty, adding a required quantitative uncertainty analysis would unnecessarily prolong and muddle issues that, for the best public health outcome, should be decided quickly (43). In summary, routine risk-based decisions should not be held hostage to meaningless analyses, although a qualitative description of the key uncertainties is welcome at all times.

The lack of public familiarity with scientific uncertainty was highlighted by Johnson & Slovic (69) in a study of response to news stories with different degrees of uncertainty. My concern about the overuse of uncertainty is also exemplified by an otherwise well-done study by Thompson et al. (124) following up on our observation that the risk of dying from an airplane hitting you while you are on the ground is about 4 in a million lifetimes (49). Our goal was to describe a low-level risk comparison for which there was no benefit to anyone and, most importantly, which could be partially avoided by lifestyle decisions (e.g., having your bedroom in the basement) but for which the risk was too low to bother with individual precautions. Thompson et al. (124) have shown that the risk varies by about 100-fold depending on geographical proximity to an airport. But I would argue that in this risk range the added information is of little or no relevance to individual or societal decisions.

PRECAUTIONARY PRINCIPLE AND/OR/VERSUS RISK ASSESSMENT

The precautionary principle has emerged in recent years as a new approach to environmental and public health risk management. Grandjean (51) thoroughly reviewed this principle last year in this series.

The precautionary principle, at least to some advocates, also provides a rationale for risk perception being as or more important than the scientific assessment of risk. (See below for a discussion of risk perception). Those most wary of the precautionary principle are North American businesses who have seen the precautionary principle used adroitly by the European Union (EU) to develop a multitude of trade barriers with little or no risk-based scientific justification (46). Carruth and I have also raised the concern that the precautionary principle will lessen the likelihood of obtaining the appropriate science needed for protecting public health and the environment (44, 47).

Public perception of risk will clearly drive political decisions as to the setting of priorities and the responsiveness of risk managers. The difference between public perception and expert ranking of risks has been frequently noted. This inherent tension is usually resolved intranationally through political and legal processes. Resolving these tensions becomes more problematic when the differences are among nations and must be dealt with through relatively weak international dispute resolution. Risk perception is one of the issues raised by the EU's use of the precautionary principle to supplant or to supplement risk assessment for the purposes of protecting their trade (48).

An example of the use of the precautionary principle to supplement risk assessment is given by Majone (83), who analyzes its use by the EU to establish the world's most stringent aflatoxin standard. Majone points out that the result of this more stringent standard is to keep out of Europe trade worth several hundred million dollars a year from sub-Saharan nations, some of the poorest nations in the world. The resultant net risk reduction is 1.4 cases of hepatocellular carcinoma in a billion people per year—or less than 1 death per year in the EU.

An example of the use by the EU of the precautionary principle to replace risk assessment is the European ban on the importation of beef from hormone-treated animals, a ban that persists despite the ruling of the World Trade Organization

(WTO) against the EU. The importance of health risk and of perception was also considered in a subsequent WTO decision on asbestos, which was particularly notable in its statement that perception of health risk by the public could be grounds for trade ban (48).

Issues related to risk assessment, the precautionary principle, and risk perception will undoubtedly be central to the forthcoming WTO decision on genetically modified foods. The case of genetic modification in general and genetically modified (GM) foods specifically has been subject to much evaluation in the risk-assessment literature. Authors have focused on a variety of different subjects, including the generally accepted idea that the Monsanto Corporation's marketing of its initial GM products frightened many Europeans, and attempts to understand differences between the European and U.S. perceptions of GM substances as being based on cultural factors and on recent causes of European distrust of government science (45, 46, 80). As with the beef hormone and other U.S.-European differences, a common U.S. perception is that Europe is simply reacting to their competitive disadvantage in the science of genetic manipulation and is using trade barriers as a means to protect their less-efficient agriculture. Those concerned with decisions made solely on risk perception without any scientific basis point out that manipulating the perception of risk is the expertise of advertising managers and politicians.

RISK COMMUNICATION

The dynamic contribution of the social sciences and social studies to risk analysis has continued to increase. This increase is most evident in the ferment of ideas guiding research into the way individuals perceive risk and how we respond to communications about risk. The distinction between social sciences and social studies is not always apparent to those outside the field. Fischhoff (29, 30, 119) has emphasized that the former primarily involves systematic data collection, statistical analysis, and hypothesis testing, whereas the latter involves more qualitative approaches to obtaining insights about underlying processes.

A major challenge to environmental public health remains the communication of expert analysis to concerned citizens and to decision makers (20). In recent years there have been significant advances in understanding risk perception and risk communication, as well as a gathering of an empirical database in which concepts can be tested and refined (8). Of note have been various attempts to bridge the gap between risk assessment and risk communication, integrating what has traditionally been seen as distinct activities. This bridging is made difficult by the different languages being spoken by social scientists and classic risk analysts and is further compounded by the many different theories that underlie discussion of risk communication.

Jasanoff (68) has eloquently described the two cultures of the multidisciplinary field of risk analysis: The quantitative side is represented primarily by engineering, mathematics, toxicology, and epidemiology; and the qualitative work is done by those in psychology, sociology, and law. She points out the persistent belief among those in the "hard" sciences that the role of the "soft" sciences is to assist in dispelling misperceptions of risk by the general public. Instead, she suggests that "qualitative studies focusing on the ethical, legal, political, and cultural aspects of risk exist conceptually on a single continuum with quantitative, model- and measurement-oriented analyses of risk" (68). This integration of risk assessment and risk perception has been central to the work of Fischhoff (29–31), Slovic (117–119), Sandman et al. (109), and many others active in the field.

Cultural Issues in Risk Perception

There continues to be much work attempting to define those aspects of risk perception that are central to all human societies and those that are culturally dependent. Not surprisingly, investigators have found that the perception of risk differs within different cultures in a single community as well as in different parts of the world and that trust is a major determinant. The importance of local cultural factors was emphasized by Earle (24) in his findings supporting a social psychological theoretical base for trust in risk management as opposed to a more normative approach of assuming that trust is based on universally relevant factors such as fairness and objectivity.

The global breadth of risk analysis has inevitably led to studies of the impact of cultural differences on the perception of risk. Two recent studies reported on the perception of risk among Chinese people. A psychometric study of 167 Hong Kong Chinese (77) who rated 25 different threats showed differences from the Western literature as to how such threats are perceived. Confucianism was proposed by the authors as the reason for the Chinese appearing to be less concerned with threats that are remote or unknown and more troubled by threats that are imminent, knowable, and controllable. Two risk-perception surveys in China by Xie et al. (133) in 1996 and 1998 were reported as showing greater concern with risks that threaten national stability and economic development and less concern with high-technology risks than reported in the Western literature.

The active work on risk analysis and perception in Japan includes a recent study by Maeda & Miyahara (82) of the determinants of trusts in industry, government, and citizens' groups. They noted a much greater reliance on consensual values in which there is bidirectional communication between the organization and the public. Study of the influence of the 1999 nuclear incident in Tokai, Japan, on public trust showed, not surprisingly, a decrease in the acceptability of nuclear power and a growing distrust of the industry, but showed no change in overall trust in the government despite the apparent failure of oversight (72).

The subculture of workers was emphasized in a "mental models" approach used by Cox et al. (14) to assess the impact of chemical risk information on workers. The focus was on a qualitative approach to the impact of the workplace culture on the perception of chemical risk with the goal of developing user-relevant risk-communication strategies.

Assessment and Communication of the Risk of Terrorism

There is inadequate space to begin to review the rapid growth in the risk-assessment and risk-communication literature related to terrorism following September 11, 2001. A number of authors have considered the applicability of quantitative risk assessment to the threat of terrorism (19, 38, 57). A dimension that has been added to standard risk analysis is that of intentionality: Environmental, chemical, and physical agents are usually considered to be free of malice or forethought. In contrast, actions to decrease risk caused by terrorists will lead terrorists to intentionally change their tactics so as to impose risk. This recognition has led to the addition of elements of game theory to standard environmental risk analysis (61).

Similarly, analysis of vulnerability as well as intent is crucial to risk analysis for terrorism. Modeling of interconnected and cascading events from a single terrorist attack includes the recognition that critical infrastructures are difficult to define, let alone to defend, in a world increasingly dependent on information technology (57). Slovic (118) has added the psychological impact of terrorism to standard vulnerability analysis. He has pointed out that terrorist acts result in an even more disturbing form of the particular dread that surrounds accidents involving chemicals and radiation, which contrast with more classic disasters such as floods, where there seems to be a specific end to the event. The boundlessness of terrorism adds to its impact on the public perception of risk. Hobbs et al. (63) consider the issue of risk communication to an alarmed public, a subject that has been explored by studies of postal workers threatened by anthrax (S. Quinn, T. Thomas & C. McAllister, manuscript in preparation).

Stakeholders' Perception

Increasing attention has been given to analyzing the factors that affect how stakeholders perceive and respond to risk as part of their involvement in decision processes. A particular rich source of study has been the stakeholder processes related to the U.S. Department of Energy's (DOE) cleanup of atom bomb production facilities and the U.S. Department of Defense's base-closure activities. The original attempts by the DOE to manage its environmental problems were handled poorly, in part representing the Cold War legacy of secrecy that surrounded anything related to nuclear weapons. The response to this poor management has been various agreements with states and to a more formalistic and open process involving citizen advisory groups. Kinney & Leschine (73) performed a procedural evaluation of the Columbia River Comprehensive Impact Assessment (CRCIA), which included a broad range of stakeholders who were charged with developing an assessment approach. Although the process is described as fitting under the analytic-deliberative model recommended by the NRC (92) various problems occurred, particularly related to achieving the elements of fairness and of competence called for under participatory models based on the work of Webler & Tuler (130) and of Habermas (55). Flynn et al. (32) noted that the technological stigma associated with the Rocky Flats DOE facility was explained reasonably well by social amplification theory to have developed from negative media coverage. Santos & Chess (110), in a study of two stakeholder groups involved in U.S. Army advisory boards, note that in addition to fairness and other aspects of process called for by the work of Habermas and Webler, community advisory committees also value outcome. Other social science theories of communication have been used as a basis for evaluating risk communication and perception at DOE sites, including Hamilton's (58) assessment of technical and cultural aspects of decisions about competing priorities for radium at the Fernald site. Trumbo & McComas (126) also utilized a variety of models of risk perception to evaluate the role of credibility in a study of citizen response to communication about cancer clusters. In particular, they explored the role of information processing in the not unexpected outcome that the higher is the credibility assigned to the state health department or to industry, the lower is the perceived risk. Study of the perception of cancer clusters in Switzerland gave further support for the theory that individuals who trust authorities are more likely to be accepting of expert explanations discounting risk, in this case the explanation that the cluster was due to random chance (116). In this study females were less trusting than males were and were more inclined to believe that the cluster was due to factors other than pure chance. Siegrist (115) has also explored the impact of expressing a risk by its probability as a decimal, as compared with its frequency as a rate, by asking the question of willingness to pay. Social contagion theory has been used to explain how social linkages within a rural community faced with a controversial threat to its water supply played a role in the different levels of risk perception within the community (111). Arvai (4) reported that a risk was deemed more acceptable if it was known that a citizen participation process had been involved, that by engaging in the process and communicating about the participatory process, industry or government may enhance public trust and the perception of legitimacy of decisions.

FOOD AND WATER SAFETY

Risk assessment has long been an approach used in food safety—in fact many of the original concepts were developed by scientists working in the United States and elsewhere at agencies responsible for food safety. There has been renewed emphasis in the use of risk analysis for food safety, in part because of the development and application of risk techniques to microbial food contamination issues and in part because of the globalization of the food industry and the need to harmonize regulatory approaches in response to trade issues (see discussion under Precautionary Principle above). Hulebak & Schlosser (64) have reviewed the Hazard Analysis and Critical Control Point (HACCP) approach that has been so effective in focusing on hazards throughout the production and distribution process. Each control point in the process can be identified, analyzed, and subjected to sensitivity analysis (37). Food safety issues in Europe have been considered in an International Life Sciences Institute (ILSI) monograph, which provides an excellent overview of risk assessment methods for chemicals in food and in the overall diet (120).

Exposure assessment for food has usually relied on questionnaires that depend on dietary recall. Despite inherent problems, such questionnaires have been useful for epidemiological studies. Tran et al. (125) developed a probabilistic method of bridging two different commonly used surveys: the daily Continuing Survey of Food Intake by Individuals, and the much larger but far more infrequent National Health and Nutrition Examination Survey.

A key issue in microbial risk assessment is defining the susceptibility of individuals. The numbers of presumably susceptible individuals are increasing as a function of the success of medical science in increasing the number of immune-compromised individuals who have survived cancer chemo- or radiotherapy; have survived immunosuppression for organ transplantation; or are alive with human immunodeficiency virus (HIV) infection. The report of a workshop on susceptibility for microbial risk assessment was notable in its call for more precise definitions of specific terms and concepts underlying understanding of microbial susceptibility (5). Makri et al. (84) have explored this important issue in a study of regional differences in cryptosporidiosis, which included acquired immunodeficiency syndrome (AIDS) status along with reported levels of *Cryptosporidium* in tap water and other exposure factors.

The existing quantitative dose-response models for population-based microbial risk assessment also have been built on to deal with issues related to the number of organisms ingested by an individual (54). Monte Carlo simulation has been used to estimate the risk of waterborne cryptosporidiosis from a given amount of oocysts of a specific strain of *Cryptosporidium parvum* (100). Using a novel approach, the variability in susceptibility to the same number of infective agents, another important consideration in microbial risk assessment, has been estimated in relation to existing anti-*Cryptosporidium* IgG levels (123). Isolates of different strains of *Cryptosporidium* had markedly different dose-response characteristics (122). Similarly, risk factors have been linked to anticryptosporidium antibodies in New Zealand (23).

An interesting approach to the abundant literature on the perception of risk of genetically modified foods noted that the opposition of the European public may be founded more on the lack of perceived benefits than on concern about the risk (39).

CUMULATIVE AND AGGREGATE RISK ASSESSMENT

Two newer risk-assessment approaches that are particularly pertinent to the complexity of human experience are aggregate risk assessment and cumulative risk assessment. Aggregate risk assessment focuses on exposure to a single agent through multiple routes (27, 65), e.g., exposure of children to chlorpyrifos through skin contact and ingestion, in this case using a model developed specifically for residential situations (134). Cumulative risk assessment is more complex. The goal is to evaluate the risks due to exposure to multiple agents by multiple routes (26, 66). Understanding the synergistic and antagonistic interaction of different chemicals, for which exposure occurs at different times and in different ratios, is crucial but still not well understood. Evidence is increasing that different agents acting by different mechanisms do not interact unless at least one of these agents is above the threshold for effect (56). Cumulative risk assessment is particularly pertinent to environmental justice considerations.

ENVIRONMENTAL JUSTICE

Risk assessment has been used to identify the problem of environmental justice, but it also has been criticized as incorporating informational biases that disproportionately underestimate risk to disadvantaged communities (67, 91). To some, the limitations of risk assessment are part of the problem, as for example the report of two community environmental justice issues in Australia (79). Other findings include reports that larger chemical facilities tended to be located in communities with larger African American populations (25) and that statistically significant differences in perceptions of risk between Caucasians and Mexican Americans in Tucson were observed only when socioeconomic variations were uncontrolled (132). Differences in the type and amount of fish consumed by black fishermen in the vicinity of the DOE's atom bomb production facility, the Savannah River Site, led to much higher risk levels than for white fishermen (9).

The issue of environmental justice has spurred new approaches to risk analysis including both aggregate and cumulative risk assessment, as described above. The literature directly related to the risk analysis and environmental justice issues is growing but all too slowly—and the findings are inconsistent. Three facts seem incontrovertible: Disadvantaged communities have more pollutant sources; disadvantaged communities have more unhealthy people; unhealthy people are more vulnerable to the adverse effects of most pollutants. The extent to which the higher levels of pollutant sources are causally related to poor health in disadvantaged communities can be debated. But those communities with the highest exposure and the most vulnerable people certainly should be the primary focus for environmental protection, including environmental research. Without such a focus, environmental justice will not be achieved.

INTERGENERATIONAL ISSUES

The risk imposed by the activities of one generation on another presents some of the more intriguing issues in risk analysis (95). The controversy has in part been sparked by concerns about long-term management of radioactive waste from nuclear energy and the residues of atom bomb production (2). Long-term stewardship of such wastes has led to questions about breakthrough of radioactivity from underground storage facilities into groundwater thousands of years from now.

Shorter-term issues include the stability of land-use restrictions when considering brownfield sites that are suitable for industrial development but not for children's playgrounds. Discussion of these long-term stewardship issues is notable for the implicit or explicit assumption that risks will not change over time. For example, the trajectory of early detection and treatment of cancer suggests that the implication of a carcinogenic mutation caused by radioactivity 1000 years from now will be of far lesser importance to our descendants than it is to us today—yet that issue has not been considered.

Intergenerational issues can be very acute. For example, Glantz & Jamieson (41) use a Honduras hurricane to point out intergenerational issues posed by the decision to spend funds on immediate relief versus strong new buildings that would protect against future hurricanes.

ACKNOWLEDGMENTS

I gratefully acknowledge the very helpful and stimulating discussions with my colleagues at the Society of Risk Analysis annual meetings. I thank Elizabeth Kim for superb technical assistance in the preparation of the manuscript.

The *Annual Review of Public Health* is online at
http://publhealth.annualreviews.org

LITERATURE CITED

1. Adgate JL, Barr DB, Clayton CA, Eberly LE, Freeman NC, et al. 2001. Measurement of children's exposure to pesticides: analysis of urinary metabolite levels in a probability-based sample. *Environ. Health Perspect.* 109:583–90

2. Ahearne JF. 2000. Intergenerational issues regarding nuclear power, nuclear waste, and nuclear weapons. *Risk Anal.* 20:759–62

3. Allen BC, Kavlock RJ, Kimmel CA, Faustman EM. 1994. Dose-response assessment for developmental toxicity. II. Comparison of generic benchmark dose estimates with no observed adverse effect levels. *Fundam. Appl. Toxicol.* 23:487–95

4. Arvai JL. 2003. Using risk communication to disclose the outcome of a participatory decision-making process: effects on the perceived acceptability of risk-policy decisions. *Risk Anal.* 23:281–89

5. Balbus J, Parkin R, Makri A, Ragain L, Embrey M, Hauchman F. 2004. Defining susceptibility for microbial risk assessment: results of a workshop. *Risk Anal.* 24:197–208

5a. Bazerman MH, Messick DM, Tenbrusel AE, Wade-Benzoni KE, eds. 1997. *Environment, Ethics and Behavior: The Psychology of Environmental Valuation and Degradation.* San Francisco: New Lexington

6. Bishop WE, Clarke DP, Travis CC. 2001. The genomic revolution: What does it mean for risk assessment? *Risk Anal.* 21:983–88

7. Bogdanffy MS, Daston G, Faustman EM, Kimmel CA, Kimmel GL, et al. 2001. Harmonization of cancer and noncancer risk assessment: proceedings of a consensus-building workshop. *Toxicol. Sci.* 61:18–31

8. Bostrom A, Löfstedt RE. 2003. Communicating risk: wireless and hardwired. *Risk Anal.* 23:241–48

9. Burger J, Gaines KF, Gochfeld M. 2001. Ethnic differences in risk from mercury

among Savannah River fishermen. *Risk Anal.* 21:533–44

10. Calabrese EJ, Baldwin LA. 2003. Toxicology rethinks its central belief. *Nature* 421(6924):691–92

11. Charnley G. 2003. How the risk commission evolved from the Red Book. *Hum. Ecol. Risk Assess.* 9:1213–17

12. Chow JC, Engelbrecht JP, Freeman NC, Hashim JH, Jantunen M, et al. 2002. Chapter one: exposure measurements. *Chemosphere* 49:873–901

13. Cohen SM, Klaunig J, Meek ME, Hill RN, Pastoor T, et al. 2004. Evaluating the human relevance of chemically induced animal tumors. *Toxicol. Sci.* 78(2):181–86

14. Cox P, Niewöhner J, Pidgeon N, Gerrard S, Fischhoff B, Riley D. 2003. The use of mental models in chemical risk protection: developing a generic workplace methodology. *Risk Anal.* 23:311–24

15. Crump K. 1995. Calculation of benchmark doses from continuous data. *Risk Anal.* 15:79–89

16. Crump KS. 2003. Quantitative risk assessment since the Red Book: Where have we come and where should we be going? *Hum. Ecol. Risk Assess.* 9:1105–12

17. Cullen AC. 1995. The sensitivity of probabilistic risk assessment results to alternative model structures: a case study of manicipal waste incineration. *J. Air Waste Manag. Assoc.* 45:538–46

18. Cunningham ML, Bogdanffy MS, Zacharewski TR, Hines RN. 2003. Workshop overview: use of genomic data in risk assessment. *Toxicol. Sci.* 73:209–15

19. Deisler PF Jr. 2002. A perspective: risk analysis as a tool for reducing the risks of terrorism. *Risk Anal.* 22:405–14

20. De Rosa CT, Hansen H. 2003. The impact of 20 years of risk assessment on public health. *Hum. Ecol. Risk Assess.* 9:1219–28

21. Dourson M, Charnley G, Scheuplein R. 2002. Differential sensitivity of children and adults to chemical toxicity. II. Risk and regulation. *Regul. Toxicol. Pharmacol.* 35(3):448–67

22. Dourson M, Patterson J. 2003. A 20-year perspective on the development of noncancer risk assessment methods. *Hum. Ecol. Risk Assess.* 9:1239–52

23. Duncanson MJ, Chang WY, Frost FJ, Muller TB, Weinstein P. 2003. Ubiquitous risk factor exposure and high prevalence of antibodies to Cryptosporidium parvum in two New Zealand communities. *Appl. Environ. Sci. Public Health* 1:111–17

24. Earle TC. 2004. Thinking aloud about trust: a protocol analysis of trust in risk management. *Risk Anal.* 24:169–83

25. Elliot MR, Wang Y, Lowe RA, Kleindorfer PR. 2004. Environmental justice: frequency and severity of US chemical industry accidents and the socioeconomic status of surrounding communities. *J. Epidemol. Community Health* 58(1):24–30

26. EPA (Environ. Prot. Agency). 2003. *Framework for Cumulative Risk Assessment.* EPA/630/P-02/001F. Risk Assess. Forum, Washington, DC http://www.epa.gov/fedrgstr/EPA-PEST/1999/November/Day-10/6043.pdf

27. EPA (Environ. Prot. Agency). 1999. *Guidance for Performing Aggregate and Risk Assessments.* Washington, DC: Off. Pestic. Programs

28. Evans JS, Wolff SK, Phonboon K, Levy JI, Smith KR. 2002. Exposure efficiency: an idea whose time has come? *Chemosphere* 49:1075–91

29. Fischhoff B. 2004. Cognitive issues in stated preference methods. In *Handbook of Environmental Economics*, ed. K-G Mäler, J Vincent. Amsterdam: Elsevier. In press

30. Fischhoff B. 2004. Decision research strategies. *Health Psychol.* http://www.pitt.edu/~super1/lecture/lec15301/index.htm

31. Fischhoff B. 1997. Ranking risks. See Ref. 5a, pp. 342–71

32. Flynn J, Peters E, Mertz CK, Slovic P.

1998. Risk, media, and stigma at Rocky Flats. *Risk Anal.* 18:715–27

33. Freeman NC, Hore P, Black K, Jimenez M, Sheldon L, et al. 2004. Contributions of children's activities to pesticide hand loadings following residential pesticide application. *J. Exp. Anal. Environ. Epidemiol.* doi:10.1038/sj.jea.7500348

34. Freeman NC, Jimenez M, Reed KJ, Gurunathan S, Edwards RD, et al. 2001. Quantitative analysis of children's microactivity patterns: the Minnesota children's pesticide exposure study. *J. Exp. Anal. Environ. Epidemiol.* 11:501–9

35. Freeman NC, Schneider D, McGarvey P. 2003. Household exposure factors, asthma, and school absenteeism in a predominantly Hispanic community. *J. Exp. Anal. Environ. Epidemiol.* 13(3):169–76

36. Freeman NC, Sheldon L, Jimenez M, Melnyk L, Pellizzari E, Berry M. 2001. Contribution of children's activities to lead contamination of food. *J. Exp. Anal. Environ. Epidemiol.* 11:407–13

37. Frey HC, Patil SR. 2002. Identification and review of sensitivity analysis methods. *Risk Anal.* 22:553–78

38. Garrick BJ. 2002. Perspectives on the use of risk assessment to address terrorism. *Risk Anal.* 22:421–24

39. Gaskell G, Allum N, Wagner W, Kronberger N, Torgersen H, et al. 2004. GM foods and the misperception of risk perception. *Risk Anal.* 24:185–94

40. Ginsberg GL. 2003. Assessing cancer risks from short-term exposures in children. *Risk Anal.* 23:19–34

41. Glantz M, Jamieson D. 2000. Societal response to hurricane Mitch and intra- versus intergenerational equity issues: Whose norms should apply? *Risk Anal.* 20:869–82

42. Goldstein BD. 1988. Risk assessment/risk management is a three-step process: in defense of EPA's risk assessment guidelines. *J. Am. Coll. Toxicol.* 7:545–49

43. Goldstein BD. 1995. Risk management will not be improved by mandating numerical uncertainty analysis for risk assessment. *Univ. Cincinnati Law Rev.* 63:1599–610

44. Goldstein BD. 1999. The precautionary principle and scientific research are not antithetical. *Environ. Health Perspect.* 107:594–95

45. Goldstein BD. 2003. Risk characterization and the Red Book. (Special issue to commemorate the 20th anniversary of the Natl. Res. Council Red Book). *Hum. Ecol. Risk Assess.* 9:1283–89

46. Goldstein BD, Carruth RS. 2003. Implications of the precautionary principle: Is it a threat to science? *Eur. J. Oncol.* 2:193–202

47. Goldstein BD, Carruth RS. 2003. Implications of the precautionary principle to environmental regulation in the United States: examples from the control of hazardous air pollutants in the 1990 Clean Air Act Amendments. *Law Contemp. Probl.* 66:247–61

48. Goldstein BD, Carruth RS. 2004. The precautionary principle and/or risk assessment in World Trade Organization decisions: a possible role for risk perception. *Risk Anal.* 24:491–99

49. Goldstein BD, Demak M, Northridge M, Wartenberg D. 1992. Risk to groundlings of death due to airplane accidents: a risk communication tool. *Risk Anal.* 12:339–41

50. Goldstein BD, Gallo MA. 2001. Paré's law: the second law of toxicology. *Toxicol. Sci.* 60:194–95

51. Grandjean P. 2004. Implications of the precautionary principle for primary prevention and research. *Annu. Rev. Public Health* 25:199–223

52. Grandjean P. 2003. The Red Book, a red herring, and the red tape: a European perspective. *Hum. Ecol. Risk Assess.* 9:1291–95

53. Greenland S. 2001. Sensitivity analysis, Monte Carlo risk analysis, and Bayesian uncertainty assessment. *Risk Anal.* 21:579–84

54. Haas CN. 2002. Conditional dose-response relationships for microorganisms: development and application. *Risk Anal.* 22:455–64

55. Habermas J. 1979. *Communication and the Evolution of Society.* Transl. T McCarthy. Boston: Beacon Press

56. Haghdoost N, Newman L, Johnson E. 1997. Multiple chemical exposures: synergism vs individual exposure levels. *Reprod. Toxicol.* 11:9–27

57. Haimes YY, Longstaff T. 2002. The role of risk analysis in the protection of critical infrastructures against terrorism. *Risk Anal.* 22:439–44

58. Hamilton JD. 2003. Exploring technical and cultural appeals in strategic risk communication: the Fernald radium case. *Risk Anal.* 23:291–302

59. Harper BL, Flett B, Harris S, Abeyta C, Kirschner F. 2002. The Spokane Tribe's multipathway subsistence exposure scenario and screening level RME. *Risk Anal.* 22:513–26

60. Hattis D, Russ A, Goble R, Banati P, Chu M. 2001. Human interindividual variability in susceptibility to airborne particles. *Risk Anal.* 21:585–600

61. Hausken K. 2002. Probabilistic risk analysis and game theory. *Risk Anal.* 22:17–27

62. Hemond HF, Solo-Gabriele HM. 2004. Children's exposure to arsenic from cca-treated wooden decks and playground structures. *Risk Anal.* 24:51–64

63. Hobbs J, Kittler A, Fox S, Middleton B, Bates DW. 2004. Communicating health information to an alarmed public facing a threat such as a bioterrorist attack. *J. Health Commun.* 9:67–75

64. Hulebak KL, Schlosser W. 2002. Guest editorial: hazard analysis and critical control point (haccp) history and conceptual overview. *Risk Anal.* 22:547–52

65. Int. Life Sci. Inst. (ILSI). 1998. *Aggregate Exposure Assessment Workshop Rep.* Washington, DC: ILSI Risk Sci. Inst.

66. Int. Life Sci. Inst. (ILSI). 1999. *A Framework for Cumulative Risk Assessment Workshop Rep.* Washington, DC: ILSI Risk Sci. Inst.

67. Israel BD. 1995. An environmental justice critique of risk assessment. *New York Univ. Environ. Law J.* 3:469–522

68. Jasanoff S. 1993. Guest editorial: bridging the two cultures of risk analysis. *Risk Anal.* 13:123–29

69. Johnson BB, Slovic P. 1995. Presenting uncertainty in health risk assessment: initial studies of its effects on risk perception and trust. *Risk Anal.* 15:485–94

70. Johnson BL, Reisa JJ. 2003. Essays in commemoration of the 20th anniversary of the National Research Council's risk assessment in the federal government: managing the process. *Hum. Ecol. Risk Assess.* 9:1093–99

71. Kaplan S, Haimes YY, Garrick BJ. 2001. Fitting hierarchical holographic modeling into the theory of scenario structuring and a resulting refinement to the quantitative definition of risk. *Risk Anal.* 21:807–19

72. Katsuya T. 2001. Public response to the Tokai nuclear accident. *Risk Anal.* 21:1039–46

73. Kinney AG, Leschine TM. 2002. A procedural evaluation of an analytic-deliberative process: the columbia river comprehensive impact assessment. *Risk Anal.* 22:83–100

74. Kinzler KW, Vogelstein B. 1996. Lessons from hereditary colorectal cancer. *Cell* 87:159–70

75. Ko G, Burge HA, Nardell EA, Thompson KM. 2001. Estimation of tuberculosis risk and incidence under upper room ultraviolet germicidal irradiation in a waiting room in a hypothetical scenario. *Risk Anal.* 21:657–74

76. Krewski D, Withey JR, Ku LF, Andersen ME. 1994. Applications of physiologic pharmacokinetic modeling in carcinogenic risk assessment. *Environ. Health Perspect.* 102:37–50

77. Lai JC, Tao J. 2003. Perception of environmental hazards in Hong Kong Chinese. *Risk Anal.* 23:669–84

78. Lioy PJ, Freeman NC, Millette JR. 2002. Dust: a metric for use in residential and building exposure assessment and source characterization. *Environ. Health Perspect.* 110(10):969–83

79. Lloyd-Williams ME, Bell L. 2003. Toxic disputes and the rise of environmental justice in Australia. *Int. J. Occup. Environ. Health* 9(1):14–23

80. Lofstedt RE. 2003. A European perspective on the NRC "Red Book," risk assessment in the federal government: managing the process. *Hum. Ecol. Risk Assess.* 9:1327–35

81. Deleted in proof

82. Maeda Y, Miyahara M. 2003. Determinants of trust in industry, government, and citizen's groups in japan. *Risk Anal.* 23:303–10

83. Majone G. 2002. The precautionary principle and its policy implications. *J. Common Mark. Stud.* 40:89–110

84. Makri A, Modarres R, Parkin R. 2004. Cryptosporidiosis susceptibility and risk: a case study. *Risk Anal.* 24:209–20

85. Mirer FE. 2003. Distortions of the "misread" book: adding procedural botox to paralysis by analysis. *Hum. Ecol. Risk Assess.* 9:1129–43

86. Moerbeek M, Piersma AH, Slob W. 2004. A comparison of three methods for calculating confidence intervals for the benchmark dose. *Risk Anal.* 24:31–40

87. Moolgavkar SH, Leubeck EG. 2003. Multistage carcinogenesis and the incidence of human cancer. *Genes Chromosomes Cancer* 38(4):302–6

88. Moschandreas DJ, Watson J, D'Abreton P, Scire J, Zhu T, et al. 2002. Chapter Three: methodology of exposure modeling. *Chemosphere* 49(9):923–46

89. Natl. Res. Council. 1993. *Pesticides in the Diets of Infants and Children.* Washington, DC: Natl. Acad. Press

90. Natl. Res. Council. 1983. *Risk Assessment in the Federal Government: Managing the Process.* Washington, DC: Natl. Acad. Press

91. Natl. Res. Council. 1999. *Toward Environmental Justice: Research, Education, and Health Policy Needs.* Washington, DC: Natl. Acad. Press

92. Natl. Res. Council. 1996. *Understanding Risk: Informing Decisions in a Democratic Society.* Washington, DC: Natl. Acad. Press

93. Natl. Res. Council. 2004. *Intentional Human Dosing Studies for EPA Regulatory Purposes.* Washington, DC: Natl. Acad. Press

94. North DW. 2003. Reflections on the red/mis-read book, 20 years after. *Hum. Ecol. Risk Assess.* 9:1145

95. Okrent D, Pidgeon N. 2000. Introduction: dilemmas in intergenerational versus intragemerational equity and risk policy. *Risk Anal.* 20:763–70

96. Omenn GS. 2003. On the significance of "the Red Book" in the evolution of risk assessment and risk management. *Hum. Ecol. Risk Assess.* 9:1155–67

97. Opiekun RE, Freeman NC, Kelly-McNeil K, Fiedler NL, Lioy PJ. 2001. Effect of vehicle use and maintenance patterns of a self-described group of sensitive individuals and nonsensitive individuals to methyl tertiary-butyl ether in gasoline. *J. Exp. Anal. Environ. Epidemiol.* 11:79–85

98. Paté-Cornell E. 2002. Risk and uncertainty analysis in government safety decisions. *Risk Anal.* 22:633–46

99. Paustenbach DJ. 2000. The practice of exposure assessment: a state-of-the-art review. *J. Toxicol. Environ. Health* 3:179–291

100. Pouillot R, Beaudeau P, Denis JB, Derouin F. 2004. A quantitative risk assessment of waterborne cryptosporidiosis in France using second-order Monte Carlo simulation. *Risk Anal.* 24:1–17

101. Pres./Congr. Comm. Risk Assess. Risk Manag. 1997. *Framework Environ. Health Risk Manag.* Final Rep. Vol. 1

102. Pres./Congr. Comm. Risk Assess. Risk Manag. 1997. *Risk Assessment and Risk*

Management in Regulatory Decision-Making. Final Rep. Vol. 2

103. Deleted in proof

104. Riley WJ, McKone TE, Hubal EAC. 2004. Estimating contaminant dose for intermittent dermal contact: model development, testing and application. *Risk Anal.* 24:73–85

105. Robinson RB, Hurst BT. 1997. Statistical quantification of the source of variance in uncertainty analyses. *Risk Anal.* 17:447–510

106. Rodricks JV. 2003. What happened to the Red Book's second most important recommendation?. *Hum. Ecol. Risk Assess.* 9:1169–80

107. Rosenkranz HS. 2003. SAR in the assessment of carcinogenesis: the MULTICASE approach. In *Quantitative Structure-Activity Relationship (QSAR) Models of Mutagens and Carcinogens*, pp. 175–206. Boca Raton, FL: CRC

108. Roy A, Georgopoulos PG, Ouyang M, Freeman N, Lioy PJ. 2003. Environmental dietary, demographic and activity variables associated with biomarkers of exposure for benzene and lead. *J. Exp. Anal. Environ. Epidemiol.* 13:417–26

109. Sandman PM, Miller PM, Johnson BB, Weinstein ND. 1993. Agency communication, community outrage, and perception of risk: three simulation experiments. *Risk Anal.* 13:585–98

110. Santos SL, Chess C. 2003. Evaluating citizen advisory boards: the importance of theory and participant-based criteria and practical implications. *Risk Anal.* 23:269–79

111. Scherer CW, Cho H. 2003. A social network contagion theory of risk perception. *Risk Anal.* 23:261–67

112. Scheringer M, Vögl T, von Grote J, Capaul B, Schubert R, Hungerbühler K. 2001. Scenario-based risk assessment of multi-use chemicals: application to solvents. *Risk Anal.* 21:481–98

113. Scheuplein RJ. 2000. The FQPA: a challenge for science policy and pesticide regulation. *Regul. Toxicol. Pharmacol.* 31:248–66

114. Schlosser PM, Lilly PD, Conolly RB, Janszen DB, Kimbell JS. 2003. Benchmark dose risk assessment for formaldehyde using airflow modeling and a single-compartment, DNA-protein cross-link dosimetry model to estimate human equivalent doses. *Risk Anal.* 23:473–87

115. Siegrist M. 1997. Communicating low risk magnitudes: incidence rates expressed as frequency versus rates expressed as probability. *Risk Anal.* 17:507–10

116. Siegrist M, Cvetkovich GT, Gutscher H. 2001. Shared values, social trust, and the perception of geographic cancer clusters. *Risk Anal.* 21:1047–54

117. Slovic P. 2003. Going beyond the Red Book: the sociopolitics of risk. *Hum. Ecol. Risk Assess.* 9:1181–90

118. Slovic P. 2002. Terrorism as hazard: a new species of trouble. *Risk Anal.* 22:425–26

119. Slovic P. 1997. Trust, emotion, sex, politics and science: surveying the risk-assessment battlefield. See Ref. 5a, pp. 277–313

120. Smith M. 2002. Food safety in Europe (FOSIE): risk assessment of chemicals in food and diet: overall introduction. *Food Chem. Toxicol.* 40:141–44

121. Tal A. 1997. A failure to engage. *The Environ. Forum* 14:13–21

122. Teunis PF, Chappell CL, Okhuysen PC. 2002. Cryptosporidium dose response studies: variation between isolates. *Risk Anal.* 22:175–83

123. Teunis PF, Chappell CL, Okhuysen PC. 2002. Cryptosporidium dose-response studies: variation between hosts. *Risk Anal.* 22:475–86

124. Thompson KM, Rabouw RF, Cooke RM. 2001. The risk of groundling fatalities from unintentional airplane crashes. *Risk Anal.* 21:1025–38

125. Tran NL, Barraj L, Smith K, Javier A, Burke TA. 2004. Combining food frequency and survey data to quantify

long-term dietary exposure: a methyl mercury case study. *Risk Anal.* 24:19–30

126. Trumbo CW, McComas KA. 2003. The function of credibility in information processing for risk perception. *Risk Anal.* 23:343–53

127. Van Landingham CB, Allen BC, Shipp AM, Crump KS. 2001. Comparison of the EU t25 single point estimate method with benchmark dose response modeling for estimating potency of carcinogens. *Risk Anal.* 21:641–56

128. Waters MD, Olden K, Tennant RW. 2003. Toxicogenomic approach for assessing toxicant-related disease. *Mutat. Res.* 544:415–24

129. Waters MD, Selkirk JK, Olden K. 2003. The impact of new technologies on human population studies. *Mutat. Res.* 244:349–60

130. Webler T, Tuler S. 2000. Fairness and competence in citizen participation, the-oretical reflections from a case study. *Admin. Soc.* 32:566–95

131. Weinstein ND, Kolb K, Goldstein BD. 1996. Using time intervals between expected events to communicate risk magnitudes. *Risk Anal.* 16:305–8

132. Williams BL, Florez Y. 2002. Do Mexican Americans perceive environmental issues differently than Caucasians: a study of cross-ethnic variation in perceptions related to water in Tucson. *Environ. Health Perspect.* 110(Suppl. 2):303–10

133. Xie XF, Wang M, Xu LC. 2003. What risks are Chinese people concerned about? *Risk Anal.* 23:685–95

134. Zartarian VG, Ozkaynak H, Burke JM, Zufa MJ, Rigas ML, Furtaw EJJr. 2000. A modeling framework for estimating children's residential exposure and dose to chlorpyrifos via dermal residue contact nad nondietary ingestion. *Environ. Health Perspect.* 108:505–14

Annu. Rev. Public Health 2005. 26:165–89
doi: 10.1146/annurev.publhealth.26.021304.144445
First published online as a Review in Advance on October 12, 2004

EMF AND HEALTH

Maria Feychting,[1] Anders Ahlbom,[1,2] and Leeka Kheifets[3]

[1]Institute of Environmental Medicine, Karolinska Institutet, S-171 77 Stockholm, Sweden; email: Maria.Feychting@imm.ki.se
[2]Division of Epidemiology, Stockholm Center of Public Health, 171 76 Stockholm, Sweden; email: Anders.Ahlbom@imm.ki.se
[3]Department of Epidemiology, School of Public Health, University of California, Los Angeles, California 90095-1772; email: kheifets@ucla.edu

Key Words childhood leukemia, electromagnetic fields, epidemiology, exposure assessment, scientific development

■ **Abstract** Electric and magnetic fields are ubiquitous in the modern society, and concerns have been expressed regarding possible adverse effects of these exposures. This review covers epidemiologic research on health effects of exposures to static, extremely low-frequency (ELF), and radio frequency (RF) fields. Research on ELF fields has been performed for more than two decades, and the methodology and quality of studies have improved over time. Studies have consistently shown increased risk for childhood leukemia associated with ELF magnetic fields, whereas ELF fields most likely are not a risk factor for breast cancer and cardiovascular disease. There are still inadequate data for other outcomes. More recently, focus has shifted toward RF exposures from mobile telephony. There are no persuasive data suggesting a health risk, but this research field is still immature with regard to the quantity and quality of available data. This technology is constantly changing and there is a need for continued research on this issue. Almost no epidemiologic data are available for static fields.

INTRODUCTION

Electric and magnetic fields (EMF) are ubiquitous in the modern society. Earth is surrounded by a static magnetic field that varies between 25 μT and 65 μT. Superimposed on the earth's magnetic field there may be manmade static magnetic fields. Power-frequency 50- and 60-Hz fields occupy the extremely low-frequency (ELF) nonionizing range of the electromagnetic spectrum (Figure 1). The ELF range includes frequencies from 3 Hz to 3000 Hz. Above 3000 Hz are, in order of increasing frequency and decreasing wavelength, radio waves, microwaves, infrared radiation, visible light, UV radiation, x-rays, and gamma rays. Microwaves have enough photon energy to heat tissue; ionizing radiation like x-rays and gamma rays can break chemical bonds, forming ions that can damage biological systems. Static and ELF electric and magnetic fields induce weak electric currents in the

0163-7525/05/0421-0165$20.00

165

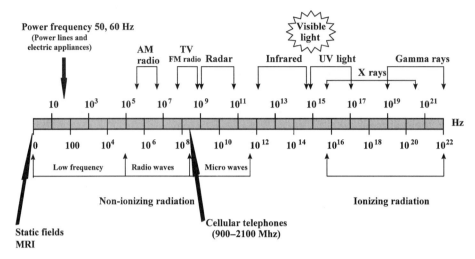

Figure 1   The electromagnetic spectrum.

body; however, they can neither break bonds nor heat tissue. Exposure guidelines for both ELF and RF fields are based on acute effects either from induced currents or from heating of tissue, respectively.

This review covers epidemiologic research on health effects of exposures to static magnetic fields, fields in the ELF range that are considerably lower than current exposure guidelines, and RF fields in the frequency ranges used for mobile telephony, which are close in magnitude to the existing guidelines but which cannot cause substantial heating of tissue (Table 1).

TABLE 1   International Commission on Non-Ionizing Radiation Protection (ICNIRP) exposure guidelines and some exposure sources

Exposure	ICNIRP's guidelines for the general population	Some exposure sources
Static fields	2 T	MRI: 1.5 or 3 T MAGLEV trains at floor level: 50 mT
50 Hz	100 μT	50 m from 400 kV power line: 0.4–1.5 μT
60 Hz	83 μT	In homes: usually <0.1 μT 0.5 m from TV: $\sim$ 0.2 μT 0.03 m from hair dryers: 6–2000 μT
900, 1800, 1900 MHz	SAR = 0.08 W/kg whole body exposure SAR = 2.0 W/kg localized exposure	Mobile phones, Specific Absorption Rate (SAR): <0.001–1.7 W/kg

STATIC FIELDS

Exposure Sources

Workers in industries such as aluminum production and chloralkali plants are exposed to static magnetic fields ranging from 4 mT to 50 mT (50), usually caused by strong rectified alternating current. Certain welding processes produce static fields, and railway workers on train systems operating from DC power supplies are exposed to static magnetic fields. Power systems for trains including magnetic levitation (MAGLEV trains) produce strong static magnetic fields, which will be an important exposure source when taken into operation in the future. Magnetic resonance imaging (MRI) systems used for medical diagnosis expose patients to flux densities as high as 2.5 T, and new machines are being developed in which exposure would be considerably higher. MRI operators are occupationally exposed to fields up to about 5 mT.

Summary of Data

Acute effects of static magnetic fields, e.g., nausea, vertigo, a metallic taste, and phosphenes, can be induced during movements in fields larger than ∼2 T. Adverse responses do not occur at field strengths below 2 T.

There is little information from animal studies regarding possible long-term effects of exposure to static magnetic fields, and there are only a few epidemiologic studies available. The majority of these have focused on cancer risks. There are also some reports on reproductive outcomes and sporadic studies of cardiovascular effects and immunological or musculoskeletal outcomes.

Cancer

A number of studies have investigated cancer risks in aluminum production workers or chloralkali workers. Most of these have focused on exposures other than static magnetic fields, e.g., polycyclic aromatic hydrocarbons, and consequently have poor or nonexistent assessment of exposure to static magnetic fields. The results from these studies are inconsistent; no patterns have emerged that can be clearly associated with effects of static magnetic field exposures. A few studies have attempted to estimate EMF exposures in broad categories (69–71, 81), but none of these found increased cancer risks related to EMF exposure.

There are a large number of studies on cancer risks among welders. However, none of these studies has estimated the exposure of welders to static magnetic fields, and it is impossible to distinguish between effects caused by welding fumes, static fields, ELF fields, or RF fields.

Other Outcomes

A few studies have reported results on reproductive outcomes among aluminum workers and MRI operators, but limitations in study designs prevent any conclusions from being drawn. Effects on immune function have been studied sporadically, producing inconsistent results, and single studies of cardiovascular or musculoskeletal outcomes have been reported.

Limitations

The available studies have several limitations apart from the crude exposure assessment. They generally compare the cancer incidence or mortality with that in the general population, which means that the "healthy worker effect" may have influenced the results. There are indeed several indications that this might be the case; many of the studies report decreased incidence or mortality rates overall. Most of the studies also have a very small number of exposed cases and do not have the power to detect modest risk increases. They also have little or no control of confounding.

A problem in occupational studies of possible health effects of static magnetic field exposure is that workers in exposed occupations are exposed also to a wide variety of other potentially harmful agents. Workers in aluminum production plants are exposed to petroleum coke and coal tar pitch volatiles, including, for example, polycyclic aromatic hydrocarbons, fluorides, sulfur dioxide, and heat (33, 34). Chloralkali workers are exposed to mercury, chlorine, and asbestos (6). Workers in both industries are exposed also to time-varying magnetic fields (mainly 50–300 Hz) ranging from 0.3 μT to 10 μT (87). Welders are exposed to welding fumes as well as high levels of ELF magnetic fields and also RF fields.

Summary of Major Reviews

Potential health effects from exposure to static fields have not received as much attention as have ELF or RF fields, and therefore few reviews have included this type of exposure in their assessments. The evaluation made by the International Agency for Research on Cancer (IARC) of static and ELF electric and magnetic fields (34) focused on ELF fields, although it reviewed epidemiologic studies of static fields also. IARC concluded that there is inadequate evidence in humans for determining the carcinogenicity of static electric or magnetic fields, and no relevant data from experimental animals is available; thus static fields were categorized as group 3, not classifiable as to their carcinogenicity to humans.

Overall Evaluation and Research Needs

The available evidence from epidemiologic studies is not sufficient to draw any conclusions about potential health effects of static magnetic field exposure at the levels encountered in the environment or the workplace. Increasing exposure to static magnetic fields in the general public is likely, e.g., with the development of new medical applications using very strong fields, and when magnetically levitated trains begin operation. Further research in this area is warranted, e.g., a cohort study of MRI workers or workers in industries where MRI systems are manufactured.

A cohort approach would allow studies with different types of outcomes. In new studies, improvement of the exposure assessment is crucial.

ELF FIELDS

Exposure Sources

Electric and magnetic fields are produced during electric power generation, transmission, and use. Electric field strength increases with increasing voltage or electric potential; magnetic field strength increases with increasing current. Both electric and magnetic fields decline rapidly with distance from their source, with a faster decline of fields from point sources such as equipment and a slower decline of fields from power lines. Electric fields are further reduced when shielded by conducting objects like buildings and have little penetrative ability; magnetic fields, in contrast, are capable of penetrating tissue and are not easily shielded.

Exposure Assessment

The early epidemiologic studies of residential magnetic fields estimated exposure through wire-codes, a categorization of homes based on distance to nearby electrical installations, e.g., power lines of different voltages (90). Subsequently, a more sophisticated method to assess magnetic field exposure from nearby power lines was developed, in which calculations were made of the fields generated by nearby power lines, on the basis of detailed information about the configuration of the lines and their historical loads (17). Also, new magnetic field meters were gradually developed, making it possible first to make spot measurements and later to assess personal or bedroom magnetic field exposure over periods of 24 or 48 h. Assessment of magnetic field exposure over a longer time period captures short-term temporal variations in the exposure levels.

A similar development of exposure assessment methods can be seen for occupational settings; early studies simply categorized certain occupational titles as "electrical occupations," whereas later studies have combined the use of systematic workplace measurements, individual job history descriptions, and the development of associated job-exposure matrices. Thus, exposure misclassification is likely to have decreased over time.

Summary of Data

Investigation of long-term ELF-EMF health effects has focused on cancer, reproductive disorders, as well as neurodegenerative and cardiovascular diseases.

In vitro studies on the possible carcinogenicity of electric and magnetic fields have investigated, under a wide range of exposure conditions, a variety of processes in a number of cell lines and tissue cultures. Because ELF EMF do not appear to initiate cancer, researchers have hypothesized that they may act as cancer promoters or progressors. In vitro research on the carcinogenicity of ELF EMF has been plagued by a lack of consistency and reproducibility. Recent reviews (34, 62, 63, 66) have concluded that cellular effects have been observed for exposures above 100 μT, although mechanisms for these effects are not known. Overall, a coherent picture is lacking. Although sporadic ELF-EMF effects have been reported in some animal studies, most results have been negative. Of the approaches to evaluating ELF EMF as a potential health hazard, toxicologic experiments provide the most consistently negative data (66). In particular, data on leukemia in experimental animals are negative (34). Epidemiologic evidence is summarized below.

Cancer

Generally studies have focused either on residential exposures or on occupational exposures; only a few studies have combined the different exposure sources (18, 20). Data on adult cancer and residential exposure to ELF EMF, including the use of appliances, are sparse and methodologically limited (56, 84). Because earlier evidence suggested that residential exposure is not a risk factor for adult cancers and because researchers expected that occupational studies would provide a more powerful test of adult cancer hypotheses than would residential ones, studies using the next generation of residential exposure assessment methods, such as long-term measurements and calculated fields, focused on children. One possible exception is breast cancer, for which several large studies with fairly sophisticated exposure assessment have been completed recently.

Effects in Children

Since the first report was published in 1979 (90), which suggested an association between residential ELF electric and magnetic fields and childhood leukemia, dozens of increasingly sophisticated studies have examined this association. In addition, there have been numerous comprehensive reviews, meta-analyses, and two recent pooled analyses. In one pooled analysis based on nine well-conducted studies, a twofold excess risk was seen for exposure above 0.4 μT (1). The other pooled analysis included 15 studies based on less-restrictive inclusion criteria and used 0.3 μT as the highest cutoff (25). A relative risk of 1.7 for exposure above 0.3 μT was reported. The two studies are closely consistent and represent the strongest association in ELF epidemiology.

No consistent relationship has been seen in studies of childhood brain tumors or other cancers and residential ELF electric and magnetic fields (44). However, these studies have generally been smaller and of lower quality, and a formal pooled analysis for brain cancer has not been done.

Several studies of the relationship between electrical appliance use and various childhood cancers have been published (56, 76). In general, these studies provide no discernable pattern of increased risk associated with increased duration and frequency of appliance use.

Effects in Adults

Data on adult cancer and residential exposure have been largely negative but fraught with limited exposure assessment and other methodological limitations. Three recently completed large breast cancer studies found no association with exposure to electric or magnetic fields (12, 53, 78).

Occupational studies conducted in the 1980s and early 1990s pointed to a possible increased risk of leukemia, brain tumors, and male breast cancer (14) in jobs with presumed exposure to ELF electric and magnetic fields above average levels. In light of a hypothesis that EMF can affect breast cancer through melatonin suppression (83), concern extended to female breast cancer and occupational exposures.

Several large studies, conducted in the 1990s, of both leukemia and brain cancer made use of improved methods for individual assessment of occupational exposure to magnetic fields and to potential occupational confounders. No consistent exposure-response relationship and no consistency in the association with specific subtypes of leukemia or brain tumors were found in either individual studies or in the meta- and pooled analyses (45–47).

Although some earlier registry-based studies provided some support for a possible association between EMF exposure and female breast cancer (48), the most recent very large study, which incorporated exposure measurements in female workers, did not find an association (20b).

Sporadic reports of elevated risk for other cancers have appeared in the literature, most notably for lung cancer (4), but none have been sufficiently suggestive to warrant presentation here.

Cardiovascular Disease

A hypothesis that EMF could affect heart rate variability (75), which in turn can influence acute cardiovascular events (13), gave Savitz et al. (77) the impetus to look at cardiovascular mortality. As postulated they observed an increased risk for acute myocardial infarction (AMI) and arrhythmia-related death but not from chronic cardiovascular disease. However, further studies specifically designed to test this hypothesis mostly failed to replicate this finding while approaching this hypothesis from different point of views: Two studies directly replicated the original study (73, 80); one study focused specifically on arrhythmia (40); and one study investigated cardiovascular morbidity and provided detailed confounding control (2).

The only support, very limited as it was, for the original observation comes from a study based on data from the Swedish twin registry (26), which observed a non-significantly increased risk for AMI. Thus only mortality studies of the association between occupational exposure to EMF and cardiovascular diseases have reported an association (26, 77). However, studies of cardiovascular diseases that rely on mortality records are questionable owing to inaccuracy of the diagnosis on the death certificates (J. Mant, S. Wilson, J. Parry, P. Bridge, R. Wilson, W. Murdoch, T. Quirke, M. Davies, M. Grammage, R. Harrison, A. Warfield, submitted manuscript). Thus, on balance, the evidence supporting an etiologic relation between occupational EMF exposures has been overturned by more focused and rigorous studies.

Neurodegenerative Diseases

Investigation of potential EMF effects on neurodegenerative diseases is still not well developed. Of the three neurodegenerative diseases that have been considered, Parkinson's disease has received the least attention. No study has provided clear evidence of an association between Parkinson's disease and above-average exposure to ELF EMF, and in the absence of laboratory evidence to the contrary, there is no good ground for believing that these fields are involved in the etiology of the disease.

The evidence relating to Alzheimer's disease is more difficult to assess. The initial reports that gave rise to the idea suggested that the increased risk could be substantial (79). Subsequent studies have been inconsistent, with no obvious pattern on the basis of study design, whether morbidity or mortality was examined, or the quality of exposure assessment. Thus the evidence that ELF EMF increases the risk of Alzheimer's disease is weak (3, 63).

More evidence is available for amyotrophic lateral sclerosis (ALS), where several studies suggested that employment in electrical occupations may increase the risk of ALS (11, 41). Currently, the most interesting suggestion is that electric shock, rather than increased exposure to EMF, may play a role in the development of ALS (63).

Reproduction

The association of electric and magnetic field exposure with human reproductive outcomes has been examined in a number of studies (32). Although several studies have reported adverse effects, more rigorous investigations have not corroborated these findings. Studies examining domestic exposures and use of electric blankets have found no increase in risk of pregnancy outcomes such as miscarriages or intrauterine growth retardation (7, 8). Two recent studies from California found an increased risk of miscarriages in women with exposures to relatively high (any exposure above 1.6 μT) intermittent fields (51, 52). In occupationally exposed groups, reported effects included congenital malformations, brain tumors, and spontaneous abortions among video display terminal operators (68). Methodological problems such as the difficulty of studying EMF exposure levels that are very close to background, possible omission of early miscarriages, and information and recall bias make firm conclusions difficult to obtain.

Limitations

Epidemiologic investigations of possible associations of EMF exposure with risk of chronic disease pose unique and substantial difficulties. Among them are difficulties specific to an outcome studied, assessment of exposure, and inter-pretation of findings.

Most of the chronic diseases considered are rare and have long latency periods for known risk factors. Thus a major challenge in EMF epidemiology is the small number of cases available in any given study and the necessity for retrospective study designs that make exposure assessment even more difficult. Small risks are notoriously difficult to evaluate, both because it is difficult to achieve enough precision to distinguish a small risk from no risk and because small risks are more vulnerable to subtle confounding and other biases that can go undetected. In particular, selection bias may account for part of the association. Case-control studies that relied on in-home measurements are especially vulnerable to this bias because of the low response rates in many studies. Studies conducted in the Nordic countries, which relied on historical calculated magnetic fields, are not subject to selection bias but suffer from very low numbers of exposed subjects.

Furthermore, the etiologies of many of the diseases studied are poorly under-stood, making difficult a search for confounding as an explanation for any observed association. For some of the more common diseases such as Alzheimer's and car-diovascular disease reliance on mortality records is particularly problematic.

EMF does not appear to be genotoxic, but biological evidence suggests that it could influence cellular function and proliferation. Therefore, it could act as a promoter or growth enhancer in carcinogenesis. The distinction between promotion and growth enhancement in cancer biology is primarily theoretical and is virtually impossible to discern in an epidemiologic study. However, the two processes can be considered as representing postinitiation events that enhance the development of cancer. As such, they can be studied by focusing on the populations that have been exposed previously to cancer initiators or who are at high cancer risk for genetic reasons. Epidemiologic studies that attempt to consider such secondary events are rare, and methodologic developments in this area are needed.

That assessment of exposure is a major weakness of epidemiologic EMF studies is not surprising because several factors make assessment of EMF exposure more difficult than assessment of many other environmental exposures. The exposure is imperceptible, ubiquitous, has multiple sources, and can vary greatly over time and short distances. Assessment of exposure to electric and magnetic fields over time has dramatically improved, yet our ability to predict exposure remains severely limited (43) and might be better for children than for adults (19).

In a 1000-person study, Zaffanella et al. (91) found that work exposures are often significantly higher and more variable than are other exposures; the highest mean and median exposures occur at work, followed by exposures at home and during travel. In contrast, in a small study of household appliance use, Mezei et al. (56) found that a large proportion of total exposure for most adults is accumulated at home. Given the large amount of time most people spend at home, ignoring either home or work exposure is likely to lead to a large misclassification.

The long latency of cancers necessitates estimation of exposure over long time periods, an exceptionally difficult task owing to the mobility and behavioral changes likely to occur over time. The situation is even worse for rapidly fatal or memory-debilitating diseases, such as brain cancer and Alzheimer's, when information is obtained from a large number of proxies.

The absence of a clearly elucidated, robust, and reproducible mechanism of interaction of EMF with biological systems deprives epidemiologic studies of focus in their measurement strategies. If some singular aspect of EMF plays a role in carcinogenesis, we have yet to identify and capture it. Given the plethora of field characteristics that could be measured, it would be difficult to undertake a truly comprehensive evaluation of exposures.

All these difficulties with EMF exposure assessment are likely to have led to substantial exposure misclassification, which is likely, in turn, to interfere with detection of an association between exposure and disease (if indeed such an association exists). If the true association is small or moderate, detecting associations with this amount of measurement error will be difficult.

Summary of Major Recent Reviews

Numerous national and international bodies have provided comprehensive reviews of this literature over the years. These reviews adhere to different philosophies: from strict focus on what is known (62), to narrative evaluation (63), to formal weight-of-evidence approach (34), to informal incorporation of prior beliefs (61). Conclusions varied somewhat with time and individuals involved; nevertheless, these reviews broadly agree that while the evidence is not conclusive, the possibility of the effect cannot be excluded and epidemiologic studies of childhood leukemia provide the strongest evidence of an association. The most formal of these, by IARC (34), concluded in 2002 that

> [t]here is limited evidence in humans for the carcinogenicity of extremely low-frequency magnetic fields in relation to childhood leukemia. There is inadequate evidence in humans for the carcinogenicity of extremely low-frequency magnetic fields in relation to all other cancers. There is inadequate evidence in experimental animals for the carcinogenicity of extremely low-frequency magnetic fields.

These evaluations have led to a classification of ELF magnetic fields as possibly carcinogenic to humans (Group 2B). The World Health Organization is developing a comprehensive risk assessment and policy recommendations with results expected in 2005.

Ongoing Work

There is little ongoing work in ELF epidemiology, and much of it relates to childhood leukemia. Of note is a cohort study in the United Kingdom, a case-control study in Italy, an evaluation of selection bias (24) (G. Mezei, L. Kheifets, manuscript in preparation), and an examination of a newly proposed contact current hypothesis (42).

Overall Evaluation and Future Research Needs

Among all the outcomes evaluated in epidemiologic studies of ELF EMF, there is most evidence of an association for childhood leukemia in relation to postnatal exposures above 0.3–0.4 μT. This association is unlikely to be caused by chance but may be partly due to bias, though it is difficult to interpret in the absence of a known mechanism or reproducible experimental support. The common chromosome translocations in childhood leukemia seem to initiate disease and often arise prenatally. However, it appears that the frequency of conversion of the preleukemic clone to overt disease is low. One or more additional postnatal event(s) is needed for leukemia development (23). Investigation of EMF as one of the postnatal exposures leading to an increased risk of childhood leukemia may prove informative.

Further studies designed to test specific hypotheses such as aspects of exposure or a possibility of selection bias are also needed. Past attempts to evaluate selection bias operating through socioeconomic status (SES) and low participation rates were largely ecological and/or focused on wire codes rather than measurements. New attempts need to focus on the interrelationship between SES and participation of cases and controls on one hand and measured fields on the other. Ultimately the question of selection bias can be resolved only in a large well-conducted cohort study or in a case-control study where exposure information can be collected independently of the included subjects. However, the rarity of both the outcome (childhood leukemia) and exposure (magnetic fields above 0.3–0.4 μT) will require either a prohibitively expensive study or an innovative study design.

Additionally, a pooled analysis of childhood brain tumors may prove informative in addressing either specificity of the association with ELF EMF or a possibility of selection bias.

Within the methodologic limitations described above, there is inadequate evidence that ELF EMF is carcinogenic to adults. Similarly, the evidence is inadequate for other diseases considered, including reproductive outcomes and cardiovascular and neurodegenerative diseases. Of all these diseases, we consider neurodegenerative disease, ALS in particular, to be the one in need of further investigation. Studies of ALS incorporating better exposure assessment methods, including assessment of contact currents, more accurate diagnosis of diseases, and adjustments for potential confounding from occupational exposures to substances such as solvents may clarify the issue.

RF FIELDS

Exposure Sources

There are different sources of RF exposure to which people may be exposed, but the most frequently discussed is exposures related to mobile telephony. This technology typically uses the frequencies from 450 to 2500 MHz, although new technology may extend this band. Other general population sources of exposure are radio and television transmitters operating at frequencies between 200 kHz and 900 MHz. Occupational exposures examples include RF PVC welding machines, plasma etchers, and military and civil radar systems, all operating at different frequencies. The main focus of this review is RF exposures related to mobile telephony. Exposure from the mobile phone is concentrated to the part of the head closest to the handset and the antenna. The exposure declines rapidly with distance to the antenna, and therefore, exposure from mobile phone base stations are several orders of magnitude lower than from the phones. Thus, most of the research has focused on mobile phone use. However, the exposure from base stations differs from that of mobile phones; base stations expose the whole body, and the exposure duration is considerably longer.

Summary of Data

There is no convincing evidence from cellular studies that RF fields are carcinogenic or promote carcinogenic agents. Isolated findings of DNA damage have not been replicated, results on micronuclei are contradictory, and the importance of the occurrence of micronuclei for human health is unclear. There is some evidence for an increase in expression of heat shock proteins after RF exposure; however, the few available studies are inconsistent. Different exposure conditions are needed to evoke the response, and the type of heat shock protein for which an increase was found has varied between models.

There have been sporadic reports of effects in animal models, but most studies have not reported dose-dependent responses in either gene expression or in increased permeability of the blood-brain barrier. Recent animal studies have not provided evidence that RF radiation below exposure guidelines could induce cancer or promote effects of known carcinogens. One earlier study reported a higher lymphoma incidence in transgenic mice (67) exposed to RF fields, but this finding was not confirmed in a recently published study (88). The comparability between these studies has been questioned (21, 22), and additional replication studies are ongoing.

Epidemiologic studies of health effects related to RF exposure from mobile telephony have primarily focused on cancer outcomes (mainly brain tumors), and a few studies focused on different types of symptoms. The mobile phone technology is relatively new, and therefore, the number of studies available is limited. Occupational studies have been performed over several decades, but the exposure frequencies may not always be relevant for an assessment of mobile telephony frequency effects. We are only beginning to measure and learn about RF exposures in various occupations.

Cancer

Handheld mobile phones have been available only since the later part of the 1980s and have become common in the general population only during recent years. In several countries, e.g., Finland and Sweden, more than 80% of the population are mobile phone users today, whereas the same statistic was less than 10% in the beginning of the 1990s. The first study of cancer in relation to mobile phone use was published in 1996 and had only a short period of follow-up (72). Subsequent studies have also been limited by short exposure durations and short latency, and no study to date has had the power to investigate potential long-term effects. Therefore, on the basis of the evidence at hand, it is possible only to evaluate short-term effects of mobile phone exposure.

Nine studies of mobile phone use and brain tumors have been published so far (5, 10, 27, 28, 37, 38, 59, 72, 89). The majority of these have found no effects on brain tumor risk. A Finnish register-based case-control study found an increased risk of glioma related to use of analog phones (5), with an increased risk found already after one to two years duration of subscription to an analog phone. This finding was not confirmed in a Danish cohort study with similar exposure assessment methods (38) or in other case-control studies. The glioma incidence in the Nordic countries, where mobile phone use in the general population started relatively early, has not increased since the introduction of handheld mobile phones (55). A Swedish case-control study reported a more-than-threefold risk increase of acoustic neuroma among users of analog mobile phones (27) but with no relation to induction period. Other studies have not provided evidence of an increased risk of acoustic neuroma (28, 37, 58) but have not had enough statistical power to adequately test the hypothesis. Two studies have investigated the risk of uveal melanoma but produced conflicting results (39, 82).

There are no studies of cancer risk related to mobile phone base stations, but a few studies have assessed cancer risk in relation to radio and TV transmitters (15, 16, 31, 57). Exposure assessment has simply been based on distance to the transmitter, and no account has been taken of the surrounding vegetation and buildings. The studies have been of an ecological design, with no data on individual exposures or confounders, and the number of observed cases has often been small. Several of the studies were conducted because of concerns for an apparent excess of cases in a certain area, and they have reported a higher incidence of leukemia close to the transmitters. However, other studies, conducted without a priori concern, have not confirmed these findings. Overall, the available data do not support the hypothesis that radiofrequency exposure from transmitters increases cancer risk; however, they do not provide strong evidence against the hypothesis either.

Occupational Studies

Occupational studies of RF exposure have been conducted for more than 20 years, and a variety of occupations have been investigated, e.g., radar technicians, radio and telegraph operators, or workers in dielectric heat sealing or in telecommunication manufacturing. The studies have several methodological weaknesses, especially regarding exposure assessment. None of the studies has made measurements of the RF exposure for the subjects included in the study, and exposure classification has often been based on the job title alone. No control or only limited control of confounding has been made. Although some increased risks have been found in certain studies, there is no consistent evidence of risk increases for any cancer sites. The exposure frequencies studied have generally been other than those used for mobile telephony.

Symptoms

All available epidemiologic studies of symptoms related either to mobile phone use (9, 65) or to exposures from mobile phone base stations (60, 74) are cross-sectional, which makes them of limited value in a health risk assessment. The subjects themselves have estimated their exposure, e.g., distance to nearest base station or amount of mobile phone use, as well as the health outcome, and no attempt has been made to verify the exposure or disease. The studies of base stations have not adequately described how subjects were selected, and there may be both selection and reporting bias. Therefore, the available epidemiologic studies on symptoms do not provide information that allows an evaluation of the effect of mobile phones or base stations on the occurrence of different types of symptoms.

Limitations

In all available mobile phone studies, exposure estimation has limitations. Exposure assessment has focused on amount of mobile phone use, with no attempt to incorporate other parameters that might influence the level of exposure while using a mobile phone, e.g., make and model of the phone or output power levels. Exposure information has been obtained either directly from the subjects included in the studies through questionnaires or interviews or from register-based information about mobile phone subscriptions. The former method may be subject to recall bias: Cases may be more prone to remember all occasions of exposure or even overestimate their exposure, whereas controls are not as motivated and may forget exposures. In contrast, a brain tumor may affect a person's memory, which could make it more difficult for cases to remember their mobile phone usage many years back in time. Thus, this type of bias can affect the risk estimates in both directions. The studies that have used register-based exposure information collected independently of case/control status do not have this potential for recall bias but have other limitations. They have not been able to identify corporate users and have no information about who is the actual user of the phone. This kind of exposure misclassification would tend to dilute risk estimates toward unity.

Some of the case-control studies used hospital controls selected among other patients at the hospitals where the brain tumor cases were treated (37, 59). It is difficult to know if these other patients are representative of the population from which the brain tumor cases come with regard to frequency of mobile phone use, and it is impossible to evaluate the potential for selection bias. Some of the case-control studies that have used population-based controls nevertheless have a large potential for selection bias because of the long time period between date of diagnosis and case recruitment, leading to a large proportion of cases having deceased before recruitment (27, 28). The remarkably high response rates (about 90% for the population-based controls) in these studies also limit the interpretability of these findings.

As described above, the occupational studies have severe limitations in the exposure assessment, and negative findings cannot be taken as evidence of a lack of an association. The limited confounding control makes positive findings hard to interpret; other exposures in the studied occupations may be responsible for increased risks observed.

Cross-sectional studies have only limited valuable information in the assessment of potential effects of RF exposure on different symptoms, and some of the available studies have severe problems with potential selection and reporting biases.

Summary of Major Reviews

During recent years the literature on potential health effects of RF exposure have been summarized and evaluated by a number of national bodies, e.g., the Royal Society of Canada (72a), the Stewart Commission in the United Kingdom (36, 64), the Health Council of the Netherlands (30), the Swedish Radiation Protection Agency (85), and the French Health General Directorate (92). These reviews come to more or less similar conclusions in their assessments of the science: The scientific evidence available does not give cause for concern, but the research has limitations and mobile telephones have been widespread only for a relatively short time. Therefore, the possibility that RF exposures from mobile telephony can have adverse health effects remains, and continued research is needed. In terms of public health recommendations, national bodies draw different conclusions; e.g., the Stewart commission in the United Kingdom recommends that children avoid unnecessary exposure, whereas the Health Council of the Netherlands finds no reason to recommend precaution.

Ongoing Work

Currently underway is a large international collaborative case-control study of brain tumors, acoustic neuroma, and parotid gland tumors in relation to mobile phone use. The study is being performed in 13 countries, and results from national analyses are expected in the near future—one has already been published (10). Results from the combined international analyses will be available in 2005 at the earliest.

Several countries have initiated research programs to clarify the question about possible health effects of mobile telecommunication. Thus, there are numerous studies ongoing, some of which are epidemiologic.

Feasibility studies have shown that establishment of a large cohort of mobile phone users is possible. Attempts are being made to establish such a cohort in several European countries. Exposure information will be based on records of incoming and outgoing calls from mobile phone operators, combined with questionnaire information. Outcomes will be determined through both questionnaires and linkage to different registries. It is urgent to begin a prospective cohort study capable of capturing rapidly changing exposures and addressing a broad range of health outcomes. Such a study, which has been identified as a high priority by WHO, will reduce scientific uncertainty and provide the most relevant data for future risk assessment.

Overall Evaluation and Future Research Needs

Although occasional significant associations between various brain tumors and mobile phone use have been found, no single association has been consistent. The few positive findings reported in two of the studies are difficult to interpret: They are either based on small numbers, have latency periods too short to be credible, or emerged only after a series of reanalyses that are reported in a way that is difficult to follow. Considering the short time period during which handheld mobile phones have been in use, and the limited use (both in terms of the number and duration of calls) among early users, it is not possible today to evaluate effects after a long induction period or for heavy use. Thus, the negative results of most of the studies cannot be taken as evidence against an effect either. The current evidence is inconclusive regarding cancer risk following RF exposure from mobile phones. The occupational studies available on cancer risks have such severe limitations that they provide little information about cancer risk related to RF exposures. Data regarding effects of RF exposure on symptoms are inadequate for an assessment.

Some investigators argue that children are more sensitive to RF exposure than are adults, and several countries (e.g., the United Kingdom) recommend special precautions for children. However, there are to date no available data on health effects in children. Mobile phone use is increasingly common among school children, and teenagers may be among the heaviest mobile phone users today. Therefore, studies assessing possible adverse health effects in children and teenagers are warranted.

Results from many ongoing case-control studies of head and neck tumors will be available in the near future, but these studies will also have limited ability to assess effects of long-term exposures. Analog mobile phones have been available for the longest time period, and some people have been users for more than 10 years. However, digital phones have been available for only ~10 years.

A large cohort of mobile phone users capable of evaluating a number of different outcomes, e.g., brain tumors, neurodegenerative diseases, cognitive effects, symptoms, and other outcomes that may become of interest as a result of experimental research or public concern, is urgently needed. Additionally, the technology is constantly changing; the third generation of mobile phones is currently being introduced, and further changes in the future are likely. Therefore, there is a need for continued research on this issue.

Exposures from base stations are only an extremely small fraction of the exposure guidelines, but the possibility of health effects from continuous whole-body exposure is an area of major public concern. The feasibility of performing epidemiologic studies on base stations is being investigated currently.

Comparative Analysis of Scientific Developments

This section focuses on research on ELF and RF fields because there are only sporadic epidemiologic studies on health effects from static field exposure. Manmade exposure to static fields has been quite limited in the past, and therefore this exposure has not attracted public concern. This may change in the future with a more widespread use of MRI and the introduction of MAGLEV trains.

There has been a longstanding scientific interest in the possibility that prolonged exposure to weak EMF, at levels far below the current exposure standards, might assert health effects through mechanisms other than the established ones (49). A new phase in this research began after the publication of an epidemiologic study that implicated an association between ELF and childhood cancer mortality in 1979 (90).

This and later studies generated a considerable interest among the public, decision makers, and scientists. Scientists were intrigued by the original results, and studies were conducted to see whether the results could be replicated and to explore the associations from various perspectives. More than two decades later, this research avenue in a way seems to have been exhausted, at least temporarily. A considerable amount of knowledge has been accumulated, and broad consensus has been reached about a number of issues involved (3).

Now the focus has shifted from power frequency fields to RF fields. For RF fields, however, the research was not initiated by an epidemiologic finding or other scientific data on the possible existence of a health risk. Instead the driving force has been a concern over the fast dissemination and penetration of new communication techniques together with the notion that the biophysical interaction between RF fields and humans may not be fully known or understood. This argument was partially based on an analogy with the ELF results.

Thus, the starting points for the ELF and the RF EMF research are rather different. Despite this difference we propose that these two scientific areas are similar with respect to the methodological challenges and several other aspects, with the caveat that the ELF research is at least a decade ahead of the RF research. We also propose that the RF research can and does learn from the ELF studies. This section assesses this tenet by conducting a comparative analysis of scientific developments.

Exposures

Because there is no known mechanism by which ELF or RF fields might assert low-level biological effects, one does not know which aspect of the fields should be measured in a particular study. Studies are therefore measuring different aspects of the EMF but are influenced by the known mechanisms for acute effects. For ELF fields the only established effect is induced currents, and the corresponding environmental quantity is the magnetic flux density, measured in μT; for various reasons the magnetic component, rather than the electrical, has been implicated. For RF fields, the only established effect is heating, and the corresponding environmental quantity is power density, measured in W/m^2. Studies have also attempted to estimate the internal dose, however, measured in W/kg, rather than the environmental levels.

Because exposure to EMF is imperceptible it does not lend itself to self-reporting by subjects in epidemiologic studies, and therefore the epidemiologist is left with two options: to use direct measurements or to use proxies based on circumstances or conditions known or thought to entail exposure. When the attempts to replicate and explore the results of the seminal study on ELF and childhood cancer began, no magnetic field meters could measure such weak fields. The development of such instrumentation began shortly afterward, and the later generation of studies has used direct field measurements. For RF fields, a meter suitable for large-scale use in epidemiologic studies has just been developed; for obvious reasons the internal dose cannot be captured directly but must be assessed on the basis of a combination of measurements and modeling.

Sources of exposure to ELF and RF fields are different. Yet for both types of fields the sources can be divided into three main categories: occupational, environmental, and personal appliances. All of these have been used as markers of exposure both in ELF and RF research.

Occupational studies have played a considerable role both in ELF and RF research (3, 64). In the early ELF studies the major limitation of this line of research was the limited knowledge about actual exposure levels and distribution in the occupations that were studied. This limitation was later rectified through extensive measurement studies within occupational groups. In the RF studies the lack of details about exposure is still a major obstacle. Measurement studies have begun recently, but the results of these efforts are not yet available.

Some early ELF studies based their exposure assessment on the presence of power lines and assessed exposure from this source according to algorithms with a varying degree of sophistication. In retrospect this approach has proven to be rather successful, partly because power lines are an important source of ELF exposure. In contrast, this avenue has not yet been successful for RF and may not be in the future either because of the complex relation between the exposure at one geographic location and the output power from the source. Another factor, however, appears to be that the environmental levels of RF exposure are very low in relation to the exposure that a subject experiences from mobile phone use, for example. Indeed, the levels may differ by a factor of one thousand. Thus, one would expect biological effects, if they exist, to be easier to detect in studies based on phone use rather than in studies based on nearby antennas. In addition, mobile phone technology is rapidly changing, which further complicates exposure assessment.

Some attempts were made to include appliance use in ELF studies (29), but they have not been successful. There are too many different appliances to consider and the patterns of usage are quite diverse, which makes exposure from the different sources difficult to combine into one parameter, which would be desirable. Assessment of exposure from appliances is rather different for RF because the obvious appliance to consider here is the mobile phone. Studies so far have used rather crude characterizations of exposure from phones, such as years of use. However, considerable efforts are currently underway to determine the relative importance of various factors related to usage that can be incorporated in epidemiologic studies. One key consideration is to what extent the degree of down-regulation of the phone can be predicted on the basis of factors such as urban/rural use or indoor/outdoor use (54).

Biological Plausibility

The fields considered here both in the ELF and the RF research are too weak for any biological effects to be explained by the known mechanisms of interaction, induced currents, or heating, respectively. In neither case is there even a good candidate for a mechanism that might explain such effects. It may be worth noting, however, that the actual exposure levels considered in the ELF research are orders of magnitude below the exposure standards, whereas for RF, exposure from mobile phone use actually may be of the same order of magnitude as the exposure standards (35).

Yet, the epidemiologic studies of ELF have shown rather consistently effects for childhood leukemia that have been considered strong enough evidence for the IARC to classify ELF in category 2B, which is translated by IARC as a possible carcinogen (34). Other evaluators have reached similar conclusions. Thus, the lack of a known or even hypothetical mechanism has not prevented evaluators from concluding that weak ELF exposure possibly may cause cancer. However, with some hints as to the mechanism, or supportive toxicologic data, the IARC classification would have been higher. For RF, the epidemiology is still immature, and it is still too early for a corresponding discussion.

ELF research has also provided examples to the contrary. For both breast cancer and cardiovascular diseases, the research began with a biological hypothesis confirmed by some early studies. More rigorous epidemiologic studies that followed showed no effect, which has led to an overall conclusion that ELF fields are not involved in the development of these diseases.

The concept of biological plausibility is vague and rather ill defined and is therefore not particularly useful in this and similar contexts. Often our understanding of what is plausible changes over time, as science makes advances and paradigms shift. If an association appears to exist, one must test every candidate for explanation and eventually perform a risk evaluation.

Quality of Research

The quality of the ELF studies have improved over time, and new study protocols were designed on the basis of prior studies' experiences. This is particularly evident with respect to exposure assessment. The earliest studies used crude proxies for

ELF as markers for exposure, whereas later studies employed sophisticated meters and measurement schemes.

The current RF studies may be best compared to the early generation of ELF studies, with respect to exposure assessment. But as knowledge advances about exposure distribution and determinants, RF research will likely follow the same track as ELF research with improving quality over time.

ELF research also showed that accusations of epidemiology as a source of many false associations are not warranted when good studies are conducted. Furthermore, although in the strictest sense one cannot prove a negative association (or a positive one for that matter), in reality the weight-of-evidence approach can provide sufficient information to conclude a negative association, provided there is comprehensive and rigorous research.

Conclusions of Reviews and Historical Changes

For ELF there are indications that the childhood leukemia association is causal, but lack of a known mechanism at such low energy levels, negative animal data, and a possibility of selection bias require explanation. For some other endpoints, such as breast cancer and cardiovascular disease, enough data now exist to conclude that ELF is most likely not a risk factor. For several other endpoints the science is considerably weaker than for childhood leukemia, so it may be too early still to discount other possible associations with ELF. To further address the childhood leukemia issue, it is possible that one must await a better general understanding of the etiology. Thus, science has been quite successful during the two decades since this research was revitalized, in that it has brought several of the issues to reasonable conclusions.

The RF situation again is very different. First, no good data thus far suggest a health risk associated with RF. Second, this research is still immature, with regard to both the amount of available data and the quality of available studies. Thus, no conclusions can be drawn yet and we must await further results.

The *Annual Review of Public Health* is online at
http://publhealth.annualreviews.org

LITERATURE CITED

1. Ahlbom A, Day N, Feychting M, Roman E, Skinner J, et al. 2000. A pooled analysis of magnetic fields and childhood leukaemia. *Br. J. Cancer* 83:692–98

2. Ahlbom A, Feychting M, Gustavsson A, Hallqvist J, Johansen C, et al. 2004. Occupational magnetic field exposure and myocardial infarction incidence in the SHEEP study. *Epidemiology* 15:403–8

3. Ahlbom IC, Cardis E, Green A, Linet M, Savitz D, Swerdlow A. 2001. Review of the epidemiologic literature on EMF and health. *Environ. Health Perspect.* 109(Suppl. 6):911–33

4. Armstrong B, Theriault G, Guenel P, Deadman J, Goldberg M, Heroux P. 1994. Association between exposure to pulsed electromagnetic fields and cancer in electric utility workers in Quebec, Canada,

and France. *Am. J. Epidemiol.* 140:805–20

5. Auvinen A, Hietanen M, Luukkonen R, Koskela RS. 2002. Brain tumors and salivary gland cancers among cellular telephone users. *Epidemiology* 13:356–59

6. Barregard L, Sallsten G, Jarvholm B. 1990. Mortality and cancer incidence in chloralkali workers exposed to inorganic mercury. *Br. J. Ind. Med.* 47:99–104

7. Belanger K, Leaderer B, Hellenbrand K, Holford TR, McSharry J, et al. 1998. Spontaneous abortion and exposure to electric blankets and heated water beds. *Epidemiology* 9:36–42

8. Bracken MB, Belanger K, Hellenbrand K, Dlugosz L, Holford TR, et al. 1995. Exposure to electromagnetic fields during pregnancy with emphasis on electrically heated beds: association with birthweight and intrauterine growth retardation. *Epidemiology* 6:263–70

9. Chia SE, Chia HP, Tan JS. 2000. Prevalence of headache among handheld cellular telephone users in Singapore: a community study. *Environ. Health Perspect.* 108:1059–62

10. Christensen HC, Schuz J, Kosteljanetz M, Poulsen HS, Thomsen J, Johansen C. 2004. Cellular telephone use and risk of acoustic neuroma. *Am. J. Epidemiol.* 159:277–83

11. Davanipour Z, Sobel E, Bowman JD, Qian Z, Will AD. 1997. Amyotrophic lateral sclerosis and occupational exposure to electromagnetic fields. *Bioelectromagnetics* 18:28–35

12. Davis S, Mirick DK, Stevens RG. 2002. Residential magnetic fields and the risk of breast cancer. *Am. J. Epidemiol.* 155:446–54

13. Dekker JM, Schouten EG, Klootwijk P, Pool J, Swenne CA, Kromhout D. 1997. Heart rate variability from short electrocardiographic recordings predicts mortality from all causes in middle-aged and elderly men. The Zutphen Study. *Am. J. Epidemiol.* 145:899–908

14. Demers PA, Thomas DB, Rosenblatt KA, Jimenez LM, McTiernan A, et al. 1991. Occupational exposure to electromagnetic fields and breast cancer in men. *Am. J. Epidemiol.* 134:340–47

15. Dolk H, Elliott P, Shaddick G, Walls P, Thakrar B. 1997. Cancer incidence near radio and television transmitters in Great Britain. II. All high power transmitters. *Am. J. Epidemiol.* 145:10–17

16. Dolk H, Shaddick G, Walls P, Grundy C, Thakrar B, et al. 1997. Cancer incidence near radio and television transmitters in Great Britain. I. Sutton Coldfield transmitter. *Am. J. Epidemiol.* 145:1–9

17. Feychting M, Ahlbom A. 1993. Magnetic fields and cancer in children residing near Swedish high-voltage power lines. *Am. J. Epidemiol.* 138:467–81

18. Feychting M, Forssén U, Floderus B. 1997. Occupational and residential magnetic field exposure and leukemia and central nervous system tumors. *Epidemiology* 8:384–89

19. Forssén UM, Ahlbom A, Feychting M. 2002. Relative contribution of residential and occupational magnetic field exposure over twenty-four hours among people living close to and far from a power line. *Bioelectromagnetics* 23:239–44

20. Forssén UM, Feychting M, Rutqvist LE, Floderus B, Ahlbom A. 2000. Occupational and residential magnetic field exposure and breast cancer in females. *Epidemiology* 11:24–29

20b. Forssén UM, Rutqvist LE, Ahlbom A, Feychting M. 2005. Occupational magnetic fields and female breast cancer: a case-control study using Swedish population registers and new exposure data. *Am. J. Epidemiol.* In press

21. Goldstein LS, Kheifets L, van Deventer E, Repacholi M. 2003. Comments on *Long-Term Exposure of Emicro-Pim1 Transgenic Mice to 898.4 MHz Microwaves Does Not Increase Lymphoma Incidence* by Utteridge et al. (Radiat. Res. 158, 357–364 2002). *Radiat. Res.* 159:275–76

22. Goldstein LS, Kheifets L, Van Deventer E, Repacholi M. 2003. Further comments on *Long-Term Exposure of Emu-Pim1 Transgenic Mice to 898.4 MHz Microwaves Does Not Increase Lymphoma Incidence* by Utteridge et al. (Radiat. Res. 158, 357–364 2002). *Radiat. Res.* 159:835

23. Greaves M. 2002. Childhood leukaemia. *BMJ* 324:283–87

24. Greenland S. 2005. Multiple-bias modelling for analysis of observational data. *J. R. Stat. Soc.: Series A.* In press

25. Greenland S, Sheppard AR, Kaune WT, Poole C, Kelsh MA. 2000. A pooled analysis of magnetic fields, wire codes, and childhood leukemia. Childhood Leukemia-EMF Study Group. *Epidemiology* 11:624–34

26. Hakansson N, Gustavsson P, Sastre A, Floderus B. 2003. Occupational exposure to extremely low frequency magnetic fields and mortality from cardiovascular disease. *Am. J. Epidemiol.* 158:534–42

27. Hardell L, Hallquist A, Mild KH, Carlberg M, Pahlson A, Lilja A. 2002. Cellular and cordless telephones and the risk for brain tumours. *Eur. J. Cancer Prev.* 11:377–86

28. Hardell L, Nasman A, Pahlson A, Hallquist A, Hansson Mild K. 1999. Use of cellular telephones and the risk for brain tumours: a case-control study. *Int. J. Oncol.* 15:113–16

29. Hatch EE, Linet MS, Kleinerman RA, Tarone RE, Severson RK, et al. 1998. Association between childhood acute lymphoblastic leukemia and use of electrical appliances during pregnancy and childhood. *Epidemiology* 9:234–45

30. Health Counc. Neth. 2002. *Mobile telephones. An evaluation of health effects.* http://www.gr.nl/pdf.php?ID=377

31. Hocking B, Gordon IR, Grain HL, Hatfield GE. 1996. Cancer incidence and mortality and proximity to TV towers. *Med. J. Aust.* 165:601–5

32. Huuskonen H, Lindbohm ML, Juutilainen J. 1998. Teratogenic and reproductive effects of low-frequency magnetic fields. *Mutat. Res.* 410:167–83

33. IARC. 1984. *Polynuclear Aromatic Compounds.* Vol. 34, Part 3: *Industrial Exposures in Aluminium Production, Coal Gasification, Coke Production, Iron and Steel Founding.* Lyon: IARC. 219 pp.

34. IARC. 2002. *Non-Ionizing Radiation.* Vol. 80, Part 1: *Static and Extremely Low-Frequency (ELF) Electric and Magnetic Fields.* Lyon: IARC. 429 pp.

35. ICNIRP. 1998. Guidelines for limiting exposure to time-varying electric, magnetic, and electromagnetic fields. *Health Physics* 74:494–522

36. IEGMP Indep. Expert Group Mob. Phones (Chairman: Sir William Stewart). 2000. *Mobile phones and health.* http://www.iegmp.org.uk/

37. Inskip PD, Tarone RE, Hatch EE, Wilcosky TC, Shapiro WR, et al. 2001. Cellular-telephone use and brain tumors. *N. Engl. J. Med.* 344:79–86

38. Johansen C, Boice J Jr, McLaughlin J, Olsen J. 2001. Cellular telephones and cancer—a nationwide cohort study in Denmark. *J. Natl. Cancer Inst.* 93:203–7

39. Johansen C, Boice JD Jr, McLaughlin JK, Christensen HC, Olsen JH. 2002. Mobile phones and malignant melanoma of the eye. *Br. J. Cancer* 86:348–49

40. Johansen C, Feychting M, Moller M, Arnsbo P, Ahlbom A, Olsen JH. 2002. Risk of severe cardiac arrhythmia in male utility workers: a nationwide Danish cohort study. *Am. J. Epidemiol.* 156:857–61

41. Johansen C, Olsen JH. 1998. Mortality from amyotrophic lateral sclerosis, other chronic disorders, and electric shocks among utility workers. *Am. J. Epidemiol.* 148:362–68

42. Kavet R, Zaffanella LE. 2002. Contact voltage measured in residences: implications to the association between magnetic fields and childhood leukemia. *Bioelectromagnetics* 23:464–74

43. Kelsh MA, Kheifets L, Smith R. 2000. The impact of work environment, utility, and sampling design on occupational magnetic field exposure summaries. *Am. Ind. Hyg. Assoc. J.* 61:174–82

44. Kheifets LI. 2001. Electric and magnetic field exposure and brain cancer: a review. *Bioelectromagnetics* 22(Suppl. 5):S120–31

45. Kheifets LI, Afifi AA, Buffler PA, Zhang ZW. 1995. Occupational electric and magnetic field exposure and brain cancer: a meta-analysis. *J. Occup. Environ. Med.* 37:1327–41

46. Kheifets LI, Afifi AA, Buffler PA, Zhang ZW, Matkin CC. 1997. Occupational electric and magnetic field exposure and leukemia. A meta-analysis. *J. Occup. Environ. Med.* 39:1074–91

47. Kheifets LI, Gilbert ES, Sussman SS, Guenel P, Sahl JD, et al. 1999. Comparative analyses of the studies of magnetic fields and cancer in electric utility workers: studies from France, Canada, and the United States. *Occup. Environ. Med.* 56:567–74

48. Kheifets LI, Matkin CC. 1999. Industrialization, electromagnetic fields, and breast cancer risk. *Environ. Health. Perspect.* 107(Suppl. 1):145–54

49. Knave B. 1994. Electric and magnetic fields and health outcomes—an overview. *Scand J. Work Environ. Health* 20(Spec. No.):78–89

50. Kowalczuk CI, Sienkiewicz ZJ, Saunders RD. 1991. *Biological Effects of Exposure to Non-Ionizing Electromagnetic Fields and Radiation. 1. Static Electric and Magnetic Fields.* Didcot, UK: NRPB

51. Lee GM, Neutra RR, Hristova L, Yost M, Hiatt RA. 2002. A nested case-control study of residential and personal magnetic field measures and miscarriages. *Epidemiology* 13:21–31

52. Li DK, Odouli R, Wi S, Janevic T, Golditch I, et al. 2002. A population-based prospective cohort study of personal exposure to magnetic fields during pregnancy and the risk of miscarriage. *Epidemiology* 13:9–20

53. London SJ, Pogoda JM, Hwang KL, Langholz B, Monroe KR, et al. 2003. Residential magnetic field exposure and breast cancer risk: a nested case-control study from a multiethnic cohort in Los Angeles County, California. *Am. J. Epidemiol.* 158:969–80

54. Lönn S, Forssén UM, Vecchia P, Ahlbom A, Feychting M. 2004. Output power levels from mobile phones in relation to the geographic position of the user. *Occup. Environ. Med.* 61:769–72

55. Lönn S, Klaeboe L, Hall P, Mathiesen T, Auvinen A, et al. 2004. Incidence trends of adult primary intracerebral tumors in four Nordic countries. *Int. J. Cancer* 108:450–55

56. Mezei G, Kheifets LI, Nelson LM, Mills KM, Iriye R, Kelsey JL. 2001. Household appliance use and residential exposure to 60-hz magnetic fields. *J. Expo. Anal. Environ. Epidemiol.* 11:41–49

57. Michelozzi P, Capon A, Kirchmayer U, Forastiere F, Biggeri A, et al. 2002. Adult and childhood leukemia near a high-power radio station in Rome, Italy. *Am. J. Epidemiol.* 155:1096–103

58. Muscat JE, Malkin MG, Shore RE, Thompson S, Neugut AI, et al. 2002. Handheld cellular telephones and risk of acoustic neuroma. *Neurology* 58:1304–6

59. Muscat JE, Malkin MG, Thompson S, Shore RE, Stellman SD, et al. 2000. Handheld cellular telephone use and risk of brain cancer. *JAMA* 284:3001–7

60. Navarro EA, Segura J, Portolés M, Gómez-Perretta de Mateo C. 2003. The microwave syndrome: a preliminary study in Spain. *Electromagn. Biol. Med.* 22:161–69

61. Neutra RR, DelPizzo V, Lee GM. 2002. *California EMF Program. An Evaluation of the Possible Risks from Electric and Magnetic Fields (EMFs) from Power Lines, Internal Wiring, Electrical*

Occupations, and Appliances. Oakland, Calif. Dep. Health Serv.

62. NRC. 1997. *Possible Health Effects of Exposure to Residential Electric and Magnetic Fields*. Washington, DC: Natl. Res. Counc., Natl. Acad. Press

63. NRPB. 2001. *ELF Electromagnetic Fields and the Risk of Cancer. Report of an Advisory Group on Non-Ionising Radiation*. Didcot, UK: NRPB. Vol. 12, No. 1

64. NRPB. 2003. *Health Effects from Radiofrequency Electromagnetic Fields. Report of an Independent Advisory Group on Non-Ionizing Radiation*. Didcot, UK: NRPB. Vol. 14, No. 2

65. Oftedal G, Wilen J, Sandstrom M, Mild KH. 2000. Symptoms experienced in connection with mobile phone use. *Occup. Med. (London)* 50:237–45

66. Portier CJ, Wolfe M. 1998. *Assessment of Health Effects from Exposure to Power-Line Frequency Electric and Magnetic Fields*. Washington, DC: NIH

67. Repacholi MH, Basten A, Gebski V, Noonan D, Finnie J, Harris AW. 1997. Lymphomas in E mu-Pim1 transgenic mice exposed to pulsed 900 MHZ electromagnetic fields. *Radiat. Res.* 147:631–40

68. Robert E. 1999. Intrauterine effects of electromagnetic fields—(low frequency, mid-frequency RF, and microwave): review of epidemiologic studies. *Teratology* 59:292–8

69. Ronneberg A. 1995. Mortality and cancer morbidity in workers from an aluminium smelter with prebaked carbon anodes—part I: exposure assessment. *Occup. Environ. Med.* 52:242–49

70. Ronneberg A, Andersen A. 1995. Mortality and cancer morbidity in workers from an aluminium smelter with prebaked carbon anodes—Part II: Cancer morbidity. *Occup. Environ. Med.* 52:250–4

71. Ronneberg A, Haldorsen T, Romundstad P, Andersen A. 1999. Occupational exposure and cancer incidence among workers from an aluminum smelter in western

Norway. *Scand J. Work Environ. Health* 25:207–14

72. Rothman KJ, Loughlin JE, Funch DP, Dreyer NA. 1996. Overall mortality of cellular telephone customers. *Epidemiology* 7:303–5

72a. R. Soc. Can. 1999. *A review of the potential health risks of radiofrequency fields from wireless telecommunication devices. An expert panel report prepared at the request of the Royal Society of Canada for Health Canada*. Ottawa, Ontario: http://www.rsc.ca/english/RFreport.html

73. Sahl J, Mezei G, Kavet R, McMillan A, Silvers A, et al. 2002. Occupational magnetic field exposure and cardiovascular mortality in a cohort of electric utility workers. *Am. J. Epidemiol.* 156:913–18

74. Santini R, Santini P, Danze JM, Le Ruz P, Seigne M. 2002. Investigation on the health of people living near mobile telephone relay stations: Incidence according to distance and sex. *Pathol. Biol. (Paris)* 50:369–73

75. Sastre A, Graham C, Cook MR. 2000. Brain frequency magnetic fields alter cardiac autonomic control mechanisms. *Clin. Neurophysiol.* 111:1942–48

76. Savitz DA, John EM, Kleckner RC. 1990. Magnetic field exposure from electric appliances and childhood cancer. *Am. J. Epidemiol.* 131:763–73

77. Savitz DA, Liao D, Sastre A, Kleckner RC, Kavet R. 1999. Magnetic field exposure and cardiovascular disease mortality among electric utility workers. *Am. J. Epidemiol.* 149:135–42

78. Schoenfeld ER, Leary ES, O'Henderson K, Grimson R, Kabat GC, et al. 2003. Electromagnetic fields and breast cancer on Long Island: a case-control study. *Am. J. Epidemiol.* 158:47–58

79. Sobel E, Davanipour Z, Sulkava R, Erkinjuntti T, Wikstrom J, et al. 1995. Occupations with exposure to electromagnetic fields: a possible risk factor for Alzheimer's disease. *Am. J. Epidemiol.* 142:515–24

80. Sorahan T, Nichols L. 2004. Mortality from cardiovascular disease in relation to magnetic field exposure: findings from a study of UK electricity generation and transmission workers, 1973–1997. *Am. J. Ind. Med.* 45:93–102

81. Spinelli JJ, Band PR, Svirchev LM, Gallagher RP. 1991. Mortality and cancer incidence in aluminum reduction plant workers. *J. Occup. Med.* 33:1150–55

82. Stang A, Anastassiou G, Ahrens W, Bromen K, Bornfeld N, Jockel KH. 2001. The possible role of radiofrequency radiation in the development of uveal melanoma. *Epidemiology* 12:7–12

83. Stevens RG, Davis S, Thomas DB, Anderson LE, Wilson BW. 1992. Electric power, pineal function, and the risk of breast cancer. *FASEB. J.* 6:853–60

84. Sussman SS, Kheifets LI. 1996. Re: *Adult Leukemia Risk and Personal Appliance Use: A Preliminary Study. Am. J. Epidemiol.* 143:743–44

85. Swed. Radiat. Prot. Auth. 2003. *Recent research on mobile telephony and cancer and other selected biological effects: first annual report from SSI's Independent Expert Group on Electromagnetic Fields.* Dnr 00/1854/02. http://www.ssi.se/english/EMF_exp_Eng_2003.pdf

86. Deleted in proof

87. Thommesen G, Bjolseth P. 1992. *Static and Low Frequency Magnetic Fields in Norwegian Alloy and Electrolysis Plants.* Oslo: Natl. Inst. Radiat. Hyg. In Norwegian

88. Utteridge TD, Gebski V, Finnie JW, Vernon-Roberts B, Kuchel TR. 2002. Long-term exposure of E-mu-Pim1 transgenic mice to 898.4 MHz microwaves does not increase lymphoma incidence. *Radiat. Res.* 158:357–64

89. Warren HG, Prevatt AA, Daly KA, Antonelli PJ. 2003. Cellular telephone use and risk of intratemporal facial nerve tumor. *Laryngoscope* 113:663–67

90. Wertheimer N, Leeper E. 1979. Electrical wiring configurations and childhood cancer. *Am. J. Epidemiol.* 109:273–84

91. Zaffanella L, Kalton GW. 1998. *Survey of Personal Magnetic Field Exposure. Phase II: 1000-Person Survey*: EMF RAPID, Program Engineering Project #6. Oak Ridge, TN: Lockheed Martin Energy Syst.

92. Zmirou D. 2001. Mobile phones, their base stations, and health. Current state-of-knowledge and recommendations. *Rep. French Health Dir.* (Chairman: D Zmirou), Paris, Dir. Générale de la Santé. http://www.sante.gouv.fr/htm/dossiers/telephon_mobil/teleph_uk.htm

Annu. Rev. Public Health 2005. 26:191–212
doi: 10.1146/annurev.publhealth.26.021304.144536
First published online as a Review in Advance on December 8, 2004

THE PUBLIC HEALTH IMPACT OF PRION DISEASES[1]

Ermias D. Belay and Lawrence B. Schonberger

*Division of Viral and Rickettsial Diseases, National Center for Infectious Diseases,
Centers for Disease Control and Prevention, Atlanta, Georgia 30333;
email: EBelay@cdc.gov*

Key Words   transmissible spongiform encephalopathy, Creutzfeldt-Jakob disease, variant Creutzfeldt-Jakob disease, bovine spongiform encephalopathy, chronic wasting disease

■ **Abstract**   Several prion disease–related human health risks from an exogenous source can be identified in the United States, including the iatrogenic transmission of Creutzfeldt-Jakob disease (CJD), the possible occurrence of variant CJD (vCJD), and potential zoonotic transmission of chronic wasting disease (CWD). Although cross-species transmission of prion diseases seems to be limited by an apparent "species barrier," the occurrence of bovine spongiform encephalopathy (BSE) and its transmission to humans indicate that animal prion diseases can pose a significant public health risk. Recent reports of secondary person-to-person spread of vCJD via blood products and detection of vCJD transmission in a patient heterozygous at codon 129 further illustrate the potential public health impacts of BSE.

INTRODUCTION

Prion diseases, also known as transmissible spongiform encephalopathies (TSEs), are a group of animal and human brain diseases that are uniformly fatal and often characterized by a long incubation period and a multifocal neuropathologic picture of neuronal loss, spongiform changes, and astrogliosis (3). Investigators believe the etiologic agents of TSEs are abnormal conformers of a host-encoded cellular protein known as the prion protein. Prion diseases do not characteristically elicit an immune response by the host, and the mechanism of brain damage is poorly understood. However, progressive neuronal accumulation of the disease-associated prions may damage neurons directly, and diminished availability of the normal prion protein may interfere with the presumed neuroprotective effect of the normal prion protein, contributing to the underlying neurodegenerative process.

---

[1]The U.S. Government has the right to retain a nonexclusive, royalty-free license in and to any copyright covering this paper.

Prion diseases attracted much attention and public concern after an outbreak of bovine spongiform encephalopathy (BSE) occurred among cattle in many European countries and scientific evidence indicated the foodborne transmission of BSE to humans (67, 74). Variant Creutzfeldt-Jakob disease (vCJD), the new form of human disease resulting from BSE transmission, is distinguished from the classic form of CJD by the much younger median age of affected patients, its clinical and neuropathologic features, and the biochemical properties of the protease-resistant prion protein (5, 7, 25, 72). The classic form of CJD was first reported in the 1920s, decades before the first BSE cases were identified in the mid-1980s (3). About 10%–15% of CJD cases occur as a familial disease associated with pathogenic mutations of the prion protein gene, and about 85% of classic CJD cases occur as a sporadic disease with no recognizable pattern of transmission. The stable, almost predictable, occurrence of the disease in many areas of the world, primarily in the elderly, led to the speculation that sporadic CJD may occur from de novo spontaneous generation of the self-replicating prions, presumably facilitated by somatic random mutations. Beginning in the 1970s, iatrogenic person-to-person transmission of the CJD agent was reported in a small percentage of CJD patients (12). This iatrogenic spread involved the use of contaminated corneal and dura mater grafts, neurosurgical equipment, and cadaver-derived human growth hormone. At present, the number of iatrogenic CJD cases is on the decline as a result of public health preventive measures implemented as the various modes of transmission were identified.

In addition to BSE and iatrogenically transmitted CJD, another prion disease of potential public health concern in the United States is chronic wasting disease (CWD) of deer and elk. CWD in free-ranging cervids has been endemic in a tricorner area of Colorado, Nebraska, and Wyoming, and new foci of infection have been detected in others parts of the United States and the Canadian province of Saskatchewan (6).

ETIOLOGIC AGENT OF PRION DISEASES

Most of the earliest studies done to identify the agents of TSEs focused on describing the causative agent of scrapie, a prion disease of sheep known to have been occurring in Europe for centuries. Lack of suitable laboratory models or cell culture systems had limited the efforts to characterize the scrapie agent; however, the successful transmission of scrapie to mice in 1961 greatly facilitated the identification and characterization of the scrapie agent (63). Several theories had been proposed to describe its characteristics. Owing to the transmissibility of the agent, retention of its infectivity after filtration, and the long incubation period before disease onset, scrapie was thought to be caused by a slow virus. The possibility that the agent could be a viroid was considered also. However, no viral particles or disease-specific nucleic acids were identified in association with scrapie infection (1, 62). Resistance of the scrapie agent to radiation, nucleases, and standard sterilization and disinfection agents and its inactivation by procedures that modify proteins led to the suggestion that the scrapie agent is not a virus but, instead, might be composed primarily of a protein (1). In 1966, Alper et al. suggested the possibility that the scrapie agent could replicate in the absence of nucleic acids. Pattison & Jones also investigated this possibility and suggested that the scrapie agent might be a basic protein or associated with such a protein, thus igniting a controversy among many of their contemporaries (62). In 1967, Griffith carefully outlined the potential pathways by which such a protein agent could support its own replication (38).

Although the protein-only hypothesis was considered almost heretical, Griffith downplayed the fear that the existence of a protein agent would cause the whole theoretical structure of molecular biology to come tumbling down. His proposal that scrapie could arise spontaneously from a host gene was later challenged by the fact that scrapie spread among sheep within a herd, indicating the infectious nature of the disease. However, his spontaneous host gene theory persisted as an explanation for the occurrence of most sporadic CJD cases and familial human prion diseases. Subsequent studies by Prusiner et al. (65) demonstrated a hydrophobic protein to be an essential component of the scrapie agent, but no specific polypeptide was identified. To underscore the requirement of a protein for scrapie infectivity, Prusiner (63) introduced the term prion in 1982 to describe the proteinaceous infectious particle. In the same year, Prusiner et al. (64) and Bolton et al. (10) reported the major success of the purification of scrapie prion and the demonstration of its relatively high resistance to proteinase K treatment.

Soon after the discovery of prions, their similarity with a normal cellular protein, which is a structural component of cell membranes, was identified (59). This cellular protein was given the name prion protein. In humans, the prion protein is encoded by genes located on the short arm of chromosome 20. Although the exact function of this protein is unknown, a protein found in such abundance in mammals, particularly in neurons, could have multiple functional roles. Several putative functions of the prion protein have been proposed, including supporting neuronal synaptic activity, binding copper, and interacting with other cell-surface proteins to provide neuroprotective functions (50). Prions are primarily distinguished from the cellular prion protein by their three-dimensional structure. The cellular prion protein is predominantly composed of the α-helix structure and is almost devoid of β-sheet, whereas about 43% of scrapie prions are composed of β-sheet (60). Other distinguishing characteristics of prions include their resistance to inactivation by proteolytic enzymes, conventional disinfectants, and standard sterilization methods (63). Prions are abnormal conformers of the cellular prion protein, the presence of which appears to be a prerequisite for the replication and propagation of prions (14). Although the exact mechanism of prion replication remains unclear, the agent is believed to promote the conversion of the cellular prion protein into the abnormal conformer by an autocatalytic or other unidentified process (66, 68).

Prions causing TSEs in different species and in some instances different disease phenotypes in the same species can be distinguished by several laboratory methods, indicating the existence of different prion strains (13, 61). In the absence of disease-specific genetic material, it is unclear how strain differences are encoded by different prions. The three-dimensional structure of prions has been suggested as a site where strain differences reside (68).

IATROGENIC CREUTZFELDT-JAKOB DISEASE

The iatrogenic transmission of CJD was first reported by Duffy et al. in 1974 (33) in a 55-year-old patient who developed autopsy-confirmed CJD 18 months after receipt of a corneal graft. Autopsy confirmed that the donor of the corneal graft also died as a result of CJD. Since then, one patient each with a probable and a possible risk of CJD transmission via corneal graft has been reported from Germany and Japan, respectively (40, 48). The German patient died at 46 years of age, 30 years after receipt of the corneal graft. The CJD transmission in this patient was considered probable primarily because her CJD illness, although, typical for the disease, it was not confirmed by neuropathologic testing. The donor of the cornea, however, died as a result of autopsy-confirmed CJD. In the Japanese case, the recipient died of confirmed CJD, but no information was available on the donor of the corneal graft.

Three additional cases of CJD (two from the United States and one from Japan) in corneal graft recipients have been reported but not published. All three cases occurred independently of each other, and investigations indicated no evidence of CJD in the cornea donors. Because of the large number of corneal transplantations carried out each year, particularly among the elderly, it is expected that sporadic CJD, not causally linked with the corneal grafts, will occur among this population.

Creutzfeldt-Jakob Disease Associated with Neurosurgical Equipment

In 1977, two unusually young patients aged 17 and 23 years were reported to have acquired CJD 16–20 months after having a stereotactic electroencephalographic (EEG) procedure in which depth electrodes were used that had been implanted 2–3 months earlier on a patient who subsequently died of autopsy-confirmed CJD (8). The heat-sensitive EEG electrodes were cleaned with benzene and disinfected with 70% ethanol and formaldehyde vapor between uses. Contamination of the EEG electrodes was demonstrated >2 years after their original use by experimentally implanting the electrodes into a brain of a chimpanzee who became ill 18 months after implantation (36).

Worldwide, four CJD patients causally linked with exposure to contaminated neurosurgical instruments have been identified (72, 75). Three of these cases occurred in the 1950s in the United Kingdom, and the patients' CJD illnesses were confirmed by neuropathology testing of autopsy brain tissues. Their neurosurgical procedures were performed within one month of craniotomy procedures in other patients who subsequently died of CJD. The fourth patient was reported in 1980 from France. The absence of recent CJD cases associated with a neurosurgical procedure was believed to be due to advances in standard hospital instrument sterilization procedures. Although these advances well may have prevented CJD transmission via contaminated neurosurgical instruments, several laboratory studies indicated that current standard sterilization procedures may not completely inactivate the CJD agent (26). Recent investigations of possible CJD transmissions via neurosurgical procedures in two U.S. patients illustrate the difficulty in identifying and linking each patient with exposure to potentially contaminated instruments used on a possible index CJD patient many years earlier. In both case-patients, closure of the hospitals and unavailability of medical records precluded an accurate assessment of the CJD risk associated with their past neurosurgical procedures.

Neurosurgical instruments used on patients suspected of having CJD should be decontaminated by using procedures recommended for reprocessing such instruments (26). Various hospital infection control professionals have consulted the Centers for Disease Control and Prevention (CDC) after CJD was confirmed in patients who underwent neurosurgical procedures with instruments that were subsequently used on other patients before being reprocessed with the appropriate CJD decontamination methods. These episodes have created several ethical and legal dilemmas, including whether potentially exposed patients should or should not be informed about any possible risk. In a minority of these instances, hospital personnel made a decision to inform the patients exposed to neurosurgical instruments that were not cleaned using the recommended CJD decontamination methods. The decision-making process may be further complicated if the contaminated instruments are mixed with other instruments during reprocessing, making identification of potentially exposed patients almost impossible. The circumstances surrounding such episodes vary and are best handled by a local hospital review board consisting of pertinent physicians, ethicists, hospital administrators, infection control professionals, and possibly others. Greater emphasis should be placed on identifying ways of preventing such episodes from occurring again. One recommended method of prevention is to consider as potentially "CJD contaminated" any neurosurgical instruments used on patients who undergo a craniotomy procedure for a condition not clearly diagnosed before the procedure (26). Those instruments could either be reprocessed using the methods recommended for CJD-contaminated instruments or quarantined until the diagnosis is clarified.

A local hospital review board may wish to consider the following factors while deliberating on the possible notification of potentially exposed patients: (a) whether autoclaving or heat was used to reprocess the instruments in question (standard autoclaving procedures seem to be superior to conventional chemical disinfection); (b) reprocessing potentially CJD-contaminated instruments numerous times using standard autoclaving methods may completely eliminate infectivity; (c) whether potentially contaminated instruments were kept moist throughout the neurosurgical procedure (drying of tissues on surgical instruments may interfere with complete inactivation of the CJD agent); (d) the ability to identify potentially contaminated neurosugical instruments and to link them to potentially exposed patients; (*e*) the potential negative impact of informing patients about possible exposure to a fatal, untreatable brain disease; (*f*) no practical CJD-specific test is currently available to screen live patients for prion infection; and (*g*) no prophylactic treatment is currently available to mitigate the risk of CJD.

Human Growth Hormone–Associated Creutzfeldt-Jakob Disease

In 1985, three U.S. patients aged 20–34 years were reported to have developed CJD after receipt of pituitary-derived human growth hormone (hGH) through the National Hormone and Pituitary Program (NHPP) (17, 37, 46). The patients received the hormone between 1963 and 1980 for growth failure secondary to hGH deficiency, and their identification led to the discontinuation of hGH use in the NHPP. A follow-up study was initiated of 6272 of the estimated total of 7700 patients who had received hGH as part of the NHPP (56). As of April 2004, 26 of the total estimated NHPP patients, including 21 of the originally identified study cohort, developed CJD. All 26 patients began their hormone treatment before a size exclusion chromatography purifying step was introduced in the extraction process in 1977 (56). The median incubation period of the U.S. hGH-associated CJD cases was estimated at 20.5 years (range, 10–30).

Worldwide, ~165 hGH-associated CJD patients were reported, including ~89 in France, 41 in the United Kingdom, and 5 in New Zealand (56, 72, 73). The cases in New Zealand and Brazil are linked to the U.S. outbreak because the patients received hGH imported from the United States. In the United States, through 2003, approximately 1 in 100 hGH recipients who began treatment before 1977 developed CJD. The risk of hGH-associated CJD varies by country primarily because of differences in the pituitary donor selection criteria and methods employed in hormone extraction and purification. The proportion of recipients developing CJD in the United Kingdom is ~2 times higher and in France is >5 times higher than that in the pre-1977 recipients in the United States (12, 72). The lower median incubation period for cases in France (10 years) and the United Kingdom (16 years) suggests that the hGH used in these countries may have contained a higher infectious dose of the CJD agent. Between 1963 and 1985, at least 140 infected pituitary glands may have been processed in the United States and randomly distributed among many hGH lots (34). The hGH-associated CJD outbreak may not completely resolve for many more years because of the relatively young age at which most recipients were treated and the long incubation period associated with TSE exposure.

Dura Mater Graft-Associated Creutzfeldt-Jakob Disease

Transmission of CJD via dura mater grafts was first reported in 1987 in a 28-year-old woman from the United States who developed the disease 19 months after a craniotomy procedure involving implantation of Lyodura, a brand of dura mater graft processed by B. Braun Melsungen AG of Germany (18, 69). In contrast to the processing procedures used by this German company, U.S. dura processors avoided commingling of dural grafts from different donors and kept records to facilitate identification and tracing of donors of each dural graft (19). The unusually young age of the 1987 U.S. case-patient, the previous association of CJD transmission with nervous tissue exposure, and the differences in processing of Lyodura compared with other dural grafts convinced public health investigators about the probable causal link of the patient's CJD illness with the Lyodura graft. In May 1987, because of this probable causal link, the Lyodura manufacturer revised its procedures for collecting and processing dura mater grafts to reduce the risk of CJD transmission. Commingling of dural grafts from different donors was discontinued and a sodium hydroxide treatment step was instituted to inactivate the CJD agent. Subsequent to widespread publication of this first case, many other Lyodura-associated CJD cases were reported worldwide, including in Germany, Italy, Japan, New Zealand, Spain, and the United Kingdom, and a second case was reported in the United States (20, 21, 47, 49, 53, 54, 57, 77).

By 2003, ~136 dura mater graft–associated CJD cases were reported worldwide (24, 72). Approximately 70% of these cases occurred in Japan, and over 90% of the cases were associated with receipt of Lyodura produced before May 1987. Japan has an unusually high number of the cases, presumably owing to the more frequent use of Lyodura in that country. On the basis of the outbreak in Japan, which appears to be ongoing, the estimated minimum risk of CJD among recipients of Lyodura within 17 years of implantation was 1 case per 1250 recipients (24). As of 2003, the median incubation period of 97 dura mater graft–associated CJD cases in Japan was about 122 months (range, 14 to 275).

In addition to the two Lyodura-associated CJD cases, two other dural graft–associated CJD cases have been reported in the United States. One of these cases was in a 39-year-old woman who had autopsy-confirmed CJD with illness onset in June 1998, 6 years after implantation of Tutoplast, a brand of dura mater graft produced by Pfrimmer-Viggo of Germany (39). The patient's young age, the time of dura implantation to CJD onset, and the report of unexplained neurologic disease in the dura mater donor indicated that the Tutoplast graft was the most likely source of CJD in the patient. This case represents the first clearly identified association of CJD with Tutoplast despite the use of >500,000 of these grafts worldwide since the early 1970s. The company's avoidance of commingling dural grafts from different donors likely played an important role in the absence of more reported CJD cases associated with Tutoplast. The fourth U.S. dural graft–associated CJD occurred in 1995 in a 72-year-old man (31). The investigation of this patient's illness indicated that the association with the dural graft used in this patient 54 months before his CJD onset may have been coincidental rather than causal.

After Japan announced the identification of 43 dural graft–associated CJD cases, Canada, Japan, and some European countries banned the use of human dura mater grafts in neurosurgical procedures (22). In the United States, the Food and Drug

Administration's (FDA) Transmissible Spongiform Encephalopathy Advisory Committee recommended that the decision to use dura mater grafts should be left to the treating neurosurgeon (24). However, the committee recognized the inherent risk of CJD transmission via dura mater grafts and encouraged the use of other alternatives whenever possible. It also recommended additional preventive measures to increase the safety margin of dural grafts processed in the United States. After the committee's recommendation, the number of dural grafts distributed for use in the United States declined to an estimated 900 grafts in 2002 from about 4500 grafts in 1997 (24).

BOVINE SPONGIFORM ENCEPHALOPATHY

United Kingdom

BSE was first recognized in the United Kingdom in 1986, where it caused a large outbreak among cattle (28, 67). The leading hypothesis for the origin of BSE is cross-species transmission of scrapie to cattle via the feeding of meat-and-bone meal that was contaminated by the inclusion of scrapie-infected sheep parts. Spontaneous occurrence of the disease in cattle, much like sporadic CJD in humans, has also been hypothesized. Although the origin of BSE remains controversial, it is widely accepted that the practice of using rendered BSE-infected carcasses for cattle feed had amplified the outbreak until a ruminant feed ban was instituted in 1988 (7, 28, 67). Because of concerns about cross-contamination of cattle feed with prohibited material intended for other species, a specified bovine offal ban (also known as specified risk material ban) was introduced in 1990 to remove the known infectious parts of cattle from all animal feed. A dramatic decline in the BSE outbreak was registered in response to these feed bans. Although the number of cattle confirmed with BSE in the United Kingdom as of 2003 is >180,000, the total estimated number of U.K. cattle potentially infected with BSE is in excess of 2 million (67). Approximately 750,000 BSE-infected cattle were estimated to have been slaughtered between 1980 and 1996 (35) and potentially consumed by millions of U.K. residents. A more recent statistical analysis incorporating data from surveillance of asymptomatic cattle >30 months of age indicated that the number of BSE-infected cattle slaughtered for human consumption in the United Kingdom may have been about twice as high as the previous estimate (32).

As the U.K. BSE outbreak progressed, several important public health preventive measures were implemented before and after evidence of BSE transmission to humans surfaced in 1996. These measures included a 1989 specified risk material ban for human food, a 1996 prohibition of the processing of cattle ≥30 months old for human food, and total ban on the feeding of mammalian protein to any farmed animals (67). The measures introduced in 1996 were intended to contain the BSE outbreak aggressively by keeping potentially BSE-contaminated feed off the farms and to remove as many BSE-infected materials as possible from the human food supply system. Unfortunately, BSE continued to be detected, albeit at a very low rate, in cattle born after the 1996 ban. The source of BSE infection in these cattle is not fully understood. Exposure to residual or imported contaminated feed or feed ingredients and unidentified nonfeed sources of transmission (e.g., maternal transmission) have been proposed as possible explanations for the occurrence of BSE among cattle born after the 1996 ban (67). Exposure to residual BSE-contaminated feed is the most favored hypothesis because as little as 10 mg of infected material has been shown to be infectious in experimental animal models.

In Other European Countries

In 1989, BSE was identified for the first time outside of the United Kingdom in the Republic of Ireland. Because many other countries, mostly within Europe, had imported cattle and meat-and-bone meal from the United Kingdom, the spread of BSE to these countries was not surprising. By the end of 1999, BSE among domestic cattle was detected in seven other European countries (Portugal and Switzerland in 1990; France in 1991; Belgium, Luxembourg, and The Netherlands in 1997; and Liechtenstein in 1998). During 2000 and 2002, indigenous BSE was reported in 11 additional European countries and, for the first time outside of Europe, in Japan and Israel (Table 1). Improved BSE surveillance particularly in the European Union contributed to the rapid increase in the number of countries with confirmed BSE. Currently, BSE surveillance in European Union countries targets all downer (nonambulatory) cattle, fallen stock (cattle who die of nonspecific causes), cattle >24 months of age slaughtered on an emergency basis, and all slaughtered cattle >30 months of age (67). The large volume of cattle tissues in these surveillance schemes are tested using rapid BSE assays, several of which were evaluated and licensed by the European Commission (58).

North America

For years, the North American continent was considered to be free of indigenous BSE primarily because of the coordinated and proactive measures taken by Canada, Mexico, and the United States to prevent introduction of the disease (45). These measures had included banning the importation of cattle and cattle products from countries known to have BSE or to be at risk of BSE and institution of ruminant feed bans, which were introduced in 1997 in Canada and the United States. BSE in a beef cow imported from the United Kingdom had been identified in 1993 in the province of Alberta, Canada. Members of the herd of the positive cow were culled and incinerated.

On May 20, 2003, BSE was confirmed in an approximately six-year-old Canadian-born Angus cow from a herd in Alberta, heralding the first report of a confirmed indigenous BSE case in North America (15). The cow had been condemned when it was presented for slaughter in January 2003 because of pneumonia. Meat from this cow did not get into the human food supply, but parts of the animal were rendered for animal feed, most likely poultry and pet food. Relevant cattle herds with potential identified risk in the trace-back and trace-forward investigations were quarantined, culled, and tested for BSE. No additional BSE cases were detected. The source of the BSE-contaminated feed likely responsible

TABLE 1   Countries with reported number of bovine spongiform encephalopathy (BSE) cases by year of first detection[a]

Country	Number of BSE cases[b]	Year BSE first detected[c]
Austria	1	2001
Finland	1	2001
Greece	1	2001
Israel	1	2002
Liechtenstein	2	1998
Luxembourg	2	1997
Canada[d]	3	1993
Slovenia	5	2001
Japan	11	2001
Czech Republic	12	2001
Denmark	14	1992
Slovakia	15	2001
Poland	16	2002
Netherlands	76	1997
Italy	117	1994
Belgium	126	1997
Germany	337	1992
Spain	462	2000
Switzerland	455	1990
Portugal	909	1990
France	914	1991
Ireland	1435	1989
United Kingdom	183,972	1986

[a]BSE cases reported to the Office International des Epizooties as of August 23, 2004; data for the United Kingdom are as of June 30, 2004 (http://www.oie.int/eng/info/en_esb.htm).

[b]Because BSE surveillance methods and testing requirements vary by country, the number of reported cases may not be comparable among the different countries.

[c]Year first BSE was detected in imported or domestic cattle.

[d]One of the BSE-positive cows was identified in the United States but was later confirmed to have been imported from Canada.

for the Canadian BSE case was not clearly identified. However, the possibility was proposed that rendered cohorts of the 1993 imported BSE cow may have been the source of infection. Rendered parts of the 1993 cohort may have entered the Alberta feed system in greater volume than it did elsewhere in Canada (15). In response to the detection of BSE in the cow, Canadian authorities implemented additional preventive measures, including a specified risk material ban for humans and increased surveillance for BSE.

Almost immediately, the identification of a native BSE case in Canada raised concern about the possible occurrence of BSE in the United States because of the continuous flow of cattle and cattle products across the U.S.-Canadian border. On the basis of the commercial flow of cattle, possible extension of BSE into the northwestern United States, rather than eastern Canada, had been suspected (15). On December 23, 2003, seven months after the identification of indigenous BSE in Canada, the U.S. Department of Agriculture (USDA) announced the preliminary diagnosis of BSE in a 6.5-year-old nonambulatory cow that was slaughtered for human food on December 9th of that year (25). On December 25th, the BSE diagnosis was confirmed by an international reference laboratory in Weybridge, England. The USDA's investigation traced the birth of the cow to a farm in Alberta, Canada. DNA testing later confirmed the Canadian origin of the cow. At the time of slaughter, meat from the BSE-positive cow had been released for human consumption, but tissues considered to be at high risk for BSE transmission (e.g., brain, spinal cord, and small intestine) were considered unfit for human consumption and, thus, sent to be rendered for other uses (e.g., to produce nonruminant animal feed) (25). The USDA issued a recall of beef from cattle slaughtered in the same plant on the same day as the BSE-positive cow. Meat products manufactured from the recalled meat were distributed primarily in Oregon and Washington, with smaller quantities distributed in California, Idaho, Montana, and Nevada. All known potentially infectious rendered products from the BSE-positive cow were located and removed from commercial distribution.

In response to the identification of BSE, the USDA announced additional safeguards to further minimize the risk of human exposure to BSE in the United States (25). These safeguards included prohibition of the use of downer cattle for human food, removal of specified risk materials from cows ≥30 months old, and withholding of the USDA "inspected and passed" mark until negative BSE results are received for any cattle tested. The USDA also proposed the implementation of a national identification system to track animals of various species through the livestock marketing chain and announced its enhancement of current BSE surveillance efforts.

VARIANT CREUTZFELDT-JAKOB DISEASE

BSE captured worldwide attention because of its impact on the farming industry and international trade and, more importantly, because strong evidence indicated its transmission to humans, causing a variant form of CJD (72, 74). The cross-species transmission of BSE was heralded by the identification in the United Kingdom of a BSE-like disease in zoo animals beginning in the late 1980s and in domestic cats beginning in 1990 (28). This resulted in the institution of national CJD surveillance in the United Kingdom, which detected an unusual clustering of ten young patients (median age, 28 years) with a unique clinical and neuropathologic profile (74). The unusually young age of the patients and their clinicopathologic homogeneity led U.K. researchers to suspect that the cases may represent an emergence of a new form of CJD resulting from BSE transmission to humans. The occurrence of this variant form of CJD (vCJD) was announced in 1996, approximately nine years after the identification of BSE in the United Kingdom. Absence of similar cases in other countries with comparable surveillance programs, their continued occurrence almost exclusively in the United Kingdom, and additional laboratory studies further strengthened the causal link between vCJD and BSE. As of November 1, 2004, a total of 151 vCJD cases had been reported from the United Kingdom (30). In addition, three cases (one each from Canada, Ireland, and the United States) among persons with potential BSE exposure in the United Kingdom because of their past U.K. residence, 8 vCJD cases from France, and 1 case from Italy have been identified (5, 7, 27).

Clinical Features

The age distribution of vCJD patients is strikingly different from that of classic CJD patients (Figure 1). Over 50% of vCJD patients died before 30 years of age, whereas only <0.2% of U.S. noniatrogenic CJD patients die before this unusually young age of 30 years. The median age at death of vCJD patients is 28 years compared with 68 years for classic U.S. CJD patients (25). In addition to differences in the age groups affected, vCJD patients also differ from classic CJD patients in the progression of clinical signs, illness duration, magnetic resonance imaging (MRI) findings, and neuropathologic lesions (Table 2) (11, 72). Characteristically, the earliest clinical manifestations in vCJD patients include psychiatric symptoms such as anxiety, depression, and withdrawal. The development of frank neurologic signs, such as myoclonus and extrapyramidal dysfunction, is often delayed for several months after illness onset. The most striking early neurologic sign in some vCJD patients is persistent dysesthesia or paresthesia (5, 7, 72). The characteristic EEG finding of periodic triphasic complexes seen in most classic CJD patients has not been reported in any of the vCJD cases to date. However, a diagnostic MRI finding of an abnormal, symmetrical, high signal intensity in the posterior thalamus, relative to that of other deep and cortical gray matter, was reported in about 87% of vCJD patients (29). In the presence of typical neurologic signs and progression, this MRI picture, designated the pulvinar sign, is considered to be highly indicative of a vCJD diagnosis. In addition, the duration of illness for vCJD patients (median, 13–14 months) is more prolonged than that for classic CJD patients (median, 4–5 months).

Neuropathologic Features

A final confirmatory diagnosis of vCJD requires histopathologic or immunodiagnostic testing (e.g., Western blot and immunohistochemistry) of brain tissues

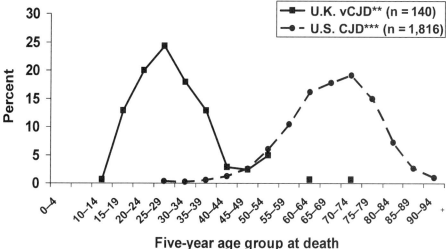

Five-year age group at death

* Excludes blood transfusion–associated vCJD and pituitary hormone- or dural graft–associated CJD

** U.K. vCJD deaths, including U.K.-related nonresident cases, 1995–2003 (R.G. Will, personal communication)

*** U.S. CJD deaths, 1995–2001.

Figure 1   Percent distribution, by age group, of noniatrogenic U.K. vCJD and U.S. CJD deaths, 1995–2003.

preferably obtained at autopsy. Frozen brain tissues are needed for Western blot testing of the protease-resistant prion protein, but immunohistochemical analysis can be done on fixed brain tissues. In addition to the neuropathologic lesions of spongiosis and neuronal loss typical for most human prion diseases, the neuropathologic findings in vCJD are distinguished by the presence of numerous deposits of kuru-type amyloid plaques that are surrounded by a halo of spongiform changes. These daisy-like amyloid deposits are designated florid plaques (44). Marked diffuse accumulation of the protease-resistant prion protein can be demonstrated in many areas of the brain by immunohistochemical staining. For some patients, immunohistochemical analysis of tonsilar biopsy tissue was used to make a premortem diagnosis of vCJD (41, 42). Prion fragments can be detected easily in the tonsils, lymph nodes, spleen, and appendix of vCJD patients but not in those of classic CJD patients (71).

Codon 129 Homozygosity for Methionine

Except for a patient with preclinical vCJD related to bloodborne transmission, all vCJD patients tested to date have been homozygous for methionine at the polymorphic codon 129 of the human prion protein gene (25, 72). Although the scientific basis for this almost exclusive occurrence of vCJD in this subgroup of the population is unknown, investigators have suggested that methionine homozygosity may be associated with a shorter incubation period, younger age distribution, and

TABLE 2   Clinical and pathologic characteristics distinguishing variant Creutzfeldt-Jakob disease (vCJD) in the United Kingdom (U.K.) from classic CJD in the United States (U.S.), 1979–2001[a]

Characteristic	vCJD, U.K.	Classic CJD, U.S.
Median age at death (years)	28 (range, 14–74)	68 (range, 23–97)[b]
Median illness duration (months)	13–14	4–5
Clinical presentation	Prominent psychiatric/ behavioral symptoms, painful sensory symptoms, delayed neurologic signs	Dementia, early neurologic signs
Periodic sharp waves on EEG	Absent	Often present
"Pulvinar sign" on MRI[c]	Present in >75% of cases	Very rare or absent
Presence of "florid plaques" on neuropathology	Present in great numbers	Rare or absent
Immunohistochemical analysis of brain tissue	Marked accumulation of PrP-res[d]	Variable accumulation
Presence of agent in lymphoid tissue	Readily detected	Not readily detected
Increased glycoform ratio on immunoblot analysis of PrP-res	Present	Not present
Genotype at codon 129 of prion protein	Methionine/methionine[e]	Polymorphic

[a]Adapted from Reference 25.
[b]U.S. CJD surveillance data 1979–2001.
[c]High signal in the posterior thalamus.
[d]Protease-resistant prion protein.
[e]One patient with preclinical vCJD related to bloodborne transmission was heterozygous for methionine and valine.

specific clinicopathologic profile. If this assumption is correct, vCJD could potentially occur in persons who are heterozygous or homozygous for valine at codon 129 after a possible longer incubation period. Studies conducted in predominantly white populations indicate that methionine homozygosity at codon 129 of the prion protein gene may be present in approximately 35%–40% of the general population (3, 72).

Statistical models have been applied to predict the eventual size of the vCJD epidemic in the United Kingdom. Some of these studies suggested that the epidemic may have already reached its peak and the eventual size may not exceed several hundred clinical cases (43, 70). However, uncertainties still exist about the influence of other factors on the size of the vCJD epidemic. These factors include the emergence of vCJD in persons with a codon 129 genotype other than methionine homozygosity, secondary spread of the vCJD agent via blood products, and the extent and contribution of subclinical infection to the potential secondary spread of the agent.

Bloodborne Transmission

A highly probable bloodborne, person-to-person transmission of vCJD was reported in the United Kingdom in a 69-year-old man who had vCJD onset in late 2002, 6.5 years after receipt of 5 units of packed red blood cells (51). One of the red blood cell units was obtained from a 24-year-old donor who developed vCJD >3 years after donation. Both the donor and recipient died of pathologically confirmed vCJD. The unusually older age of the recipient, appropriate latency period, and the remote likelihood that confirmed vCJD in a donor and recipient pair would have occurred by chance alone indicates that this episode represents a highly probable bloodborne transmission of vCJD. The patient was identified as part of a cohort study of 48 patients who received blood components during 1980–2003 from 15 donors who subsequently died of vCJD. None of the 27 recipients who died within approximately 10 years after transfusion had a death certificate diagnosis of a neurodegenerative disease (51); the cause of death in 3 recipients was unknown. Of the remaining 17 patients under follow up, one elderly patient was recently diagnosed with preclinical vCJD on the basis of detection of the agent in the spleen and cervical lymph node. The patient died of a ruptured abdominal aortic aneurysm five years after transfusion, and no pathologic lesions were detected in the brain. This latter case represented a second episode of vCJD transmission via blood transfusion, which indicates that this mode of spread may be more frequent than previously appreciated. Most significantly, the patient was the first ever with methionine and valine heterozygosity at the polymorphic codon 129 of the prion protein gene, which indicates that persons who are not homozygous for methionine can be susceptible to infection by the BSE agent.

The bloodborne transmission of vCJD had long been suspected as possible because of some unusual features of the disease. These features included the ease by which the vCJD agent was detected in lymphoid tissues, raising the possibility that it could also be found in circulating lymphocytes, and the existence of a possible blood phase, or prionemia, of the agent as it travels from the original site of infection in the gut to the brain (71). The FDA, on recommendation from its Transmissible Spongiform Encephalopathy Advisory Committee and with support from the CDC and the National Institutes of Health, had recommended a blood donor deferral policy to exclude donors who have spent specific periods of time in the United Kingdom and other European countries (7). This policy was implemented in 1999 despite considerable criticism by people who focused more on the potential negative impact on the blood supply and on the mere theoretical nature of the risk of bloodborne transmission of vCJD. In hindsight, the reports of bloodborne spread of vCJD in the United Kingdom appear to justify the precautionary deferral policy recommended by the FDA.

Multiple BSE Strains

Unlike scrapie or classic CJD, BSE is likely caused by a single strain of an infectious agent that has a strikingly stable molecular property after natural or experimental transmission to other species. In 2004, however, researchers in Italy reported that the brain lesions of two of eight cattle they studied were distinguished from BSE by the presence of amyloid plaques and distribution of protease-resistant prion protein in the brain (16). On Western blot analysis, the prion fragment in the two cases had a lower molecular mass than that of the classic form of BSE. The researchers suggested that the difference in neuropathology and molecular mass indicates the existence of a second strain of BSE. To distinguish the disease in the two cows from the classic form of BSE, the researchers coined the name bovine amyloidotic spongiform encephalopathy (BASE). Three BSE cases with distinct molecular phenotype among cattle routinely diagnosed in a BSE surveillance system were independently reported in France also (9). Whether the findings from Italy and France do or do not represent new strains of widely circulating BSE should be confirmed through identification of more cases and additional laboratory studies.

No scientific evidence exists to causally link any form of BSE with a sporadic CJD-like illness in humans. Concerns about BSE causing a sporadic CJD-like illness have persisted after BSE-infected transgenic mice expressed prions with a molecular phenotype consistent with a subtype of sporadic CJD (2). The transgenic mice were designed to produce the human prion protein, which is homozygous for methionine at codon 129. If BSE causes a sporadic CJD-like illness in humans, an increase in sporadic CJD cases would be expected to occur in the United Kingdom first, where the vast majority of vCJD cases have been reported. However, in the period following the first published description of vCJD in 1996, there was no increasing trend in the reported annual number of U.K. sporadic CJD deaths (52). Furthermore, surveillance in the United Kingdom has shown no increase in the proportion of sporadic CJD cases that are homozygous for methionine.

CHRONIC WASTING DISEASE

Distribution

CWD (chronic wasting disease), a prion disease of North American deer and elk, was first identified as a fatal wasting syndrome of captive mule deer in the late 1960s in research facilities in Colorado (76). It was first recognized as a TSE in 1978. The occurrence of CWD among wild cervids was first identified in 1981 when a free-ranging elk from Colorado was diagnosed with the disease. Subsequent surveillance studies demonstrated the endemic occurrence of CWD among free-ranging deer and elk in a contiguous area in northeastern Colorado, southeastern Wyoming, and, most recently, in western Nebraska (76). Epidemic modeling suggested that CWD might have been present among free-ranging animals in some portions of the endemic area several decades before it was initially recognized (55).

After 2000, new foci of CWD have increasingly been identified in Illinois, New Mexico, South Dakota, Utah, Wisconsin, and non-CWD-endemic areas of Colorado and Wyoming (6, 76). The identification of CWD in these new areas seems to be related to increased surveillance and spread of the disease as a result of natural migration of deer and elk or translocation of infected cervids by humans. Currently, two largely independent outbreaks, one in free-ranging deer and elk and another in the captive elk and deer industry, are occurring in Canada and the United States (6).

Risk to Humans

The increasing spread of CWD in the United States and the zoonotic transmission of BSE raised concerns about the possible transmission of CWD to humans (6). Several CJD cases or apparent CJD clusters with suspect CWD transmission have been reported in the United States (4, 6, 23). Epidemiologic and laboratory investigations of these isolated cases and clusters did not provide convincing evidence for a link between CWD and the patients' illnesses. However, the studies seeking evidence for a possible link between CWD and human illness have been limited. Additional epidemiologic and laboratory studies should be conducted before the CWD agent can be exonerated as a possible human pathogen. Because persons who hunted deer and elk in the known CWD-endemic areas of Colorado and Wyoming are more likely to have been exposed to the CWD agent over many years, a follow-up study of these hunters has been initiated to monitor the possible zoonotic transmission of CWD. A transgenic mice study, involving humanized and cervidized mice, is also in progress to determine the susceptibility of these mice to the CWD agent (6).

CONCLUSION

Three distinct prion disease–related human health risks from environmental sources of infection can be identified in the United States. These include the iatrogenic transmission of CJD, occurrence of vCJD from exposure to BSE-contaminated cattle products in the United States or other countries with BSE, and possible transmission of CWD to humans. The iatrogenic transmission of CJD appears to be on the decline following appropriate preventive measures that were instituted as the different iatrogenic modes of spread were identified. Additional iatrogenic CJD cases, however, can be anticipated primarily because of the long incubation period associated with prion diseases.

To date, only one vCJD patient has been identified as a resident of the United States (25). This patient is believed to have contracted the disease while growing up in her native country of Britain during the height of human exposure to the BSE outbreak. Although the public health preventive measures recently instituted by the USDA should further reduce the risk of BSE exposure to the U.S. population, the possibility that domestically acquired vCJD may appear in the

United States cannot be totally dismissed. However, this possibility is probably much smaller than the risk of contracting vCJD as a result of BSE exposure during any previous travel or residence in countries where a much higher rate of BSE has been documented. Recent reports of vCJD transmission via blood products obtained from donors who were incubating the disease are of concern because of a potentially large number of blood donors who might have been exposed to BSE and are incubating the disease. Theoretically, these persons might transmit the vCJD agent if they donate blood while they are clinically asymptomatic. The blood donor deferral policy instituted by the FDA is expected to greatly minimize this possible risk of bloodborne transmission of vCJD in the United States. The findings of vCJD transmission in a patient who was heterozygous at codon 129 may have implications for the eventual size of the vCJD outbreak. Heterozygous patients may develop vCJD after a longer incubation period and at an older age than methionine homozygous patients, potentially resulting in a more protracted course for the vCJD outbreak.

To date, no convincing evidence of CWD transmission to humans has been reported. Because the decade-long occurrence of CWD had been relatively limited to a small geographic area, it is possible that not enough human exposure with the appropriate latency period has occurred for the agent to overcome the species barrier and cause disease in humans. There is a concern that the level of human exposure to CWD might increase over time with the increasing spread of CWD to new areas. Continued surveillance for possible human CWD among high-risk populations (e.g., persons hunting for many years in the CWD-endemic areas of Colorado and Wyoming) and evaluation of the zoonotic potential of the CWD agent in transgenic animal models should be conducted to monitor the possibility that the CWD agent can cause disease in humans.

Suspected cases of iatrogenic CJD, vCJD, or human CWD cases should be reported to the CDC through local and state health departments. To facilitate surveillance for emerging forms of prion diseases such as vCJD and human CWD, the CDC, in collaboration with the American Association of Neuropathologists, established a National Prion Disease Pathology Surveillance Center. This pathology center is located at Case Western Reserve University, in Cleveland, Ohio, and provides state-of-the-art diagnostic support free of charge to U.S. physicians and develops laboratory methods to detect emerging human prion diseases. Autopsies should be sought in all clinically suspected and diagnosed human prion disease cases. Brain tissues from these cases should be sent to the National Prion Disease Pathology Surveillance Center to confirm the diagnosis of CJD and determine the CJD subtype. Increased testing of brain tissues from suspected case-patients would facilitate detection of the emergence of any new prion diseases, such as vCJD or possible human CWD, in the United States.

ACKNOWLEDGMENT

The authors thank Claudia Chesley for editing the manuscript.

The *Annual Review of Public Health* is online at
http://publhealth.annualreviews.org

LITERATURE CITED

1. Alper T, Haig DA, Clarke MC. 1966. The exceptionally small size of the scrapie agent. *Biochem. Biophys. Res. Commun.* 22:278–84

2. Asante EA, Linehan JM, Desbruslais M, Joiner S, Gowland I, et al. 2002. BSE prions propagate as either variant CJD-like or sporadic CJD-like prion strains in transgenic mice expressing human prion protein. *EMBO J.* 21:6358–66

3. Belay ED. 1999. Transmissible spongiform encephalopathies in humans. *Annu. Rev. Microbiol.* 53:283–314

4. Belay ED, Gambetti P, Schonberger LB, Parchi P, Lyon DR, et al. 2001. Creutzfeldt-Jakob disease in unusually young patients who consumed venison. *Arch. Neurol.* 58:1673–78

5. Belay ED, Maddox RA, Gambetti P, Schonberger LB. 2003. Monitoring the occurrence of emerging forms of Creutzfeldt-Jakob disease in the United States. *Neurology* 60:176–81

6. Belay ED, Maddox RA, Williams ES, Miller MW, Gambetti P, Schonberger L. 2004. Chronic wasting disease and potential transmission to humans. *Emerg. Infect. Dis.* 10:977–84

7. Belay ED, Schonberger LB. 2002. Variant Creutzfeldt-Jakob disease and bovine spongiform encephalopathy. *Clin. Lab. Med.* 22:849–62

8. Bernoulli C, Siegfried J, Baumgartner G, Regli F, Rabinowicz T, et al. 1977. Danger of accidental person-to-person transmission of Creutzfeldt-Jakob disease by surgery. *Lancet* 1:478–79

9. Biacabe AG, Laplanche JL, Ryder S, Baron T. 2004. Distinct molecular phenotypes in bovine prion diseases. *EMBO Rep.* 5:110–15

10. Bolton DC, McKinley MP, Prusiner SB.
1982. Identification of a protein that purifies with the scrapie prion. *Science* 218: 1309–11

11. Brown P, Gibbs CJ, Rodgers-Johnson P, Asher DM, Sulima M, et al. 1994. Human spongiform encephalopathy: the National Institutes of Health series of 300 cases of experimentally transmitted disease. *Ann. Neurol.* 35:513–29

12. Brown P, Preece M, Brandel JP, Sato T, McShane L, et al. 2000. Iatrogenic Creutzfeldt-Jakob disease at the millennium. *Neurology* 55:1075–81

13. Bruce ME. 2003. TSE strain variation. *Br. Med. Bull.* 66:99–108

14. Büeler H, Aguzzi A, Sailer A, Greiner RA, Augenried P, et al. 1993. Mice devoid of PrP are resistant to scrapie. *Cell* 73:1339–47

15. Can. Food Insp. Agency. 2003. *Narrative background to Canada's assessment of and response to the BSE occurrence in Alberta.* http://www.inspection.gc.ca/english/anima/heasan/disemala/bseesb/evale.shtml

16. Casalone C, Zanusso G, Acutis P, Ferrari S, Capucci L, et al. 2004. Identification of a second bovine amyloidotic spongiform encephalopathy: molecular similarities with sporadic Creutzfeldt-Jakob disease. *Proc. Natl. Acad. Sci. USA* 101:3065–70

17. Cent. Dis. Control. 1985. Fatal degenerative neurologic disease in patients who received pituitary-derived human growth hormone. *MMWR* 34:359–60, 365–66

18. Cent. Dis. Control. 1987. Rapidly progressive dementia in a patient who received a cadaveric dura mater graft. *MMWR* 36:49–50, 55

19. Cent. Dis. Control. 1987. Update: Creutzfeldt-Jakob disease in a patient receiving a cadaveric dura mater graft. *MMWR* 36:324–25

20. Cent. Dis. Control. 1989. Update: Creutzfeldt-Jakob disease in a second patient who received a cadaveric dura mater graft. *MMWR* 38:37–38, 43

21. Cent. Dis. Control Prev. 1993. Creutzfeldt-Jakob disease in patients who received a cadaveric dura mater graft—Spain, 1985–1992. *MMWR* 42:560–63

22. Cent. Dis. Control Prev. 1997. Creutzfeldt-Jakob disease associated with cadaveric dura mater grafts—Japan, January 1979–May 1996. *MMWR* 46:1066–69

23. Cent. Dis. Control Prev. 2003. Fatal degenerative neurologic illnesses in men who participated in wild game feasts — Wisconsin, 2002. *MMWR* 2:125–27

24. Cent. Dis. Control Prev. 2003. Update: Creutzfeldt-Jakob disease associated with cadaveric dura mater grafts—Japan, 1979–2003. *MMWR* 52:1179–81

25. Cent. Dis. Control Prev. 2004. Bovine spongiform encephalopathy in a dairy cow—Washington state, 2003. *MMWR* 52: 1280–85

26. Cent. Dis. Control Prev. 2004. *Questions and answers regarding Creutzfeldt-Jakob disease infection-control practices.* http://www.cdc.gov/ncidod/diseases/cjd/cjd_inf_ctrl_qa.htm

27. Chazot E, Broussolle E, Lapras CI, Blattler T, Aguzzi A, Kopp N. 1996. New variant of Creutzfeldt-Jakob disease in a 26-year-old French man. *Lancet* 347:1181

28. Collee JG, Bradley R. 1997. BSE: a decade on—part 1. *Lancet* 349:636–41

29. Collie DA, Summers DM, Sellar RJ, Ironside JW, Cooper S, et al. 2003. Diagnosing variant Creutzfeldt-Jakob disease with the pulvinar sign: MR imaging findings in 86 neuropathologically confirmed cases. *Am. J. Neuroradiol.* 24:1560–69

30. Dep. Health, United Kingdom. 2004. *Monthly Creutzfeldt-Jakob disease.* http://www.dh.gov.uk/PolicyAndGuidance/HealthAndSocialCareTopics/CJD/CJDGeneralInformation/CJDGeneralArticle/fs/en?CONTENT_ID = 4032396&chk = 5shT1Z

31. Dobbins JG, Belay ED, Malecki J, Buck BE, Bell M, et al. 1998. Creutzfeldt-Jakob disease in a recipient of a dura mater graft processed in the US: cause or coincidence? *Neuroepidemiology* 19:62–66

32. Donnelly CA, Ferguson NM, Ghani AC, Anderson RM. 2002. Implications of BSE infection screening data for the scale of the British BSE epidemic and current European infection levels. *Proc. R. Soc. London B* 269:2179–90

33. Duffy P, Wolf J, Collins G, DeVoe AG, Streeten B, Cowen D. 1974. Possible person-to-person transmission of Creutzfeldt-Jakob disease. *N. Engl. J. Med.* 290:692–93

34. Fradkin JE, Schonberger LB, Mills JL, Gunn WJ, Piper JM, et al. 1991. Creutzfeldt-Jakob disease in pituitary growth hormone recipients in the United States. *JAMA* 265:880–84

35. Ghani AC, Ferguson NM, Donnelly CA, Anderson RM. 2000. Predicted vCJD mortality in Great Britain. *Nature* 406:583–84

36. Gibbs CJ, Asher DM, Kobrine A, Amyx HL, Sulima MP, Gajdusek DC. 1994. Transmission of Creutzfeldt-Jakob disease to a chimpanzee by electrodes contaminated during neurosurgery. *J. Neurol. Neurosurg. Psychiatry* 57:757–58

37. Gibbs CJ Jr, Joy A, Heffner R, Franko M, Miyazaki M, et al. 1985. Clinical and pathological features and laboratory confirmation of Creutzfeldt-Jakob disease in a recipient of pituitary-derived human growth hormone. *N. Engl. J. Med.* 313:734–38

38. Griffith JS. 1967. Self-replication and scrapie. *Nature* 215:1043–44

39. Hannah EL, Belay ED, Gambetti P, Krause G, Parchi P, et al. 2001. Creutzfeldt-Jakob disease after receipt of a previously unimplicated brand of dura mater graft. *Neurology* 56:1080–83

40. Heckmann JG, Lang CJG, Petruch F, Druschky A, Erb C, et al. 1997. Transmission of Creutzfeldt-Jakob disease via a corneal transplant. *J. Neurol. Neurosurg. Psychiatry* 63:388–90

41. Hill AF, Butterworth RJ, Joiner S, et al.

1999. Investigation of variant Creutzfeldt-Jakob disease and other human prion diseases with tonsil biopsy samples. *Lancet* 353:183–89

42. Hill AF, Zeidler M, Ironside J, Collinge J. 1997. Diagnosis of new variant Creutzfeldt-Jakob disease by tonsil biopsy. *Lancet* 349:99–100

43. Huillard d'Aignaux JN, Cousens SN, Smith PG. 2001. Predictability of the UK variant Creutzfeldt-Jakob disease epidemic. *Science* 294:1729–31

44. Ironside JW. 1998. Neuropathological findings in new variant CJD and experimental transmission of BSE. *FEMS Immunol. Med. Microbiol.* 21:91–95

45. Kellar JA, Lees VW. 2003. Risk management of the transmissible spongiform encephalopathies in North America. *Rev. Sci. Tech. Off. Int. Epizoot.* 22:201–25

46. Koch TK, Berg BO, DeArmond SJ, Gravina RF. 1985. Creutzfeldt-Jakob disease in a young adult with idiopathic hypopituitarism. Possible relation to the administration of cadaveric human growth hormone. *N. Engl. J. Med.* 313:731–33

47. Lane KL, Brown P, Howell DN, Crain BJ, Hulette CM, et al. 1994. Creutzfeldt-Jakob disease in a pregnant woman with an implanted dura mater graft. *Neurosurgery* 34:737–40

48. Lang CJG, Heckmann JG, Neundörfer B. 1998. Creutzfeldt-Jakob disease via dural and corneal transplants. *J. Neurol. Sci.* 160:128–39

49. Lang CJG, Schüler P, Engelhardt A, Spring A, Brown P. 1995. Probable Creutzfeldt-Jakob disease after a cadaveric dural graft. *Eur. J. Epidemiol.* 11:79–81

50. Lasmézas CI. 2003. Putative functions of PrP^C. *Br. Med. Bull.* 60:61–70

51. Llewelyn CA, Hewitt PE, Knight RSG, Amar K, Cousens S, et al. 2004. Possible transmission of variant Creutzfeldt-Jakob disease by blood transfusion. *Lancet* 363:417–21

52. Maddox RA, Belay ED, Schonberger LB. 2003. *Re-monitoring the occurrence of emerging forms of Creutzfeldt-Jakob disease in the United States (letter).* http://www.neurology.org/cgi/eletters/60/2/176

53. Martinez-Lage JF, Sola J, Poza M, Esteban JA. 1993. Pediatric Creutzfeldt-Jakob disease: probable transmission by a dural graft. *Child's Nerv. Syst.* 9:239–42

54. Masullo C, Pocchiari M, Macchi G, Alema G, Piazza G, Panzera MA. 1989. Transmission of Creutzfeldt-Jakob disease by dural cadaveric graft. *J. Neurosurg.* 71:954–55

55. Miller MW, Williams ES, McCarty CW, Spraker TR, Kreeger TJ, et al. 2000. Epizootiology of chronic wasting disease in free-ranging cervids in Colorado and Wyoming. *J. Wildl. Dis.* 36:676–90

56. Mills JL, Schonberger LB, Wysowski DK, Brown P, Durako SJ, et al. 2004. Long-term mortality in the United States cohort of pituitary-derived growth hormone recipients. *J. Pediatr.* 144:430–36

57. Miyashita K, Inuzuka T, Kondo H, Saito Y, Fujuta N, et al. 1991. Creutzfeldt-Jakob disease in a patient with a cadaveric dural graft. *Neurology* 41:940–41

58. Moynagh J, Schimmel H. 1999. Tests for BSE evaluated. *Nature* 400:105

59. Oesch B, Westaway D, Wälchli M, McKinley MP, Kent SBH, et al. 1985. A cellular gene encodes scrapie PrP 27–30 protein. *Cell* 40:735–46

60. Pan KM, Baldwin M, Nguyen J, Gasset M, Serban A, et al. 1993. Conversion of ∀-helices into ∃-sheets features in the formation of the scrapie prion proteins. *Proc. Natl. Acad. Sci. USA* 90:10962–66

61. Parchi P, Castellani R, Capellari S, Ghetti B, Young K, et al. 1996. Molecular basis of phenotypic variability in sporadic Creutzfeldt-Jakob disease. *Ann. Neurol.* 39:767–78

62. Pattison IH, Jones KM. 1967. The possible nature of the transmissible agent of scrapie. *Vet. Rec.* 80:2–9

63. Prusiner SB. 1982. Novel proteinaceous infectious particles cause scrapie. *Science* 216:136–44

64. Prusiner SB, Bolton DC, Groth DF, Bowman KA, Cochran P, McKinley MP. 1982. Further purification and characterization of scrapie prions. *Biochemistry* 21:6942–50

65. Prusiner SB, McKinley MP, Groth DF, Bowman KA, Mock NI, et al. 1981. Scrapie agent contains a hydrophobic protein. *Proc. Natl. Acad. Sci. USA* 78:6675–79

66. Prusiner SB, Scott M, Foster D, Pan PK, Groth D, et al. 1990. Transgenic studies implicate interactions between homologous PrP isoforms in scrapie prion replication. *Cell* 63:673–86

67. Smith PG, Bradley R. 2003. Bovine spongiform encephalopathy (BSE) and its epidemiology. *Br. Med. Bull.* 66:185–98

68. Telling GC, Parchi P, DeArmond SJ, Cortelli P, Montagna P, et al. 1996. Evidence for the conformation of the pathologic isoform of the prion protein enciphering and propagating prion diversity. *Science* 274:2079–82

69. Thadani V, Penar PL, Partington J, Kalb R, Janssen R, et al. 1988. Creutzfeldt-Jakob disease probably acquired from cadaveric dura mater graft. *J. Neurosurg.* 69:766–69

70. Valleron AJ, Boelle PY, Will R, Cesbron JY. 2001. Estimation of epidemic size and incubation time based on age characteristics of vCJD in the United Kingdom. *Science* 294:1726–28

71. Wadsworth JDF, Joiner S, Hill AF, Campbell TA, Desbruslais M, et al. 2001. Tissue distribution of protease resistant prion protein in variant Creutzfeldt-Jakob disease using highly sensitive immunoblotting assay. *Lancet* 358:171–80

72. Will RG. 2003. Acquired prion disease: iatrogenic CJD, variant CJD, kuru. *Br. Med. Bull.* 66:255–65

73. Will RG, Alper MP, Dormont D, Schonberger LB. 2004. Infectious and sporadic prion diseases. In *Prion Biology and Diseases*, ed. SB Prusiner, 13:629–72. Cold Spring Harbor, NY: Cold Spring Harbor Lab. Press

74. Will RG, Ironside JW, Zeidler M, Cousens SN, Estibeiro K, et al. 1996. A new variant of Creutzfeldt-Jakob disease in the UK. *Lancet* 347:921–25

75. Will RG, Matthews WB. 1982. Evidence for case-to-case transmission of Creutzfeldt-Jakob disease. *J. Neurol. Neurosurg. Psychiatry* 45:235–38

76. Williams ES, Miller MW, Kreeger TJ, Khan RH, Thorne ET. 2002. Chronic wasting disease of deer and elk: a review with recommendations for management. *J. Wildl. Manage.* 66:551–63

77. Willison HJ, McLaughlin JE. 1991. Creutzfeldt-Jakob disease following cadaveric dura mater graft. *J. Neurol. Neurosurg. Psychiatry* 54:940

Annu. Rev. Public Health 2005. 26:213–37
doi: 10.1146/annurev.publhealth.24.100901.140910
First published online as a Review in Advance on November 11, 2004

WATER AND BIOTERRORISM: Preparing for the Potential Threat to U.S. Water Supplies and Public Health

Patricia L. Meinhardt

Center for Occupational and Environmental Medicine, Arnot Ogden Medical Center, Elmira, New York 14905; email: pmeinhardt@aomc.org

Key Words   water terrorism, waterborne disease, intentional water contamination, biowarfare agents, biotoxins

■ **Abstract**   Water supplies and water distribution systems represent potential targets for terrorist activity in the United States because of the critical need for water in every sector of our industrialized society. Even short-term disruption of water service can significantly impact a community, and intentional contamination of a municipal water system as part of a terrorist attack could lead to serious medical, public health, and economic consequences. Most practicing physicians and public health professionals in the United States have received limited training in the recognition and evaluation of waterborne disease from either natural or intentional contamination of water. Therefore, they are poorly prepared to detect water-related disease resulting from intentional contamination and may not be adequately trained to respond appropriately to a terrorist assault on water. The purpose of this review is to address this critical information gap and present relevant epidemiologic and clinical information for public health and medical practitioners who may be faced with addressing the recognition, management, and prevention of water terrorism in their communities.

INTRODUCTION

Recent terrorist activity in the United States has forced the public health community, federal regulatory agencies, and local water utilities to consider the possibility of intentional contamination of U.S. water supplies as part of an organized effort to disrupt and damage important elements of our national infrastructure (19, 39, 59). Water supplies and water distribution systems represent potential targets for terrorist activity in the United States because of the essential role that water plays in every segment of our industrialized society (39). Even short-term disruption of the provision of water can have a significant impact on a community, and intentional contamination of a municipal water system as part of a terrorist attack could lead to sobering medical, public health, and economic consequences. In the past, protection of potable water supplies from intentional contamination with biological agents and biotoxins was a concern primarily of the military, which was tasked with protecting troops from bioweapons exposure in the field (9, 42, 62). Since September 11, 2001, there is growing concern that biological warfare agents may be used against the U.S. civilian population, with water as one possible vehicle of transmission or mode of dispersal of weaponized compounds (19, 21, 35, 39, 59).

The plausibility of intentional contamination of water supplies as part of an overt or covert terrorist act has been reinforced by recent congressional testimony, a consensus statement by a governmental review panel, and a joint Centers for Disease Control and Prevention (CDC) and Environmental Protection Agency (EPA) water advisory health alert (15, 47). As part of their 2002 congressional report, the National Research Council of the National Academy of Sciences concluded that water supply system contamination and disruption should be considered a possible terrorist threat in the United States (47). On February 7, 2003, the National Terrorism Threat Level was increased to a "high risk" threat level on the basis of information received and analyzed by the federal intelligence community. Subsequent to this heightened alert, the CDC and the EPA issued a *Water Advisory in Response to the High Threat Level* describing the need for enhanced vigilance by the public health and water utility community regarding the risk of a terrorist attack on the nation's water infrastructure (15) (Figure 1). Apprehension regarding a terrorist assault on drinking water systems has also been reinforced by news reports and recent arrests of suspects charged with threatening to contaminate municipal water supplies in the United States (46, 59). In addition, President George Bush noted in his 2002 State of the Union Address (49) that captured Al Qaeda documents included detailed maps of several U.S. municipal public drinking water systems.

A review of two recent examples of waterborne disease outbreaks resulting from accidental contamination of municipal drinking water systems illustrates the potential consequences of an intentional act of water terrorism (45). The massive outbreak of waterborne cryptosporidiosis in Milwaukee, Wisconsin, in 1993 is an example of how contaminated water distributed through a municipal water system can result in significant medical, public health, and economic consequences in a community. An estimated 403,000 Milwaukee residents developed diarrhea, which reflected an attack rate of 52% of the population served by the affected municipal water system. In addition, more than 4000 Milwaukee residents were hospitalized during the waterborne outbreak, and cryptosporidiosis was listed as the underlying or contributory cause of death in 54 residents following the outbreak. Investigators estimate that 725,000 productive days were lost as a result of the water contamination event, at a cost in excess of $54 million in lost work time or additional expenses to residents and local authorities in Milwaukee. In 2000, the municipal water supply of Walkerton, Ontario, was contaminated with *E. coli* O157:H7, resulting in 2300 symptomatic residents and 7 deaths attributed to the waterborne disease outbreak. More than $11 million was required to reconstruct the community municipal water system and install temporary filtration after the contamination event. Current estimates of the total cost of the Walkerton,

This is an official
CDC HEALTH ADVISORY

Distributed via Health Alert Network
February 07, 2003, 20:56 EDT (8:56 PM EDT)
CDCHAN-000113-03-02-07-ADV-N

CDC and EPA Water Advisory in Response to High Threat Level

Today, the Department of Homeland Security upgraded the Homeland Security Advisory System from yellow level (elevated risk of terrorist attack) to orange level (high risk of terrorist attack).

While there are no data to indicate that water has been specifically targeted, our nation's water infrastructure remains at risk to terrorist attacks, or acts intended to substantially disrupt the ability of a water system to provide a reliable supply of water. Therefore, public health agencies and water utilities are encouraged to continue to work together, keep each other informed of any unusual activities, and confirm the proper operation of notification channels in emergency response plans.

Public health agencies should immediately notify local water utilities and the state's drinking water administrator in the event of an unusual number of cases of gastrointestinal illnesses or other indications of illness that may suggest water contamination by a biological, chemical or radiological agent.

Water utilities should immediately notify public health agencies 24/7 emergency operations number, and the state's drinking water administrator in the event of specific threats received at a water facility, customer complaints in water quality, or if circumstances lead the utility to believe that the water has been or will be contaminated with a biological, chemical or radiological agent.

The Centers for Disease Control and Prevention (CDC) and the U.S. Environmental Protection Agency (EPA) issue this advisory jointly.

Categories of Health Alert messages:
Health Alert: conveys the highest level of importance; warrants immediate action or attention.
Health Advisory: provides important information for a specific incident or situation; may not require immediate action.
Health Update: provides updated information regarding an incident or situation; unlikely to require immediate action.
===

You have received this message based upon the information contained within our emergency notification data base. If you have a different or additional e-mail or fax address that you would like us to use please notify us as soon as possible by e-mail at healthalert@cdc.gov.

=======================================

Figure 1 CDC and EPA *Water Advisory in Response to High Threat Level* distributed as part of the emergency notification Health Alert Network (HAN) on February 7, 2003 (15).

Ontario, waterborne disease outbreak and municipal water contamination event have reached $155 million.

Both overt and covert acts of terrorism involving weaponized biological pathogens and biotoxins pose an intimidating public health threat and a significant challenge to our healthcare infrastructure, as was demonstrated following the intentional release of *Bacillus anthracis* spores through the U.S. postal system in 2001 (31). Most public health and law enforcement authorities consider a successful attack using weaponized biological agents in the United States as "simply a matter of time" (30). Although significant progress has been made to improve the terrorism preparedness of the medical and public health community in the United States, most healthcare providers and public health professionals have a limited working knowledge of the skills necessary to recognize and manage waterborne biological agents that terrorists may use to threaten the U.S. civilian population (46). Therefore, the purpose of this review is to summarize relevant epidemiologic and clinical information and highlight valuable diagnostic and management tools for public health and medical practitioners who may be faced with addressing the recognition, management, and prevention of acts of water terrorism in their communities.

THE PUBLIC HEALTH CHALLENGE OF WATER TERRORISM

Although public health and medical practitioners may not be able to prevent the first cases of illness or injury resulting from a bioterrorism attack, they are positioned to play a critical role in minimizing the impact of such an event by practicing public health with an increased index of suspicion that such an attack may occur in their communities (7, 30). Even if the probability of occurrence remains low, the public health consequences of a successful overt or covert terrorist attack with biological agents would be serious (37). With prompt diagnosis and proper management including preventive and therapeutic measures, prepared medical and public health professionals may make the difference between a controlled response to a terrorist incident and a public health crisis (33).

Therefore, early detection and rapid response to biological terrorist assaults on the nation's infrastructure, including U.S. water supplies, are critical elements to any effective terrorism response strategy. This is particularly important when addressing the possibility of intentional water contamination resulting from bioterrorism. In a water terrorism scenario, early detection will be critical to diminish (*a*) the public health impact of the contamination event, (*b*) the secondary disruption to potable water distribution and availability, and (*c*) the psychological impact of the public's lack of confidence in water safety and quality following a water terrorism event (39, 46).

Recognizing and managing a waterborne disease outbreak and the health effects of exposure to water contamination are diagnostic challenges in the best of circumstances. These challenges would be even more significant in an emergency situation resulting from waterborne exposure to potentially weaponized biological agents (46). The public health and medical challenges associated with waterborne disease resulting from an act of water terrorism include but are not limited to the following.

1. Prompt identification of waterborne disease resulting from water terrorism may be confounded by difficulties in early diagnosis. Many diseases resulting from exposure to weaponized biological agents present with vague, nonspecific symptoms in the early phase of illness and may be difficult to differentiate from naturally occurring disease in a community (23). In addition, the signs and symptoms of waterborne disease and the health effects of water contamination are often nonspecific and mimic more common medical conditions and disorders unrelated to water contaminant exposure (45).

2. Many weaponized biological agents display a significantly different clinical picture when the route of exposure is ingestion. Using food and water as a mode of dispersion for weaponized biological agents (7, 23) may confound diagnosis, delay treatment, and impede protective public health measures if epidemiologic investigations and clinical assessments are restricted to evaluation of inhalation and cutaneous routes of exposure alone (9, 28, 30).

3. A bioterrorist attack on water supply systems may not first occur in a populous community usually considered as a preferred target. A small outbreak of terrorism-related waterborne disease may act as a warning of a more large-scale attack. Water systems in small rural communities may represent testing grounds for larger-scale attacks in metropolitan municipal water systems (46). This potential scenario reinforces the need for incorporation of possible terrorism-related waterborne disease into the daily differential diagnosis of every public health and medical practitioner in practice in the United States, no matter how small or large the community (51, 58).

4. Medical and public health practitioners will play a critical role as front-line responders in detecting water-related disease resulting from biological terrorism. Although environmental detection and water-quality testing methods for recognizing intentional contamination of water are improving (59), the most likely initial indication that a water contamination event has occurred in a community will be a change in disease trends and illness patterns. Early recognition, timely outbreak investigations, accurate diagnosis, and conscientious reporting by the medical and public health community of suspected waterborne terrorism disease cases will be essential to maintaining water security and safety (46).

5. Water-related disease resulting from intentional contamination with biological agents may present as benign symptoms or self-limited illness in a healthy patient population, whereas the same waterborne exposure in a vulnerable patient population may result in significant morbidity and mortality. The

impact of a terrorist attack depends on not only the type of agent used or method and efficiency of dispersal but also on the type of population exposed and their level of immunity or vulnerability (9, 36). Individual vulnerability to weaponized biological compounds including waterborne agents may vary widely, and differences in host susceptibility factors may complicate recognition of an intentional water contamination event.

6. A coordinated and effective response to acts of water terrorism will depend on cooperation among a multidisciplinary team of professionals. As in the case of any type of antiterrorism preparedness (38, 55), a coordinated and effective response to mitigate the negative consequences of an intentional act of water terrorism will depend on cooperation among a multidisciplinary team of health care providers, public health and water utility practitioners, law enforcement professionals, and community leaders. The medical and public health community will need to develop and foster new partnerships and working relationships with water utility practitioners to protect the public's health and ensure water safety (46).

7. Medical and public health practitioners will be faced with providing credible and timely risk communication and public notification of a suspected water contamination event. As a result of heightened public awareness regarding the potential for additional terrorist activity, the medical and public health community will be required to play a leading role in risk communication with the public, if an act of waterborne terrorism occurs in the United States. Health care providers are among the most trusted sources of information for the general public regarding drinking water quality and safety in the United States (45), and community residents will immediately turn to their health care providers and public health leaders for advice regarding the safety of their drinking water during and after an intentional water contamination event.

Effective risk communication by the medical and public health community will play a critical role in a coordinated response to intentional acts of water terrorism and will be essential to prevent panic and hysteria in the community experiencing the terrorism event (7, 46). Risk communication will be challenging since there will be pressure from the public and media to provide information before confirmatory evidence is available. Incorporating the public and media as key partners in risk communication efforts during and after a terrorism event can help modulate the ultimate impact on a community. Health care providers will need to embrace the concept that providing timely information and effective risk communication may be as important as providing medical care in the event of a water terrorism attack (46).

Any effective response to the public health threat of water terrorism must include targeted education and terrorism preparedness training for the medical and public health community (46). Critical elements of any antiterrorism preparedness training for public health and medical practitioners include prompt recognition, treatment, and prevention of the public health consequences of weaponized biological agent exposure in a community population (5, 38). However, public health officials and health care providers must become familiar with not only the clinical presentation, diagnosis, management, and prevention of terrorism-related disease but also the appropriate mechanisms for communicating with law enforcement agencies, public utilities, the media, and the concerned public (1, 60).

A thorough understanding of the recognition and management of waterborne disease resulting from intentional contamination of U.S. water supplies and distribution systems will be essential for several reasons if an effective response to acts of water terrorism is to be implemented by the public health and medical community. The illness and injury resulting from community exposure to weaponized biological agents would not be part of any health care provider or public health practitioner's routine clinical or public health practice experience (38, 53, 57). Most practicing physicians and public health professionals in the United States have received limited training in the recognition and evaluation of waterborne disease from either natural or intentional contamination of water. Therefore, they are poorly prepared to detect water-related disease resulting from intentional contamination and may not be adequately trained to respond appropriately to a terrorist assault on water (45, 46). The remainder of this review attempts to address this critical information gap and presents relevant epidemiologic and clinical information for public health and medical practitioners who may be faced with addressing the recognition, management, and prevention of water terrorism in their communities.

WATER AS A DISPERSAL MECHANISM FOR BIOTERRORISM

The deliberate contamination of the wells, reservoirs, and other water sources of civilian populations has been employed as a method of attack by opposing military forces throughout the history of war (18). Many armies have resorted to using this method of biowarfare, including the Romans who contaminated the drinking water of their enemies with diseased cadavers and animal carcasses (18, 65). With enhanced technology and modern scientific advances, the mechanisms of biowarfare agent dispersal have expanded considerably.

In addition, terrorist attacks on the U.S. population with deliberate release of biological warfare agents may be difficult to identify quickly and reliably in the environment (65). Intentional contamination of water with a biological pathogen or biotoxin that is colorless, odorless, tasteless, and therefore not detectable by human senses presents a serious challenge for those responsible for environmental detection of such a biological compound in water (21, 23).

As part of a collaborative effort, water utilities and several federal public health agencies have undertaken a major effort to improve and enhance their ability to detect and characterize deliberate contamination of water systems in the United States (24–27, 59). As a result, U.S. water systems are currently more physically secure with multiple layers of enhanced protection. However, there remain several potential points in the U.S. water supply and distribution systems that could be vulnerable to intentional contamination. In their congressional report addressing infrastructure vulnerability to acts of terrorism, the National Research Council of the National Academy of Sciences outlined a series of these potential points of contamination in the U.S. water supply (47). Other public health and water utility specialists have also addressed this issue and presented other possible points of intentional contamination. This information is summarized in Table 1 and can be a resource for health care providers and public health professionals to use when evaluating an unusual symptoms complex or an atypical illness pattern, which may represent a case of waterborne terrorism (20, 21, 23, 39, 47, 48, 61).

TABLE 1   Possible points of contamination of U.S. water from acts of water terrorism[a,b]

Upstream of a community water supply system or collection point—Water supply systems are composed of small streams and bodies of water, rivers, service reservoirs, aquifers, wells, and dams that may act as points of deliberate contamination of water.

Community water supply intake access point or at the water treatment plant—Many water supply systems are designed to receive water from source water reserves at a central intake point; this source water is subsequently filtered and sanitized at the community water treatment facility for eventual distribution as potable water. Both water-intake points and community water treatment plants may be targeted for terrorist activity and deliberate water contamination.

Selected points in the posttreatment water distribution system—Treated water is distributed to water consumers or end-users through transmission pipelines to homes and businesses. Selected portions of a water distribution system or water main are also potential points of water contamination that may be targeted by terrorists and could affect a subdivision, specific neighborhood, school, medical center, or nursing home.

Private home or office building water supply connection, individual building water supply, water tanks, cisterns, or storage tanks—Treated water stored very close to the water consumer or end-user as well as individual house or building connections may serve as points of water contamination by terrorists.

Water used in food processing, bottled water production, or commercial water—Water used for food processing or preparation as well as bottled water production also represent points of potential water contamination by terrorists.

Deliberate contamination of recreational waters and receiving waters—Both treated and untreated recreational waters may serve as points of potential contamination of water, including swimming pools, water parks, and natural bodies of water (small lakes and ponds). Receiving waters such as rivers, estuaries, and lakes may be secondarily contaminated with wastewater from sanitary and storm sewer systems that may have been environmentally contaminated by biological warfare agents.

[a]A number of the potential points of contamination of water outlined above are more probable terrorist targets than others (19, 47). However, all health care providers and public health practitioners should consider these potential sources of water contamination and unusual modes of delivery of biowarfare agents when evaluating a suspected case of terrorism-related disease (20, 21, 23, 39, 47, 48, 61).
[b]Modified and reprinted with permission from the author and Arnot Ogden Medical Center (46).

DISSEMINATION OF BIOWARFARE AGENTS THROUGH MULTIPLE MODES OF DISPERSAL INCLUDING WATER

Possible Water-Related Exposure Scenarios

Following the release of a biological warfare compound, the nature and extent of the medical and public health consequences resulting from the intentional exposure depend on a multitude of factors (66):

- the method by which the biowarfare agent is dispersed,
- the biowarfare agent characteristics profile including toxicity and virulence,
- the amount of biowarfare compound released and level of infective dose,
- the state of the exposed individual's host susceptibility and level of personal protection,
- the routes of exposure used to disperse the biowarfare agent, and
- the movement and dilution of the biowarfare agent in the environment.

Public health practitioners and healthcare providers faced with evaluating a suspected case of terrorism-related disease will rarely have access to the type of extensive exposure information detailed above when completing an epidemiologic investigation or when questioning exposed patients, most of whom may be unaware of biowarfare agent contact prior to presentation of their symptoms. Therefore, public health and medical practitioners, particularly communicable disease control epidemiologists and other surveillance experts, must become familiar with the various modes of dispersal or methods of dissemination that may be utilized to disperse biological warfare agents to effectively recognize cases of terrorism-related exposure and prevent additional cases from occurring in their community. Several important exposure scenarios should be noted during an outbreak investigation or during a clinician's evaluation of a suspicious case of intentional exposure to biological agents that may include water as one exposure pathway.

1. Intentional contamination of water may occur with nonweaponized, naturally occurring agents. In many cases, terrorism-related disease produced by biowarfare agents mimics naturally occurring disease because the illness may be caused by the same pathogen found in nature (23). Naturally occurring waterborne diseases can cause significant morbidity and mortality in a community as well (1, 2, 6, 12, 14, 22, 50). Therefore, intentional contamination of water supplies with nonweaponized, naturally occurring pathogens or contaminants should also be considered a credible exposure source when completing an exposure history of a suspicious case of terrorism-related disease.

2. Patients may present with a different clinical picture when the route of exposure is ingestion rather than inhalation or dermal absorption. Using food and water supplies as a mode of dispersal for biological warfare (7, 23)

may confound diagnosis, delay treatment, and impede protective public health measures if exposure histories are restricted exclusively to questions regarding inhalation and cutaneous routes of exposure (9, 28). Many biological warfare agents display a significantly different clinical picture when the route of exposure is ingestion rather than inhalation or cutaneous absorption, and this unusual exposure pathway must not be overlooked by public health or medical practitioners.

3. Patients may be exposed to multiple biowarfare agents and coinfections may be common. A terrorist attack on the U.S. population may take place with multiple biological agents, resulting in exposed patients presenting with both acute and delayed symptoms and short- and long-term medical sequelae from mixed biological agent exposure (23, 52). Multiple biowarfare agent exposures could lead to the presence of coinfections and confusing syndromes associated with different biological pathogens and biotoxins. Coinfections with multiple waterborne pathogens is a typical scenario during waterborne outbreaks resulting from natural or accidental water contamination (45). Therefore, when evaluating a suspected case of terrorism-related disease, the exposure history and differential diagnosis must include the possibility of multiple warfare agent exposures and coinfections (46).

4. Water may act as an exposure pathway from both direct contamination as well as environmental contamination from secondary sources. Waterborne exposure to biological warfare agents may result from deliberate direct contamination of water supplies, recreational waters, and receiving waters. However, water may also become indirectly contaminated by biowarfare agents through environmental contamination of wastewater from such sources as sanitary and storm sewer systems receiving the run-off from an aerosolized terrorist attack. In addition, patient decontamination procedures that include flushing contaminated skin surface with water may generate decontamination wastewater and indirect contamination of water systems after a terrorist event (43, 46).

Intentional Dispersal of Bioweapons Using Multiple Exposure Pathways or Portals of Entry

Biological warfare may include the use of unusual biological agents as weapons delivered through unconventional mechanisms of dispersal via unexpected exposure pathways (23, 46, 66). The diversity of dispersal mechanisms for weaponized biological agent release is extensive, ranging from deliberate release of pathogens that may contaminate food supplies or infect livestock to intentional contamination of community water systems in a targeted population (66). The various modes of delivery of biowarfare agents include aerosols or aerial sprays, foodborne and waterborne vehicles, vectorborne and dermal delivery, and intentional injection (23, 61).

Biowarfare agents may enter the body through portals of entry of naturally oc-curring disease or through biotoxin exposure. Appropriate terrorism preparedness skills for the public health and medical community must include familiarity with the various routes of exposure of biological warfare agents to prevent a missed diag-nosis and complete an effective outbreak investigation in the event of a bioterrorist attack. To protect the public's health, working knowledge of the multiple routes of biowarfare agent exposure is essential (23, 61, 66). Possible routes include

1. the natural reservoirs of the biological pathogen or biotoxin,
2. the potential vehicles of transmission of the biological pathogen or biotoxin, and
3. the possible biological warfare or weaponized modes of delivery of the biological pathogen or biotoxin.

Many difficult diagnostic challenges are inherent, for even the most experienced medical or public health practitioner, in evaluating a suspicious case of waterborne terrorism (46). A key factor in the accurate diagnosis and appropriate management of waterborne disease resulting from water terrorism is inclusion of water by medi-cal and public health practitioners as one possible exposure pathway of biowarfare agents at the time of initial case presentation. The biological agents and biotox-ins that have been designated as potential bioterrorist weapons arise from varied biological compounds and can be dispersed through multiple exposure pathways including water (7, 23, 28, 30, 35, 39, 42, 44).

A summary of selected biological pathogens and biotoxins that have been des-ignated as possible bioterrorist agents of public health concern is presented in Table 2 for reference and includes the natural reservoirs, potential vehicles of transmission, and possible warfare modes of delivery for each biological agent. The waterborne route of exposure to these potential biowarfare agents has been placed in context with other exposure pathways of clinical and public health sig-nificance when terrorist activity is suspected. The selected biological pathogens and biotoxins presented in Table 2 have been identified by multiple governmental, military, and medical organizations as possible biowarfare agents that pose a direct threat to public health.

CLINICAL APPROACH TO DIAGNOSING WATERBORNE BIOWARFARE AGENT EXPOSURE AND DISEASE

Clinical Challenges of Evaluating Waterborne Biowarfare Agent Exposure and Disease

Early recognition of unusual illness patterns and rare diseases resulting from in-tentional dispersal of weaponized biological pathogens and biotoxins is a seri-ous challenge facing every health care provider and public health practitioner in the United States. The medical and public health consequences of this difficult

TABLE 2 Selected biological agents and biotoxins of public health concern that include water as a potential mode of dispersal[a,b]

| Etiologic agent | Natural reservoirs | Bacterial pathogens | |
		Potential vehicles of transmission	Possible biological warfare modes of delivery
Anthrax *Bacillus anthracis*	Soil with worldwide distribution	Airborne, foodborne, vectorborne, cutaneous contact with infected tissue	Aerosolized spores during a biowarfare attack, food contamination, and direct or incidental water contamination
Brucellosis *Brucella melitensis, Brucella suis, Brucella abortus, Brucella canis* (undulant or Malta fever)	Cattle, swine, goats, sheep, camels, dogs, coyotes	Airborne, foodborne, entry through cutaneous or mucosal abrasion	Aerosolized release during a biowarfare attack, possible food and water contamination
Cholera *Vibrio cholerae*	Aquatic environments worldwide	Waterborne, foodborne, wound infections from exposure to contaminated water	Intentional contamination of potable water and food
Clostridium perfringens	Soil, gastrointestinal tract of healthy humans and animals	Foodborne, waterborne	Possible aerosolized release during a biowarfare attack, intentional contamination of food or water
Glanders *Burkholderia mallei* (formerly *Pseudomonas mallei*)	Horses, mules, donkeys	Airborne, entry through abraded or lacerated skin, ingestion	Possible aerosolized release, possible water contamination
Melioidosis *Burkholderia pseudomallei* (formerly *Pseudomonas pseudomallei*)	Soil and water throughout the world	Inoculation of skin lesion from contact with contaminated soil or water, aspiration or ingestion of contaminated water, inhalation of contaminated dust	Presumably aerosolized release during a biowarfare attack

Plague *Yersinia pestis*	Wild and domestic rodents, lagomorphs	Vectorborne, airborne	Intentional aerosolized release, release of contaminated vectors (fleas), contamination of water and food
Salmonella *Salmonella typhimurium* and *Salmonella typhi* (acute gastroenteritis and typhoid fever)	Wide range of domestic and wild animals, humans contaminating food and drinking water	Foodborne, waterborne, person-to-person and animal-to-person transmission	Contamination of drinking water, intentional food poisoning
Shigellosis *Shigella dysenteriae* and other *Shigella* sp.	Humans contaminating food and water	Foodborne, waterborne, person-to-person transmission	Contamination of potable water supplies
Tularemia *Francisella tularensis*	Diverse mammalian and tick reservoirs, rodent-mosquito cycle possible	Vectorborne, foodborne, waterborne, airborne	Weaponized aerosolized form, contamination of water
Parasitic pathogens			
Cryptosporidiosis *Cryptosporidium parvum* and other *Cryptosporidium* sp.	Humans, diverse range of animals including cattle and other domestic animals	Foodborne, waterborne, person-to-person, animal-to-person transmission, possibly airborne	Contamination of potable water supplies
Viral pathogens			
Hepatitis A virus (HAV)	Humans, rarely other nonhuman primates	Person-to-person transmission, waterborne, foodborne	Possible intentional contamination of potable water supplies
Smallpox *Variola major*	Humans (eradicated), only in designated laboratories officially	Person-to-person, airborne, direct contact with skin lesions or contaminated objects	Dissemination through aerosol cloud or contaminated items, possible water threat

(Continued)

TABLE 2 (*Continued*)

Etiologic agent	Natural reservoirs	Potential vehicles of transmission	Possible biological warfare modes of delivery
Viral pathogens			
Viral Encephalitides including Venezuelan equine encephalomyelitis (VEE)	Rodents, mosquitoes, horses as amplifying hosts	Arthorpodborne	Weaponized aerosolized form
Viral Hemorrhagic Fevers including Ebola, Marburg, Lassa fever, Rift Valley fever, Yellow fever, Hantavirus and Dengue fever	Rodents, mosquitoes, ticks, primates, humans	Arthorpodborne, aerosol or fomites from slaughtering infected animals	Delivery by aerosol release
Rickettsial and Rickettsial-like Pathogens			
Psittacosis *Chlamydia psittaci*	Birds, poultry	Inhalation of infected droppings and secretions	Presumably aerosolized release, possible water treat
Q Fever *Coxiella burnetti*	Sheep, goats, cattle, dogs, cats, some wild animals, ticks, birds	Airborne, inhalation of dust from infected tissue, direct contact with infected animals	Aerosolized form, contamination of food, possible water threat
Typhus *Rickettsia prowazekii*	Humans	Louse-borne	Aerosol dissemination
Bacterial biotoxins			
***Clostridium botulinum* toxins** (collectively BTX)	Soil, animals, fish	Foodborne with consumption of food contaminated by *C. botulinum* toxin; wound infection from exposure to toxin spores	Primarily aerosol release during biowarfare attack; intentional contamination of food and water possible

***Clostridium perfringens* toxins**	Soil and gastrointestinal tract of healthy humans and animals	Foodborne with clostridial food poisoning, wound contamination with *C. perfringens* spores	Primarily as aerosol threat during biowarfare attack, toxin may be delivered in combination with other toxins, waterborne contamination conceivable but unlikely
Staphylococcus enterotoxin B (SEB)—including protein toxin from *Staphylococcus aureus*	Humans, contaminated milk and milk products	Foodborne through ingestion of food, milk, and milk products containing the preformed toxin	Primary threat as an aerosol release, intentional contamination of food and water also possible
Fungal-derived biotoxins (mycotoxins)			
Aflatoxin Metabolite of *Aspergillus flavus*	Variety of agricultural plants including peanuts	Foodborne through ingestion of contaminated food	Potential intentional water and food contamination
T-2 mycotoxin Extract from *Fusarium* spp.	Grain infected with *Fusarium* mold	Foodborne through ingestion of food prepared with moldy grain	Probable water threat, intentional infection of agricultural products, release in aerosolized form
Anatoxin A Product of cyanobacteria, *Anabaena flos-aquae*	Freshwater cyanobacteria (blue-green algae)	Waterborne	Possible water threat
Microcystins Products of cyanobacteria, *Microcystis* spp.	Freshwater blooms of cyanobacteria (blue-green algae)	Waterborne	Aerosolized release during a biowarfare attack, possible water threat

(Continued)

TABLE 2 *(Continued)*

Etiologic agent	Natural reservoirs	Potential vehicles of transmission	Possible biological warfare modes of delivery
Plant- and algae-derived biotoxins			
Ricin Extract from castor bean	Castor bean (*Ricinus communis*)	Airborne through inhalation during industrial operations, foodborne through ingestion of castor bean meal	Potential aerosol threat, delivery through injection, possible contamination of food and water
Marine biotoxins			
Saxitoxin [Paralytic shellfish poisoning (PSP)]—product of dinoflagellate, *Gonyaulax*	Shellfish	Foodborne by ingesting bivalve mollusks with accumulated dinoflagellates	Primary threat through aerosol release, delivery by injection or projectiles, contamination of food and water supplies
Tetrodotoxin Neurotoxin from pufferfish sp.	Pufferfish	Foodborne through consumption of improperly prepared pufferfish	Possible aerosol form, possible water contamination threat

[a]This summary table is a compilation of information from several resources (9, 13, 17, 23, 28, 30, 37–39, 42, 44, 46, 59, 62) and is intended for educational purposes only. This resource is not intended to be an exhaustive or comprehensive review of the epidemiologic or medical features of each biological agent nor is it intended to be construed as a definitive list of potential biowarfare threats.

[b]Modified and reprinted with permission from the author and Arnot Ogden Medical Center (46).

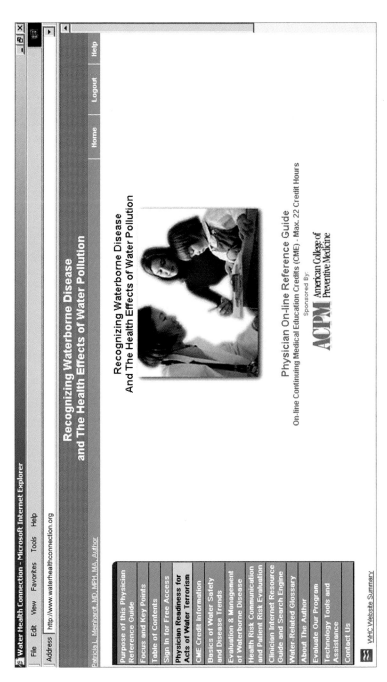

Figure 2 *Recognizing Waterborne Disease and the Health Effects of Water Pollution: Physician On-line Reference Guide* is accessible at http://www.WaterHealthConnection.org (45).

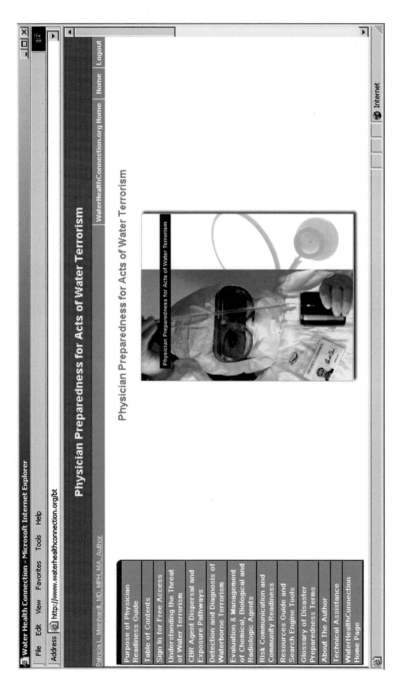

Figure 3 *Physician Preparedness for Acts of Water Terrorism: Physician On-line Readiness Guide* is accessible at http://www. WaterHealthConnection.org (46).

diagnostic challenge were apparent after the deliberate release of weaponized *Bacillus anthracis* via the U.S. postal system in 2001 (31). With 22 confirmed cases and five deaths, this biological attack necessitated a change in the approach to the practice of medicine and public health in the United States. The following sections of this review provide a synopsis of the clinical approach and enhanced knowledge base necessary to diagnose waterborne disease resulting from intentional biological pathogen and biotoxin exposure.

DIAGNOSIS OF WATERBORNE DISEASE RESULTING FROM BIOLOGICAL PATHOGEN EXPOSURE   In theory, any microbial pathogen could be used as a biological weapon, but in reality, the list of weaponized biological pathogens that pose a significant public health threat is restricted. However, the threat list will continue to be dynamic (37, 42, 46), and the changing nature and number of potential biological pathogens that could be used to intentionally contaminate water also remains uncertain, which adds to the clinical challenge of accurate and timely diagnosis. Health care and public health practitioners will face many diagnostic dilemmas when attempting to accurately diagnose and appropriately manage waterborne disease resulting from intentional contamination of water supplies and the water environment with biological pathogens. Although weaponized biological pathogens are most effectively delivered as aerosolized particles, alternative modes of delivery and routes of exposure include intentional contamination of food and water systems and supplies (7, 9, 23, 30, 35, 39, 42). Biological pathogens that have been identified as potential biowarfare agents and that may cause waterborne disease include bacterial, parasitic, viral, and rickettsial and rickettsial-like pathogens (see Table 2).

DIAGNOSIS OF WATERBORNE DISEASE RESULTING FROM BIOTOXIN EXPOSURE   Biological toxins or biotoxins are also attractive biological warfare weapons owing to their severe toxicity and comparative ease of production (5). Biological toxins are an important and complex group of potential biowarfare agents that result from natural metabolites of bacteria, fungi, plant and algal, or marine species (42). These natural biotoxins are considered to be some of the most toxic substances known to man; lethal doses are often expressed in nanograms of exposure (5, 23). In general, most weaponized biotoxins have been developed primarily for aerosolized application and dissemination in military and civilian populations (62). However, many biotoxins are considered to be potential waterborne threats and would be effective contaminants in drinking water under suitable conditions (42, 62). The potential range of biotoxins available for direct and indirect contamination of water supply systems is significant (39). Many of the biotoxins of public health concern are stable in water and may not produce readily detectable changes in the physical characteristics of water (42, 62). Biotoxins that have been identified as potential biowarfare agents and that may cause waterborne disease include bacterial biotoxins, mycotoxins, fungal-, plant-, or algal-derived biotoxins, and marine biotoxins (see Table 2).

Many biotoxins are very stable under normal environmental conditions and produce serious symptoms when ingested, inhaled, or introduced into the body by other methods (23). Biological toxins display a broad range of physical and chemical characteristics and varied mechanisms of action, which results in a diverse spectrum of health effects ranging from minor illness to death in humans (5, 23).

Biological toxins including aflatoxins, botulinum toxins, and ricin have already been weaponized, and possible weaponization of other biotoxins may have been accomplished including microcystins, saxitoxin, T-2 mycotoxin, staphylococcal enterotoxins, and tetradotoxin (9, 62). There is evidence to suggest that natural production of microcystins found in stagnant bodies of water could produce enough biotoxin to cause illness in human populations if these bodies of water are used for public drinking water consumption (28, 40). Biotoxins are complex chemical compounds with varying solubilities, reaction rates, and degradation products in the water environment (28, 64). In addition, a specific toxin may display varying environmental stability and toxicity in water even within species type, such as for botulinum toxin with variation among types A, B, C, D, and E (56).

Biotoxin exposure and subsequent disease may be easily misdiagnosed if the diagnosis is not strongly suspected early during initial case presentation and in the early evaluation phase of a waterborne outbreak investigation (10). Biotoxins such as botulinum toxin may be stable for several days in untreated water or beverages, and, to prevent misdiagnosis, these potential contaminant sources should be included in an exposure history as a possible mode of dispersal of the biotoxin (3). Naturally occurring toxic blooms of cyanobacterial biotoxins have created potential health hazards in both drinking and recreational water (63). Therefore, recreational water exposure will also need to be included in a thorough exposure history to prevent a missed diagnosis of a possible intentional contamination event with certain biotoxins.

Use of Diagnostic Indicators and Epidemiologic Patterns to Diagnose Biowarfare Agent Exposure and Waterborne Disease

Even though specific detection methods for recognizing intentional contamination of water systems are improving rapidly (59), the most likely initial indication that a water contamination event has occurred will be a change in disease trends and illness patterns and possibly a community-wide waterborne disease outbreak. Therefore, the first indication of a terrorist attack may be an increased number of patients presenting to their health care provider or hospital emergency department with unusual or unexplained illness or injury (23, 29, 35). Frequently, humans are the most sensitive or only detectors, in many cases, of an intentional bioterrorist agent release, including the route of waterborne exposure (21, 29, 48). Consequently, the medical and public health community may provide the initial warning of intentional contamination of water and must understand their critical role as front-line responders in detecting water-related disease resulting from biological terrorism. Early presenting symptoms of waterborne biological warfare agents may be nonspecific and mimic more common endemic diseases and medical disorders. However, certain clinical manifestations and disease syndromes may be characteristic of a terrorist attack using the route of waterborne exposure to biological warfare agents.

Several published epidemiologic patterns and clinical sentinel clues provide a valuable resource for both the medical and public health community facing the challenges of diagnosing terrorism-related illness and injury (8, 11, 23, 34, 38, 44, 48, 51). These epidemiologic indicators may result from multiple exposure pathways including water and have universal application in a clinical and public health setting (see Table 3).

Use of Syndromic Surveillance and Disease Trends to Assist in the Diagnosis of Waterborne Terrorism

Although diagnostic laboratory testing, public health surveillance, and notifiable disease reporting have been enhanced since September 11, 2001, these systems may not be able to detect an evolving terrorist event or emerging outbreak (8). One method to supplement these traditional sources of public health "intelligence" is to employ syndromic surveillance, which utilizes the recognition of characteristic signs and symptoms of large groups of presenting patients usually at hospital emergency departments (8, 30, 51, 54). Embracing the use of syndromic surveillance as a diagnostic tool has the potential for enhancing early recognition of suspected cases of terrorism-related waterborne disease or waterborne outbreaks resulting from intentional water contamination (8, 30, 38, 51).

The benefit of using this approach to detect terrorism-related waterborne disease is based on the fact that syndromic surveillance monitors disease trends by grouping cases into syndromes rather than by specific diagnoses. Several state and local health departments are developing and implementing syndromic surveillance systems to complement traditional diagnosis-based surveillance systems (4). For the medical community, syndromic surveillance systems may augment emergency room and hospital diagnosis-based surveillance by adding the ability to quickly identify clusters of acute illness resulting from potential terrorism exposure (41).

Medical and public health practitioners should maintain a high level of suspicion for the following types of syndromes or clusters of disease in their patient populations or public health districts, which may indicate possible biowarfare agent exposure (8, 30, 54), including the use of water as a potential exposure route (46):

- gastroenteritis of an apparent infectious etiology or acute biotoxin exposure;
- upper and lower respiratory disease with fever and sudden death of previously healthy patients;
- rash of synchronous vesicular or pustular lesions and fever;
- suspected meningitis, encephalitis, and encephalopathy;
- sepsis or nontraumatic shock;
- unexplained death with a history of fever; and

TABLE 3 Epidemiologic indicators and sentinel clues indicating possible biowarfare agent exposure and illness[a,b]

Point source illness and injury patterns with record numbers of severely ill or dying patients presenting within a short period of time

Very high attack rates with 60%–90% of potentially exposed patients displaying symptoms or disease from possible biological agent exposure

Severe and frequent disease manifestations in previously healthy patients

Increased and early presentation of immunocompromised patients and vulnerable population patients with debilitating disease because the dose of inoculum or biotoxic exposure required to cause disease may be less than for the general healthy population

"Impossible epidemiology" with naturally occurring diseases diagnosed in geographic regions where the disease has not been encountered previously

Higher than normal numbers of patients presenting with gastrointestinal, respiratory, neurologic, and fever diagnoses

Record number of fatal cases with few recognizable signs and symptoms, indicating lethal doses near a point of dissemination or dispersal source of biological pathogen or biotoxin

Localized areas of disease epidemics that may occur in a specific neighborhood or sector, possibly indicating contamination of a selected point in a posttreatment water distribution system

Multiple infections at a single location (school, hospital, nursing home) with an unusual or rare biological pathogen

Lack of response or clinical improvement of presenting patients to traditional treatment modalities

Near simultaneous outbreaks of similar or different epidemics at the same or different locations, indicating an organized pattern of intentional biological agent release

Endemic disease presenting in a community during an unusual time of the year or found in a community where the normal vector of transmission is absent

Unusual temporal or geographic clustering of cases with patients attending a common public event, gathering, or recreational venue

Increased patient presentation with acute neurologic illness or cranial nerve impairment with progressive generalized weakness

Unusual or uncommon route of exposure of a disease such as illness resulting from a waterborne agent not normally found in the water environment

[a]Several epidemiologic patterns are presented above that have been identified as possible sentinel clues of a terrorist attack from several public health and military sources (8, 11, 23, 34, 38, 44, 48, 51). None of these indicators alone is pathognomonic for terrorism-related disease, but they are presented as an educational tool for use by health care providers and public health practitioners as possible disease trends that may warrant further investigation.
[b]Modified and reprinted with permission from the author and Arnot Ogden Medical Center (46).

- advancing cranial nerve impairment with progressive generalized weakness.

None of these indicators alone are pathognomonic for terrorism-related disease but represent disease trends that may warrant further investigation.

WEB-BASED RESOURCES AND CLINICAL TOOLS FOR WATERBORNE DISEASE AND WATER TERRORISM

Quick access to constantly updated and credible clinical information could assist most health care providers and public health practitioners to rapidly evaluate, manage, and prevent disease resulting from exposure to biowarfare agents (32, 38), including exposure from water sources (46). Results of a national survey of approximately 1000 family physicians conducted in 2002 revealed that the greatest predictor of responding appropriately to bioterrorism was "knowing how to get information in the event of a suspected attack"—this includes clinical information (16). The need of the medical and public health community for immediate access to specialized information and reference materials is extremely important when addressing the recognition and managment of acts of water terrorism, particularly if a public drinking water system is contaminated. In addition, the initial medical and public health response required to address an act of water terrorism will be inherently a local or regional challenge until external resources become available to a community (46). The American Medical Association estimates that local medical and public health responders may need to function unassisted for up to 6–8 hours until outside resources arrive, in the event of a terrorist attack (1).

An online clinical resource guide and management tool has been developed for health care practitioners and public health specialists faced with addressing the evaluation and management of water-related disease resulting from terrorist activity (45, 46). This free resource is posted as part of the physician online guide, *Recognizing Waterborne Disease and the Health Effects of Water Pollution* (http://www.WaterHealthConnection.org; Figures 2 and 3, see color insert). The primary purpose and educational intent of the terrorism preparedness tool, *Physician Preparedness for Acts of Water Terrorism*, is to provide the medical and public health community with streamlined access to resources that will help guide them through the recognition, management, and prevention of water-related disease resulting from intentional acts of water terrorism. This web-based educational program has been peer-reviewed by medical, public health, and military experts and has received, in the first 18-month period online, more than 7 million hits or requests for information from members of the medical and public health community from across the United States. Sustained use of these types of terrorism preparedness resources and targeted education of the medical and public health community are essential strategies for the continued protection and security of water supplies in the United States and for the prevention of waterborne disease resulting from intentional acts of water terrorism.

ACKNOWLEDGMENTS

The author thanks the Environmental Protection Agency, Arnot Ogden Medical Center, and the American Water Works Association for providing funding during the development and ongoing maintenance of the http://www.WaterHealth Connection.org Web site highlighted in this review. The author also extends a special thanks to Ms. Laura Campbell for her extremely valuable assistance and extraordinary expertise during the preparation of this manuscript.

The *Annual Review of Public Health* is online at
http://publhealth.annualreviews.org

LITERATURE CITED

1. Am. Med. Assoc. 2003. *Medical preparedness for terrorism and other disasters (1-00).* Counc. Sci. Aff. Rep. http://www.ama-assn.org/ama/pub/article/2036-5419.html (accessed 15 Jan. 2003)

2. Anda P, del Pozo JS, Diaz Garcia JM, Escudero R, Garcia Pena FJ, et al. 2001. Waterborne outbreak of tularemia associated with crayfish fishing. *Emerg. Infect. Dis.* 7:575-82

3. Arnon SS, Schechter R, Inglesby TV, Henderson DA, Bartlett JG, et al. 2001. Botulinum toxin as a biological weapon. *JAMA* 285:1059-70

4. Begier EM, Sockwell D, Branch LM, Davies-Cole JO, Jones LH, et al. 2003. The national capital region's emergency department syndromic surveillance system: Do chief complaint and diagnosis yield different results? *Emerg. Infect. Dis.* 9:393-96

5. Blazes DL, Lawler JV, Lazarus AA. 2002. When biotoxins are tools of terror: early recognition of intentional poisoning can attenuate effects. *Postgrad. Med.* 112:89-92

6. Boccia D, Tozzi AE, Cotter B, Rizzo C, Russo T, et al. 2002. Waterborne outbreak of Norwalk-like virus gastroenteritis at a tourist resort, Italy. *Emerg. Infect. Dis.* 8:563-68

7. Brachman PS. 2002. Bioterrorism: an update with a focus on anthrax. *Am. J. Epidemiol.* 155:981-88

8. Burkle FM. 2002. Mass casualty management of a large-scale bioterrorist event: an epidemiological approach that shapes triage decision. *Emerg. Med. Clin. N. Am.* 20:409-36

9. Burrows WD, Renner SE. 1999. Biological warfare agents as threats to potable water. *Environ. Health Perspect.* 107:975-84

10. Cent. Dis. Control Prev. 1998. Botulinum in the United States, 1899-1996. *Handbook for Epidemiologists, Clinicians, and Laboratory Workers.* Atlanta, GA: Cent. Dis. Control Prev. 66 pp.

11. Cent. Dis. Control Prev. 2001. Recognition of illness associated with the intentional release of a biologic agent. *Morb. Mortal. Wkly. Rep.* 50:893-97

12. Cent. Dis. Control Prev. 2002. Surveillance for waterborne disease outbreaks—United States, 1999-2000. *Morb. Mortal. Wkly. Rep.* 51:1-48

13. Cent. Dis. Control Prev. 2002. *Biological agents/diseases. Public health emergency preparedness and response.* http://www.bt.cdc.gov/agent/agentlist.asp (accessed 1 March 2003)

14. Cent. Dis. Control Prev. 2002. Tularemia-United States, 1990-2000. *Morb. Mortal. Wkly. Rep.* 51:181-84

15. Cent. Dis. Control Prev. Environ. Prot. Agency. 2003. *Water advisory in response to high threat level.* CDC Health Advis., Health Alert Netw. http://www.

phppo.cdc.gov/HAN/Index.asp (accessed 7 Feb. 2003)

16. Chen FM, Hickner J, Fink KS, Galliher JM, Burstin H. 2002. On the front lines: family physicians' preparedness for bioterrorism. *J. Fam. Pract.* 51:745–50

17. Chin J. 2000. *Control of Communicable Disease Manual.* Washington, DC: Am. Public Health Assoc. 624 pp.

18. Christopher GW, Cieslak TJ, Pavlin JA, Eitzen EM Jr. 1997. Biologic warfare—a historical perspective. *JAMA* 278:412–17

19. Clark RM, Deininger RA. 2000. Protecting the nation's critical infrastructure: the vulnerability of US water supply systems. *J. Conting. Crisis Manag.* 8:73–80

20. Daniels JI, Gallegos GM. 1990. *Evaluation of Military Field Water Quality:* Volume 1—*Executive Summary, No. UCRL-21008*, Rep. U.S. Army Med. Res. Dev. Command, Fort Detrick, Frederick, MD

21. Deininger RA. 2000. *The threat of chemical and biological agents to the public drinking water supply systems.* Water Pipeline Database, Sci. Appl. Int. Corp., MacLean, VA

22. Dennis TD, Inglesby TV, Henderson DA, Bartlett JG, Ascher MS, et al. 2001. Tularemia as a biological weapon. *JAMA* 285:2763–73

23. Dep. Army, Navy Air Force Command. Marine Corp. 2000. *Treatment of Biological Warfare Agent Casualties Field Manual.* No. FM 8–284/NAVMED P-5042/AFMAN (I) 44–156/MCRP 4–11.1C. Washington, DC

24. Environ. Prot. Agency. 2001. *EPA actions to safeguard the nation's drinking water supplies.* http://cfpub.epa.gov/safewater/watersecurity/index.cfm (accessed 31 Oct. 2001)

25. Environ. Prot. Agency. 2002. *EPA announces homeland security strategic plan, one of many efforts to ensure agency's ability to protect, respond and recover.* http://www.epa.gov/cgi-bin/epapr intonly.cgi (accessed on 2 Jan. 2003)

26. Environ. Prot. Agency. 2002. *ORD national homeland security research center.* http://www.epa.gov/nhsrc (accessed 2 Jan. 2003)

27. Environ. Prot. Agency. 2003. *EPA water protection program.* Natl. Homeland Secur. Res. Cent. http://www.epa.gov/ordnhsrc/programs.htm (accessed 19 March 2003)

28. Franz DR. 2002. *Defense against toxin weapons.* U.S. Army Med. Res. Inst. Infect. Dis., Fort Detrick, Frederick, MD. http://www.nbc-med.org (accessed 28 Sept. 2002)

29. Franz DR, Jahrling PB, Friedlander AM, McClain DJ, Hoover DL, et al. 1997. Clinical recognition and management of patients exposed to biological warfare agents. *JAMA* 278:399–411

30. Franz DR, Jahrling PB, McClain DJ, Hoover DL, Byrne WR, et al. 2001. Clinical recognition and management of patients exposed to biological warfare agents. *Clin. Lab. Med.* 21:435–73

31. Gerberding JL, Hughes JM, Koplan JP. 2002. Bioterrorism preparedness and response: clinicians and public health agencies as essential partners. *JAMA* 287:898–99

32. Greenough PG. 2002. Infectious diseases and disasters. See Ref. 34a, pp. 23–33

33. Henderson DA. 2003. Bioterrorism as a public health threat. *Emerg. Infect. Dis* 4:488–92. http://www.cdc.gov/ncidod/eid/vol4no3/hendrsn.htm (accessed 21 Jan. 2003)

34. Henretig FM, Cieslak TJ, Eitzen EM. 2002. Biological and chemical terrorism. *J. Pediatr.* 141:743–46

34a. Hogan DE, Burstein JL, eds. 2002. *Disaster Medicine*. Philadelphia, PA: Lippincott Williams & Wilkins

35. Inglesby TV, O' Toole T. 2003. *Medical aspects of biological terrorism.* Am. Coll. Physicians. http://www.acponline.org/bioterro/medicalaspets.htm (accessed 15 Jan. 2003)

36. Kaufmann AF, Meltzer MI, Schmid GP.

2003. The economic impact of a bioterrorist attack: Are prevention and postattack intervention programs justifiable? *Emerg. Infect. Dis.* 3:83–94. http://www.cdc.gov/ncidod/EID/vol3no2/kaufman.htm (accessed 21 Jan. 2003)

37. Kortepeter MG, Parker GW. 2003. Potential biological weapons threats. *Emerg. Infect. Dis.* 5:523–7. http://www.cdc.gov/ncidod?EID/vol5no4/kortepeter.htm (accessed 21 Jan. 2003)

38. Kortepeter MG, Rowe JR, Eitzen EM. 2002. Biological weapon agents. See Ref. 34a, pp. 350–63

39. Krieger G. 2003. Water and food contamination. In *Terrorism: Biological, Chemical and Nuclear from Clinics in Occupational and Environmental Medicine*, ed. KH Chase, MJ Upfal, GR Krieger, SD Phillips, TL Guidotti, D Weissman, pp. 253–62. Philadelphia, PA: Saunders

40. Layton DW, Mallon BJ, McKone TE, Ricker YE, Lessard PC. 1988. Evaluation of military field-water quality, volume 2-constituents of military concern from natural and anthropogenic sources. *Final Rep. APO 82PP2817.* U.S. Army Med. Res. Dev. Command, Fort Detrick, Frederick, MD

41. Lazarus R, Kleinman K, Dashevsky I, Adams C, Kludt P, et al. 2002. Use of automated ambulatory-care encounter records for detection of acute illness clusters, including potential bioterrorism events. *Emerg. Infect. Dis.* 8:753–60 http://www.cdc.gov/ncidod/EID/vol8no8/02–0239.htm (accessed 7 May 2003)

42. Linstren DC. 1987. Nuclear, biological and chemical (NBC) contamination to army field water supplies. *Rep. 2438, ADB109393.* U.S. Army Belvoir Res., Dev. Eng. Cent. Fort Belvoir, VA

43. Macintyre AG, Christopher GW, Eitzen E Jr, Gum R, Weir S, et al. 2000. Weapons of mass destruction events with contaminated casualties: effective planning for health care facilities. *JAMA* 283:242–49

44. McGovern TW, Christopher GW, Eitzen EM. 1999. Cutaneous manifestations of biological warfare and related threat agents. *Arch. Dermatol.* 135:311–22

45. Meinhardt PL. 2002. *Recognizing waterborne disease and the health effects of water pollution: physician on-line reference guide.* Am. Water Works Assoc./Arnot Ogden Med. Cent. http://www.waterhealthconnection.org (accessed 3 Jan. 2003)

46. Meinhardt PL. 2003. *Physician preparedness for acts of water terrorism: physician on-line readiness guide.* Environ. Prot. Agency/Arnot Ogden Med. Cent. http://www.waterhealthconnection.org (accessed 5 July 2003)

47. Natl. Res. Counc. 2002. *Making the Nation Safer: The Role of Science and Technology in Countering Terrorism.* Comm. Sci. Technol. Count. Terror. Washington, DC: Natl. Acad. Press

48. N. Atlantic Treaty Org. 1996. *NATO Handbook on the Medical Aspects of NBC Defensive Operations.* MedP-6(B) http://www.fas.org/nuke/guide/usa/doctrine/dod/fm8-9/toc.htm (accessed 21 Jan. 2003)

49. Off. Press Secretary. 2002. *President delivers state of the union address. Whitehouse Off. Press Secretary* http://www.whitehouse.gov/news/releases/2002/01/20020129–11.html (accessed 14 Sept. 2002)

50. Olsen SJ, Miller G, Breuer T, Kennedy M, Higgins C, et al. 2002. A waterborne outbreak of *Escherichia coli* O157:H7 infections and hemolytic uremic syndrome: implications for rural water systems. *Emerg. Infect. Dis.* 8:370–75

51. Pavlin JA. 2003. Epidemiology of bioterrorism. *Emerg. Infect. Dis.* 5:528–30. http://www.cdc.gov/ncidod/EID/vol5no4/pavlin.htm (accessed 21 Jan. 2003)

52. Pile JC, Malone JD, Eitzen EM, Friedlander AM. 1998. Anthrax as a potential biological warfare agent. *Arch. Intern. Med.* 158:429–34

53. Rohr R, Stapleton DR. 2002. The response

of health systems to bioterrorism. *The Guthrie J.* 71:138–46

54. Sauri M. 2002. Bioterrorism treatment information. *Md. Med.* 3:40–42

55. Sharp TW, Brennan RJ, Keim M, Williams RJ, Eitzen E, Lillibridge S. 1998. Medical preparedness for a terrorist incident involving chemical or biological agents during the 1996 Atlanta Olympic games. *Ann. Emerg. Med.* 32:214–23

56. Siegel LS. 1993. Destruction of botulinum in food and water. In *Clostridium Botulinum: Ecology and Control in Foods,* ed. HW Hauschild, K Dodds, pp. 45–57. New York: M. Dekker

57. Sifton DW, ed. 2002. *PDR Guide to Biological and Chemical Warfare Response,* pp. vii–xii. Montvale, NJ: Thomson/Physicians' Desk Ref.

58. Smith C. 2002. Biological warfare and bioterrorism. *J. Med. Assoc. Ga.* 91 (Summer):12–15

59. States S, Scheuring M, Kuchta J, Newberry J, Casson LW. 2003. Utility-based analytical methods to ensure public water supply security. *J. Am. Water Works Assoc.* 95:103–15

60. Straight TM, Lazarus AA, Decker CF. 2002. Defending against viruses in biowarfare: how to respond to smallpox, encephalitides, and hemorrhagic fevers. *Postgrad. Med.* 112:75:75–76

61. Uniformed Serv. Univ. Health Sci. 1995. *Proc. Semin. Responding to the Consequences of Chemical and Biologic Terrorism.* Bethesda, MD

62. U.S. Army Center Health Promot. Prev. Med. 1998. Biological warfare agents as potable water threats. *Med. Issues Inf. Pap.*, No. IP-31–017

63. Vasconcelos VM, Sivonen K, Evans WR, Carmichael WW, Namikoshi M. 1996. Hepatotoxic microcystin diversity in cyanobacterial blooms collected in Portuguese freshwaters. *Water Res.* 30:2377–84

64. Warner JS. 1990. Review of reactions of biotoxins in water. *Final Rep. CBIAC Task 152.* U.S. Army Med. Res. Dev. Command, Fort Detrick, Frederick, MD

65. Weinstein B. 2003. *Uncovering bioterrorism.* http://www.llnl.gov/str/Weinstein. html (accessed 15 Jan. 2003)

66. WHO. 2001. *Public health response to biological and chemical weapons-WHO guidance.* http://www.who.int/emc/pdfs/ BIOWEAPONS_exec_sum2.pdf (accessed 5 Jan. 2003)

Annu. Rev. Public Health 2005. 26:239–57
doi: 10.1146/annurev.publhealth.26.021304.144628
Copyright © 2005 by Annual Reviews. All rights reserved
First published online as a Review in Advance on November 1, 2004

ECONOMIC CAUSES AND CONSEQUENCES
OF OBESITY

Eric A. Finkelstein,[1] Christopher J. Ruhm,[2]
and Katherine M. Kosa[1]

[1]*RTI International*, Research Triangle Park, North Carolina 27709;*
email: finkelse@rti.org, kkosa@rti.org
[2]*Bryan School, University North Carolina, Greensboro, North Carolina 27402-6165;*
email: c_ruhm@uncg.edu

Key Words   costs, expenditure, technology, wages, intervention

■ **Abstract**   Obesity is not only a health but also an economic phenomenon. This chapter (*a*) examines underlying economic causes, such as technological advancements, behind the obesity epidemic; (*b*) describes economic consequences of obesity, including increasing obesity-related medical expenditures; and (*c*) discusses the role of government in combating the obesity epidemic. Because of the high costs of obesity, and the fact that the majority of these costs are financed by taxpayers, there is a clear motivation for government to try to reduce these costs. However, because obesity may result from poor information and addictive behavior and/or as a result of living in an increasingly obesogenic environment, interventions will need to be multifaceted to ensure the best chance of success.

INTRODUCTION

As shown in Figure 1, the rapid rise in obesity rates began in the 1980s. Between 1960 and 1980, obesity prevalence rates in the United States increased less than 2 percentage points to 15% (23).[1] In the past 25 years, obesity rates have more than doubled. During the late 1980s and early 1990s, obesity prevalence climbed to 23% and reached 31% by 2000. Grade III obesity (BMI ≥ 40.0 kg/m^2) grew even more rapidly, rising from 1.3% in the late 1970s to 4.7% in 2000 (22, 23).

As the prevalence of obesity has increased, so too has the incidence of obesity-related diseases, including type 2 diabetes, cardiovascular disease, several types of

---

*RTI International is a trade name of Research Triangle Institute.
[1]Adults are classified as obese if their body mass index (BMI) is ≥ 30 kg/m^2 (48, 78). These prevalence rates are age-adjusted using the 2000 Census population.

239

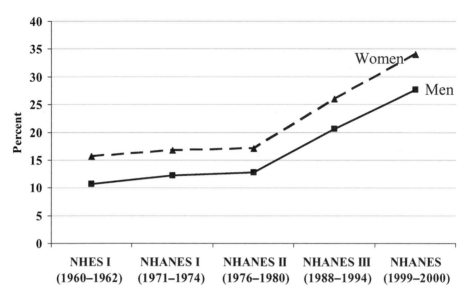

Figure 1   Adult obesity trends by gender, United States, 1960–2000 (Source: Reference 23). NHANES, National Health and Nutrition Examination Survey.

cancer (endometrial, postmenopausal breast, kidney, and colon cancers), musculoskeletal disorders, sleep apnea, and gallbladder disease (19, 45, 75). As a result, obesity now accounts for approximately 400,000 deaths per year, second only to tobacco (44).

Obesity is not only a health but also an economic phenomenon. Several economic factors affect our food consumption and physical activity decisions, and ultimately our weight. The first section of this chapter provides a review of articles attempting to explain the underlying economic causes of the obesity epidemic. Without a better understanding of these causes, it is difficult to identify effective strategies that might help stem the rise in obesity rates. The second half of the review focuses on the economic consequences of obesity, including the increase in medical and other obesity-related expenditures and the relationship between obesity and wages. We conclude with a summary and discussion of the government's role in reducing obesity rates.

This review is meant to be selective rather than exhaustive. We conducted a systematic exploration of computerized scientific literature databases of economic (EconLit), medical (Medline), and agricultural (AGRICOLA) citations. Our search started with a list of key words established by the investigators. The key words included body weight terms (e.g., BMI, overweight, and obesity) and various economic indicators, including food prices, employment, income, direct medical costs, and productivity loss.

CAUSES OF OBESITY

Taking a historical perspective, obesity was a rare phenomena until the latter part of the twentieth century (11). Because the majority of the population was more likely to suffer from weight deficits, increased body weight was typically associated with improved health. This view changed when obesity rates skyrocketed during the past 25 years.

At the most basic level, the cause of increased body weight is well understood: Individuals gain weight when calories consumed exceed those expended. Why this imbalance changed so abruptly in the early 1980s and continues today remains an open question. Shifts in economic factors that substantially pre- or postdate the rise in obesity rates are unlikely to explain a large portion of the trend; however, identifying economic factors that changed around the time that obesity prevalence markedly increased may help identify underlying causes of the epidemic. A complicating factor, as pointed out by Hill et al. (37), is that the rise in obesity rates could be explained by as little as an average net increase of 50–100 calories per day, which is less than half the calories in a 16-ounce carbonated beverage.

Reductions in Energy Expenditure

Philipson (53) and Lakdawalla & Philipson (40) argued that technological change is responsible for the obesity epidemic largely because of its effect of reducing energy expenditure in the workplace. Advancements in workplace technology may have been responsible for a portion of the increase in obesity in the 1980s, but the majority of the shift away from manual employment predated this time period.

Consider employment in goods-producing (versus service-providing) industries as an approximation of the strenuousness of market work. The fraction of wage and salary workers employed in goods-producing industries fell from 27% in 1980 to 19% in 2000 (12); however, this decline represents the continuation of a longer-term trend: 35% of jobs were in goods-producing industries in 1960. This gradual decline in manual labor began well before the rapid rise in obesity rates and suggests that other factors are more likely to be responsible for the rise in obesity. This evidence is not intended to be comprehensive, since goods-producing jobs have also become more sedentary over time. However, this too is likely to represent a longer trend, with little reason to suspect that sharp changes have occurred since the late 1970s. Even when expanded to include labor-saving devices in the home, the same story can be told. For example, the portion of homes with washing machines and dishwashers rose from 55% to 77% and from 7% to 43%, respectively, between 1960 and 1979, but only slightly further to 79% and 54%, respectively, by 2001 (72, 73).

More generally, the available evidence, although prone to considerable error, suggests that reductions in calorie expenditures are unlikely to explain the majority of the rise in obesity observed during the last quarter-century. For example, using data from time use diaries presented by Robinson & Godbey (58), Cutler et al. (13) reported that energy expenditure fell substantially from 1.69 to 1.57 kcal/min/kg between 1965 and 1975 but has remained fairly constant since that time.

Moreover, Robinson & Godbey (58) provided evidence that leisure-time activities have become more active. For instance, the time individuals spent in "active" sports, outdoor recreation, or walking/hiking/exercise rose from 7 to 24 min per day between 1965 and 1995. Similarly, survey data indicate the percentage of adults who engage in light-to-moderate physical activity rose from 22% to 30%, and the percentage who participate in vigorous activities rose from 12% to 14% between 1985 and 1998 (47).[2] Conversely, the fraction of adults who engage in no leisure-time physical activity declined from 31% in 1988 to 25% in 2002 (9). Finally, the rapid rise in obesity rates among children and adolescents, who are presumably less affected by labor-saving technology, suggests that other factors are responsible for the obesity epidemic.

Increases in Energy Intake

Table 1 summarizes the results of five studies examining trends in energy intake. These data suggest that the number of calories consumed has risen markedly during the same time period as the increase in obesity, and that the growth in energy intake is of sufficient magnitude to explain the rise in body weight. For instance, Putnum et al. (54) showed that, after remaining roughly constant between 1910 and 1985, caloric intake rose by roughly 12% (300 calories per day) between 1985 and 2000, mainly because of increased consumption of grains, added fats, and added sugars. The Centers for Disease Control and Prevention (CDC) (10) indicated that caloric consumption remained essentially unchanged between 1971–1974 and 1976–1980 but increased 7.3% (179 calories per day) for men and 23.3% (355 calories per day) for women between 1976–1980 and 1999–2000 (10). Nielsen & Popkin (49) did not show any change in energy consumption from 1977–1978 through 1989–1991 but found an 11% (190 kcal per day) increase from 1989–1991 to 1994–1996.

Much of the rise in energy intake is related to increased consumption of carbohydrates. In 1976–1980, adult men and women aged 20–74 years consumed daily 1039 and 700 kcal of carbohydrates, respectively. In 1999–2000, these numbers increased to 1283 and 969 kcal (10). Beverages, particularly fruit and soft drinks, are also responsible for a surprising number of calories. In 1997, the average American consumed 53 gallons of soft drinks and 17 gallons of fruit juices or drinks, a

---

[2]Individuals are defined as engaging in light-to-moderate physical activity if the activities last for at least 30 min on 5 or more days per week and cause light sweating or slight-to-moderate increases in heart rate. Vigorous activities require heavy sweating or large increases in heart rate for at least 20 min on 3 or more days per week.

TABLE 1 Trends in energy intake

Study	Data[a]	Results
Centers for Disease Control and Prevention (2004) (10)	NHANES: 1971–1974, 1976–1980, 1988–1994, 1999–2000	Daily energy intake of males and females aged 20–74 years increased from 2439 kcals and 1522 kcals in 1976–1980 to 2618 and 1877, respectively, in 1999–2000. The increase is due primarily to a rise in the intake of carbohydrates, which accounted for 42.6% and 46.0% of the total calories consumed in 1976–1980 for men and women, respectively, and 49.0% and 51.6%, respectively, in 1999–2000.
Cutler et al. (2003) (13)	CSFII: 1977–1978, 1994–1996	Daily energy intake for males and females increased from 2080 kcals and 1515 kcals in 1977–1978 to 2347 kcals and 1658 kcals in 1994–1996, respectively.
Nielsen & Popkin (2003) (49)	NFCS: 1977–1978; CSFII: 1989–1991 and 1994–1996	Daily energy intake for persons aged 2 years and older increased from 1795 kcals in 1989–91 to 1985 kcals in 1994–1996.
Putnum et al. (2002) (55)	USFSS: 1985–2000	Average daily energy intake rose 12% (approximately 300 kcal) between 1985 and 2000. Grains, added fats, and added sugars accounted for 46%, 24%, and 23%, respectively, of the increase.
Troiano et al. (2000) (70)	NHANES: 1971–1974, 1976–1980, 1988–1994 (12 to 19 year olds)	Daily energy intake of males and females aged 12–19 years increased from 2789 kcals and 1751 kcals in 1976–1980 to 2864 kcals and 1975 kcals in 1988–1994, respectively.

[a] Abbreviations: CSFII: Continuing Survey of Food Intake by Individuals; NHANES: National Health and Nutrition Examination Survey; NFCS: Nationwide Food Consumption Surveys; USFSS: U.S. Food Supply Series.

51% and 40% increase since 1980 (55).[3] During the 1988–1994 period, 20%–24% of the calories consumed by children came from beverages of all types and, among 12- to 19-year-olds, 8% came from soft drinks, and 4% came from fruit juices and drinks (70).[4]

The increase in energy intake has been accompanied by changes in eating patterns; snacking has become more prevalent over time. Cutler et al. (13) found that higher snack calories are responsible for the entire rise in energy intake among females between 1977–1978 and 1994–1996 and for 90% of the increase among males. Nielsen & Popkin (49) showed that 76% of the growth in calories between these two periods resulted from increased snacking. Related studies highlight the increases in the prevalence of snacking, number of snacks per day, and energy density of snacks for children and young adults (38, 80). There is some variation across studies in the trends in calories consumed per snack. Jahns et al. (38) found that this has remained relatively constant for 2- to 18-year-olds, whereas Zizza et al. (78) indicated a 26% increase over the past two decades for adults between the ages of 19 and 29 years.

Causes of Increased Consumption

Economists' first law of demand implies that a decrease in the price of food will cause consumption to increase (43). Moreover, if the price of calorie-dense, prepackaged, and/or prepared foods (e.g., fast food) falls faster than for less calorie-dense foods (e.g., vegetables), then individuals will shift their consumption toward these cheaper alternatives.

Consumer price index (CPI) data indicate that food prices rose 3.4% per year from 1980 to 2000, which is slower than the 3.8% average rise in the inflation rate over the same period (12). Although this difference may not seem large, it implies that the relative price of food fell 14% over this time period. Interestingly, from 1960 through 1980, when the prevalence of obesity did not change, food prices actually rose slightly faster than the overall inflation rate (5.5% versus 5.3% per year). Moreover, the relative prices of calorie-dense foods and beverages (i.e., those made from added sugars and fats) decreased since the early 1980s, compared with less energy-dense foods, like fruits and vegetables. Between 1985 and 2000, the price of fresh fruits and vegetables, fish, and dairy products increased by 118%, 77%, and 56%, respectively, whereas sugar and sweets, fats and oils, and carbonated beverages (54) increased at lower rates—46%, 35%, and 20%,

---

[3]Consumption of fruit drinks was not reported in 1980. The percentage increase in fruit juices and drinks was therefore calculated by assuming that the ratio of fruit juices to drinks consumed was the same in 1980 as in 1987, the first year in which fruit drink consumption was identified. This probably overstates the consumption of fruit drinks in the earlier year, implying that the trend growth for the entire category is likely to be underestimated.

[4]For children aged 2–5 years and 6–11 years, 27% and 4%, respectively, of calories came from soft drinks and 8% and 5%, respectively, came from fruit juice/drinks.

respectively (55). These trends in relative prices are consistent with rapid increases in the consumption of products made with added sugars and fats (15). As a result, Cutler et al. (13) hypothesized that the rise in caloric intake and obesity primarily resulted from changes in food production technology that reduced the price of mass-produced, calorie-dense foods. In addition, evidence from a randomized experiment conducted by Devitt & Mattes (14) suggested that among subjects given equal-sized meals (measured by weight), those receiving foods with the highest energy densities consume more calories because they do not materially change the amount of food eaten.

Reductions in the relative price of energy-dense foods and an increased prevalence of marginal cost pricing (i.e., "supersizing") have resulted not only in an increase in food consumption between meals, but also in an increase in the amount of food consumed at each meal (i.e., larger portion sizes). Young & Nestle (79) provided evidence that serving sizes of virtually all food eaten away from home have increased over time. Nielsen & Popkin (49) found similar growth in portion sizes for the majority of foods examined, with the largest increases seen for French fries and sweetened beverages. Serving sizes, which began to increase in the 1970s, continued to increase in the 1980s and 1990s at the same time that obesity rates rose. In fact, classic cook books, such as *Joy of Cooking*, now specify fewer servings from the same recipes than did older editions, which suggests that portion sizes have also increased for meals eaten at home. Moreover, serving sizes are also larger in the United States than in Europe.

In addition to affecting the strenuousness of most activities and reducing the relative price of food, technological advancements have also resulted in an increase in real wages for those in many occupations. For example, between 1982 and 2002, the average hourly wage of workers in private nonagricultural industries rose by approximately 5% (12). Several studies (29–33) influenced by Becker's seminal work (5) have shown that changes in wage rates affect both employment and "household production."

A rise in wages will presumably result in more hours worked, which could lead to an increase in the consumption of restaurant and prepackaged foods, and ultimately increased weight. Lakdawalla & Phillipson (40) used data from the National Longitudinal Survey of Youth (NLSY) to test the relationship between wages and weight. They found no statistically significant effects of wages on men's weight but find that higher wages are associated with lower weight for women. As discussed in the following section, however, the direction of causality in the relationship between wages and weight remains an open question.

Although not addressed in the Lakdawalla & Phillipson (40) analysis, higher wage opportunities for women have also led to a dramatic increase in female labor force participation, which may have independently increased obesity rates. From 1970 to 1990, the typical two-income family increased annual market work by 600 hours (6). This trend may partly explain why the consumption of food away from home increased from 18% to 32% of total calories between 1977–1978 and 1994–1996 and from 32% to 38% of food expenditures between 1980 and 2000 (17,

35).[5] Foods eaten away from home, particularly fast food, are associated with high levels of fat and calorie intake. In 1995, 27% of meals included away-from-home foods, and 34% of calories came from these foods (25).

Chou et al. (10a) linked the rise in body weight to the increase in the availability of fast-food and full-service restaurants, which they interpret as a reduction in time costs that occur in response to an increase in the value of household time.[6] Similarly, Anderson et al. (2) and Ruhm (62) provided evidence that increases in maternal employment may account for some of the rise in childhood obesity and suggest that children of working mothers eat home-cooked meals less frequently. One caveat, however, is that the number of women in the labor force increased well before the rise in obesity began.[7]

Investigators have posited many other factors as at least partly responsible for the rise in obesity rates. These factors may have independent effects or interact with the economic factors discussed above. For example, urban sprawl has been correlated with obesity (18). Although urban sprawl began prior to the obesity epidemic and has changed fairly gradually over time, an increase in sprawl likely acts to attenuate the effects of the economic factors detailed above.

Television has also received a great deal of attention for its role in promoting a sedentary lifestyle. However, there is some evidence that the largest growth in viewing hours occurred during the early 1960s and mid-1970s, when color televisions first became widely available at relatively low prices. For example, time diary evidence summarized by Cutler et al. (13) indicated that daily television viewing increased 21% (from 158 to 191 min) between 1965 and 1975 but just 11% from 1975 to 1995 (to 212 min). Although Nielsen data suggested much higher levels of television viewing during this time period (48a), it is unlikely that television viewing alone is responsible for the obesity epidemic. In fact, total screen time, including time spent in front of computers, video games, and other media devices, all of which increased dramatically since the 1980s, may better explain the rise in obesity rates than television viewing alone. However, only television viewing has been shown to increase snacking, portion sizes, the percentage of calories from fat, and calories (25), and these effects are likely to be more pronounced when calorie-dense foods are cheaper and more widely available. Moreover, since children are exposed to ~10 food commercials per hour of viewing, most for fast foods, soft drinks, sweets, and sugar-sweetened cereals (16), television may increase demand for these products more than computer or video game use.

---

[5]Nielsen et al. (50) showed that the dramatic increases in food consumption away from home occurred fairly uniformly across age groups rather than being concentrated among the young as is often believed.

[6]Ruhm (61, 63) showed that obesity becomes more prevalent during macroeconomic upturns, in part because higher time costs lead to reductions in health-preserving activities such as exercise.

[7]The fraction of females aged 16 years and over who were employed rose from 36% in 1960 to 48% in 1980 and to 58% in 2000 (12).

CONSEQUENCES OF OBESITY

The rapid rise in body weight has been associated with a commensurate increase in obesity-related medical treatments and expenditures. Between 1988 and 1994, there was an 88% increase in the number of physician office visits resulting from obesity (77). Two papers, Quesenberry et al. (56) and Thompson et al. (68), presented statistics detailing obesity-attributable utilization and cost differences for specific medical services.

Compared with individuals of normal weight (20 kg/m^2 ≤ BMI ≤ 24.9 kg/m^2), Quesenberry et al. (56) estimated that individuals who are moderately obese (30 kg/m^2 ≤ BMI ≤ 34.9 kg/m^2) and severely obese (BMI ≥ 35 kg/m^2) have 14% and 25% more physician visits, respectively. Thompson et al. (68) found that obese adults (BMI ≥ 30 kg/m^2) have 38% more visits to primary care physicians. Quesenberry et al. (56) reported that moderately and severely obese individuals have 34% and 74%, respectively, more inpatient days than those of normal weight, and Thompson et al. (68) reported that obese individuals average 48% more inpatient days per year. They also reported that individuals with a BMI greater than 30 kg/m^2 had 1.84 times the annual number of pharmacy dispenses, including 6 times the number of dispenses for diabetes medication and 3.4 times the number of dispenses for cardiovascular medications (68).

Annual Medical Costs

Two recent nationally representative studies compare the annual obesity-attributable medical costs for obese and normal-weight individuals; the findings are nearly identical. Sturm (66) used nationally representative data from the 1997–1998 Healthcare for Communities survey and found that obese adults aged 18–65 years incur annual medical expenditures that are 36% higher than expenditures of normal-weight individuals. Similarly, Finkelstein et al. (20) used data from the 1998 Medical Expenditure Panel Survey (MEPS) linked to the National Health Interview Survey (NHIS) and found that the average increase in annual medical expenditures associated with obesity is 37.4% ($732) and ranges between 26.1% ($125) for out-of-pocket expenses, 36.8% ($1486) for Medicare recipients, and 39.1% ($864) for Medicaid recipients.

Several studies (67, 76, 77) that combined prevalence and cost data to produce aggregate obesity cost estimates revealed similar results. Early studies rely mostly on epidemiologic methods. Using this approach, Thompson et al. (67) found that total spending attributable to obesity accounts for approximately 5% of health insurance expenditures among businesses with employer-provided health insurance. Wolf & Colditz (76, 77) published several papers that suggest aggregate costs of obesity range from 5.5% to 7.0% of annual medical expenditures. In two papers that use an econometric approach to quantify costs of obesity, Finkelstein et al. (20, 21) produced cost estimates ranging from 5.3% to 5.7% of annual medical expenditures. These papers provide evidence that the aggregate annual obesity-attributable medical costs in the United States are between 5% and 7% of annual health care expenditures.

These two papers were the first to show the percentage of obesity costs financed by taxpayers (20, 21). Because many obese individuals will inevitably be covered by Medicare, and because the Medicaid population has a 50% higher prevalence of obesity, the government finances roughly half the total annual medical costs attributable to obesity. As a result, the average taxpayer spends approximately $175 per year to finance obesity-related medical expenditures among Medicare and Medicaid recipients (20, 21).

Lifetime Medical Costs

Policy makers have used the high annual cost of obesity as a justification for governmental intervention (74). Although annual health care costs among the obese are higher, investigators have suggested that lifetime costs may be lower because obese individuals have shorter life expectancies (24, 65). Three papers address lifetime medical costs of obesity and find no "savings" (1, 27, 69). In the only paper to quantify aggregate costs, Allison et al. (1) reported that 4.3% of lifetime costs are attributable to obesity, compared with an annual estimate between 5.6% and 7.0% (20, 21, 76, 77).

Nonmedical Expenditures

The increase in medical expenditures is not the only cost associated with obesity. Although results vary considerably, many studies have shown that obese individuals, especially women, are more likely to be absent from work than are their normal-weight coworkers (7, 41, 46, 67, 71). After controlling for confounders, Tucker & Friedman (71) reported obese employees (percent body fat $\geq 25\%$ and 30% for men and women, respectively) are 1.74 and 1.61 times more likely to experience high (7 or more absenses due to illness per 6 months) and moderate (3–6 more absenses due to illness per 6 months) levels of absenteeism, respectively, than were their lean counterparts (percent body fat $\leq 15\%$ and 20% for men and women, respectively). Thompson et al. (67) estimated obesity-attributable absenteeism cost employers $2.4 billion in 1998 ($2.95 billion in 2003 dollars). In addition to medical expenditures and absenteeism, Wolf & Colditz (77) estimated that obesity (in aggregate) resulted in 239 million restricted activity days and 89.5 million bed days in 1995.

Occupational Choice and Wages

Some evidence exists that obese individuals' occupations, primarily women's, differ from those of normal-weight individuals. Pagan & Davila (52) reported that obese women work mostly in relatively low-paying occupations and are largely excluded from high-paying managerial/professional and technical occupations. Haskins & Ransford (36), using data from one employer in the aerospace industry, reported that 65% of normal-weight women are in managerial/professional positions compared with only 39% of overweight women (defined as 10% or more over the upper limit of ideal body weight range). Sarlio-Lahteenkorva et al. (64) found that obese women are 2.5 times more likely to report long-term unemployment and have higher rates of poverty. Even for those in similar occupations, obese individuals may earn less than their normal-weight counterparts do.

Eight studies (3, 4, 8, 28, 42, 43, 52, 57) have used nationally representative data from the NLSY to quantify the effect of obesity on wages. Although most studies found a negative correlation between women's wages and weight (3, 8, 43, 52, 57), they were unable to determine whether lower wages result from higher weight or vice versa. Gortmaker et al. (28) attempted to solve this problem by focusing on the effects of weight in adolescence on wages seven years later. They found that women who are overweight (BMI > 95th percentile for age and sex) in adolescence have 22% ($6710) lower annual household incomes than do women of normal weight.

The effect of weight on women's wages may differ by race. Averett & Korenman (4) reported that white obese (BMI $\geq$ 30 kg/m^2) women earn 17% less than do white women of normal weight (19 kg/m^2 < BMI < 25 kg/m^2). Cawley (8) reported that an increase in weight of two standard deviations (roughly 65 pounds) is associated with a 7% decrease in wages of white women. Neither of the studies found a significant effect of weight on wages of black women.

There is less compelling evidence of a negative relationship between earnings and weight for men; three studies (43, 52, 57) found no relationship, and one study (42) found a positive relationship. When Averett & Korenman (3) examined the effect of obesity in 1981 on the wages of men in 1988, they found a statistically significant negative relationship; however, the effect becomes insignificant when differences for social class and family background are controlled. Gortmaker et al. (28) reported that men overweight (BMI > 95th percentile for age and sex) in adolescence have 9% ($2876) lower annual household incomes seven years later than do men of normal weight. The results from these studies for both males and females are summarized in Table 2.

CONCLUSION

The published evidence, although not conclusive, suggests that technology may be primarily responsible for the obesity epidemic. Technological advancements have allowed us to be increasingly productive at work and at home while expending fewer calories and have also reduced food prices, especially prices for energy-dense foods. These changes directly increase net calories and may interact with other factors (e.g., television, the built environment) to further promote weight gain.

The obesity epidemic has deleterious economic consequences. Obesity is responsible for between 5% and 7% of the total annual medical expenditures in the United States or $75 billion per year (20). Updated to 2003 dollars, the 2001 U.S. Surgeon General's report on obesity stated that annual indirect costs of obesity

TABLE 2 Findings on the effect of body weight on earnings for males and females

Study	Obesity measure	Findings Males	Findings Females
Register & Williams (1990) (57)	Obesity (relative weight $\geq$ 20% above the standard)	No effect	Obese females earn 12% less than nonobese females.
Gortmaker et al. (1993) (28)	Overweight (BMI $\geq$ 95th percentile for age and sex)	Men overweight in adolescence have 9% lower annual household incomes 7 years later.	Women overweight in adolescence have 22% lower annual household incomes 7 years later.
Loh (1993) (42)	Obesity (relative weight $\geq$ 20% above the standard)	Men who weigh 10% more than their ideal weight earn 1.4% more.	No effect
Averett & Korenman (1996) (3)	Overweight (BMI is 25–29 kg/m^2) and Obesity (BMI $\geq$ 30 kg/m^2)	Obese males in 1981 earned 8% less in 1988 in the cross-sectional specifications. In the sibling-differenced specifications, the wage effect on weight is insignificant.	Obese females earn 10% less and overweight females earn 5% less than normal-weight women in the cross-sectional specifications. In the sibling-differenced specifications, the wage effect of weight is insignificant.
Pagan & Davila (1997) (52)	Continuous BMI	No effect	A one point increase in BMI is associated with a decrease in wages ranging from 0.1% in the precision production/craft/repair operators occupation to 1.5% in the technical and assemblers/inspectors/machine occupations.

Study		Measure	Results
Averett & Korenman (1999) (4)	Not in the sample	Overweight (BMI is 25–29 kg/m^2) and Obesity (BMI $\geq$ 30 kg/m^2)	White obese women earn 17% less than white women of recommended weight. The effect of weight is insignificant for black women.
Cawley (2000) (8)	Not in the sample	Continuous BMI or weight in pounds controlled for height in inches	An increase in weight of two standard deviations (roughly 65 pounds) is associated with a 7% decrease in wages for white women. No effect of weight is found for Hispanic or black women.
Mitra (2001) (43)	No effect	Continuous weight in pounds controlled for height in inches	A one-pound increase in weight is associated with a 2% decrease in wages of women in professional and managerial occupations. A one-pound increase in weight is associated with a 1% decrease in wages of women with below-average mathematical skills. No effect of weight on wages is found among women with above-average mathematical skills.

total $64 billion (74), which suggests that the total (direct and indirect) costs of obesity may now be as high as $139 billion per year.

The published literature reveals a negative correlation between wages and weight, primarily among white women; however, two questions need to be answered. First, do lower wages result in weight gain, or does excess weight lead to lower wages? Second, are earnings lower because of discrimination, as suggested (3, 4, 28, 36, 43, 52, 57), or productivity differences?[8]

Given the changes in our environment that have occurred over the past 30 years, it has become increasingly more difficult for individuals to maintain a healthy weight. It is not surprising, therefore, that the prevalence of obesity has increased. Many people who could have maintained a healthy weight in decades past find it too difficult to do so today. Even with full information about the benefits of physical activity, the nutrient content of food, and the health consequences of obesity, some fraction of the population will optimally choose to engage in a lifestyle that leads to weight gain because the costs (in terms of time, money, and opportunity costs) of not doing so are just too high. Because much of the monetary costs of obesity are financed by taxpayers, the physical activity and food consumption decisions of these individuals are not optimal from a broader societal perspective, implying a role for government in attempting to reduce obesity. It should be acknowledged, however, that for many individuals information-based interventions or other interventions that do not affect the costs or benefits of physical activity and food consumption decisions are unlikely to be effective. For some individuals, additional incentives may be needed to encourage them to lose weight.

An emerging class of economic models emphasizes how suboptimal outcomes will be obtained by individuals with self-control problems, either because of genetics or other factors (34, 39, 51). These individuals would like to make different choices but are not able to do so.[9] Given self-control problems associated with food consumption (59, 60), many individuals consume more food than they would like. This notion receives support from the existence of the more than $40 billion-per-year diet industry currently serving nearly 55 million Americans who attempt to lose weight each year (26). The trend toward larger portion sizes, perhaps due to falling food prices, only serves to exacerbate this problem. Similar to those who optimally choose to be overweight, for individuals with self-control problems, provision of additional information is also unlikely to be effective because these individuals are unable to take advantage of their newfound knowledge.

---

[8]Results in the Occupational Choice and Wages section indicate that obese women miss more days from work, raising the possibility that lower wages are not caused by discrimination, which presumably would also affect men and nonwhite women, but that employers are paying lower wages to compensate for increased absenteeism or other factors resulting from obesity.

[9]For example, Gruber & Koszegi (34) considered tobacco policies with time-inconsistent preferences and Cutler et al. (13) briefly considered the effects of self-control problems on policies related to obesity.

Moreover, for those with self-control problems, analogous to those addicted to smoking, changes in costs and benefits of behaviors related to weight may also be ineffective. However, other strategies, such as limiting portion sizes, may be desirable.

This discussion suggests that information-based strategies to combat obesity will have a limited impact. Some subset of the population, even with this information, will still choose a lifestyle that leads to excess weight gain. Those with self-control problems are also unlikely to benefit from the information. For the remainder of the population, these strategies may be effective. Individuals require accurate information to make decisions. Thus, policies such as nutrition labeling laws that increase access to information may allow individuals to make better food consumption choices. Those who are unaware of the consequences of obesity may also benefit from public health education efforts, although the number of individuals who will benefit and the cost-effectiveness of such types of interventions remain largely unexplored. Regardless, this discussion reveals that interventions will need to be multifaceted to have the best chance of success. Given current trends, a concerted effort by individuals, employers, and the government will be needed to prevent obesity rates and related expenditures from rising in the foreseeable future.

ACKNOWLEDGMENT

The authors gratefully acknowledge Olga Khavjou of RTI for her research assistance on this chapter.

The *Annual Review of Public Health* is online at
http://publhealth.annualreviews.org

LITERATURE CITED

1. Allison DB, Zannolli R, Narayan KM. 1999. The direct health care costs of obesity in the United States. *Am. J. Public Health* 89(8):1194–99
2. Anderson PM, Butcher KF, Levine PB. 2003. Maternal employment and overweight children. *J. Health Econ.* 22(3): 477–504
3. Averett S, Korenman S. 1996. The economic reality of the beauty myth. *J. Hum. Resour.* 31(2):304–30
4. Averett S, Korenman S. 1999. Black-white differences in social and economic consequences of obesity. *Int. J. Obes.* 23: 166–73

5. Becker G. 1965. A theory of the allocation of time. *Econ. J.* 75:493–517
6. Bluestone B, Rose S. 1997. Overworked and underemployed: unraveling an economic enigma. *Am. Prospect.* 8(31):58–69
7. Burton WN, Chen CY, Schultz AB, Edington DW. 1998. The economic costs associated with body mass index in a workplace. *J. Occup. Environ. Med.* 40(9): 786–92
8. Cawley J. 2000. *Body weight and women's labor market outcome.* Work. Pap. No. 7841, National Bur. Econ. Res., Cambridge, MA

9. Cent. Dis. Control Prev. 2004. Prevalence of no leisure-time physical activity—35 states and the District of Columbia, 1988–2002. *Morb. Mortal. Wkly. Rep.* 53(4):82–86

10. Cent. Dis. Control Prev. 2004. Trends in the intake of energy and macronutrients—United States, 1971–2000. *Morb. Mortal. Wkly. Rep.* 53(4):80–82

10a. Chou S-Y, Grossman M, Saffer H. 2004. An economic analysis of adult obesity: results from the Behavioral Risk Factor Surveillance System. *J. Health Econ.* 23(3):565–87

11. Costa DL, Steckel RH. 1997. Long-term trends in U.S. health, welfare, and economic growth. In *Health and Welfare During Industrializaton*, ed. RH Steckel, R Floud, pp. 47–89. Chicago: Univ. Chicago Press, NBER Project Rep. Ser.

12. Counc. Econ. Advis. 2004. *Economic Report of the President, 2004.* Washington, DC: U.S. Gov. Print. Off.

13. Cutler DM, Glaeser EL, Shapiro JM. 2003. Why have Americans become more obese? *J. Econ. Perspect.* 17(3):93–118

14. Devitt AA, Mattes RD. 2004. Effects of food unit size and energy density on intake in humans. *Appetite* 42(2):213–20

15. Drewnowski A, Specter SE. 2004. Poverty and obesity: the role of energy density and costs. *Am. J. Clin. Nutr.* 791:6–16

16. Ebbeling CB, Pawlak DB, Ludwig DS. 2002. Childhood obesity: public-health crisis, common sense cure. *Lancet* 360 (9331):473–82

17. Econ. Res. Serv. 2004. Food CPI, Prices, and Expenditures (Table 7), Economic Research Service Briefing Room. http://www.ers.usda.gov/Briefing/CPIFoodAndExpenditures/Data/table7.htm

18. Ewing R, Schmid T, Killingsworth R, Zlot A, Raudenbush S. 2003. Relationship between urban sprawl and physical activity, obesity, and morbidity. *Am. J. Health Promot.* 18(1):47–57

19. Field A, Coakley EH, Must A, Spadano JL, Laud N, et al. 2001. Impact of over-weight on the risk of developing common chronic diseases during a 10-year period. *Arch. Intern. Med.* 161(13):1581–86

20. Finkelstein EA, Fiebelkorn IC, Wang G. 2003. National medical spending attributable to overweight and obesity: how much, and who's paying? *Health Aff.* Suppl. W3-219–26

21. Finkelstein EA, Fiebelkorn IC, Wang G. 2004. State-level estimates of annual medical expenditures attributable to obesity. *Obes. Res.* 12:18–24

22. Flegal KM, Carroll MD, Kuczmarski RJ, Johnson CL. 1998. Overweight and obesity in the United States: prevalence and trends, 1960–1994. *Int. J. Obes.* 22(1):39–47

23. Flegal KM, Carroll MD, Ogden CL, Johnson CL. 2002. Prevalence and trends in obesity among U.S. adults, 1999–2000. *JAMA* 288(14):1723–27

24. Fontaine KR, Redden DT, Wang C, Westfall AO, Allison DB. 2003. Years of life lost due to obesity. *JAMA* 289(2):187–93

25. French SA, Story M, Jeffery RW. 2001. Environmental influences on eating and physical activity. *Annu. Rev. Public Health* 22:309–35

26. Goodstein E. 2004. 10 Secrets of the Weight-Loss Industry. http://www.bankrate.com/brm/news/advice/20040113a1.asp

27. Gorsky R, Pamuk E, Williamson D, Shaffer P, Koplan J. 1996. The 25-year health care costs of women who remain overweight after 40 years of age. *Am. J. Prev. Med.* 12:388–94

28. Gortmaker SL, Must A, Perrin JM, Sobol AM, Dietz W. 1993. Social and economic consequences of overweight in adolescence and young adulthood. *N. Eng. J. Med.* 329(14):1008–12

29. Gronau R. 1973. The intrafamily allocation of time: the value of the housewives' time. *Am. Econ. Rev.* 63(4):634–51

30. Gronau R. 1977. Leisure, home production, and work: the theory of the allocation of time revisited. *J. Polit. Econ.* 85(6):1099–124

31. Gronau R. 1980. Home production—a forgotten industry. *Rev. Econ. Stat.* 62(3): 408–16

32. Gronau R. 1997. The theory of home production: the past ten years. *J. Labor Econ.* 15(2):197–205

33. Grossman M. 2000. The human capital model. In *Handbook of Health Economics*, ed. J Culyer, JP Newhouse, pp. 347–408. New York: Elsevier

34. Gruber J, Koszegi B. 2001. Is addiction rational? Theory and evidence. *Q. J. Econ.* 116(4):1261–303

35. Guthrie JF, Lin BH, Frazao E. 2002. Role of food prepared away from home in the American diet, 1977–78 versus 1994–96: changes and consequences. *J. Nutr. Educ. Behav.* 34(3):140–50

36. Haskins K, Ransford HE. 1999. The relationship between weight and career payoffs among women. *Sociol. Forum* 14(2): 295–318

37. Hill JO, Wyatt HR, Reed GW, Peters JC. 2003. Obesity and the environment: Where do we go from here? *Science* 299(5608):853–55

38. Jahns L, Siega-Riz AM, Popkin BM. 2001. The increasing prevalence of snacking among U.S. children from 1977 to 1996. *J. Pediatr.* 138(4):493–98

39. Laibson D. 1997. Golden eggs and hyperbolic discounting. *Q. J. Econ.* 112(2):443–77

40. Lakdawalla D, Philipson T. 2002. *The growth of obesity and technological change: a theoretical and empirical examination.* Natl. Bur. Econ. Res. Work. Pap. No. 8946, Cambridge, MA

41. Leigh JP. 1991. Employee and job attributes as predictors of absenteeism in a national sample of workers: the importance of health and dangerous working conditions. *Soc. Sci. Med.* 33:127–37

42. Loh ES. 1993. The economic effect of physical appearance. *Soc. Sci. Q.* 74(2): 420–37

42a. Mankiw NG. 1998. The market forces of supply and demand. In *Principles of Microeconomics*, 4:61–87. Orlando, FL: Harcourt Brace. 64 pp.

43. Mitra A. 2001. Effects of physical attributes on the wages of males and females. *Appl. Econ. Lett.* 8:731–35

44. Mokdad AH, Marks JS, Stroup DF, Gerberding JL. 2000. Actual causes of death in the United States. *JAMA* 291:1238–45

45. Must A, Spadano J, Coakley EH, Field AE, Colditz G, Dietz WH. 1999. The disease burden associated with overweight and obesity. *JAMA* 282(16):1523–29

46. Narbro K, Jonsson E, Larsson B, Waaler J, Wedel H, Sjostrom L. 1996. Economic consequences of sick-leave and early retirement in obese Swedish women. *Int. J. Obes. Relat. Metab. Disord.* 20:895–903

47. Natl. Cent. Health Stat. 2001. *Healthy People 2000 Final Review.* Hyattsville, MD: Public Health Serv.

48. Natl. Heart Lung Blood Inst. 1998. *Clinical Guidelines on the Identification, Evaluation, and Treatment of Overweight and Obesity in Adults.* Bethesda, MD: Natl. Inst. Health

48a. Nielsen Media Res. 2004. Average Daily Viewing: 1949–2003. http://www.nielsenmedia.com

49. Nielsen SJ, Popkin BM. 2003. Patterns and trends in food portion sizes, 1977–1998. *JAMA* 289(4):450–53

50. Nielsen SJ, Siega-Riz AM, Popkin BM. 2002. Trends in energy intake in the U.S. between 1977 and 1996: similar shifts seen across age groups. *Obes. Res.* 10(5):370–78

51. O'Donohue T, Rabin M. 1999. Doing it now or later. *Am. Econ. Rev.* 89(1):103–24

52. Pagan JA, Davila A. 1997. Obesity, occupational attainment, and earnings. *Soc. Sci. Q.* 78(3):756–70

53. Philipson T. 2001. The world-wide growth in obesity: an economic research agenda. *Health Econ.* 10(1):1–7

54. Putnum JJ, Allshouse JE. 1999. *Food Consumption, Prices, and Expenditures,*

1970–97. Econ. Res. Serv., USDA, Stat. Bull. No. 965. Washington, DC

55. Putnum JJ, Allshouse JE, Kantor LS. 2002. U.S. per capita food supply trends: more calories, refined carbohydrates, and fats. *Food Rev.* 25(3):2–15

56. Quesenberry CP Jr, Caan B, Jacobson A. 1998. Obesity, health services use, and health care costs among members of a health maintenance organization. *Arch. Intern. Med.* 158(5):466–72

57. Register CA, Williams DR. 1990. Wage effects of obesity among young workers. *Soc. Sci. Q.* 71(1):130–41

58. Robinson JP, Godbey G. 1997. *Time for Life: The Surprising Ways Americans Use Their Time.* University Park: Penn. State Univ. Press

59. Rolls BJ, Morris EL, Roe LS. 2002. Portion size of food affects energy intake in normal-weight and overweight men and women. *Am. J. Clin. Nutr.* 76(6):1207–13

60. Rolls BJ, Roe LS, Kral TVE, Meengs JS, Wall DE. 2004. Increasing portion size of a packaged snack increases energy intake in men and women. *Appetite* 42(1):63–69

61. Ruhm CJ. 2000. Are recessions good for your health? *Q. J. Econ.* 115(2):617–50

62. Ruhm CJ. 2003. *Maternal employment and adolescent development.* Work. Pap. w10691, Univ. N.C., Greensboro

63. Ruhm CJ. 2005. Healthy living in hard times. *J. Health Econ.* In press

64. Sarlio-Lahteenkorva S, Lahelma E. 1999. The association of body mass index with social and economic disadvantage in women and men. *Int. J. Epidemiol.* 28(3):445–49

65. Stevens J, Cai J, Pamuk ER, Williamson DF, Thun MJ, Wood JL. 1998. The effect of age on the association between body-mass index and mortality. *N. Engl. J. Med.* 338(1):1–7

66. Sturm R. 2002. The effects of obesity, smoking, and drinking on medical problems and costs. Obesity outranks both smoking and drinking in its deleterious effects on health and health costs. *Health Aff.* 21:245–53

67. Thompson D, Edelsberg J, Kinsey KL, Oster G. 1998. Estimated economic costs of obesity to U.S. business. *Am. J. Health Promot.* 13(2):120–27

68. Thompson D, Brown JB, Nichols GA, Elmer PJ, Oster G. 2001. Body mass index and future healthcare costs: a retrospective cohort study. *Obes. Res.* 9(3):210–18

69. Thompson D, Edelsberg J, Colditz GA, Bird AP, Oster G. 1999. Lifetime health and economic consequences of obesity. *Arch. Intern. Med.* 159(18):2177–83

70. Trioiano RP, Briefel RR, Carroll MD, Bialostosky K. 2000. Energy and fat intakes of children and adolescents in the United States: data from the National Health and Nutrition Examination survey. *Am. J. Clin. Nutr.* 72(Suppl. 5):1343–53

71. Tucker LA, Friedman GM. 1998. Obesity and absenteeism: an epidemiologic study of 10,825 employed adults. *Am. J. Health Promot.* 12(3):202–7

72. US Census Bur. 1982. *Statistical Abstract of the United States: 1982–83.* Washington, DC: US Census Bur. 103rd ed.

73. US Census Bur. 2003. *Statistical Abstract of the United States: 2003.* Washington, DC: US Census Bur. 123rd ed.

74. US Dep. Health Hum. Serv. 2001. *The Surgeon General's Call to Action to Prevent and Decrease Overweight and Obesity.* Rockville, MD: US Dep. Health Hum. Serv., Public Health Serv., Off. Surg. Gen.

75. Visscher T, Seidell J. 2001. The public health impact of obesity. *Annu. Rev. Public Health* 22:355–75

76. Wolf AM, Colditz GA. 1994. The cost of obesity: the US perspective. *Pharmacoeconomics* 5(Suppl. 1):34–37

77. Wolf AM, Colditz GA. 1998. Current estimates of the economic cost of obesity in the United States. *Obes. Res.* 6(2):97–106

78. World Health Organ. 1997. Obesity: preventing and managing the global epidemic. *Rep. WHO Consult. Obesity.* World Health Organ., Geneva, Switz.

79. Young LR, Nestle M. 2002. The contribution of expanding portion sizes to the US obesity epidemic. *Am. J. Public Health* 97(2):246–49

80. Zizza C, Siega-Riz AM, Popkin BM. 2001. Significant increase in young adults' snacking between 1977–1978 and 1994–1996 represents a cause for concern! *Prev. Med.* 32(4):303–10

Annu. Rev. Public Health 2005. 26:259–79
doi: 10.1146/annurev.publhealth.26.021304.144652

MAGNITUDE OF ALCOHOL-RELATED MORTALITY AND MORBIDITY AMONG U.S. COLLEGE STUDENTS AGES 18–24: Changes from 1998 to 2001

Ralph Hingson,[1] Timothy Heeren,[1] Michael Winter,[1] and Henry Wechsler[2]
[1]*Boston University School of Public Health, Center to Prevent Alcohol Problems Among Young People, Boston, Massachusetts 02118;*
email: rhingson@bu.edu, tch@bu.edu, mwinter@bu.edu
[2]*Harvard School of Public Health, Boston, Massachusetts 02115;*
email: hwechsle@hsph.harvard.edu

Key Words   injury, prevention, enforcement, screening, counseling

■ **Abstract**   Integrating data from the National Highway Traffic Safety Administration, the Centers for Disease Control and Prevention, national coroner studies, census and college enrollment data for 18–24-year-olds, the National Household Survey on Drug Abuse, and the Harvard College Alcohol Survey, we calculated the alcohol-related unintentional injury deaths and other health problems among college students ages 18–24 in 1998 and 2001. Among college students ages 18–24 from 1998 to 2001, alcohol-related unintentional injury deaths increased from nearly 1600 to more than 1700, an increase of 6% per college population. The proportion of 18–24-year-old college students who reported driving under the influence of alcohol increased from 26.5% to 31.4%, an increase from 2.3 million students to 2.8 million. During both years more than 500,000 students were unintentionally injured because of drinking and more than 600,000 were hit/assaulted by another drinking student. Greater enforcement of the legal drinking age of 21 and zero tolerance laws, increases in alcohol taxes, and wider implementation of screening and counseling programs and comprehensive community interventions can reduce college drinking and associated harm to students and others.

INTRODUCTION

National surveys have focused attention on the heavy drinking patterns of many college students. In 1993, 1997, and 1999, the Harvard School of Public Health College Alcohol Surveys (CAS) monitored among college students heavy or binge drinking, defined as five or more drinks in a single drinking session for males and four or more for females (77–79). In 1999, of 14,138 full-time students randomly selected at 128 4-year colleges and universities, 44% reported at least one heavy drinking episode in the previous year, the same percentage as in 1993 (79). About one fourth (23%) frequently drank in this manner (3 or more times in the past 2 weeks), up from 20% in 1993. Similarly, the national Monitoring the Future study (36) reported 40% of 1440 full-time 2- and 4-year college students surveyed in 1999 consumed 5 or more drinks on a single occasion at least once in the previous 2 weeks, a greater proportion than found among same-age noncollege peers (35%) and high school seniors (31%).

In 1998 the National Advisory Council of the National Institute on Alcohol Abuse and Alcoholism (NIAAA), one of the Institutes of the National Institutes of Health, created a task force to review the research on college drinking to advise administrators and the NIAAA on implementing and evaluating college programs and future research directions. This study resulted in a 2002 report: *A Call to Action: Changing the Culture of Drinking on U.S. College Campuses* (57). Background papers appeared in "College Drinking, What Is It and What to Do About It? A Review of the State of the Science" in the *Journal of Studies for Alcohol* (23).

One of the 24 articles commissioned for this panel (30) estimated that in 1998 more than 1400 students ages 18–24 enrolled in 2- and 4-year colleges died from alcohol-related injuries including motor vehicle crashes. Further, of the 8 million college students in the United States more than 2 million drove under the influence of alcohol and over 3 million rode with a drinking driver. More than 500,000 full-time 4-year-college students were unintentionally injured under the influence of alcohol, and more than 600,000 were hit or assaulted by and more than 70,000 experienced a date rape caused by another student who had been drinking.

The purpose of this review is to assess whether the magnitude of alcohol-related morbidity and mortality among U.S. college students ages 18–24 changed from 1998 to 2001. We also outline interventions, identified by rigorous research in the 2002 NIAAA report and the recent *National Academy of Science Report to Congress Preventing Under Age Drinking: A Collective Responsibility*, to reduce college drinking problems (52).

METHODS: CALCULATING CHANGES IN ALCOHOL-RELATED MORTALITY

This review compares the number of alcohol-related traffic and other unintentional injury deaths in 1998 and 2001 among 18–24-year-olds in the United States who are full- or part-time college students attending either 2- or 4-year colleges. Information was integrated from multiple data sets because the U.S. Department of Transportation Fatality Analysis Reporting System (FARS): NHTSA (56) does not routinely record whether persons who die in motor vehicle crashes are college students. In addition, people who die from other types of unintentional injuries are not systematically tested for blood alcohol concentrations (BACs). The data sources consulted are described below.

First, the Centers for Disease Control and Prevention (CDC) annually records the numbers and ages of unintentional injury deaths (5), but they do not record whether these deaths are alcohol related. Second, a recent meta-analysis of 331 medical examiner studies (65) from 1975 to 1995 revealed that 84% of unintentional nontraffic fatalities were tested for BACs. Of those tested, 38% had positive BACs, and 31% had BACs of 0.10% or higher, exceeding legal limits for intoxication nationwide (65). This analysis provides the best available estimates for alcohol involvement in injury deaths (other than motor vehicle crash deaths), but it does not provide information on annual changes in the proportions of those deaths that are alcohol related.

Third, the National Highway Traffic Safety Administration's (NHTSA) FARS records all motor vehicle crash deaths in the United States (55, 56) and the proportion that are alcohol related, defined as involving a driver or pedestrian with a positive BAC. The ages of decedents are recorded, as are their blood alcohol concentrations. Because BACs are not drawn on all motor vehicle crash deaths, an imputational formula projects the likelihood of alcohol involvement in those crashes for which test results are not available.

Fourth, the Department of Education's National Center for Education Statistics (53) reports the number of undergraduate college students in the United States. In 1998, of the 26,058,760 18–24-year-olds living in the United States (17), 8,670,000 (33%) were enrolled as full- or part-time students in either 2- or 4-year colleges: 24% ($n = 6,106,000$) in 4-year colleges and 10% ($n = 2,564,000$) in 2-year colleges. Of students enrolled in 4-year colleges, 74% were ages 18–24, as were 60% of those enrolled in 2-year colleges. In 2001, of the 27,918,979 18–24-year-olds living in the United States, 8,894,000 (32%) were enrolled as either full- or part-time college students: 23% 6,381,000 (23%) in 4-year colleges and 9% 2,518,000 (9%) in 2-year colleges. Of students enrolled in 4-year colleges 74% were age 18–24, as were 61% of those enrolled in 2-year colleges.

Fifth, the National Household Survey of Drug Abuse in 1999 and 2002 surveyed 18–24-year-olds regardless of whether they were college students (66, 67). In both surveys, college students were more likely than same-age noncollege respondents to report drinking five or more drinks on at least one occasion in the past month and driving under the influence in the past year. On the basis of those survey results, we projected that the proportions of traffic and other unintentional injury decedents testing positive for alcohol would be as high among college 18–24-year-olds as noncollege-year-olds same-age persons. Because college students comprised 33% of the 18–24-year-old population in 1998 and 32% in 2001, we estimated that in 1998 18–24-year-old college students accounted for 33% and in 2001 32% of traffic and other unintentional injury deaths experienced by the 18–24-year-old U.S. population.

Calculation of other Alcohol-Related Risks

Two national surveys conducted in 1999 and 2002 (66, 67) asked students about their experiences with alcohol in the previous year. Using their responses and data on the numbers of college students in the United States during those years, we estimated the annual numbers of college students ages 18–24 who drive under the influence of alcohol, were injured because of drinking, and experienced other alcohol-related problems.

The National Household Survey on Drug Abuse (NHSDA) (67) is the primary source of statistical information on illegal drug use in the United States. Sponsored by the Substance Abuse and Mental Health Services Administration (SAMHSA) (66), computer-assisted interviews are conducted with a representative sample of the United States: residents of households and noninstitutional group quarters (e.g., shelters, rooming houses, dormitories) and civilians living on military bases.

The 1999 and 2002 NHSDA used an independent multistage area probability sample for each of the 50 states and the District of Columbia. Youth and young adults were oversampled so that each state's sample was approximately equally distributed among people ages 12–17, 18–25, and 26 and older.

In 1999, 169,166 addresses across the United States were screened, and 66,706 persons were interviewed within screened addresses. Weighted response rates for households screened and interviewed were 89.6% and 68.6%, respectively. The sample included 19,438 respondents ages 18–24, of whom 6930 (36%) were enrolled in college, 5796 (30%) as full-time students and 1134 (6%) as part-time students.

In 2002, 68,126 persons were interviewed within the screened addresses. Weighted response rates for households screened and persons interviewed were 91% and 79%. In the survey 20,478 respondents were ages 18–24, of whom 8041 (39%) were enrolled in college.

Respondents were asked how often they drank 5 or more alcoholic drinks on any one occasion in the past 30 days. They were also asked, reflecting on the previous 12 months, Has your use of alcohol caused you to have any health problems?, Have you driven a vehicle under the influence of alcohol only?, and Have you received treatment or counseling for your use of alcohol?

The Harvard School of Public Health CAS began in 1993 (77) with a sample of 140 colleges selected from a list of all accredited 4-year colleges provided by the American Council on Education, using probability sampling proportionate to the size of undergraduate enrollment at each institution. At each college, a random sample of 225 undergraduates was drawn from the total enrollment of full-time students. In 1999 (79), another survey was conducted with 128 of the original 140 colleges. The inability of 10 colleges in 1997 and 2 colleges in 1999 to provide a random sample of students and their mailing addresses resulted in the attrition of those schools. In 1999, 12,317 full-time students, ages 18–24 and having come from 40 states, were surveyed; nearly half of these students lived in dormitories, college housing, fraternities, or sororities (response rate 60%) (79).

In 2001, 215 full-time students ages 18–24 were randomly selected for the survey from each of 119 colleges and universities that had been part of the 1999 sample, response rate 52% (80). Respondents were asked their frequency and usual quantity of drinking, whether during the current school year they experienced a variety of health and social problems because of their drinking, and whether the drinking of other college students posed any of a series of social and health problems for them.

Statistical Analyses of Surveys

For both surveys we present weighted results that consider their respective designs and nonresponse. All statistical estimates of percentages for the survey data were conducted using the SUDAAN statistical package to account for each survey's design (63). The SUDAAN package accounts for sampling weights in calculating both estimates and standard errors, using first-order Taylor series approximations to provide standard errors that approximately account for sampling design.

Using the information above, we identified the percentage of 2- and 4-year college students ages 18–24 who responded affirmatively to the survey questions regarding alcohol problems and then calculated 95% confidence intervals for those responses. To estimate the numbers of 18–24-year-old college students who experienced those problems, we then multiplied those percentages and confidence intervals by the appropriate population count from the Department of Education of students 18–24 years enrolled in 2- and 4-year colleges in the United States. Data from the Department of Education are considered to be true population totals; therefore, our confidence intervals reflect only the sampling variability in the percentage estimates. We also made projections from the CAS responses to the full-time 4-year college population using the same analytic strategy.

Percentages of responses with 95% confidence intervals were calculated from survey data accounting for the sampling design. Changes in numbers of events and rates of events per 100,000 population were described through relative risks, and 95% confidence intervals were calculated using the Poisson model. These percentages and confidence intervals are available on request.

RESULTS

Motor Vehicle Crash Deaths

The NHSDA surveys in both 1999 and 2002 revealed that in the year prior to the survey, a significantly greater percentage of 18–24-year-old college students compared with same-age noncollege respondents drank 5 or more drinks on a single occasion in the past month (41.7% versus 36.5% in 1999 and 43.2% versus 39.8% in 2002) and drove under the influence of alcohol in the previous year (26.5% versus 19.8% in 1999 and 31.4% versus 23.7% in 2002). The percentage in both groups of 18–24-year-olds who drank 5 or more drinks in the past 30 days did not significantly increase from 1999 to 2002. However, the percentage of college students who drove under the influence in the past year increased significantly [RR $= 1.18$ (95% CI 1.13, 1.25)].

In 1998, in the United States, among persons ages 18–24, 3783 (51%) of 7452 traffic deaths were alcohol related. On the basis of a deliberately conservative assumption that college students (33% of the U.S. population ages 18–24 in 1998) experienced alcohol-related fatalities at the same rate as the entire 18–24-year-old population, 1248 (33%) of the alcohol-related traffic deaths in that age group would have been college students. (Note this figure is somewhat higher than reported by Hingson et al. (30) because the Census Bureau revised its estimate of college students in 1998 from 8 million to 8.67 million.)

In 2001, in the United States, among persons ages 18–24, 4216 (51%) of the 8242 traffic deaths were alcohol related. Assuming that college students (32% of the U.S. population ages 18–24 in 2001) experienced alcohol-related fatalities at the same rate as the entire 18–24-year-old population, 1349 (32%) of the alcohol-related traffic deaths in that age group would have been college students (Table 1).

From 1998 to 2001 the U.S. population ages 18–24 increased 7%, whereas alcohol-related traffic deaths increased 11%. Thus the increase in alcohol-related traffic deaths per 18–24-year-old population was 4%. The U.S. college population ages 18–24 increased 3%, but the number of alcohol-related traffic deaths among 18–24-year-old students increased 8%. The 5% increase in the rate of alcohol-related traffic deaths from 14.4 to 15.2 per 100,000 college students approached, but did not reach, statistical significance [RR $=$ 1.05 (95% CI 0.98, 1.14)].

Unintentional Nontraffic Deaths

In the NHSDA survey, 18–24-year-olds in college and not in college were equally likely to report alcohol-related health problems (1.9% versus 2.0% in 1999 and 2.1% versus 2.3% in 2002). According to the CDC there were 10,052 unintentional injury deaths among 18–24-year-olds in 1998 and 11,272 in 2001 (5). Subtracting 7444 traffic deaths in 1998 from the total unintentional injury deaths among 18–24-year-olds that year and 8242 from the total in 2001 yielded 2608 nontraffic injury unintentional deaths in 1998 and 3030 in 2001. If 38% were alcohol related, as reported in national analyses of coroner studies (64), then 991 persons ages 18–24 in 1998 and 1151 in 2001 died from alcohol-related nontraffic injuries. If 33% of those deaths were among college students in 1998 and 32% in 2001, then 327 students in 1998 and 368 in 2001 died from alcohol-related nontraffic unintentional injuries.

From 1998 to 2001, the rate of these deaths showed a non-significant 10% increase from 3.8 to 4.1 per 100,000 college students, RR $=$ 1.10 (95% CI 0.95, 1.27). Among 18–24-year-old college students, deaths from all alcohol-related unintentional injuries, including traffic and other unintentional injury deaths, increased from 1575 in 1998 to 1717 in 2001, corresponding to an increase in the rates of these deaths from 18.2 to 19.3 per 100,000 students, a 6% increase that approached statistical significance (RR $=$ 1.06, 95% CI 0.99, 1.14). From 1998

TABLE 1   Estimated U.S. alcohol-related injury deaths among 18–24-year-olds, 1998 and 2001

	1998	2001	Change (95% CI)	Change/ population (95% CI)
Alcohol-related motor vehicle crash deaths				
Number of alcohol-related motor vehicle crash deaths	3783	4216	↑11% (↑7%, ↑16%)	↑4% (↓0.5%, ↑9%)
Percentage who are college students	33%	32%		
Number of college-student alcohol-related motor vehicle crash deaths	1248	1349	↑8% (↑0.1%, ↑16%)	↑6% (↓2%, ↑14%)
Alcohol-related unintentional nontraffic deaths				
Number of unintentional deaths	10,052	11,272	↑12% (↑9%, ↑15%)	↑5% (↑2%, ↑8%)
Number of motor vehicle crash deaths	7452	8242		
Number of unintentional nontraffic injury deaths	2608	3030		
Percentage of nontraffic injury deaths that are alcohol related	38%	38%		
Number of nontraffic injury deaths that are alcohol related	991	1151	↑16% (↑7%, ↑25%)	↑8% (↓0.5%, ↑18%)
Percentage who are college students	33%	32%		
Number of college-student alcohol-related unintentional injury deaths	327	368	↑13% (↓3%, ↑28%)	↑10% (↓5%, ↑27%)
All alcohol-related unintentional deaths	4771	5367	↑12% (↑8%, ↑17%)	↑5% (↑1%, ↑9%)
Total alcohol-related unintentional injury death				
Total alcohol-related unintentional injury deaths among college students	1575	1717	↑9% (↑2%, ↑16%)	↑6% (↓1%, ↑14%)

to 2001 the total population of persons ages 18–24, including college students and others, increased 7%, and alcohol-related unintentional injury deaths increased 12% from 4771 to 5367, a significant 5% increase per population [RR = 1.05 (95% CI 1.01, 1.09)].

Heavy Episodic Drinking

From 1999 to 2002, the proportion of college students ages 18–24 who drank 5 or more drinks on an occasion in the previous 30 days increased from 41.7% to 43.2%, a nonsignificant increase. The number of college students ages 18–24

TABLE 2   Interventions demonstrated to reduce college drinking problems

	References
Individually oriented onterventions	See Larimer & Cronce 2002 (43)
Brief motivational interventions	Baer et al. 1992 (3), Borsari & Carey 2000 (4), Marlatt et al. 1998 (48)
Mailed graphic feedback	Agostinelli et al. 1995 (1); Aubrey 1998 (2); Dimeff 1997 (18); Monti et al. 1999 (49); Walters et al. 1999, 2000 (75, 76)
Self-monitoring self-assessment	Garvin et al. 1990 (21), Marlatt et al. 1998 (48)
Expectancy challenge	Darkes & Goldman 1993 (14)
Life skills training	Murphy 1986 (50), Rohsenow et al. 1985 (60)
Environmental interventions	D'Amico & Fromme 2000 (13)
Raising the minimum legal drinking age to 21	Shults et al. 2001 (64), Wagenaar & Toomey 2002 (74)
Zero-tolerance laws	Hingson et al. 1994 (28), Wagenaar & Toomey 2002 (74)
Increased price of alcohol	See Wagenaar & Toomey 2002 (74); Chaloupka et al. 2002 (6); Chesson 2000 (9); Coate & Grossman 1988 (10); Cook & Moore 1999 (11); Cook & Tauchen 1982 (12); Dee & Evans 2001 (16); Godfry 1997 (22); Grossman et al. 1997 (25); Kenkel 1993 (39); Laixuthai & Chaloupka 1993 (42); Manning et al. 1995 (45); Markowitz & Grossman 1998 (46); Natl. Acad. Sci. 2004 (52); Ruhm 1996 (61); Saffer & Grossman 1987 (62); Sutton & Godfrey 1995 (68)
Comprehensive community intervention	Hingson et al. 1996 (34), Hingson & Howland 2002 (32), Holder et al. 2000 (35), Wagenaar et al. 2000 (71, 72), Weitzman et al. 2004 (83)

who consumed at least 5 drinks on an occasion in the previous month increased from 3,615,550 to 3,842,208, a nonsignificant 4% increase per college student population. The increase in the proportion who reported a health problem related to alcohol, from 1.9% to 2.1%, was also not significant. However, the proportion of college students ages 18–24 who in the past year reported driving under the influence of alcohol increased significantly from 26.5% to 31.4%, RR = 1.18% (95% CI 1.13, 1.25); the proportion of students who were arrested for an alcohol-related offense or who were receiving treatment for an alcohol or drug problem increased from 1.4% to 2.2%, RR = 1.37 (95% CI 1.22, 2.01). The number of students who drove under the influence of alcohol in the previous year increased from 2,297,550 to 2,792,716, a highly significant 18% increase per college student population.

Other Alcohol-Related Health Problems

From 1998 to 2001 the number of full-time 4-year college students ages 18–24 in the United States increased 4% from 5,496,000 to 5,709,000. Because the proportion of students who in the CAS reported being hurt or injured or having unprotected sex did not significantly change from 1999 to 2001, the projected number of students with these experiences increased at rates similar to the proportional population increase. In 2001, 599,000 (10.5%) were injured because of drinking and 474,000 (8%) had unprotected sexual intercourse as a result of their drinking. Although in 2001 slightly smaller proportions reported being assaulted or hit by another drinking college student, more than 696,000 (12%) experienced that problem in 2001, and 97,000 (2%) were alcohol-related sexual assault or date rape victims.

DISCUSSION: ESTIMATES OF THE MAGNITUDE OF COLLEGE DRINKING PROBLEMS

From 1998 to 2001 the nationwide number of alcohol-related deaths among 18–24-year-olds rose at a rate that significantly exceeded that age group's proportional population increase. Whereas the population increased 7% from 26,058,760 to 27,918,979, alcohol-related unintentional injury deaths rose 12% from 4771 to 5367. Thus, alcohol-related deaths per population of 18–24-year-olds rose 5% from 1998 to 2001.

From 1998 to 2001, among college students ages 18–24 the population increased 3% from 8,670,000 to 8,894,000, whereas unintentional alcohol-related injury deaths increased 9% from 1575 to 1717. Thus, similar to the overall 18–24-year-old group, among college students alcohol-related unintentional injury deaths per population rose 6%, an increase that approached statistical significance. In 2001, nearly 600,000 college students were injured because of drinking, and 696,000 were assaulted by another drinking college student.

Although the numbers are disturbingly high, we believe our estimates of alcohol-related college deaths are conservative. First, we focused only on unintentional injury deaths, not homicides and suicides, many of which are also alcohol related. Second, the proportion of 18–24-year-olds who engage in heavy episodic drinking and driving under the influence of alcohol is higher among persons that age who are enrolled in college. Consequently, our projection that college and noncollege 18–24-year-olds experience traffic alcohol-related injury deaths at the same rate per population in each group was intentionally conservative.

Third, the meta-analysis of coroner studies (65) did not provide age-specific estimates of alcohol involvement in nontraffic unintentional injury deaths. We estimated the proportion of nontraffic unintentional injury deaths was the same among 18–24-year-old college students as among adults all ages, even though persons 18–24 are known to drink more than other adults. A higher proportion of traffic fatalities are alcohol related in the 18–24-year-old population (51%)

than among all age groups (38%). It is therefore possible, if not likely, that our estimates of the number of unintentional alcohol-related nontraffic injury deaths among 18–24-year-olds are also conservative.

Fourth, if respondents underreport illegal behaviors like driving under the influence of alcohol, our estimate of the numbers of students who engage in those behaviors may be low.

Fifth, response rates for the NHSDA and CAS were low. Thus, students may under- or overrepresent problems associated with alcohol. In 1999 a short form of the CAS was sent to nonresponding students, and there was no significant difference in rates of previous year alcohol use for those answering the short survey compared with the full questionnaire. Of note, the estimates of heavy episodic drinking reported by college students in the NHSDA and the CAS are very similar to those obtained by other major national surveys that include college students e.g., the Monitoring the Future Survey (36, 37).

Sixth, this analysis focused only on college students ages 18–24. In 1998 only 74% of 4-year college students and 60% of students at 2- or 4-year colleges were ages 18–24. In 2001, 74% of 4-year college students and 61% at 2-year colleges were in that age group. We have calculated the overall numbers of college students all ages who drink heavily and experience alcohol-related health problems. These numbers are larger than those reported here and are available on request.

IMPLICATIONS

The magnitude of problems posed by excessive drinking among college students should stimulate both improved measurement of these problems and efforts to reduce them. We believe every unnatural death in the United States should be tested for alcohol. The average cost of such testing would be approximately $50 per deceased person or an annual cost of $1.1 million if all injury deaths of those under 21 were tested or $7.2 million for 144,374 unintentional deaths, homicides, and legal intervention and suicide deaths of all ages recorded in 2001. In comparison, the National Academy of Sciences (52) reports $71.1 million are spent annually to reduce underage drinking. Even though this review used cautious assumption to estimate the numbers of alcohol-related deaths among college students and other 18–24-year-olds, direct systematic alcohol test results would be preferable. Also, mortality data sets (e.g., the Department of Transportation's FARS and CDC's Vital Statistics Mortality File) should include occupation and student status categories so that the absolute number of annual college student deaths can be tabulated.

Progress has been made over the past two decades to reduce alcohol-related crash deaths. This process has occurred in part because a sufficiently high and consistent level of fatally injured drivers in crashes are tested for alcohol that statistical models based on crash factors, vehicle factors, and person factors have been developed and used to estimate the annual numbers of alcohol-involved fatal crashes in all states (40). The data on the numbers of alcohol-related fatal crashes annually in each state has proven invaluable to researchers seeking to study the effects of state-level legislative interventions to reduce alcohol-related traffic deaths.

Unfortunately, without comprehensive testing for alcohol and determination of college student status of all persons who die from unnatural deaths, we lack the most dependable yardstick by which to measure the magnitude of alcohol-related injury death among college students, and whether this figure is changing over time.

INTERVENTIONS TO REDUCE COLLEGE DRINKING

The increase in the past 3 years in alcohol-related traffic and other unintentional injury deaths among 18–24-year-olds both in college and not in college underscores the need for colleges and their surrounding communities to expand and strengthen interventions demonstrated to reduce excessive drinking among college students and their same-age noncollege counterparts.

Of note, heavy-drinking college students not only place their own health at risk, but also they jeopardize the well-being of others. As many as 46% of the 4553 people killed in 2001 in crashes involving 18–24-year-old drinking drivers are persons other than the drinking driver, and the total deceased has increased 33% from 3425 to 4553 between 1998 and 2001. Further, surveys both in 1999 and again in 2001 indicate annually over 600,000 college students nationwide were hit or assaulted by a drinking college student, and in 2001 97,000 students were the victim of a date rape or assault perpetrated by a drinking college student. Colleges and surrounding communities have an obligation to protect people from potential harm contributed by excess college drinking.

The recent report on college drinking (57) and its background reports (23) and the National Academy of Sciences Report on Underage Drinking (52) identified numerous individually oriented counseling approaches, environmental interventions, and comprehensive community interventions that can reduce drinking and related problems among college students and the college age population. These documents summarize scientifically valid approaches for effective prevention, and some believe they establish a new legal standard by which the adequacy of any college or university's efforts can be judged (44). See Table 2.

Individually Oriented Interventions

Larimer & Cronce (43) reviewed individually oriented strategies to reduce problematic alcohol consumption by college students from 1984 to 1999. Studies were included in this review if they had a control or comparison group and had at least one change in drinking or alcohol consequences outcome. A total of 34 separate studies were identified. The reviewers found little evidence for the effectiveness of information-based and values-clarification programs. Several skills-based interventions (13, 50, 60) resulted in decreases in alcohol consumption, including self-monitoring/self-assessment (21, 48) as well as expectancy-challenge procedures (14) involving alcohol/placebo administration. Brief motivational interventions had demonstrated effectiveness in a variety of contexts including selected high-risk freshmen, high school classrooms, fraternity organizations, outpatient counseling centers, and emergency rooms. Mailed graphic feedback alone in three studies (1, 75, 76) resulted in reductions in alcohol consumption equivalent or superior to skills-based interventions with combined feedback.

Environmental Interventions: Legal Drinking Age of 21

The most powerful environmental intervention to reduce drinking among college students is the minimum legal drinking age of 21. In 1984, when 25 states had a legal drinking age of 21, the U.S. Congress passed legislation that would withhold highway construction funds from states that did not make it illegal to sell alcohol to people younger than 21. By 1988, all states adopted this law. A review of more than 49 studies of legal drinking age changes revealed that in the 1970s and 1980s, when many states lowered the drinking age, alcohol-related traffic crashes increased 10%. In contrast, when states increased the legal drinking age to 21, alcohol-related crashes among people younger than 21 decreased an average of 16% (64). Wagenaar & Toomey (74) reviewed more than 48 studies of the effects of drinking age changes on drinking and 57 studies on traffic crashes. They concluded that increases in the age of legal alcohol purchase and consumption have been the most successful intervention to date in reducing drinking- and alcohol-related crashes among persons under 21. One national study of laws raising the drinking age to 21 indicated that persons who grew up in states with a drinking age of 21 relative to those with lower legal drinking ages drank less not only when they were younger than 21, but also when they were ages 21–25 (58). NHTSA (54) estimates that a legal drinking age of 21 saves 700–1000 lives annually, and that more than 21,000 traffic deaths have been prevented by such laws since 1976.

Zero tolerance laws, which make it illegal in every state for persons under 21 to drive after any drinking, have also contributed to declines in alcohol-related traffic deaths among people younger than 21. A comparison of the first 8 states to adopt zero tolerance laws with nearby states without such laws revealed a 21% greater decline in zero tolerance law states in the proportion of fatal crashes among drivers younger than 21 that were of the type most likely to involve alcohol (i.e., single-vehicle fatal crashes at night) (28). Wagenaar et al. (73) found that in the first 30 states to adopt zero tolerance laws, relative to the rest of the nation, there was a 19% decline in the proportion of people younger than 21 who drove after any drinking and a 23% decline in the proportion who drove after 5 or more drinks.

Unfortunately, despite their demonstrated benefits, legal drinking age and zero tolerance laws generally have not been vigorously enforced (38). Young drivers are substantially underrepresented in the driving while intoxicated (DWI) arrest population relative to their contributions to the alcohol crash problem (59, 70). Younger drivers may be more likely to drink at locations where DWI enforcement resources are less likely to be deployed. Young drivers with high BACs also are more likely to be missed by police at sobriety checkpoints (82).

Stepped-up enforcement of alcohol purchase laws aimed at sellers and buyers can be effective (59, 69, 72) if resources are made available for this purpose. Enforcement of zero tolerance laws is hindered in some states because their implied consent laws require either an arrest for DWI or probable cause for a DWI arrest before the evidentiary test can be done to prove a zero tolerance violation (19). Thus in practice zero tolerance laws often are not enforced independently of DWI. In states such as New Mexico, where this situation exists, most teenagers are unaware that there is a zero tolerance law (20).

Price of Alcohol

The National Academy of Sciences (52) reviewed the literature on price of alcohol and alcohol-related problems and recommended that Congress and state legislators raise excise taxes to reduce underage alcohol consumption and to raise additional revenues to reduce underage drinking problems.

With rare exceptions (8, 15) research since the early 1980s generally has concluded that increases in the price of alcohol beverages lead to reductions in drinking and heavy drinking, as well as reductions in the adverse consequences of alcohol use and abuse (6). Higher alcohol prices have also been found to reduce alcohol-related problems such as motor vehicle fatalities (16, 39, 62), robberies, rapes, liver cirrhosis deaths (11, 12, 61), sexually transmitted diseases (9), and child abuse (46, 47). Among moderate drinkers, investigators have estimated that a 1% price increase results in a 1.19% decrease in consumption (45). Younger, heavier drinkers tend to be more affected by price than older, heavier drinkers (7, 22, 39, 68), perhaps because younger drinkers have less discretionary income. Laixuthai & Chaloupka (42), Grossman et al. (25), and Coate & Grossman (10) all found increasing the price of alcohol reduces the percent of youths who drink infrequently and produces even greater percentage declines in youths who drink frequently.

Research taking into account the addictive nature of alcohol shows that the long-term price elasticity is well above short-term elasticity (24). Kenkel (39) reported a 10% increase in the price of alcohol would reduce DWI 7% among men and 8% among women, and among persons under 21 this action would produce a 13% decrease among men and a 21% decrease among women.

If, as recommended by the National Academy of Sciences Report (52), revenues generated by alcohol tax increases to raise beverage prices are in turn earmarked for programs and enforcement of policies known to reduce underage drinking, reductions in underage drinking problems could exceed deductions associated with alcohol price increases alone.

Other Environmental Interventions

Alcohol outlet density has been associated with alcohol-related problems (26) and reducing outlet density may in turn reduce drinking-related problems. Wechsler et al. (81) found that students who attend colleges in states that have more restrictions on underage drinking, high volume consumption, and sales of alcohol beverages and which devote more resources to enforce drunk-driving laws, report less drinking and driving. Laws in these states included prohibitions against using a false identification, restrictions on attempting to buy or consume for those under the legal drinking age, enforcement of a clerk age minimum, and maintenance of minimum mandatory postings of warning signs in retailers to potential underage buyers. Laws pertaining to volume alcohol sales were keg registration, a statewide 0.08 g/dl per se BAC law, and restrictions on happy hours, open alcohol containers, beer sold in a pitcher, and billboards and advertising. The availability of large volumes of alcohol (24- and 30-can cases of beer, kegs, party balls), low sale prices, and frequent promotions and advertisements at both on- and off-premise establishments were also associated with higher binge drinking rates on the college campuses (41).

Shults (64) also reviewed 19 studies of states lowering legal blood alcohol limits for persons above 21 to 0.08% and reported that this law cut alcohol-related fatalities on average by 7% and concluded that there is strong evidence in favor of such a change.

Comprehensive Community Interventions

Several carefully conducted community-based initiatives have had particular success in reducing drinking- and/or alcohol-related problems among young people (32). These programs typically coordinate efforts of city officials from multiple departments of city government, school, health, police, alcohol beverage control, etc.; concerned private citizens and their organizations; students; parents; and merchants who sell alcohol. Often multiple intervention strategies are incorporated into the programs, including school-based programs involving students, peer leaders, and parents; media advocacy; community organizing and mobilization; environmental policy change to reduce alcohol availability to youth; and heightened enforcement of laws regulating sales and distribution of alcohol and laws to reduce alcohol-related traffic injuries and deaths.

Three comprehensive community programs in particular have shown reduction in alcohol problems among college-age youth: the Communities Mobilizing for Change Program (71, 72), the Community Trials Program (35), and the Saving Lives Program (34). Two programs (35, 71, 72) concentrated program efforts on underage alcohol purchase attempt surveys with feedback to alcohol sales merchants and the community about the proportion of attempts that resulted in sales and penalties for continued violations. Two programs (34, 35) focused on publicized police enforcement of drinking driver laws and alcohol service laws, and one (34) targeted risky motorist behaviors—such as speeding, running red lights, failing to wear safety belts, and yielding to pedestrians in crosswalks—engaged in disproportionally by drinking drivers.

Relative to the comparison communities, the Communities Mobilizing for Change communities achieved a 17% increase in outlets checking the age identification of youthful-appearing alcohol purchasers, a 24% decline in sales by bars and restaurants to potential underage purchasers, a 25% decrease in the proportion of 18–20-year-olds seeking to buy alcohol, a 17% decline in the proportion of older teens who provided alcohol to younger teens, and a 7% decrease in the percentage of respondents younger than 21 who drank in the previous 30 days (71). Further, drinking and driving arrests declined significantly among 18–20-year-olds, and disorderly conduct violators declined among 15–17-year-olds (72).

In the Community Trials Program, single-vehicle crashes at night, a measure of alcohol-related crashes, declined 11% more in program than in comparison communities. Alcohol-related trauma visits to emergency departments declined 43% (35).

In the Saving Lives Program (34) the proportion of drivers younger than 20 who reported in telephone surveys driving after drinking declined from 19% to 9% over the course of the program. The proportion of vehicles observed speeding through use of radar was cut in half, and there was a 7% increase in safety belt use. Minimal change in these outcomes occurred in comparison areas. Fatal crashes declined from 178 during the 5 preprogram years to 120 during the 5 program years, a 25% greater reduction than in the rest of Massachusetts. Fatal crashes involving alcohol declined 42%, and the number of fatally injured drivers with positive BACs declined 47%, relative to the rest of Massachusetts. Visible injuries per 100 crashes declined 5% more in Saving Lives cities than in the rest of the state during the program period. The fatal crash declines were greater in all six program cities relative to comparison areas, particularly among drivers ages 15–25.

Weitzman et al. (83) recently evaluated the impact of college/community partnerships implementing environmentally based interventions to reduce drinking and related problems specifically among college students. Interventions included in the A Matter of Degree (AMOD) program included keg registration, mandatory responsible beverage service, increased enforcement of community police collaboration or wild party enforcement, substance-free residence halls, and a variety of alcohol bars advertising environment with change. Of the ten AMOD programs, the five that most vigorously implemented these interventions achieved significant reductions in binge and frequent binge drinking, frequent intoxication, driving after drinking, alcohol-related injury, and a variety of other alcohol-related problems. Relative to control colleges, significant reductions were observed also in the proportion of students who reported being assaulted by another drinking college student.

CONCLUSIONS

Binge drinking and particularly DWI among college students and others in the 18–24 age group has increased since 1998, and alcohol-related deaths have increased significantly more than the population totals for that age. Colleges and the communities in which they are located have an obligation to control the harms to others posed by college-age drinkers, regardless of whether these drinkers are college students. Although a high percentage of 18–24-year-old college students drink heavily and engage in behaviors, such as driving a motor vehicle after drinking, that pose risk to themselves and others, there are so many more 18–24-year-olds not in college that this population actually accounts for more heavy drinkers, drinking drivers, and alcohol-related deaths. In 2001, while 3.8 million college students ages 18–24 engaged in heavy (5+ drinks) drinking episodes, so too did 7.6 million 18–24-year-olds who were not in college. While 2.8 million college students this age drove under the influence of alcohol, so too did 4.5 million persons that age who were not in college. While in 2001 nearly 1349 18–24-year-old college students died in alcohol-related motor vehicle crashes, among all 18–24-year-olds, there were 4216 of these deaths in 2001. While more than 300 college students ages 18–24 died from other unintentional alcohol-related injuries, among all 18–24-year-olds, 1151 individuals died from alcohol-related nontraffic unintentional injuries in 2001.

Moreover, while young adults ages 18–24 have the highest rates of binge drinking (5+ drinks at a time) than do other adults, persons over age 26 account for two thirds of all binge drinking episodes (51). Also, while the highest rates of alcohol-related traffic deaths are among 18–24-year-olds, they accounted for only 24% of alcohol-related traffic deaths and 9% of all other alcohol-related unintentional deaths in 2001; this fact suggests that efforts are needed to reduce alcohol-related traffic and unintentional injury deaths among persons of all ages, including college students.

Further, new research indicates that persons who drink to excess even before they enter college are more likely to experience alcohol-related problems both in high school and in college (33). According to the CDC National Youth Risk Behavior Survey, in 2001 47% of high school students (over 7 million) drank alcohol in the previous 30 days and 34% (over 5 million) drank at least 5 drinks within a 2-hour period at least once in the previous 30 days. Thirteen percent or 1.9 million individuals drove after drinking in the previous 30 days, and 31% (4.6 million) rode with a drinking driver (27). Further, the average age of starting to drink is declining (66). In 2001, 29% of high school students reported that they began drinking before age 13 (27). Analyses of the 1999 CAS among college students 19 and older revealed that the younger college students were when they first drank to intoxication (got drunk), the more likely they were to experience alcohol dependence in college, to engage in frequent heavy episodic drinking, to drive after drinking and heavy (5+ drinks) drinking, to ride with drunk drivers, to be injured under the influence of alcohol (31), and to have unplanned and unprotected sex after drinking (29). Community alcohol policy enforcement targeting high school students may have carryover effects in college years.

Because increased efforts to enforce underage drinking laws at the community level have reduced underage drinking, alcohol-related assault, emergency department visits, and alcohol-related fatal crashes involving people of college age (34, 35, 71, 72), it is important that colleges and their surrounding communities collaborate in these efforts. These efforts can include individually oriented screening and counseling strategies of proven efficiency among college and adolescent populations as well as environmental interventions such as alcohol tax increases, heightened education, and enforcement of minimum legal drinking age and zero tolerance laws. College crackdowns on campus drinking absent community support may drive problematic drinking off campus. Community crackdowns without college support may similarly drive drinking problems back onto campus. Moreover, community efforts to reduce underage drinking are needed to prevent the development of unsafe underage drinking practices before they spill over into the college setting.

ACKNOWLEDGMENTS

This article is dedicated to Brad McCue, a Michigan State junior who died from alcohol poisoning on his 21st birthday. The 2002 National Survey on Drug Use and Health data was provided in a special tabulation by the Office of Applied Statistics at Substance Abuse and Mental Health Services Administration (SAMHSA). The college alcohol survey data were collected under grants from the Robert Wood Johnson Foundation.

The *Annual Review of Public Health* is online at
http://publhealth.annualreviews.org

LITERATURE CITED

1. Agostinelli G, Brown JM, Miller WR. 1995. Effects of normative feedback on consumption among heavy drinking college students. *J. Drug Educ.* 25:31–40

2. Aubry LL. 1998. *Motivational interviewing with adolescents presenting for outpatient substance abuse treatment*. PhD. diss. Univ. New Mexico, Albuquerque

3. Baer JS, Marlatt GA, Kivlahan DR, Fromme K, Larimer ME, Williams E. 1992. An experimental test of three methods of alcohol risk reduction with young adults. *J. Cons. Psychol.* 60:974–79

4. Borsari B, Carey KB. 2000. Effects of a brief motivational intervention with college student drinkers. *J. Cons. Clin. Psychol.* 68: 728–33

5. Cent. Dis. Control Prev. Natl. Cent. Injury Prev. Control. 2003. *Web-Based Injury Statistics Query and Reporting System* (*WISQARS*). http://www.cdc.gov/ncipc/wisqars

6. Chaloupka FJ, Grossman M, Saffer H. 2002. The effects of price on alcohol consumption on alcohol related problems. *Alcohol Res. Health* 26(1):22–33

7. Chaloupka FJ, Saffer H, Grossman M. 1993. Alcohol-control policies and motor vehicle fatalities. *J. Legal Stud.* 22(1): 161–86

8. Chaloupka FJ, Wechsler H. 1996. Binge drinking in college: the impact of price, availability, and alcohol control policies. *Contemp. Econ. Policy* 14(4):112–24

9. Chesson H, Harrison P, Kassler WJ. 2000. Sex under the influence: the effect of alcohol policy on sexually transmitted disease rates in the United States. *J. Law Econ.* 43(1):215–38

10. Coate D, Grossman M. 1998. Effects of alcoholic beverage prices and legal drinking ages on youth alcohol use. *J. Law Econ.* 31(1):145–71

11. Cook PJ, Moore MJ. 1993. Economic perspectives on reducing alcohol-related

violence. Alcohol and interpersonal violence: fostering multidisciplinary perspectives. *NIH Pub. No. 93–3496, 1939–212*

12. Cook PJ, Tauchen G. 1982. The effect of liquor taxes on heavy drinking. *Bell J. Econ.* 13(2):379–90

13. D'Amico E, Fromme K. 2000. Implementation of the risk skills training program: a brief intervention targeting adolescent participation in risk behaviors. *Logist. Beh. Pract.* 7:101–17

14. Darkes J, Goldman MS. 1993. Expectancy challenge and drinking reduction: experimental evidence for a meditational process. *J. Cons. Clin. Psychol.* 61:344–53

15. Dee TS. 1999. State alcohol policies, teen drinking and traffic accidents. *J. Public Econ.* 72(2):289–15

16. Dee TS, Evans WN. 2001. Teens and traffic safety. In *Risky Behavior Among Youth: An Economic Perspective*, ed. J Gruber, pp. 121–65. Chicago: Univ. Chicago Press

17. Dep. Commer. Bur. Census. 2003. http://www.census.gov/

18. Dimeff LA. 1997. *Brief intervention for heavy and hazardous college drinkers in a student primary health care setting.* PhD diss. Univ. Wash., Seattle

19. Ferguson SA, Fields M, Voas RB. 2000. Enforcement of zero tolerance laws in the United States. *Proc. 15th ICADTS. Swed. Natl. Road Adm. Borlänge, Sweden.* CD-ROM

20. Ferguson SA, Williams AF. 2002. Awareness of zero tolerance laws in three states. *J. Safety Res.* 33:293–99

21. Garvin RB, Alcorn JD, Faulkner KK. 1990. Behavioral strategies for alcohol abuse prevention with high-risk college males. *J. Alcohol Drug Educ.* 36(1):23–34

22. Godfrey C. 1997. Can tax be used to minimize harm? A health economist's perspective. In *Alcohol: Minimizing the Harm: What Works?*, ed. M Plant, E Single, T Stockwell, pp. 29–42. London, UK: Free Assoc. Books

23. Goldman M, Boyd G, Faden V. 2002. College Drinking. What is it and What to do

About it? A Review of the State of the Science. *J. Stud. Alcohol Suppl.* 14:1–250

24. Grossman M, Chaloupka FJ, Sirtalin I. 1998. An empirical analysis of alcohol addiction results from monitoring the future panels. *Econ. Inq.* 36(1):39–48

25. Grossman M, Coate D, Anluck GM. 1997. Price sensitivity of alcoholic beverages in the United States. In *Control Issues in Alcohol Abuse Prevention: Strategies for States and Communities*, ed. MH Moore, DR Gerstein, pp. 169–98. Greenwich, CT: JAI Press

26. Gruenewald PJ, Ponicki WR, Holder HD. 1993. The relationship of outlet densities to alcohol consumption: a time series cross-sectional analysis. *Alcohol. Clin. Exp. Res.* 17:38–47

27. Grunbaum JA, Kahn L, Kindum S, Williams B, Ross R, Koelbe L. 2002. Youth risk behavior surveillance United States 2001. *MMWR* 51(5504):1–64

28. Hingson R, Heeren T, Winter M. 1994. Lower legal blood alcohol limits for young drivers. *Public Health Rep.* 109:738–44

29. Hingson R, Heeren T, Winter M, Wechsler H. 2003. Early age of first drunkenness as a factor in college students' unplanned and unprotected sex attributable to drinking. *Pediatrics* 111(1):34–41

30. Hingson R, Heeren T, Zakocs R, Kopstein A, Wechsler H. 2002. Magnitude of alcohol-related mortality and morbidity among U.S. college students ages 18–24. *J. Stud. Alcohol.* 63:136–44

31. Hingson R, Heeren T, Zakocs R, Winter M, Wechsler H. 2003. Age of first intoxication, heavy drinking, driving after drinking and risk of unintentional injury among U.S. college students. *J. Stud. Alcohol.* 64(1):23–31

32. Hingson R, Howland J. 2002. Comprehensive community interventions to promote health: implications for college-age drinking problems. *J. Stud. Alcohol* (Suppl.) 14:226–40

33. Hingson R, Kenkel D. 2003. Social, health and economic consequences of underage

drinking. *Natl. Acad. Sci. CD-ROM Backgr. Pap.*, pp. 351–82

34. Hingson R, McGovern T, Howland J, Heeren T, Winter M, Zakocs R. 1996. Reducing alcohol-impaired driving in Massachusetts: the Savings Lives program. *Am. J. Public Health* 86:791–97

35. Holder H, Gruenewald PJ, Ponicki WR, Treno AJ, Grube JW, et al. 2000. Effects of community-based interventions on high risk driving and alcohol-related injuries. *JAMA* 284(18):2341–47

36. Johnston L, O'Malley P, Bachman J. 2000. Monitoring the future: national survey results on drug use 1975–1999, Volume II: college students and adults ages 19–40. *NIH Publ. No. 00–480*, Natl. Inst. Drug Abuse

37. Johnston L, O'Malley P, Bachman J. 2001. Monitoring the future: national survey results on drug use 1975–1999. Volume II: college students and adults ages 19–40. *NIH Publ. No. 02–5107*, Natl. Inst. Drug Abuse

38. Jones RK, Lacey JH. 2001. Alcohol and highway safety 2001, a review of the state of knowledge. *Report No. DOT HS—809—383,* Natl. Highway Traffic Safety Adm., Washington, DC

39. Kenkel DS. 1993. Drinking, driving and deterrence: the effectiveness and social costs of alternative policies. *J. Law Econ.* 36(2):877–14

40. Klein T. 1986. Methods for estimating posterior BAC distribution for persons involved in fatal crashes. *DOT HS 807 904*, Natl. Highway Traffic Safety Adm.

41. Kuo M, Wechsler H, Greenberg P, Lee H. 2003. The marketing of alcohol to college students: the role of low prices and special promotions. *Am. J. Prev. Med.* 25(3)204–11

42. Laixuthai A, Chaloupka FJ. 1993. Youth alcohol use and public policy. *Contemp. Policy Issues* 11(4):70–81

43. Larimer M, Cronce J. 2002. Identification, prevention and treatment: a review of individual-focused strategies to reduce problematic alcohol consumption by college students. *J. Stud. Alcohol* 14(Suppl.): 148–64

44. Lake P. 2002. *Keynote address.* Presented at College Alcohol Summit, Penn. Liquor Control Board, Harrisburg, PA

45. Manning WG, Blumberg L, Moulton LH. 1995. The demand for alcohol: the differential response to price. *J. Health Econ.* 14(2):123–48

46. Markowitz S, Grossman M. 1998. Alcohol regulation and domestic violence towards children. *Contemp. Econ. Policy* 16(3): 309–20

47. Markowitz S, Grossman M. 2002. The effects of beer taxes on physical child abuse. *J. Health Econ.* 19(2):271–82

48. Marlatt GA, Baer JS, Kivlahan DR, Dimeff LA, Larimer ME, et al. 1998. Screening and brief intervention for high-risk college student drinkers: results from a two-year follow-up assessment. *J. Cons. Clin. Psychol.* 66:604–15

49. Monti PM, Colby SM, Barnett NP, Spirito A, Rohsenow DJ, et al. 1999. Brief intervention for harm reduction with alcohol-positive older adolescents in a hospital emergency department. *J. Cons. Clin. Psychol.* 67:989–94

50. Murphy TJ, Pagano RR, Marlatt GA. 1986. Lifestyle modification with heavy alcohol drinkers: effects of aerobic exercise and meditation. *Addict. Behav.* 11:175–86

51. Naimi T, Brewer R, Mokdas A, Denny L, Serdula M, Marks J. 2003. Binge drinking among U.S. adults. *JAMA* 289(1):70–74

52. Natl. Acad. Sci. 2004. *Reducing Underage Drinking: A Collective Responsibility*, ed. RJ Bonnie, ME O'Connell. Washington, DC: NAS

53. Natl. Cent. Educ. Stat. 2004 [2001]. *Integrated Post Secondary Education Data System Fall Enrollment, 1999.* http://www.census.gov/population/socdemo/school/p20-533/tab09.pdf

54. Natl. Highway Traffic Safety Adm. 2003. Traffic safety facts 2002: alcohol.

DOT HS 809–6061, NHTSA, Washington, DC

55. Natl. Highway Traffic Safety Adm. US Dep. Transp. 2002. Traffic safety facts. *DOT HS 809–470*

56. Natl. Highway Traffic Safety Adm. US Dep. Transp. 2002. Transitioning to multiple imputation: a new method to estimate missing blood alcohol concentration values in FARS. *DOT HS 809–403*

57. Natl. Inst. Alcohol Abuse and Alcoholism Natl. Advis. Counc. 2002. A call to action: changing the culture of drinking at U.S. colleges, *NIH Publ. No. 02–5010*

58. O'Malley P, Wagenaar AC. 1991. Effects of minimum drinking age laws on alcohol use, related behavior and traffic crash involvement among American youth. *J. Stud. Alcohol* 52:478–91

59. Preusser DF, Ulmer RB, Preusser CW. 1992. Obstacles to enforcement of youthful (under 21) impaired driving. *Rep. No. DOT HS-807–878,* Natl. Highway Traffic Safety Adm., Washington, DC

60. Rohsenow DJ, Smith RE, Johnson S. 1985. Stress management training as a prevention program for heavy social drinkers: cognitions, affect, drinking and individual differences. *Addict Behav.* 10:45–54

61. Ruhm CJ. 1996. Alcohol policies and highway vehicle fatalities. *J. Health Econ.* 15(4):435–54

62. Saffer H, Grossman M. 1987. Beer taxes, the legal drinking age, and youth motor vehicle fatalities. *J. Legal Stud.* 16(2):351–74

63. Shah BU, Barnwell BG, Bieller GS, Suda AN. 1996. *User's Manual Release 7.* Research Triangle Park, NC: Res. Triangle Inst.

64. Shults RA, Elder RW, Sleet DA, Nichols JL, Alao MO, et al. 2001. Reviews of evidence regarding interventions to reduce alcohol-impaired driving. *Am. J. Prev. Med.* 21(4)(Suppl.):66–68

65. Smith G, Branings KC, Miller T. 1999. Fatal non traffic injuries involving alcohol, a meta-analysis. *Ann. Emerg. Med.* 33:699–02

66. Subst. Abuse Mental Health Serv. Adm. Off. Appl. Stud. 2000. Summary of findings of the 1999 National Household Survey on Drug Abuse. *DHHS Publ. No. (SMA) 00–3466*

67. Subst. Abuse Mental Health Serv. Adm. Off. Appl. Stud. 2002. Results of the 2001 National Household Survey on Drug Abuse: Volume 1. Summary of national findings. *NHSDA Ser. H-17, DHHS Publ. No. (SMA) 02–3758*

68. Sutton M, Godfrey C. 1995. A grouped data regression approach to estimating economic and social influences on individual drinking behavior. *Health Econ.* 4:237–47

69. Voas RB, Tippets A, Fell J. 2000. The relationship of alcohol safety laws to drinking drivers in fatal crashes. *Accid. Anal. Prev.* 32:483–92

70. Voas RB, Williams AF. 1986. Age difference of arrested and crash-involved drinking drivers. *J. Stud. Alcohol.* 47:244–48

71. Wagenaar AC, Murray DM, Gehan JP, Wolfson M, Forster JL, et al. 2000. Communities mobilized for change on alcohol effects of a randomized trial on arrests and traffic crashes. *Addiction* 95:209–17b

72. Wagenaar AC, Murray DM, Gehan JP, Wolfson M, Forster J, et al. 2000. Communities mobilizing for change: outcomes from a randomized community trial. *J. Stud. Alcohol* 161(1):85–94

73. Wagenaar AC, O'Malley PM, LaFond C. 2001. Lowered legal blood alcohol limits for young drivers: effects on drinking, driving and driving after drinking behaviors in 30 states. *Am. J. Public Health* 91:801–4

74. Wagenaar AC, Toomey TL. 2002. Effects of minimum drinking age laws: review and analyses of the literature from 1960 to 2000. *J. Stud. Alcohol.* (Suppl. 14):206–25

75. Walters ST, Bennett ME, Miller JH. 2000. Reducing alcohol use in college students: a controlled trial of two brief interventions. *J. Drug Educ.* 30:361–72

76. Walters ST, Martin JE, Noto J. 1999. *A controlled trial of two feedback-based interventions for heavy drinking college students.* Poster presented at the Annu. Meet. Res. Soc. Alcoholism, Santa Barbara, CA

77. Wechsler H, Davenport A, Dowdall G, Moeykins B, Castillo S. 1994. Health and behavioral consequences of binge drinking in college, a national survey of students at 140 campuses. *JAMA* 272(21):1672–77

78. Wechsler H, Dowdall GW, Maenner G, Gledhill-Hoyt J, Lee H. 1998. Changes in binge drinking and related problems among American college students between 1993 and 1997. *J. Am. College Health* 47:57–68

79. Wechsler H, Lee JE, Kuo M, Lee H. 2000. College binge drinking in the 1990's: a continuing problem. *J. Am. College Health* 48:199–210

80. Wechsler H, Lee JE, Kuo M, Seibring M, Nelson TF, Lee H. 2002. Trends in alcohol use, related problems and experience of prevention efforts among U.S. college students 1993–2001: results from the Harvard School of Public Health College Alcohol Study. *J. Am. College Health* 5:203–17

81. Wechsler H, Lee JE, Nelson TF, Lee H. 2003. Drinking and driving among college students: the influence of alcohol-control policies. *Am. J. Prev. Med.* 25(3):212–18

82. Wells JK, Greene MA, Foss RD, Ferguson SA, Williams AF. 1997. Drinking drivers missed at sobriety checkpoints. *J. Stud. Alcohol* 58:513–17

83. Weitzman ER, Nelon TF, Lee H, Wechsler H. 2004. Reducing drinking and related harms in college: evaluation of the Matter of Degree program. *Am. J. Prev. Med.* 27:187–96

Annu. Rev. Public Health. 2005. 26:281–302
doi: 10.1146/annurev.publhealth.26.021304.144522
Copyright © 2005 by Annual Reviews. All rights reserved
First published online as a Review in Advance on September 28, 2004

NEW MICROBIOLOGY TOOLS FOR PUBLIC HEALTH AND THEIR IMPLICATIONS[1]

Betty H. Robertson and Janet K.A. Nicholson

*National Center for Infectious Diseases, Centers for Disease Control and Prevention,
Atlanta, Georgia 30333; email: bjr1@cdc.gov; jkn1@cdc.gov*

Key Words   polymerase chain reaction, flow cytometry, pulsed field gel
electrophoresis, multi-locus variable number tandem repeat analysis, time-resolved
fluorescence, microarrays

■ **Abstract**   The realm of diagnostic assays for detection of acute infections is
rapidly changing from antibody detection to pathogen detection, from clinical laboratory based to point-of-care based, from single analyte detection to multiple analyte
detection, and is more focused on detection using less invasive approaches for collecting biological samples. New assays are typically more sensitive than are conventional
assays and have the capability of providing more information that characterizes the
pathogen or the host response to the pathogen. From a public health perspective, the advent of molecular epidemiology, which allows tracking of pathogens based on unique
genetic sequences or antigenic properties, has revolutionized how epidemiologists investigate and evaluate epidemics and assess endemic diseases. In addition, the use of
point-of-care (POC) devices can impact the detection and surveillance of infections
and will enhance our ability to accurately identify the causes of illnesses.

INTRODUCTION

Over the past 20 years, a number of scientific discoveries and technologies have
converged to change the approach to diagnostic laboratory procedures for infectious diseases and have altered the landscape for detection and characterization of
infectious diseases within public health. Most of these discoveries have involved
nucleic acid technology, starting with the polymerase chain reaction (PCR) and
culminating in cDNA/oligonucleotide microarrays. PCR technology generates exponential amplification of genome sequences, which enhances detection limits
(46), whereas microarray technology facilitates the parallel analysis of multiple
markers (genetic or protein) from a single sample (16). During this same time
frame, the complete sequence of many genomes, including the complete human

---

[1]The U.S. Government has the right to retain a nonexclusive, royalty-free license in and to
any copyright covering this paper.

genome (35, 59), was obtained and microfluidic technology was developed, which allows investigators to use submicroliter volumes for testing (3, 17). In addition, flow cytometry, once relegated to identifying cells, particularly lymphocytes, has been revolutionized by the introduction of microarray bead technology, which promises to allow detection of multiple analytes in a single tube (multiplexing).

This chapter describes the major changes in microbiological detection resulting from these and associated findings and how they have been used for public health research and disease prevention. The current use of nucleic acid detection (especially PCR detection) and the future use of microassay technology, multiplexed assays, point-of-care assays, and the use of noninvasive techniques to obtain specimens for testing have resulted and will result in a rapidly evolving scenario that has major implications for diagnostic laboratories and public health practitioners who focus on control of infectious diseases.

TRANSITION FROM PROTEIN DETECTION
TO NUCLEIC ACID DETECTION ASSAYS

Twenty years ago, the major diagnostic assays used to support microbiologic public health decisions were primarily based on enzyme immunoassays (EIA) for detection of antigen or antibodies or based on colorometric determination of biochemical products. As we entered the 1980s, nucleic acid cloning, sequencing, and expression of the cloned products in bacteria were rapidly becoming common laboratory procedures. The most important infectious disease event of the early 1980s was the discovery of human immunodeficiency virus (HIV) (4, 18), which ultimately resulted in an EIA to detect antibodies against the viral antigens (10). However, this assay lacked perfect sensitivity and specificity, and confirmatory assays including Western blotting or indirect immunofluorescence (IFA) were necessary to evaluate indeterminate or equivocal EIA reactions. The use of two assays, a simple, less expensive screening assay followed by a more complex, more expensive confirmatory assay, became the standard for identification of new and prevalent HIV cases.

The Western blot assay relied on producing purified HIV antigens derived from cell cultures, which varied with HIV strain and culture conditions. This problem was solved using a technology called recombinant immunoblotting assay (RIBA), in which individual recombinant viral antigens were deposited as a line on a nitrocellulose filter followed by detection using specific antibody binding and colorimetric labels (7). The discovery of hepatitis C virus (HCV) (11) also rapidly resulted in the development of an EIA for diagnosis (34) using recombinant antigens as targets since the virus did not grow in cell culture. As was done for HIV, recombinant viral antigens were used to develop an RIBA confirmatory assay.

In the situations described above, the assays detect an antibody response to a pathogen. Detection of antibody does not provide information about the presence of pathogen and, if present, about the amount of the pathogen. For HIV, virus detection could be ascertained by prolonged cocultivation of peripheral blood mononuclear cells with a susceptible cell line (15), but this method was far from sensitive. In contrast, HCV cannot be grown in cell culture. In HIV (as with other viral infections), measurement of viral load has been extremely helpful in characterizing the stage of infection, as viral loads are high in both acute and end-stage disease with much lower levels in the months or years in between. Therefore, treatment decisions may be based on viral load and treatment effectiveness as measured in large part by the decrease in viral load (9).

NUCLEIC ACID TECHNOLOGY

Molecular Epidemiology and Surveillance

Concurrent with these classic EIA diagnostic approaches to measure viral infection, polymerase chain reaction (PCR) entered the world of science and rapidly began to impact the investigator's ability to detect and characterize the genetic features of pathogens. This discovery (Table 1; 46), which would transform molecular biology and science, changed diagnostic testing and approaches to the identification and classification of infectious agents. PCR amplification is achieved using two oligonucleotide primers that flank an intervening region of dsDNA (Figure 1). After binding the primers, DNA polymerase generates replicas of the targeted sequence. Using the ability of DNA to denature at high temperatures, and then re-anneal when the temperature is lowered, multiple cycles of DNA synthesis provide incredible amplification of the targeted sequence. PCR technology paved the way for the use of nucleic acid technology in diagnostics and public health research and is the foundation on which many of the subsequent technological and public health science advances are based.

The same year the first publication describing PCR technology appeared, Ou et al. (41) used this technology to amplify and detect HIV sequences from seropositive individuals (Table 1). Subsequently, PCR amplification and sequence analysis of HIV amplicons represented the first use of comparative nucleic sequence information in an outbreak setting (40). Comparative analysis of the HIV sequences from a group of patients and their dentist (who was accused of transmitting HIV during dental procedures) confirmed a close genetic relationship between the HIV isolates, consistent with a common source of infection. This investigation provided the first demonstration of the power of nucleic acid sequence information to answer issues related to transmission and heralded the beginning of the field of molecular epidemiology.

Sequence analysis has provided the foundation for molecular surveillance in addition to providing valuable information for outbreak investigations. In 1987, the concept of sequencing selected regions of the poliovirus genome (Table 1; 45) from temporally and geographically separated isolates provided the model for a sequence database that is currently used as a molecular surveillance tool. The practical application of this information is most elegantly illustrated in the

TABLE 1   Milestones in technology and public health research application

Year	Technology advance	Public health research application
1983		HIV identified by growth in cell culture
1984		
1985		
1986		
1987		Comparative sequence database model developed for poliovirus
1988	PCR technology published	Identification of HIV by PCR amplification
1989		HCV identified by expression cloning and genome sequencing; diagnostic EIA and RIBA confirmatory assay developed
1990		
1991	PFGE technique published Microarray technology published	RIBA confirmation assay for HIV developed
1992		
1993		Molecular epidemiology used in HIV outbreak Respiratory hantavirus identified by PCR amplification
1994		
1995		PFGE used as standard for bacterial foodborne disease outbreaks
1996	Real-time PCR technology published	Microarrays used to evaluate HIV sequences
1997		
1998		
1999	Use of microfluidics for biological applications published	
2000		
2001	Human genome sequence completed	Real-time PCR used to test anthrax samples
2002		Microarray technology applied to viral pathogens
2003		Microarray technology used to identify SARS CoV

current campaign to eradicate poliovirus. A database of sequence information from isolates all over the world has allowed investigators to ascertain importation of wild poliovirus into polio-free regions (14), to characterize transmission patterns during an outbreak (50), and to determine that attenuated vaccine strain virus can remain undetected and circulate for years before suddenly causing an outbreak if sufficient numbers of a nonimmunized cohort are available (30).

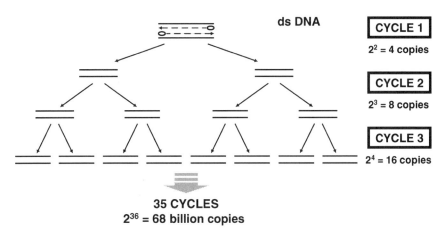

Figure 1 Schematic illustration of PCR amplification. Solid lines represent double-stranded DNA (dsDNA). Primer binding sites are illustrated by the ovals adjacent to the ends of the initial dsDNA fragment. The dashed lines illustrate the synthesis of the complementary sequence, which then results in two exact replicas of the original sequence. Each cycle results in an exponential doubling of the previous population. This figure also illustrates the amount of amplification that can occur from a single dsDNA target sequence.

However, about the same time, the first description was published of a technique to characterize bacterial isolates based on genetic approaches (1). This technology, called pulsed-field gel electrophoresis (PFGE), utilizes restriction enzymes that cut genomic DNA into 10–20 restriction fragments. These fragments are resolved by a process termed PFGE, in which the differential migration of large DNA fragments is mediated by constantly changing the direction of the electrical field during electrophoresis. A schematic representation of PFGE-separated fragments is shown in Figure 2. Uniform guidelines for performing PFGE and the interpretation of data (55) have resulted in the maturation of this technology such that it has resulted in an international consortium of researchers who share data electronically to follow outbreaks of food-borne illness (*Camplyobacter*, *E. coli* 0157, *Listeria monocytogenes*, *Salmonella*, and *Shigella*). Investigators enter the PFGE fingerprint into PulseNet's electronic database at the Centers for Disease Control and Prevention (CDC), where it is compared with other bacterial DNA patterns. Identical or highly similar patterns suggest that samples represent a common source outbreak (http://www.cdc.gov/pulsenet).

Nucleic Acid Technology and Identification of Unknown Agents

PCR takes advantage of the investigator's ability to amplify DNA through the action of DNA polymerase. DNA pieces are amplified under the correct conditions using primers that are complementary to the sequences of interest, and detection

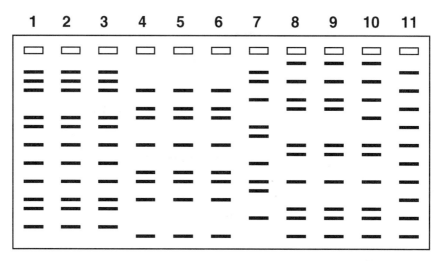

Figure 2 Hypothetical PFGE patterns. The origin for application of the restriction-digested fragments is indicated by the rectangle at the top of each lane. Lanes 1–3, 4–6, 7, and 8–10 illustrate four separate PFGE patterns. Lane 11 contains a standard DNA ladder used as a reference.

is accomplished using probes that carry detectable signals (e.g., fluorescence or light). Variations on this theme have been developed to increase the sensitivity and specificity of the methodology and are included below.

The use of PCR and nucleic acid technology for detection and characterization of agents, in which sequence information is known, is relatively straightforward. Primers can be selected easily based on known sequences and amplification of the targeted region performed. However, for unknown agents, the use of nucleic acid technology also provides a powerful tool that has facilitated rapid identification by complementing classical approaches to disease identification.

The combination of classic serology combined with the use of PCR technology to address unknown infections is strikingly illustrated (39) by the discovery and characterization of the hantavirus associated with acute respiratory distress syndrome in 1993 (Table 1). When this outbreak was recognized, a broad approach to determine the cause was initiated, including microbiological, environmental, and chemical investigations. Preliminary serology assays suggested that the agent was related to hantaviruses causing hemorrhagic fevers with renal syndromes (43). On the basis of this clue, scientists selected conserved sequences to use as PCR primers that flanked highly conserved regions of known hantaviruses and used these primers to amplify genetic fragments from the unknown agent. Sequencing of the intervening region identified the new hantaviral agent and provided information on the potential reservoir (mice) and approaches to control the transmission of disease.

During the recent severe acute respiratory syndrome (SARS) outbreak, PCR technology was used once again to assist in the identification of the unknown agent in conjunction with classical virological approaches. Inoculation of patient samples onto tissue culture cells resulted in cytopathic effects, and negative stained electron micrographs were consistent with the morphology of a coronavirus. Once again, highly conserved primers for coronavirus were selected and PCR amplification of a selected genome region, followed by sequencing of the intervening region, revealed the presence of a previously undescribed coronavirus (33).

Nucleic Acid Technology and Diagnostic Assays

Direct sequence data can provide detailed information over large stretches of genomes, but it is a highly labor-intensive and expensive approach for clinical applications and limits the rapid turnaround of results for diagnostic purposes. An alternative, which was developed for the HIV, HCV, and HBV fields, is an application termed the line immunoprobe assay (LIPA) (51–54). This assay is a nucleic acid RIBA assay: Selected oligonucleotides that differentiate different genetic variants (genotypes or drug-resistant mutants) are applied as a line on a nitrocellulose strip. As shown in Figure 3, PCR is performed from the clinical sample using primers that are chosen to amplify the selected genome region containing nucleotide differences. These differences provide a unique signature that differentiates genotypes or drug-resistant mutants. Hybridization followed by detection using a colorimetric monitor is used to detect binding and positive reactivity. These assays are among the first commercial assays to use nucleic acid hybridization for diagnostic purposes.

Investigators used a similar approach in another early commercial application of PCR technology. Biotinylated primers are used for PCR amplification, and the product is subsequently purified by hybridization to magnetic beads containing specific sequences and detected using conventional EIA colorimetric substrates (COBAS AMPLICOR PCR, Roche Diagnostics). This technology currently supports detection of agents that are difficult or impossible to grow in culture (HCV, HBV, cytomegalovirus, *Chlamydia trachomatis*, *Neisseria gonorrhoeae*, *Mycobacterium tuberculosis*, *Mycobacterium avium*, *Mycobacterium intracellulare*) and has been proposed as a reasonable alternative for detection of these agents (29).

A third approach for rapid turnaround detection of nucleic acid derived from infectious organisms is real-time PCR. This technology is based on the detection and quantitation of a fluorescent reporter, which is measured at each cycle of the PCR. Two approaches for following and quantitating fluorescent reporters are used. The first is fluorescent probes [TaqMan probes (22) and molecular beacons (57)], which involve sequence-specific hybridization to the target amplicon and fluorescence readout based on the hybridization. Figure 4 illustrates the reaction process for Taqman probes. Molecular beacons are single-stranded hybridization probes that form a stem loop structure; the loop contains the probe sequence, whereas the stem contains the reporter and quencher adjacent to each other. Hybridization of the loop to the target sequence separates the reporter and quencher, and the resulting fluorescence is measured. The other detection method measures dye (such as

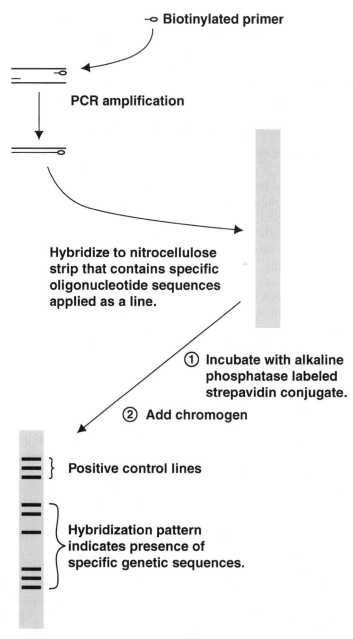

Figure 3   Flow diagram of LIPA assay. One of the primers used for PCR amplification is biotinylated; this primer targets the sequence that is complementary to the oligonucleotides that have been applied to the nitrocellulose test strip. The biotinylated PCR product is subsequently hybridized to the oligonucleotides on the test strip and detected using conventional EIA technology.

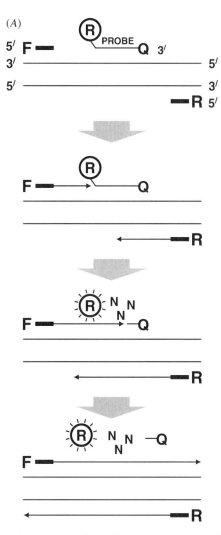

Figure 4   (*A*) Schematic representation of Taqman real-time PCR detection. Double-stranded DNA is represented by parallel lines. Forward (F₋) and reverse (R₋) primers are indicated by the bold lines adjacent to the 3′ ends. The probe containing the fluorescent reporter (*circled R*) and the adjacent quencher (Q) is illustrated as binding to the strand being copied by the forward primer. As the Taq polymerase proceeds toward the 5′ end, nuclease activity digests the hybridized probe, releasing the fluorescent reporter from the influence of the quencher molecule. *N* indicates the release of free nucleotides caused by the nuclease activity. As amplification proceeds, the amount of free fluorescent reporter increases, with a resulting increase in signal. (*B*) Representative graph illustrating the fluorescent signal generated during a real-time PCR reaction. C_t is the threshold cutoff, and the dotted line and arrow indicate the threshold level at which fluorescent is detected and quantitated.

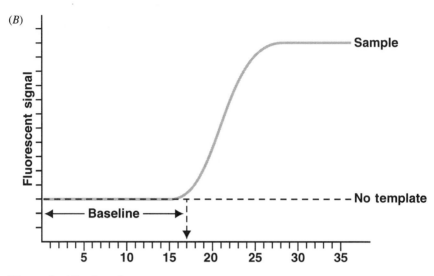

Figure 4 (*Continued*)

SYBER Green I) binding to double-stranded DNA, which quantitates the amplicon accumulation. Both methods result in quantitative measures and have been useful for determining viral load, for example.

Fluorescent probes labeled with different reporter dyes can be multiplexed, allowing for detection of multiple amplicons within the same reaction mixture, whereas detection of double-stranded DNA is limited to a single product per reaction. Multiplexing such assays has had to overcome technical challenges and, as a result, is generally less sensitive than are conventional molecular assays. Nevertheless, these technologies provide the basis for detection and quantitation of nucleic acid in the diagnostic and public health fields, and a number of commercial laboratories now offer this service for detection and quantitation of agents such as HIV, HCV, and HBV.

Given the sensitivity of detection and the development of real-time PCR detection, the CDC and its affiliated Laboratory Response Network (LRN) have implemented real-time PCR reagents and protocols to identify the biothreat agents of greatest concern. This technology was used by the CDC and LRN in a highly effective manner in the U.S. anthrax event of 2001, where thousands of samples were tested using a real-time assay (Table 1; 26). The use of common equipment, reagents, and protocols, and the sensitivity of the technology, facilitates the investigator's ability to rapidly implement sensitive testing for new agents in a public health emergency, such as the recent global SARS coronavirus (CoV) outbreak.

Nucleic acid methodology has been used primarily to detect viruses, in part because of their small size compared with bacteria. Molecular characterization of bacteria is a growing field. Methods to distinguish strains of bacteria have mostly relied on serological assays. More recently, identification of unique sequences in bacterial strains have led to the development of assays that have the potential for strain subtyping. One of these assays, the multi-locus variable-number tandem repeat analysis (MLVA), was particularly useful in determining the source of anthrax delivered in letters to Florida, New York, and Washington, D.C., in the fall of 2001 (25). This assay determines the copy number of variable-number tandem repeats at a number of different genetic loci (eight loci in the anthrax example). Expansion of the number of genetic loci targeted increases the specificity of the assay, and the use of 20 or more loci is currently under development.

Controls and Standards

The biggest challenge that has plagued nucleic acid detection methods, particularly those where sequences are amplified, is contamination of reagents and the extraction and PCR work areas with nucleic acid. Because of this problem, some investigators have been reluctant to include positive controls within the assay format. Novel ways to provide assurance that the assay was performed correctly, while avoiding contamination by the positive control, must be included in assay formats. Self-contained assay systems have helped overcome this problem, and development of nucleic acid assays that are simple and easy to use must ensure contamination is avoided.

FLOW CYTOMETRY

Flow cytometry was developed in the 1970s (24) and was originally termed fluorescence-activated cell sorting (FACS) after the first commercial instrument that was developed to analyze individual fluorescently tagged cells as they passed through a laser light for detection. Cells are typically identified on the basis of size and granularity characteristics, and the presence and quantity of fluorescence is characterized for each cell. On the heels of the development of this new technology, monoclonal antibodies were developed (31), and what we now know as HIV infection was first recognized in the developed world (20, 37). This combination of flow cytometry and monoclonal antibodies quickly led to the application of flow cytometry in the identification of patients with low numbers and percentages of CD4 lymphocytes, whom investigators ultimately found to be infected with HIV. Since that time, flow cytometry has moved from the research laboratory into clinical practice and, in infectious diseases, has been relegated primarily to identifying T and B lymphocyte subsets in HIV and other viral infections, such as cytomegalovirus and Epstein-Barr infection, that result in changes in these cell populations (8, 44). Other applications include assessing cancer patients, particularly those with lymphoma and leukemia, for type and grade of disease. In all cases, flow cytometry is considered an adjunct to other clinical tests because it helps stage patients (for cancer and HIV infection) and assesses therapy effectiveness (for transplant and cancer patients).

Multiplexed Assays Using Flow Cytometry

More recently, the basic concepts of flow cytometry (detection of fluorescently tagged particles) have been exploited in the development of fluorescent microbeads that can be used as surfaces onto which antibodies, antigens, or nucleic acid sequences can be attached for the detection of antigens, antibodies, and peptides, respectively (28, 36). Because it is possible to imbed the microbeads with a wide variety of fluorescent colors, each bead can become an individual assay and multiple beads can be combined in a tube, thus comprising multiple assays in a single tube (multiplexed assay). A schematic illustrating this concept is shown in Figure 5. This is attractive to infectious agents for the detection of a wide variety of antibodies or cytokines, for detection of a variety of antigens or antigenic components, and for detection of nucleic acid sequences.

The practical application of this technology is still in its pubescent stage. Relatively inexpensive instrumentation is available, but commercial kits with built-in quality control have yet to become available for common use.

Flow Cytometry for Use in Microbiology

Although flow cytometers analyze particles (cells, typically), they can also detect and analyze some bacteria. Because the size of the bacteria is often similar to that of debris in the sample preparation, the detection of bacteria based on size is of limited use. Identification of bacteria based on cellular antigens holds promise, but at this time reagents are limited for not only detecting but also characterizing (typing or subtyping) bacteria. As more reagents become available and instruments become less expensive, and the sensitivity of the assay is increased to detect lower levels of fluorescence, bacteria may be quickly identified in urine or other body fluids using flow cytometry.

Controls and Standards

Flow cytometry instrumentation has become more simplified over the past 25 years; however, like most instrument-based technologies, if the instrument is not properly calibrated, there is a risk of obtaining poor data. Small, relatively inexpensive instruments are becoming available for specific applications such as multiplexing. Controls and standardization of the test are less problematic for multiplexed assays than with flow cytometry used for cellular characterization, including that for bacteria.

Other Antigen Detection Methods

Further developments in antigen detection have focused on increasing the level of detection of antigens, and ultimately organisms. One of these new developments is time-resolved fluorescence (TRF). TRF is an assay system that also takes advantage of characteristics of fluorescent molecules and the fact that some fluorochromes have a large Stokes shift (e.g., Europium), and therefore it has a time

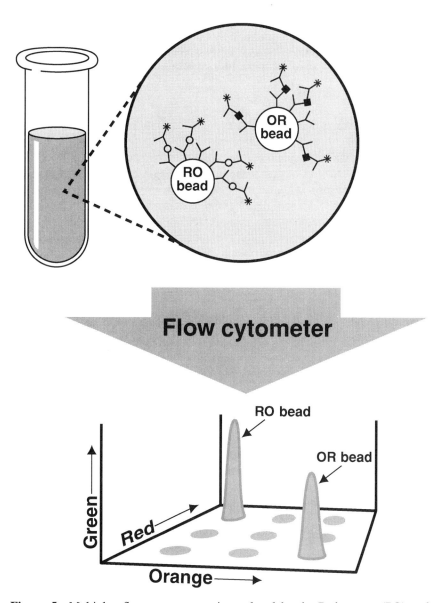

Figure 5 Multiplex flow cytometry using colored beads. Red-orange (RO) and orange-red (OR) beads have two different antibodies (indicated by Y) attached that recognize different antigens: One is illustrated by the open circles, and the other is depicted by the closed square. Subsequent reaction with a detector antibody containing a green fluorescence tag identifies the positive reaction. Histogram readouts from the flow cytometer provide information about the positive (green) and negative (no green signal) results from each bead set (RO and OR in this example).

delay between excitation and emission, which allows for a longer time to detect the fluorescence; thus greater signals are being detected. The types of assays to which this methodology is applied are similar to that of an EIA, but special instrumentation is required for TRF. This method has been used for antibodies as well as antigens (2, 38, 47).

MICROARRAY TECHNOLOGY

The next wave of technology for diagnostic and public health laboratories will entail the use of microarrays and microfluidics. Nucleic acid microarrays consist of rows and rows of unique oligonucleotides, or cDNA, lined up on a miniature silicone chip or glass slide. These immobilized pieces of nucleic acid are then hybridized with fluorescent-labeled cDNA from the sample of interest; the bound label identifies the corresponding unique sequences found in the sample of interest. A schematic illustrating the principles used in this technology is shown in Figure 6. This technology was first introduced in a 1991 *Science* manuscript (16), which described its ability to generate up to a 1024-member array of peptides using photolithography and its ability to synthesize oligonucleotides in situ using the same technology. Since this first description of microarray technology, the number of publications that focus on this technology have increased rapidly. This technology has been used to tackle identification of nucleic acid arrays (48), to address gene expression in human cancer (13), to evaluate human genome analysis (49), and to detect inflammatory disease–related genes (23).

DNA Microarrays in Infectious Diseases

DNA microarray technology is highly flexible and use of this technology has barely scratched the surface within infectious diseases. One of the first applications of this technology was once again in the field of HIV, in which a high-density oligonucleotide array was used to evaluate polymorphisms within the protease gene to detect drug resistance (32).

However, the technology is easily adapted to identify pathogens and, depending on the strategy used to design the array, could focus on specific groups of pathogens. The first description of such an approach, focusing on the detection and genotyping of viral pathogens, used an array with approximately 1600 long oligonucleotides (70 mers) representing 140 sequenced viral genomes (60). During the SARS epidemic, this group expanded this prototype DNA microarray to cover approximately 1000 different viruses (61). They tested nucleic acid from cells experimentally infected with SARS material (autopsy tissues, etc.), and the data using this microarray indicated that the unknown agent had sequences common to coronaviruses and astroviruses and provided crucial information to help investigators identify the SARS coronavirus. These findings indicated that it was not a currently known viral agent (33).

From a commercial perspective, the initial efforts focused on identifying drug-resistant HIV (32, 58) and identifying mycobacteria and rifampicin resistance (19,

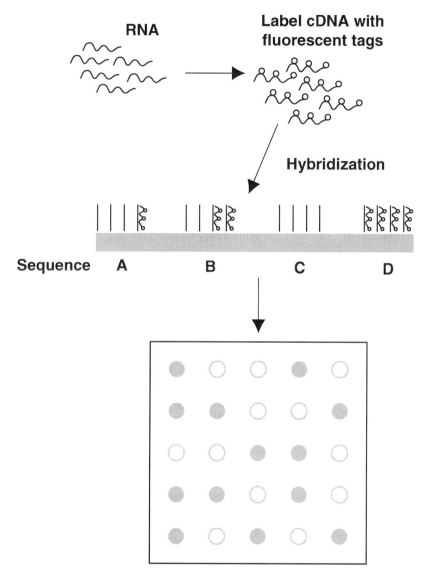

Figure 6   Microarray hybridization and detection. This figure illustrates the generation of cDNA from RNA for use as hybridization probes (*wavy lines*) that are chemically labeled with multiple fluorescent tags (*open circles*) per molecule. These are then hybridized to different oligonucleotide or cDNA targets (*straight lines, indicating sequence A, B, C, and D*) that are affixed to a solid support such as a glass slide, silicon chip, or nitrocellulose (*open rectangle*). As shown in the cross-sectional view, the relative amount of different RNA molecules can determine the amount of probe bound and influence the amount of fluorescence. A representative array, viewed from the top, is shown below the cross-sectional view.

56). Industry is currently evaluating the market for the use of "gene chips" in the diagnosis of infectious diseases, although all these chips are only for research use at this time. Since their market will be clinical laboratories, the focus for commercialization might encompass a broad spectrum of respiratory pathogens (including bacterial and viral) or enteric pathogens. Currently, Prodesse (Milwaukee, Wisconsin) markets multiplex assays that detect the seven most common respiratory viruses, human metapneumovirus, and adenoviruses and the three most common bacterial causes of atypical pneumonia: mycoplasma, *Chlamydia*, and *Legionella*. They have recently entered into a collaboration with Nanogen, Inc. (San Diego, California) to develop a microarray-based product that will detect all these agents in addition to herpes viruses, West Nile Virus, and SARS CoV (http://prodesse.com/news/article20.htm).

DNA Microarrays to Evaluate Host-Microbe Interactions and Chronic Diseases

Microarrays can dramatically change how host genomic data is evaluated in the arena of chronic diseases. Since many chronic diseases result in changes in the host genome, the information derived from sequencing the human genome has provided the framework for the development of microarrays that are specific for host genetic changes and can identify host changes that occur during chronic infections. Evaluation of changes over time within an individual can provide information about disease progression and efficacy of treatment. Expression profiling (evaluation of mRNA) in *Plasmodium falciparum*, the most lethal form of human malaria, in the schizont and trophozoite stage were evaluated and revealed selective gene expression at these two stages of the organism, which may result in future drug targets or vaccine candidates (6). In other situations, such as chronic infection with hepatitis C, evaluation of host cell products will illustrate the host response to this virus and provide information that can be used to improve viral therapy.

In addition, from an infectious disease perspective, this technology has potential use in the characterization of host-microbe interactions that result in chronic diseases. Increasing numbers of infections leading to chronic disease are being recognized, including *Chlamydia pneumonia* and atherosclerosis (5, 12); *Helicobacter pylori* and stomach cancer (42); HBV, HCV, and hepatocellular carcinoma; and borna disease virus and behavioral disorders (21, 27). The ability to evaluate host and microbial markers in situations such as these infectious diseases may lead to methods for treatment or prevention.

Controls and Standards

The field of microarray technology within infectious diseases and pathogen detection is young; however, with science moving at the current pace, the use of this technology will rapidly move into the diagnostic arena. As identified within Table 2, five major steps are involved in microarray detection. At each point, critical features must be addressed for technology to mature fully and be implemented within a diagnostic laboratory. Assuming investigators can collect the appropriate

TABLE 2 Basic steps for microarray analysis

Step	Technique
1	Target cDNA/oligonucleotide spotted/printed onto substrate
2	Sample RNA is isolated
3	cDNA is synthesized and labeled
4	Hybridization of substrate and target
5	Results are imaged and analyzed

biological sample to be tested, i.e., sputum or bronchial washings for respiratory pathogens or stool samples for enteric pathogens, optimization and standardization of the steps in Table 2 will help ensure reproducible results.

In addition, three more general issues that affect the overall results and reliability of the assay need to be resolved. Reproducibility between laboratories, and sometimes within the same laboratory, is a core feature of reliability that dramatically affects interpretation of results. Because the technology is highly sensitive, conditions for processing have to be followed rigidly. The second area that needs to be addressed is the potential for data overload. Because multiple data points can be generated from each array, computer algorithms are needed to analyze the data. A related issue is the assay's ability to perform statistical analysis to assess the significance of differences detected within or between arrays. The third issue currently being addressed by the commercial microarray community is standardization for best practices and standard controls. With standardization and controls in place, this technology has great potential to revolutionize public health practice.

POINT-OF-CARE ASSAYS AND NONINVASIVE TECHNIQUES FOR SPECIMEN COLLECTION

Another area that will change as a result of these advances in technology is the development of simple, inexpensive, point-of-care (POC) assays and the use of noninvasive techniques for specimen collection. Simple, rapid assays for the detection of HIV antibody in oral fluid have found their way into clinical laboratories and, more importantly, into drug-treatment centers and other settings where transient patients can obtain results in fewer than 30 min. Rapid tests for flu and streptococcus infections are now commonly available in doctor's offices.

Advances in microarray technology will be coupled with the implementation of microfluidic technology in many applications. This combination of microarray and microfluidic technology will lead to the possibility of self-contained handheld point-of-care assays for detection of infectious or other diseases. In such situations, there will be a need for samples that can be self-collected, such as saliva, urine, stools, or blood spots. The point-of-care assays and self-collected biologic samples are not necessarily "high-tech" endeavors, but implementation of these technologies could further revolutionize diagnostics and public health research. Though these methods are becoming simpler to the point of requiring little to no expertise to perform, care must be taken to ensure their appropriate use. In particular, because of simplicity, minimal training of the assay performer is needed, and therefore quality assurance is a concern. In addition, if assays are available over the counter (for example, for HIV), there must be assurances that positive test findings will result in appropriate medical care. These are challenges that the field of public health must address and overcome.

THE FUTURE

Maintaining control of the rising health care costs in the United States has had a serious impact on diagnostic testing. Reimbursement for the cost of laboratory tests has resulted in lower investments in highly trained medical technologists and the purchase of less expensive methodologies. Diagnostic tests are sought by medical providers that are simple to perform, are at least as sensitive and specific as conventional assays, and are inexpensive. Many of the new technologies described here potentially meet these objectives; however, for some of these technologies, more innovation is needed to accomplish this.

The assays described above are predominately research or commercial-based assays and are performed in specialized laboratories with trained personnel using varying types of sophisticated equipment. Nucleic acid–based assays, either PCR based or assays that rely on detection of the microbial nucleic acid in the absence of amplification, use microliter volumes of sample and, for the most part, have an extremely labor-intensive extraction phase that necessitates carefully trained personnel. Assays of the future will utilize nanoliter volumes, and the major input of technical personnel will be to arrange the specimens for application to the supporting media that will be used for testing. The remainder of the steps involved in testing will be performed in situ with automatic readout occurring. The four diagnostic areas that will probably change over the next ten years include increased use of the detection of nucleic acid compared with antibody detection currently used; the use of microliter or nanoliter volumes concurrent with the focus on microtechnology; multiplexing assays to detect more than one analyte in a single assay; and the use of noninvasive methods for collection of biological specimens used for testing. In addition, a transition will occur from central specialized laboratories to prepackaged, POC assays that can be used at the physician's office or in the privacy of one's home.

SUMMARY

Over the past 20 years, the leading edge of public health research has focused on nucleic acid detection technologies. The impact of PCR amplification and the ability of investigators to detect and characterize the genetic features of pathogens are starting to transform diagnostic testing and change approaches to identification and classification of infectious agents. Additional enhancements to conventional assays and the development of more sensitive methods to detect smaller numbers of organisms are becoming the norm. These changes have resulted in development of the field of molecular epidemiology and molecular surveillance of organisms, thereby changing the face of public health control and prevention strategies.

The *Annual Review of Public Health* is online at
http://publhealth.annualreviews.org

LITERATURE CITED

1. Anderson DJ, Kuhns JS, Vasil ML, Gerding DN, Janoff EN. 1991. DNA fingerprinting by pulsed field gel electrophoresis and ribotyping to distinguish *Pseudomonas cepacia* isolates from a nosocomial outbreak. *J. Clin. Microbiol.* 29:648–49
2. Aggerbeck H, Norgaard-Pedersen B, Heron I. 1996. Simultaneous quantitation of diphtheria and tetanus antibodies by double antigen, time-resolved fluorescence immunoassay. *J. Immunol. Methods* 190:171–83
3. Barker SL, Ross D, Tarlov MJ, Gaitan M, Locascio LE. 2000. Control of flow direction in microfluidic devices with polyelectrolyte multilayers. *Anal. Chem.* 72:5925–29
4. Barre-Sinoussi F, Chermann JC, Rey F, Nugeyre MT, Chamaret S, et al. 1983. Isolation of a T-lymphotropic retrovirus from a patient at risk for acquired immune deficiency syndrome (AIDS). *Science* 220:868–71
5. Belland RJ, Ouellette SP, Gieffers J, Byrne GI. 2004. *Chlamydia pneumoniae* and atheroscerosis. *Cell. Microbiol.* 6:117–27
6. Bozdech Z, Zhu J, Joachimiak MP, Cohen FE, Pulliam B, DeRisi JL. 2003. Expression profiling of the schizont and trophozoite stages of *Plasmodium falciparum* with a long-oligonucleotide microarray. *Genome Biol.* 4:R9.1–9.15
7. Busch MP, el Amad Z, McHugh TM, Chien D, Polito AJ. 1991. Reliable confirmation and quantitation of human immunodeficiency virus type 1 antibody using a recombinant antigen immunoblot assay. *Transfusion* 31:129–37
8. Carney WP, Iacoviello V, Hirsch MS. 1983. Functional properties of T lymphocytes and their subsets in cytomegalovirus mononucleosis. *J. Immunol.* 130:390–93
9. Cavert W. 1998. In vivo detection and quantitation of HIV in blood and tissues. *AIDS* 12(Suppl. A):S27–34
10. Chase RA, Kessler HA, Landay AL, Vahey A, Blaauw B, et al. 1986. Sensitivity and specificity of an HIV antibody assay. *AIDS Res.* 2:369–75
11. Choo QL, Kuo G, Weiner AJ, Overby LR, Bradley DW, Houghton M. 1989. Isolation of a cDNA clone derived from a bloodborne non-A, non-B viral hepatitis genome. *Science* 244:359–62
12. Davidson M, Kuo C-C, Middaugh JP, Campbell LA, Wang S-P, et al. 1998. Confirmed previous infection with *Chlamydia pneumoniae* (TWAR) and its presence in early coronary atherosclerosis. *Circulation* 98:628–33
13. DeRisi J, Penland L, Brown PO, Bittner ML, Meltzer PS, et al. 1996. Use of a cDNA microarray to analyse gene expression in human cancer. *Nat. Genet.* 14:457–60
14. Drebot MA, Mulders MN, Campbell JJ, Kew OM, Fonseca KK, et al. 1997. Molecular detection of an importation of type 3 wild poliovirus into Canada from The Netherlands in 1993. *Appl. Environ. Microbiol.* 63:519–23

15. Feorino PM, Kalyanaraman VS, Haverkos HW, Cabradilla CD, Warfield DT, et al., 1984. Lymphadenopathy associated virus infection of a blood donor–recipient pair with acquired immunodeficiency syndrome. *Science* 225:69–72

16. Fodor SP, Read J, Pirrung MC, Stryer L, Lu AT, Solas D. 1991. Light-directed, spatially addressable parallel chemical synthesis. *Science* 251:767–73

17. Folch A, Ayon A, Hurtado O, Schmidt MA, Toner M. 1999. Molding of deep polydimethylsiloxane microstructures for microfluidics and biological applications. *J. Biomech. Eng.* 121:28–34

18. Gallo RC, Sarin PS, Gelmann EP, Robert-Guroff M, Richardson E, et al. 1983. Isolation of human T-cell leukemia virus in acquired immune deficiency syndrome (AIDS). *Science* 220:865–67

19. Gingeras TR, Ghandour G, Wang E, Berno A, Small PM, et al. 1998. Simultaneous genotyping and species identification using hybridization pattern recognition analysis of generic *Mycobacterium* DNA arrays. *Genome Res.* 8:435–48

20. Gottlieb MS, Schroff R, Schanker HM, Weisman JD, Fan PT, et al. 1981. *Pneumocystis carinii* pneumonia and mucosal candidiasis in previously healthy homosexual men. *N. Engl. J. Med.* 305:1425–31

21. Hatalski CG, Lewis AJ, Lipkin WI. 1997. Borna disease. *Emerg. Infect. Dis.* 3:129–35

22. Heid CA, Stevens J, Livak KJ, Williams PM. 1996. Real time quantitative PCR. *Genome Res.* 6:986–94

23. Heller RA, Schena M, Chai A, Shalon D, Bedilion T, et al. 1997. Discovery and analysis of inflammatory disease-related genes using cDNA microarrays. *Proc. Natl. Acad. Sci. USA* 94:2150–55

24. Herzenberg LA, Sweet RG, Herzenberg LA. 1976. Fluorescence-activated cell sorting. *Sci. Am.* 234:108–17

25. Hoffmaster AR, Fitzgerald CC, Ribot E, Mayer LW, Popovic T. 2002. Molecular subtyping of *Bacillus anthracis* and the 2001 bioterrorism-associated anthrax outbreak, United States. *Emerg. Infect. Dis.* 8:1111–16

26. Hoffmaster AR, Meyer RF, Bowen MP, Marston CK, Weyant RS, et al. 2002. Evaluation and validation of a real-time polymerase chain reaction assay for rapid identification of *Bacillus anthracis*. *Emerg. Infect. Dis.* 10:1178–82

27. Hornig M, Weissenbock H, Horscroft N, Lipkin WI. 1999. A infection-based model of neurodevelopmental damage. *Proc. Natl. Acad. Sci. USA* 96:12102–7

28. Iannone MA. 2001. Microsphere-based molecular cytometry. *Clin. Lab. Med.* 21:731–42

29. Jungkind D, Direnzo S, Beavis KG, Silverman NS. 1996. Evaluation of automated COBAS AMPLICOR PCR system for detection of several infectious agents and its impact on laboratory management. *J. Clin. Microbiol.* 34:2778–83

30. Kew O, Morris-Glasgow V, Landaverde M, Burns C, Shaw J, et al. 2002. Outbreak of poliomyelitis in Hispaniola associated with circulating type 1 vaccine-derived poliovirus. *Science* 296:356–59

31. Kohler F, Milstein C. 1976. Derivation of specific antibody-producing tissue culture and tumor lines by cell fusion. *Eur. J. Immunol.* 6:511–19

32. Kozal MJ, Shah N, Shen N, Yang R, Fucini R, et al. 1996. Extensive polymorphisms observed in HIV-1 clade B protease gene using high-density oligonucleotide arrays. *Nat. Med.* 2:753–59

33. Ksiazek TG, Erdman D, Goldsmith CS, Zaki SR, Peret T, et al. 2003. A novel coronavirus associated with severe acute respiratory syndrome. *N. Engl. J. Med.* 348:1953–66

34. Kuo G, Choo QL, Alter HJ, Gitnick GL, Redeker AG, et al. 1989. An assay for circulating antibodies to a major etiologic virus of human non-A, non-B viral hepatitis genome. *Science* 244:362–64

35. Lander ES, Linton LM, Birren B, Nusbaum C, Zody MC, et al. 2001. Initial sequencing

and analysis of the human genome. *Nature* 409:860–921

36. Mandy FF, Nakamura T, Bergeron M, Sekiguchi K. 2001. Overview and application of suspension array technology. *Clin. Lab. Med.* 21:713–29

37. Masur H, Michelis MA, Greene J, Onorato I, Stouwe RA, et al. 1981. An outbreak of community-acquired *Pneumocystis carinii* pneumonia: initial manifestation of cellular immune dysfunction. *N. Engl. J. Med.* 305:1431–38

38. Meurman OH, Hemmila IA, Lovgren TN, Halonen PE. 1982. Time-resolved fluoroimmunoassay: a new test for rubella antibodies. *J. Clin. Microbiol.* 16:920–25

39. Nichol ST, Spiropoulou CF, Morzunov S, Rollin PE, Ksiazek TG, et al. 1993. Genetic identification of a hantavirus associated with an outbreak of acute respiratory illness. *Science* 262:914–17

40. Ou CY, Ciesielski CA, Myers G, Bandea CI, Luo CC, et al. 1992. Molecular epidemiology of HIV transmission in a dental practice. *Science* 256:1165–71

41. Ou CY, Kwok S, Mitchell SW, Mack DH, Sninsky JJ, et al. 1988. DNA amplification for direct detection of HIV-1 in DNA of peripheral blood mononuclear cells. *Science* 239:295–97

42. Parsonnnet J, Friedman GD, Vandersteen DP, Chang Y, Vogelman JH, et al. 1991. *Helicobacter pylori* infection and the risk of gastric carcinoma. *N. Engl. J. Med.* 325:1127–31

43. Peters CJ, Olshaker M. 1997. *Virus Hunter: Thirty Years of Battling Hot Viruses Around the World*. New York: Doubleday. 323 pp.

44. Reinherz EL, O'Brien C, Rosenthal P, Schlossman SF. 1980. The cellular basis for viral-induced immunodeficiency: analysis by monoclonal antibodies. *J. Immunol.* 125:1269–74

45. Rico-Hesse R, Pallansch MA, Nottay BK, Kew OM. 1987. Geographic distribution of wild poliovirus type 1 genotypes. *Virology* 160:311–22

46. Saiki RK, Gelfand DH, Stoffel S, Scharf SJ, Higuchi R, et al. 1988. Primer-directed enzymatic amplification of DNA with a thermostable DNA polymerase. *Science* 239:487–91

47. Scalia G, Gerna G, Halonen PE. 1989. Detection of rubella virus antigen by one-step time-resolved fluoroimmunoassay and by enzyme immunoassay. *J. Med. Virol.* 29:164–69

48. Schena M, Shalon D, Davis RW, Brown PO. 1995. Quantitative monitoring of gene expression patterns with a complementary DNA microarray. *Science* 270:368–69

49. Schena M, Shalon D, Heller R, Chai A, Brown PO, Davis RW. 1996. Parallel human genome analysis: microarray-based expression monitoring of 1000 genes. *Proc. Natl. Acad. Sci. USA* 93:10614–19

50. Shulman LM, Handsher R, Yang CF, Yang SJ, Manor J, et al. 2000. Resolution of the pathways of poliovirus type 1 transmission during an outbreak. *J. Clin. Microbiol.* 38:945–52

51. Stuyver L, Van Geyt C, De Gendt S, Van Reybroeck G, Zoulim F, et al. 2000. Line probe assay for monitoring drug resistance in hepatitis B virus-infected patients during antiviral therapy. *J. Clin. Microbiol.* 38:702–7

52. Stuyver L, Wyseur A, Rombout A, Louwagie J, Scarcez T, et al. 1997. Line probe assay for rapid detection of drug-selected mutations in the human immunodeficiency virus type 1 reverse transcriptase gene. *Antimicrob. Agents Chemother.* 41:284–91

53. Stuyver L, Wyseur A, van Arnhem W, Hernandez F, Maertens G. 1996. Second-generation line probe assay for hepatitis C virus genotyping. *J. Clin. Microbiol.* 34:2259–66

54. Stuyver L, Wyser A, van Arnhem W, Lunel F, Laurent-Puig P, Pawlotsky J-M. 1995. Hepatitis C virus genotyping by means of 5'UR/core line probe assays and molecular analysis of untypeable samples. *Virus Res.* 38:137–57

55. Tenover FC, Arbeit RD, Goering RV, Mickelsen PA, Murray BE, et al. 1995. Interpreting chromosomal DNA restriction patterns produced by pulsed-field gel electrophoresis: criteria for bacterial strain typing. *J. Clin. Microbiol.* 33:2233–39

56. Troesch A, Nguyen H, Miyada CG, Desvarenne S, Gingeras TR, et al. 1999. *Mycobacterium* species identification and rifampin resistance testing with high-density DNA probe arrays. *J. Clin. Microbiol.* 37:49–55

57. Tyagi S, Kramer FR. 1996. Molecular beacons: probes that fluoresce upon hybridization. *Nat. Biotech.* 14:303–8

58. Vahey M, Nau ME, Barrick S, Cooley JD, Sawyer R, et al. 1999. Performance of the Affymetrix GeneChip HIV PRT 440 platform for antiretroviral drug resistance genotyping of human immunodeficiency virus type 1 clades and viral isolates with length polymporphisms. *J. Clin. Microbiol.* 37:2533–37

59. Venter JC, Adams MD, Myers EW, Li PW, Mural RJ, et al. 2001. The sequence of the human genome. *Science* 291:1304–51

60. Wang D, Coscoy L, Zylberberg M, Avila PC, Boushey HA, et al. 2002. Microarray-based detection and genotyping of viral pathogens. *Proc. Natl. Acad. Sci. USA* 99: 15687–92

61. Wang D, Urisman A, Liu YT, Springer M, Ksiazek TG, et al. 2003. Viral discovery and sequence recovery using DNA microarrays. *PLoS Biol.* 1:257–60

Annu. Rev. Public Health 2005. 26:303–18
doi: 10.1146/annurev.publhealth.26.021304.144647

THE PUBLIC HEALTH INFRASTRUCTURE AND OUR NATION'S HEALTH[1]

Edward L. Baker, Jr.

The North Carolina Institute for Public Health, The University of North Carolina School of Public Health, Chapel Hill, North Carolina 27599-8165; email: elbaker@email.unc.edu

Margaret A. Potter

Center for Public Health Practice, University of Pittsburgh, Pittsburgh, Pennsylvania 15260; email: potterm@edc.pitt.edu

Deborah L. Jones

The Interfaith Health Program, Rollins School of Public Health, Emory University, Atlanta, Georgia 30322; email: djones9@sph.emory.edu

Shawna L. Mercer

Public Health Practice Program Office, Department of Health and Human Services, Centers for Disease Control and Prevention, Atlanta, Georgia 30341; email: zhi5@cdc.gov

Joan P. Cioffi

Public Health Practice Program Office, Department of Health and Human Services, Centers for Disease Control and Prevention, Atlanta, Georgia 30341; email: vzc1@cdc.gov

Lawrence W. Green

School of Public Health, University of California, Berkeley, California 94720; email: lwgreen@comcast.net

Paul K. Halverson

University of Arkansas for Medical Sciences, Little Rock, Arkansas, 72205; email: phalverson@healthyarkansas.com

Maureen Y. Lichtveld

Institute of Public Health, Georgia State University, Atlanta, Georgia 30302; email: mlichtveld@gsu.edu

David W. Fleming

Global Health Strategies, Bill & Melinda Gates Foundation, Seattle, Washington 98102; email: davidf@gatesfoundation.org

---

[1]The U.S. Government has the right to retain a nonexclusive, royalty-free license in and to any copyright covering this paper.

0163-7525/05/0421-0303$20.00

Key Words organizational capacity, workforce development, information systems, public health preparedness

■ **Abstract**   Threats to Americans' health—including chronic disease, emerging infectious disease, and bioterrorism—are present and growing, and the public health system is responsible for addressing these challenges. Public health systems in the United States are built on an infrastructure of workforce, information systems, and organizational capacity; in each of these areas, however, serious deficits have been well documented. Here we draw on two 2003 Institute of Medicine reports and present evidence for current threats and the weakness of our public health infrastructure. We describe major initiatives to systematically assess, invest in, rebuild, and evaluate workforce competency, information systems, and organizational capacity through public policy making, practical initiatives, and practice-oriented research. These initiatives are based on applied science and a shared federal-state approach to public accountability. We conclude that a newly strengthened public health infrastructure must be sustained in the future through a balancing of the values inherent in the federal system.

INTRODUCTION

The nation's public health system is vigorous in some places but weak in many others. The terrorist attacks of September 2001 forcefully drew widespread attention to this fact, but it was not news to public health professionals (5). For more than a decade the scientific literature, government reports, and even popular media had been documenting numerous signs of weakness (11, 22, 36). Two recent Institute of Medicine (IOM) reports, *The Future of the Public's Health in the 21st Century* (37) and *Who Will Keep the Public Healthy?* (38), both published in 2003, provide compelling assessments of the state of the public health system along with specific recommendations that outline an agenda for action. These reports contend that the public health infrastructure that was "in disarray" in 1988 is "still in disarray today" (37). The same infrastructure that supports routine public health activities is also essential for emergency preparedness. The first lines of defense for deliberate attacks—a skilled workforce, robust information systems, and strong organizational capacity—are also those that stand against infectious diseases, injuries, chronic diseases, natural disasters, and high-risk behaviors. Building the national capacity for domestic protection against, and response to, hostile biological or chemical attacks serves as well against naturally occurring threats.

Federal funding priorities have begun to address these challenges. Starting with the Public Health Improvement Act of 2000, the U.S. Congress called for a plan to assure the preparedness of every community in the nation. In fiscal year (FY) 2002, the federal budget allocated $1.1 billion for state and local infrastructure to begin the process of upgrading health system capabilities; in FY 2003, $1.4 billion was allocated through the Center for Disease Control and Prevention (CDC) and the Health Resources and Services Administration (HRSA). Although these funds will help to improve some elements of the public health infrastructure, their application in scale and scope is not adequate to address national needs (30).

Unfortunately, recent cuts in state funding (1) threaten the gains that have occurred to date and create uncertainty about future support. This uncertainty, in turn, weakens commitment, particularly in local and state government public health, to permanently staff critical positions. Further, funding cuts and uncertainties jeopardize partnership development at a time when strong and effective partnerships are critical to assure public health preparedness.

In this review, we begin with a description of the current and foreseeable threats to the health of Americans and an assessment of weaknesses in the current public health infrastructure relative to those threats. We describe approaches to correcting the deficits and conclude with recommendations for maintaining a strong public health infrastructure, drawing heavily on our collective experiences, as well as on the recent IOM reports and other published literature.

THREATS TO AMERICANS' HEALTH

Serious and constantly evolving threats face the health of Americans. These include a major burden of chronic disease and disability (10); injury and illness due to occupational and environmental hazards; infectious diseases, both familiar and newly emerging; threats related to terrorism; and other preventable problems (12). Taken as a whole, these behavior-related, environmentally caused, and deliberately imposed dangers to health and well-being frame the existing challenge to our nation's public health infrastructure. Most of the advances in the health of Americans achieved over the past century (9) are largely attributable to prevention strategies falling within the domain of the nation's public-sector, population-oriented health agencies. The vigor and effectiveness of these agencies continue to be important factors in the nation's health because some of the twentieth-century threats to health have returned or persist, and emerging threats will require similar prevention strategies of these same agencies (39).

Perhaps Americans' most perilous threat is that local and state public health agencies lack the capacity to respond to predictable and unpredictable threats (61).

These public health agencies do not act alone and must participate with private-sector partners in collaborative efforts to build trust in communities and to provide objective data on health issues. If government agencies are not strong, their ability to form these strategic partnerships is jeopardized, thus further compromising a fragile public health system (31).

THE PUBLIC HEALTH INFRASTRUCTURE

The functional supports for executing the essential services in the formal, public-sector framework constitute the public health infrastructure: the workforce competencies, the communication and information systems, and the organizational capacities (6) (Figure 1). This infrastructure is the base that enables the various

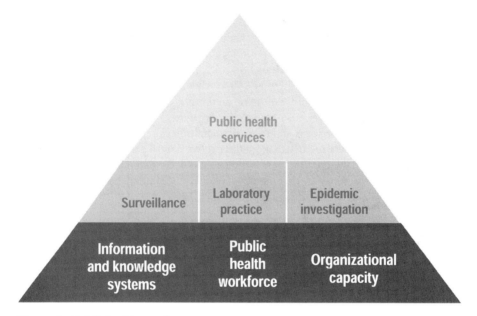

Figure 1   Public health practice.

entities within the public health system—including private-sector entities—to function both independently and in partnerships (58).

On this base rest certain key capacities: surveillance, epidemiology, and laboratory practice. The entire structure relies on strong science and ongoing research, including sound evaluation studies.

The science base for public health informs all stages of conceptualizing, implementing, maintaining, and adapting public health services and programs. Research questions arise from the practice of public health functions (30, 43). Each infrastructure component is both a subject of and a predicate for practical research. In terms of workforce capacity and competency, research defines the numbers and characteristics of professionals optimal to carry out the essential services. As the end-users of research, practitioners participate in defining their research needs and then engage resources (e.g., funding, experts, facilities) to assist them in meeting these needs.

WEAKNESSES IN THE CURRENT PUBLIC HEALTH INFRASTRUCTURE

When the components of public health infrastructure are strong, the system can carry out its core functions and essential services with uniform effectiveness. But when the components are weak, inconsistent, or deficient, the system's capacity to function is likewise at risk. Today's public health system will be able to withstand existing and potential threats to Americans' health only if its supporting infrastructure is strengthened (11). Unfortunately, major challenges confront those committed to assuring a strong infrastructure, and the research base needed for well-informed infrastructure development is sparse.

Fragmented and Precarious Public Funding

The public health infrastructure is seriously and systematically underfunded owing to its low priority among state and federal policy makers, and unfortunately, a sound estimate of the level of funding for infrastructure and the resources needed to assure its strength does not yet exist (37, 44). Systematic studies are lacking, but media and professional organizations have reported that the post–September 11, 2001, infusion of federal funds to state health departments was coupled with a reduction of funds for routine public health functions (20).

The levels of funding necessary or appropriate for carrying out essential public health services at the state and local levels has not been established. However, the Community Health Status Indicators Project (cosponsored by the Public Health Foundation, ASTHO, NACCHO, and HRSA) produced some tools and measures for collecting and analyzing expenditure data from state and local health agencies (54). Some methods developed through this project were piloted in three separate studies involving various state and local health agencies between 1995 and 1999 (4). Analyzed together, these studies showed that no state was spending more on population-based services than on personal health services. These studies also revealed a range of total per-capita spending on essential public health services of $37–$102 among local agencies and of $86–$232 in state agencies (4).

Uneven and Antiquated Legal Foundation

No single entity—governmental or otherwise—has comprehensive authority and responsibility for creation, maintenance, and oversight of the nation's public health infrastructure. To some extent, this aspect of federalism has encouraged the creativity celebrated in Justice Brandeis' famous observation that the states serve as "laboratories of democracy." It is manifest, however, that the division of authority among governments at the state, federal, and local levels has often led to inconsistency, ineffective resource allocation, and uncertainty about their respective roles and responsibilities (27, 28). Fifty separate state governments each hold the "police power" and the *parens patriae* power, on which public health laws are based. When each of the states ratified the U.S. Constitution, it delegated powers, including limited authority for public health matters, to the federal government. The Constitution permits Congress to regulate commerce among the states and—important for public health—to tax and spend for the general welfare. Through legislation, Congress exercises its power to allocate duties and resources among federal executive agencies and even to redelegate some responsibilities back to the states through spending programs. Further, each state internally delegates public health powers to its own counties, municipalities, and other local authorities. Finally, through licenses, contracts, and specific laws, each state also chooses whether, when, and how to delegate certain health responsibilities to private-sector organizations and professionals.

A social value related to this division of legal authority is personal and local self-determination. This characteristic of the public health infrastructure flows directly from a core value of the federal system: state and local preference for autonomy and/or control, especially in matters closely affecting personal rights and private interests. Such concerns are deeply rooted in public health matters: consider tobacco advertising (72), firearms control (65, 71), and HIV/AIDS (6, 29), to name only a few. The central value of self-determination is embodied in policies and programs that prefer to "devolve" authority to smaller and more local jurisdictions—those closest to individual persons. But this policy preference is a double-edged sword. Although it tends to enhance local control, appropriateness, and flexibility of programs to meet the needs of local populations, it can also lead to fragmentation and unevenness in the quality and the distribution of services. Because of their inherent autonomy in matters of public health, each of the fifty states is unique in the particulars of its political culture, its civil service rules, its budgetary and appropriations processes and constraints, its authorizing statutes, and more.

These differences in turn lead inevitably to vast differences among local public health agencies in services, available resources, staffing, and performance capacity. In a 1999–2000 national survey of 1000 local health agencies, the National Association of County and City Health Officials (45) found that service priorities that were broadly consistent among agencies included communicable disease control, environmental health, and child health; however, many agencies lacked other services such as primary care, chronic disease treatment, behavioral health, programs for the homeless, and veterinary public health. Annual expenditures varied from $0 to more than $836 million, with a median of $621,100. Staff sizes varied widely, with a mean of 67 full-time equivalent positions (FTEs) contrasted with a median of only 1 FTE per agency. Only 55% of responding agencies had conducted an assessment of community health in the preceding three years; and, of the remainder, only half planned to do so in the next three years. The respondents cited inadequate funding and workforce issues among their biggest challenges.

Thus, American health policy and its legal foundations have shaped and determined the quality, extent, and vitality of the public health infrastructure. The outcomes have been all too frequently unfavorable to the public's health and safety.

Inadequate Workforce

A 2000 enumeration study estimated the public health workforce at 448,254 salaried persons in local, state, and federal agencies as well as some private organizations, such as academic institutions (17). Over the 30-year period beginning in 1970, the ratio of public health workers to U.S. residents had fallen from 1:457 to 1:635. Given the rising challenges to Americans' health over this period, this decline in workforce numbers indicates a serious erosion of functional capacity in the public health system (55, 66).

Moreover, the decline is projected to continue and perhaps to accelerate. In 2002, the Council of State Governments and the National Association of State Personnel Executives reported that, on the basis of a national survey, health departments were identified by 34 states as being most likely among the departments of state government to be most affected by a worker shortage (18). In 2003, the Association of State and Territorial Health Officials (ASTHO) conducted a survey of its members, which found that 24% of respondents' workforce were eligible for retirement, a 20% average vacancy rate, and a 14% annual average turnover rate (3). ASTHO's survey report found that low salaries, lack of qualified applicants, and relocation requirements contributed to these shortages, which were found most frequently for the occupations of nurse, epidemiologist, laboratory worker, and environmental health specialist.

Validated standards for workforce FTE levels needed to effectively perform the essential public health services do not exist yet; however, the example of decline in the numbers of one key public health occupation illustrates how detrimental to performance these declining workforce numbers may be. In 2003, the Council of State and Territorial Epidemiologists (CSTE) reported that the number of epidemiologists had fallen in the preceding decade from 1700 to 1400 (18)—a decline of almost 18% during a period of increasing need due to emerging infections and terrorism. To put this number into perspective, a rough estimate of the number of epidemiologists needed for the U.S. population, on the basis of an expert-consensus ratio of 1.1 FTEs per 50,000 residents, yields an optimal number of about 6160 (50). This analysis suggests that the shortage of epidemiologists at the state level may be three times greater than the present number of employed epidemiologists.

Lack of both formal graduate training and professional certification in the public health field hampers individuals' career development and weakens the performance capability of agencies and organizations that employ these individuals (8). Economics plays a big role here. The graduates of schools and programs of public health in colleges and universities tend to find employment elsewhere than in relatively low-paying state and local agencies (2). According to a 1989 estimate, only 44% of public health workers had any formal, academic training in public health; and those with graduate public health degrees were an even smaller percentage (34). This was true at all levels and in all areas of expertise within public health, including its top leadership. As of 1997, 78% of local health department executives had no graduate degree in public health (26). Furthermore, periodic hiring freezes and rigid personnel policies tend to hinder the ability of public health departments at the state and local levels to recruit and retain talented public health professionals. The average tenure of a state health department's chief executive—who increasingly is a political appointee—is two years (69).

Instead of preparing for their jobs through professional education, public health workers tend to learn on the job (63). CSTE reports that 42% of the current epidemiology workforce lacks formal training in this field (18). In nursing, the largest professional group of the public health workforce, entry-level education varies. Nurses may enter practice upon completing either a two-year associate degree, a hospital diploma program, or a four-year undergraduate program. Because ~60% of public health nurses lack a baccalaureate degree and have no formal training in community-based nursing, they are typically ineligible to pursue a Master of Public Health degree (35). Self-assessments of public health competency by agency workers and their supervisors consistently show gaps between mastery and what is needed for effective practice. For example, in 1999, Florida's state public health agency served as a testing ground for a new national program of performance standards based on the ten essential services (57). This agency, in many ways typical of its counterparts nationwide, had spent the previous decade working on carefully designed, quality-improvement efforts. Nevertheless, among all the measures included in this performance appraisal, scores for the measures for workforce systems ranked the lowest. State officials attributed this ranking to the lack of available training in basic and essential service-related competencies for the agency's employees.

Professional certification in many health-related fields is associated with competency standards, career-path development, and enhanced recognition in the forms of prestige and compensation. Certification is common for professions represented in the public health workforce (such as medicine, nursing, health education, and engineering); however, the field of public health lacks its own standards for educational attainment, continuing competency, and career achievement (62). The twentieth century saw a series of academic, philanthropic, and governmental reports documenting the low compensation, poor educational preparation, and high turnover of public health officers throughout the country; many of the reports took specific note of the low prestige attached to these positions (21). Few states require professional credentialing of local public health officials (68), and little research has focused on the impact of professional development on the quality of public health services (8, 42).

Inconsistent Application of Information Technology

The present infrastructure for information and data systems is inconsistent: excellent in some jurisdictions, outdated in some, and virtually nonexistent in others (11, 48). In a world where microbes and disease vectors move quickly around the world through tourism, immigration, and commerce, many public health surveillance systems in the United States have been late to replace their time-consuming, resource-intensive, paper-based or telephone-based reporting systems (58). In the early 1990s, some public health laboratories—often the first to detect a new pathogen—were reporting their results by surface mail with lag times of up to 10–14 days (40).

Recently, the CDC conducted several informal tallies to explore the quality of public health's information infrastructure. For example, in response to a 1998 survey about infrastructure problems, one local health department admitted to not reporting diseases to avoid the cost of long-distance phone calls. In 1999, CDC and the National Association of County and City Health Officials (NACCHO) conducted an email test to determine how quickly they could contact local health departments in the event of a health alert or bioterrorist emergency. For a variety of reasons, only 35% of these messages were delivered successfully. In another 1999 survey, CDC found that only 45% of local health departments had the capacity to broadcast alerts via facsimile to labs, physicians, state health agencies, the CDC, and others; fewer than half had high-speed continuous access to the Internet; and 20% lacked email capability.

Organizational Deficits

Against an ideal picture of intra- and interorganizational effectiveness, what do we know about the current performance capacity of the public health system? First, it is misleading to assume that a strong local public health organization serves every U.S. community. Though every state and many, if not most, major cities have a public health agency, the levels of staffing and the breadth of services available among them are highly variable (23, 45, 66). Moreover, in other (typically rural) communities, there may be no officially designated local public health authority, but rather only one or more state agencies and a more or less organized and monitored collection of private entities, under contracts, offering a patchwork of public health services (49).

Second, the performance capacities of state health departments and their existing local counterparts appear to be inadequate. In 1993, Turnock et al. (70) studied the performance of local health departments and concluded that only a third of the U.S. population was being served effectively, using adequate performance of the 10 essential public health services as the standard (33). A 1998 study conducted by researchers at the University of North Carolina (UNC) found that the nation's largest health departments scored an average of only 64% in assessments of the quality of their 10 essential public health services, on the basis of 20 performance measures (30). Through field-testing of the National Public Health Performance Standards Program, the CDC found that three state public-health systems had performance levels of 51%, 40%, and 56% and that 131 local public health systems in these three states scored on average 55%, 62%, and 53% (32).

Improvements in organizational capacity have occurred between the fall of 2001 and 2004. In surveys conducted by the NACCHO (46) shortly after September 11, 2001, local public health officials reported that their departments were not well prepared to carry out their key roles in public health response, did not have comprehensive response plans, and had difficulty in answering some frequent public inquires. A year later, however, NACCHO's survey of local health agencies found that these agencies had become better equipped to handle bioterrorist attacks:

84% of the 500 respondents indicated that they were better off than 1 year previous, but still lack the capacity for effective response to specific threats.

INFRASTRUCTURE IMPROVEMENT INITIATIVES

The 1988 IOM report (36) launched a decade of dialogue and stimulated national policy making on the need to develop the public health infrastructure (56). The results included a series of initiatives beginning in the early 1990s in which CDC and HRSA moved to improve workforce capacity, enhance information and communication systems, and strengthen organizational capacity. During the 1990s, federal Public Health Service agencies devoted considerable attention to the workforce component of infrastructure. CDC created the Public Health Training Network for national distance-learning capacity, established the National Public Health Leadership Institute, and supported the development of state and regional leadership institutes as well as the National Laboratory Training Network. An evaluation at the Public Health Leadership Institute revealed that 68% of participants improved their community leadership skills, including developing coalitions and collaborations; 51% reported improvement in their ability to accomplish agency missions. The Management Academy for Public Health, another innovative workforce development program, funded by the Robert Wood Johnson Foundation, the W.K. Kellogg Foundation, HRSA, and the CDC, and managed by UNC–Chapel Hill School of Public Health, has trained more than 60 managers and generated $6 million in projects from an initial $2 million investment. HRSA funded 15 training centers at schools of public health focused on enhancing the access of employed public health workers to continuing education opportunities. CDC began its support for Centers for Public Health Preparedness in 2000 and now sponsors 34 academic sites for training and education in public health competencies and in bioterrorism and infectious-disease preparedness and response. The W.K. Kellogg Foundation and the Robert Wood Johnson Foundation launched the Turning Point Initiative in 1997 to enhance local and state public health capacity across the nation (60, 67).

Programs initiated recently are also beginning to address information-system deficits (48). In 1999, with Congressional support and funding, CDC launched the national Health Alert Network (HAN) initiative to improve information access, training, and organizational capacity in local health departments. In partnership with state and local agencies, HAN has now grown to include all states and three large cities funded to begin basic implementation of Internet connectivity, broadcast communications, and distance-learning capacity at the local level. In addition, three local health departments have been funded as Centers for Public Health Preparedness to develop more advanced applications for sister agencies nationwide. In 2000, again with Congressional support and funding, CDC launched the National Electronic Disease Surveillance System (NEDSS) by providing support to states and large metropolitan areas. NEDSS provides national standards, specifications, and working prototypes so that critical information collected by the local health departments and supported by the Health Alert Network initiative can be used to detect and manage outbreaks that affect more than one local or state jurisdiction. Evaluation of the impact of the Health Alert Network program revealed that 89% of local health agencies had developed continuous high-speed Internet access by 2003; 5 years earlier, less than 40% had this capability (46).

Additionally, federal programs directed to state and local health agencies are focused on evaluating and building organizational capacity. Starting in the late 1990s, the CDC collaborated with a range of partners to design a set of performance standards and metrics based on the ten essential services (16, 32). Launched in pilot tests at the state and local levels, this National Public Health Performance Standards Program provided a uniform, outcome-based model for evaluating public health programs. Following the investigation of a national commission funded by the Pew Charitable Trust, CDC has launched a major national effort to enhance environmental health capacity at the state and local level.

Congress recognized the importance of building organizational capacity in the Frist-Kennedy Public Health Threats and Emergencies Act of 2000 and subsequently through much-increased funding after the fall 2001 terrorist attacks. In both 2002 and 2003, the Department of Health and Human Services through the CDC made awards to the 50 states for bioterrorism preparedness and response. This cooperative agreement program provided almost $1 billion to address critical and enhanced capacities in six focus areas: preparedness planning and readiness; surveillance and epidemiology capacity; biological laboratory capacity; the Health Alert Network and other initiatives for communications and information technology; public information and communications; and education and training. The first awards in 2002 allowed each state to develop a plan for infrastructure building and to begin implementing its plan. The second awards in 2003 supported ongoing implementation and technical assistance.

In the past three years, numerous research and development initiatives focused on building up the three components of public health infrastructure. Examples include the following:

- A broadly based partnership of federal, state, and local practitioners as well as academicians convened to address specific barriers to improving the workforce component, and this group produced a National Implementation Plan for Public Health Workforce Development (41).

- Another partnership of federal agencies, professional public health associations, and academicians developed schematics for core competencies in bioterrorism and public health emergency preparedness to add to the universal competencies previously cited for routine public health (25).

- Academic sponsors of workforce-development programs turned competency definitions into assessment protocols (14, 53), strategic training plans (19, 51), and evaluation models (52).

- The project Public Health Ready, a collaboration of NACCHO and CDC, is developing a model for assuring workforce competency within the context of a high-quality local health agency (47).

- The National Committee on Vital and Health Statistics has recommended the development of a National Health Information Infrastructure, with public health as one of its three key components (48, 64).

WHERE DO WE STAND TODAY?

Despite this recent progress, serious gaps continue to weaken the nation's public health infrastructure. As mentioned above, a recent survey (3) by ASTHO revealed a rapidly aging state agency workforce, high retirement eligibility rates, high vacancy rates, and high annual staff turnover rates. These findings are indicative of a critical workforce shortage related in part to the largest state budget cuts in 60 years (3). The ASTHO report indicated that some strategies such as increased access to advanced education, competitive pay and benefits, and flexible work arrangements may help address the crisis.

Further, information and communications systems, though growing in sophistication and geographic coverage, do not operate seamlessly across the continuum of federal, state, and local authorities (73). Finally, especially at the local level, public health still lacks a verified set of standards and criteria for performance; and, in part for that very reason, local agencies remain a low priority for policy makers, are unevenly staffed, and are organized on models based on historical circumstance and antiquated laws rather than on efficiency or effectiveness criteria.

PRIORITIES FOR ACTION

In light of this assessment, we recommend six priorities for building and sustaining the public health infrastructure:

1. assure a sound financial base;
2. update antiquated public statutes;
3. accredit public health agencies;
4. certify the competency of public health professionals;
5. invest in public health research; and
6. strengthen public health communications (59).

Public health has historically given too little attention to the theory and practice of financing the public health enterprise (44). As a result, we know relatively little about best practices and innovative approaches in public health finance (4). A concerted attempt to develop a body of scientific knowledge followed by translation of knowledge into practice is vital to financing a strong infrastructure.

Progress has been made in recent years in the scholarship surrounding public health law (27, 28). Now, this knowledge base related to model statutes and exemplary legal practices management must be conveyed to our nation's legal practitioners and used to update and improve public health statutes (13).

Many states are exploring accreditation of local public health agencies using performance standards as a template for action. NACCHO has developed a proposed operational definition of a local health agency. Strong local public health agencies form the bedrock of public health practice; a system for accrediting them is essential for assuring adequate organizational capacity (37). Further, similar actions at the state and federal levels will be needed to complete the task of assuring strong public health organizations.

Although quite challenging, a comprehensive system to credential public health workers, building on existing efforts (15, 42, 68), will help to assure workforce competency. Given the complexity of the workforce, this task is daunting but necessary to provide public health workers comparable status to other health professions and to improve quality of service delivery (24).

Needs for investment in public health research have been highlighted recently in the course of the development of the *Guide to Community Preventive Services* (7). Research into the impact of selected approaches to disease prevention and health promotion is needed to provide public health leaders with an evidence base for decision making.

Finally, we must constantly strive to communicate effectively with our colleagues and, more importantly, with the broader community of policy makers and the general public about what public health is and what it does (69). At times of national crisis, attention is drawn to the need for a strong public health system, but attention and effort are often short-lived. Sustained investment in communication systems and in the expertise needed for effective communication will be crucial to the success of public health for decades to come.

The *Annual Review of Public Health* is online at
http://publhealth.annualreviews.org

LITERATURE CITED

1. Am. Public Health Assoc. 2004. Shift in preparedness funds undermines readiness efforts. *Nation's Health* 36(6):1

2. Assoc. Sch. Public Health, Counc. Pract. Coord. 2000. Demonstrating excellence in academic public health practice. *J. Public Health Manag. Pract* 6(1):10–24

3. Assoc. State Territ. Health Off. 2004. *State Public Health Employee Worker Shortage Report: A Civil Service Recruitment and Retention Crisis*. Washington, DC: Assoc. State Territ. Health Off.

4. Atchison C, Barry MA, Kanarek N, Gebbie K. 2000. The quest for an accurate accounting of public health expenditures. *J. Public Health Manag. Pract.* 6(5):93–102

5. Baker EL, Koplan JP. 2002. Strengthening the nation's public health infrastructure: historic challenge, unprecedented opportunity. *Health Aff.* 21(6):15–27

6. Bayer R, Toomey KE. 1992. HIV prevention and the two faces of partner notification. *Am. J. Public Health* 82:1158–64

7. Briss PA, Brownson RC, Fielding JE, Zaza S. 2004. Developing and using the guide to community preventive services: lessons learned about guidance-based public health. *Annu. Rev. Public Health* 25: 281–302

8. Cary A. 2000. Data driven policy: the case for certification research. *Policy Polit. Nurs. Pract.* 1(3):165–71

9. Cent. Dis. Control Prev., Dep. Health Hum. Serv. 1999. Ten great public health achievements—United States 1900–1999. *MMWR* 48(50):241–43

10. Cent. Dis. Control Prev., Dep. Health Hum. Serv. 2000. *Chronic Diseases and Their Risk Factors: The Nation's Leading Causes of Death*. Natl. Cent. Chronic Dis. Prev. Health Promot. Atlanta, GA: Cent. Dis. Control Prev.

11. Cent. Dis. Control Prev., Dep. Health Hum. Serv. 2001. *Public Health Infrastructure, A Status Report*. Atlanta, GA: Cent. Dis. Control Prev.

12. Cent. Dis. Control Prev., Dep. Health Hum. Serv. 2002. Surveillance Summaries, June 28, 2002. *MMWR* 51(SS04):1–64

13. Cent. Law Public's Health, Georgetown and Johns Hopkins Univ. 2001. The Model State Emergency Health Powers Act. http://www.publichealthlaw.net/MSEHPA/MSEHPA2.pdf

14. Chauvin SW, Anderson AE, Bowdish BE. 2001. Assessing the professional development needs of public health professionals. *J. Public Health Manag. Pract.* 7(4):23–37

15. Cioffi JP, Lichtveld M, Thielen L, Miner K. 2003. Credentialing the public health workforce: an idea whose time has come. *J. Public Health Manag. Pract.* 9(6):451–58

16. Corso LC, Weisner PJ, Halverson PK, Brown CK. 2000. Using the essential services as a foundation for performance measurement and assessment of local public health systems. *J. Public Health Manag. Pract.* 6(5):1–18

17. Counc. Link. Between Public Health Pract. Acad. 2002. Competencies Project. http:www.trainingfinder.org/competencies/list.htm

18. Counc. State Territ. Epidemiol. 2003. *National Assessment of Epidemiologic Capacity in Public Health: Findings and Recommendations*. Washington, DC: Counc. State Territ. Epidemiol.

19. Dato VM, Potter MA, Fertman CI. 2001. Training readiness of public health agencies: a framework for assessment. *J. Public Health Manag. Pract.* 7(4):91–95

20. Elliott VS, Amednews.com. 2002. Public Health Funding: Feds Giveth but the States Taketh Away. http://www.ama-assn.org/amednews/2002/10/28/h1121028.htm

21. Fee E. 1991. Designing schools of public health for the United States. In *A History of Education in Public Health*, ed. E Fee, RM Acheson, 2:155–94. New York: Oxford Univ. Press

22. Garrett L. 2000. *Betrayal of Trust: The Collapse of Global Public Health*. New York: Hyperion

23. Gebbie K. 2000. *The Public Health Workforce Enumeration 2000*. New York: Cent. Health Policy, Columbia Univ. Sch. Nurs.

24. Gebbie K, Hwang I. 1998. *Preparing Currently Employed Public Health Professionals for Changes in the Health System*. New York: Cent. Health Policy, Columbia Univ. Sch. Nurs.

25. Gebbie K, Merrrill J. 2002. Public health worker competencies for emergency response. *J. Public Health Manag. Pract.* 8(3):73–81

26. Gerzoff RB, Richards TB. 1997. The education of local health department top executives. *J. Public Health Manag. Pract.* 3(4):50–56

27. Gostin LO. 2000. *Public Health Law. Power, Duty, and Restraint*. Berkeley: Univ. Calif. Press

28. Gostin LO. 2002. *Public Health Law and Ethics*. New York: Univ. Calif. Press, Milbank Mem. Fund

29. Gostin LO, Curran WJ. 1987. The case against compulsory casefind in controlling AIDS: testing, screening and reporting. *Am. J. Law Med.* 12:1–47

30. Green LW, Mercer SL. 2001. Can public health researchers and agencies reconcile the push from funding bodies and the pull from communities? *Am. J. Public Health* 91(12):1926–29

31. Halverson P. 2002. Embracing the strength of the public health system: why strong government public health agencies are vitally necessary but insufficient. *J. Public Health Manag. Pract.* 8(1):90–100

32. Halverson P, Mays G. 2001. Public health assessment. In *Public Health Administration: Principles for Population-Based Management*, ed. LE Novick, GP Mays, p. 288. Gaithersburg, MD: Aspen

33. Harrell JA, Baker EL. 1994. The essential services of public health. *Leadersh. Public Health* 3(3):27–31

34. Health Resour. Serv. Adm., Dep. Health Hum. Serv. 1994. *A Report to President and Congress on the Status of Health Professions Personnel in the United States, 1978–1990.* Washington, DC: Bur. Health Manpower, Manpower Anal. Branch

35. Health Resour. Serv. Adm., Dep. Health Hum. Serv. 1996. *Sample Survey of the Registered Nurse Workforce.* Washington, DC: Div. Nurs.

36. Inst. Med. 1988. *The Future of Public Health.* Washington, DC: Natl. Acad. Press

37. Inst. Med. 2003. *The Future of the Public's Health in the 21st Century.* Washington, DC: Natl. Acad. Press

38. Inst. Med. 2003. *Who Will Keep the Public Healthy? Educating Public Health Professionals for the 21st Century.* Washington, DC: Natl. Acad. Press

39. Koplan JP, Fleming DW. 2000. Current and future public health challenges. *JAMA* 284(13):1696–98

40. Lederberg J, Shope R, Oaks S. 1992. *Committee on Emerging Microbial Threats to Health.* Washington, DC: Inst. Med.

41. Lichtveld MY, Cioffi JP, Baker EL Jr, Bailey SBC, Gebbie K, et al. 2001. Partnership for front-line success: a call for a national agenda on workforce development. *J. Public Health Manag. Pract.* 7(4):1–7

42. Livingood WC, Woodhouse H, Godin S. 1995. The feasibility and desirability of public health credentialing: a survey of public health leaders. *Am. J. Public Health* 8(6):765–70

43. Mays G, Halverson P, Scutchfield FD. 2003. Behind the curve? What we know and need to learn from public health systems research. *J. Public Health Manag. Pract.* 9(3):179–82

44. Moulton AD, Halverson PK, Honore PA, Berkowitz B. 2004. Public health finance: a conceptual framework. *J. Public Health Manag. Pract.* 10(5):377–82

45. Natl. Assoc. County City Health Off. 2001. *Local Public Health Agency Infrastructure: A Chartbook (October).* Washington, DC: NACCHO. http://www.naccho.org/prod111.cfm

46. Natl. Assoc. County City Health Off. 2003. *Local Public Health Agencies Better Equipped to Handle Bioterrorist Attacks.* Res. Brief No. 8 (Jan.). Washington, DC: NACCHO

47. Natl. Assoc. County City Health Off. 2003. Project Public Health Ready. http://www.naccho.org/project83.cfm

48. Natl. Comm. Vital Stat. 2001. Information for health: a strategy for building the national health information infrastructure. http://www.nevhs.hhs.gov/nhiilayo.pdf

49. Potter MA. 2003. Public Health Emergencies: Agencies with Authority in Pennsylvania Counties and Cities. Univ. Pittsburgh Cent. Public Health Preparedness. http://www.cphp.pitt.edu/upcphp/resources.htm

50. Potter MA. 2003. Reuniting Schools of Public Health and Public Health Practice, presented to the Institute of Medicine Forum on Emerging Infections. http://www.cphp.pitt.edu ("resources")

51. Potter MA, Barron G, Cioffi JP. 2003. A model for public health workforce development using the national public health performance standards program. *J. Public Health Manag. Pract.* 9(3):199–207

52. Potter MA, Ley CE, Fertman CI, Eggleston MM, Duman S. 2003. Evaluating workforce development: perspectives, processes, and lessons learned. *J. Public Health Manag. Pract.* 9(6):489–95

53. Potter MA, Pistella CL, Fertman CI, Dato VM. 2000. Needs assessment and a model

agenda for training the public health work-force. *Am. J. Public Health* 90(8):1294–96

54. Public Health Found. 2003. Public Health Data and Infrastructure. http://www.phf.org/data-infra.htm

55. Public Health Funct. Proj. 1995. *The Public Health Workforce: An Agenda for the 21st Century*. Washington, DC: US Dep. Health Hum. Serv.

56. Public Health Funct. Steer. Comm. 1994. *Public Health in America*. Washington, DC: US Public Health Serv.

57. Reid WM, Beitsch LM, Brooks RG, Mason KP, Mescia ND, Webb SC. 2001. National public health performance standards: workforce development and agency effectiveness in Florida. *J. Public Health Manag. Pract.* 7(4):67–73

58. Richet HM, Mohammed J, McDonald LC, Jarvis WR. 2001. Building communication networks: international network for the study and prevention of emerging antimicrobial resistance. *J. Emerg. Infect. Dis.* 7(2):319–22

59. Roper WL, Baker EL. 2003. The state of the public health system: Where do we go from here? In *America's Health: State Health Rankings-2003*. St. Paul, MN: United Health Found.

60. Sabol B. 2002. Innovations in collaboration for the public's health through the turning point initiative: the W.K. Kellogg Foundation perspective. *J. Public Health Manag. Pract.* 8(1):6–12

61. Salinsky E. 2002. *Public Health Emergency Preparedness: Fundamentals of the System*, Natl. Health Policy Forum Backgr. Pap. Washington, DC: George Washington Univ.

62. Somer A, Akhter MN. 2000. It's time we became a profession. *Am. J. Public Health* 90:845–46

63. Sorensen AA, Bialek RG, eds. 1991. *Public Health Faculty/Agency Forum: Linking Graduate Education and Practice*. Gainesville: Univ. Press Fla.

64. Teich JM, Wagner MM, Mackenzie CF, Schafer KO. 2002. The informatics response in disaster, terrorism, and war. *J. Am. Med. Informatics Assoc.* 9:97–104

65. Teret S, Webster DW, Vernick JS, Smith TW, Leff D, et al. et al. 1998. Support for new policies to regulate firearms: results of two national surveys. *New Engl. J. Med.* 339:813–18

66. Tilson H, Gebbie KM. 2004. The public health workforce. *Am. Rev. Public Health* 25:341–56

67. Turning Point. 2003. Public Health Statute Modernization. http://www.turningpointprogram.org/Pages/publichealth2.html

68. Turnock BJ. 2001. Competency-based credentialing of public health administrators in Illinois. *J. Public Health Manag. Pract.* 7(4):74–82

69. Turnock BJ. 2004. *Public Health—What it is and How it Works*. Sudbury, MA: Jones and Bartlett. 3rd ed.

70. Turnock BJ, Handler AS, Hall W, Potsic S, Nalluri R, Vaught EH. 1994. Local health department effectiveness in addressing the core functions of public health. *Public Health Rep.* 109(5):653–58

71. Vernick JS, Teret SP, Webster DW. 1997. Regulating firearm advertisements that promise home protection. *JAMA* 277(17):1391–97

72. Warner KE. 1986. *Selling Smoke: Cigarette Advertising and Public Health*. Washington, DC: Am. Public Health Assoc.

73. Yasnoff W, Overhage JM, Humphreys BL, LaVenture M, Goodmark W, et al. 2001. A national agenda for public health informatics. *J. Am. Med. Informatics Assoc.* 8:535–45

Annu. Rev. Public Health 2005. 26:319–39
doi: 10.1146/annurev.publhealth.26.021304.144610
Copyright © 2005 by Annual Reviews. All rights reserved
First published online as a Review in Advance on October 12, 2004

SOCIAL MARKETING IN PUBLIC HEALTH

Sonya Grier[1] and Carol A. Bryant[2]

[1]*The University of Pennsylvania, Colonial Penn Center, Philadelphia,
Pennsylvania 19104; email: griers@wharton.upenn.edu*
[2]*University of South Florida, Florida Prevention Research Center, Tampa,
Florida 33609; email: cbryant@hsc.usf.edu*

Key Words audience segmentation, consumer research, consumer orientation,
theory, evaluation

■ **Abstract** Social marketing, the use of marketing to design and implement programs to promote socially beneficial behavior change, has grown in popularity and
usage within the public health community. Despite this growth, many public health
professionals have an incomplete understanding of the field. To advance current knowledge, we provide a practical definition and discuss the conceptual underpinnings of
social marketing. We then describe several case studies to illustrate social marketing's
application in public health and discuss challenges that inhibit the effective and efficient
use of social marketing in public health. Finally, we reflect on future developments in
the field. Our aim is practical: to enhance public health professionals' knowledge of
the key elements of social marketing and how social marketing may be used to plan
public health interventions.

INTRODUCTION

Societies worldwide face an ever-increasing array of health challenges, heighten-
ing the importance of social change efforts. Social marketing, the use of marketing
to design and implement programs to promote socially beneficial behavior change,
has grown in popularity and usage within the public health community. In recent
years, the Centers for Disease Control and Prevention (CDC), the U.S. Department of Agriculture (USDA), the U.S. Department of Health and Human Services
(USDHHS), and other governmental and nonprofit organizations have used social
marketing to increase fruit and vegetable consumption, promote breastfeeding,
decrease fat consumption, promote physical activity, and influence a wide variety
of other preventive health behaviors (12). State and local communities are using
social marketing to increase utilization of the Supplemental Food and Nutrition
Program for Women, Infants, and Children (WIC), prenatal care, low cost mammograms, and other health services (9). Internationally, social marketing has been
used to improve access to potable water (42), eliminate leprosy in Sri Lanka (55),
increase tuberculosis medicine adherence (37), and promote immunizations and

universal iodization legislation (15, 31), among other applications. Social marketing has enormous potential to affect other health problems such as observed health disparities between members of ethnic minority and majority groups (54).

There also has been increasing professional activity in the field by academics, nonprofit organizations, and governmental agencies. New textbooks and workbooks, multiple annual conferences, the inclusion of social marketing in national public health conferences, training programs, including CDCynergy–Social Marketing Edition and other materials developed by the Turning Point Program (available online at http:/www.turningpointprogram.org), and a certificate program for graduate trained public health professionals have emerged in the past decade. [See Andreasen (4) for a review of social marketing's history.] Public health has been important in the field's growth, with the promotion of condom use internationally being among social marketing's first applications (22).

The widespread adoption of social marketing in public health has garnered important successes. Among these is VERB$_{TM}$, a national, multicultural, social marketing program coordinated by CDC (56). The VERB$_{TM}$ program encourages "tweens" (young people ages 9–13) to be physically active every day. The program was based on extensive marketing research with tweens, their parents, and other influencers. Results were used to design an intervention that combines mass-media advertising, public relations, guerrilla (i.e., interpersonal) marketing, and partnership efforts with professional sports leagues and athletes, as well as well-known sporting-goods suppliers and retailers, to reach the distinct audiences of tweens and adult influencers. VERB$_{TM}$ also partners with communities to improve access to outlets for physical activity and capitalize on the influence parents, teachers, and other people have on tweens' lives. After just one year, this award-winning program resulted in a 34% increase in weekly free-time physical activity sessions among 8.6 million children ages 9–10 in the United States. In communities that received higher levels of VERB$_{TM}$ interventions, the increases in physical activity were more dramatic (45). Another well-known example is the TRUTH$_{TM}$ campaign, which contributed to the reduction of smoking among teenagers nationwide (16).

Despite its popularity and influence, many public health professionals have an incomplete understanding of social marketing (28, 36, 38). In Hill's (28) review of the health promotion literature between 1982 and 1996, he concluded that health promoters' views of marketing differed considerably from how the marketing discipline is usually defined. Specifically, he found that many health promoters perceive social marketing as a predominantly promotional or, even more narrowly, a communication activity. Other common problems he noted were neglect of the exchange process and a lack of integration of the marketing mix in planning program interventions. These misunderstandings persist today as evidenced by the large number of abstracts submitted to the Social Marketing in Public Health conference and manuscripts submitted to *Social Marketing Quarterly*, which use the social marketing label to describe social advertising or communication activities not developed with marketing's conceptual framework. In this chapter, we provide an overview of social marketing in hopes of overcoming misconceptions about its key elements and advancing current knowledge. First, we provide a practical definition, discuss social marketing's conceptual underpinnings, and present case studies to illustrate its application in public health. Next, we discuss challenges that may inhibit the effective and efficient use of social marketing by public health professionals. Finally, we reflect on future developments needed in the field. Our objective is to enhance public health professionals' understanding of the key elements of social marketing and their ability to use social marketing to design public health interventions.

Defining Social Marketing

Although a variety of definitions have been proposed by social marketers, and debate continues (49), social marketing is typically defined as a program-planning process that applies commercial marketing concepts and techniques to promote voluntary behavior change (1, 34). Social marketing facilitates the acceptance, rejection, modification, abandonment, or maintenance of particular behaviors (34) by groups of individuals, often referred to as the target audience. Although social marketing's target audience is usually made up of consumers, it is used also to influence policy makers who can address the broader social and environmental determinants of health (15, 48). Hastings & Saren's (27) definition of social marketing includes also the analysis of the social consequences of commercial marketing policies and activities, e.g., monitoring the effects of the tobacco or food industries' marketing practices.

The defining features of social marketing emanate from marketing's conceptual framework and include exchange theory, audience segmentation, competition, "the marketing mix," consumer orientation, and continuous monitoring. Although social marketing shares many features with other related public health planning processes, it is distinguished by the systematic emphasis marketers place on the strategic integration of the elements in marketing's conceptual framework.

THE NOTION OF EXCHANGE   The field of marketing attempts to influence voluntary behavior by offering or reinforcing incentives and/or consequences in an environment that invites voluntary exchange (47). Exchange theory (6) views consumers acting primarily out of self interest as they seek ways to optimize value by doing what gives them the greatest benefit for the least cost. Contrary to commercial exchanges, in which consumers receive a product or service for a cash outlay, in public health situations, there is rarely an immediate, explicit payback to target audiences in return for their adoption of healthy behavior (47). Nevertheless, exchange theory reminds social marketers that they must (*a*) offer benefits that the consumer (not the public health professional) truly values; (*b*) recognize that consumers often pay intangible costs, such as time and psychic discomfort associated with changing behaviors; and (*c*) acknowledge that everyone involved in the exchange, including intermediaries, must receive valued benefits in return for their efforts (15).

AUDIENCE SEGMENTATION   Social marketers know it is not possible to be "all things to all people." Rather, marketing differentiates populations into subgroups or segments of people who share needs, wants, lifestyles, behavior, and values that make them likely to respond similarly to public health interventions. Public health professionals have long recognized intragroup differences within populations, but they typically use ethnicity, age, or other demographics as the basis for identifying distinct subgroups. Social marketers are more likely to divide populations into distinct segments on the basis of current behavior (e.g., heavy versus light smoking), future intentions, readiness to change, product loyalty, and/or psychographics (e.g., lifestyle, values, personality characteristics). Compared with other systematic planning processes, social marketing devotes greater attention and resources to segmentation research, the identification of one or more segments as the target audience to receive the greatest priority in program development, and development of differential marketing strategies (e.g., in how products will be positioned, placed, or promoted) for selected population segments (17).

The VERB$_{TM}$ program initially segmented its target population by age (e.g., youth aged 9–13 and parents/influencers) and then conducted research that identified important differences among specific segments within the tween audience on the basis of activity level, receptivity to physical activity, ethnicity, and gender. Segmentation and target marketing increase program effectiveness and efficiency by tailoring strategies to address the needs of distinct segments (17) and helping to make appropriate resource allocation decisions.

COMPETITION   In commercial marketing, competition refers to products and companies that try to satisfy similar wants and needs as the product being promoted. In social marketing, the term refers to the behavioral options that compete with public health recommendations and services, e.g., bottle-feeding versus breastfeeding (23). The marketing mindset asks, what products (behaviors, services) compete with those we are promoting, and how do the benefits compare to those offered by competing behaviors? Answers to these questions enable social marketers to offer benefits that best distinguish healthy behaviors from the competition and develop a sustainable competitive advantage that maximizes their products' attractiveness to consumers (23).

An assessment of the competition also may be useful in determining which behaviors are best to promote and which segments are best to target. As Novelli (43) explains, "Thinking about where, how, and with whom to compete is important— you might do that analysis and decide not to compete because the foe is too formidable. And that is okay: "we need to have the courage not to compete." We may also decide to compete for specific population segments in which we can provide better value than the competition (25).

THE MARKETING MIX   Another core concept adopted from the commercial sector is the marketing mix, also known as the four Ps: product, price, place, and promotion. These key elements of social marketing are central to the planning and implementation of an integrated marketing strategy.

Product refers to the set of benefits associated with the desired behavior or service usage. Kotler et al. (34) distinguish between the core product (what people will gain when they perform the behavior) and the actual product (the desired behavior). They also use the concept of the augmented product to refer to any tangible objects and services used to facilitate behavior change. However, it is important to note that pamphlets and other promotional activities are designed to facilitate adoption of the behavior and are not the actual product.

To be successful, social marketers believe the product must provide a solution to problems that consumers consider important and/or offer them a benefit they truly value. For this reason, research is undertaken to understand people's aspirations, preferences, and other desires, in addition to their health needs, to identify the benefits most appealing to consumers. For instance, the VERB$_{TM}$ program positioned physical activity as a way to have fun, spend time with friends, and gain recognition from peers and adults rather than to prevent obesity or chronic disease later in life. The marketing objective is to discover which benefits have the greatest appeal to the target audience and design a product that provides those benefits. In some cases, public health professionals must change their recommendations or modify their programs to provide the benefits consumers value most.

Price refers to the cost or sacrifice exchanged for the promised benefits. This cost is always considered from the consumer's point of view. As such, price usually encompasses intangible costs, such as diminished pleasure, embarrassment, loss of time, and the psychological hassle that often accompanies change, especially when modifying ingrained habits. In setting the right price, it is important to know if consumers prefer to pay more to obtain "value added" benefits and if they think that products given away or priced low are inferior to more expensive ones. Consumer research conducted by Population Services International, for instance, revealed that many teens did not trust condoms that were given away by public health agencies. But even a small, affordable monetary price (25 cents) was sufficient to reassure them that the condoms were trustworthy.

Place refers to the distribution of goods and the location of sales and service encounters. In social marketing, place may be thought of as action outlets: "where and when the target market will perform the desired behavior, acquire any related tangible objects, and receive any associated services" (34). Place includes the actual physical location of these outlets, operating hours, general attractiveness and comfort, and accessibility, e.g., parking and availability by public transportation (15). It also includes intermediaries—organizations and people—that can provide information, goods, and services and perform other functions that facilitate the change process. Research may be necessary to identify the life path points—places people visit routinely, times of the day, week, or year of visits, and points in the life cycle—where people are likely to act so that products and supportive services or information can be placed there. In the Kentucky Youth Nutrition and Fitness Program, a community coalition offered numerous opportunities for tweens to try out new forms of physical activity (or VERBS) at multiple times and locations throughout the summer months. The public parks, YWCAs, Children's Museum, neighborhood associations, retail outlets, university and high school athletic clubs, the Lexington Legends (a minor league baseball team), and other organizations designed action outlets where tweens could have a summer scorecard validated each time they tried a new VERB. Tweens that participated in a designated number of activities received special recognition and eligibility to win prizes (13). A key element in this project's placement strategy is providing sufficient incentive to the intermediaries to provide opportunities, consistent with the VERB$_{TM}$ program's exciting and edgy brand attributes, for tweens to be physically active.

Promotion is often the most visible component of marketing. Promotion includes the type of persuasive communications marketers use to convey product benefits and associated tangible objects and services, pricing strategies, and place components (34). Promotional strategy involves a carefully designed set of activities intended to influence change and usually involves multiple elements: specific communication objectives for each target audience; guidelines for designing attention-getting and effective messages; and designation of appropriate communication channels. Promotional activities may encompass advertising, public relations, printed materials, promotional items, signage, special events and displays, face-to-face selling, and entertainment media. In public health, policy changes, professional training, community-based activities, and skill building usually are combined with communication activities to bring about the desired changes.

An integrated marketing mix is essential. Though promotion, one of the four Ps, is generally what people think of when considering social marketing, marketers use their understanding of consumers to develop a carefully integrated strategy addressing all four Ps. By integration, we mean that each element has been planned systematically to support clearly defined goals, and all marketing activities are consistent with and reinforce each other. For instance, a program offering the emotional benefits associated with breastfeeding would use a warm, emotional appeal rather than one that instills fear, and advertisements for a breastfeeding advice program would not be aired until those support services were readily available. In similar fashion, the VERB$_{TM}$ program uses a tone consistent with its positioning of physical activity as fun and exciting rather than using a serious, factual description of the health benefits of physical activity.

The emphasis marketers place on understanding the exchange process and competition, and the development of an integrated marketing strategy based on the 4 Ps, are social marketing's most distinctive features.

CONSUMER ORIENTATION AND THE IMPORTANCE OF RESEARCH   Marketing's conceptual framework demands a steadfast commitment to understanding consumers, the people whose behavior we hope to change. The premise is that all program planning decisions must emanate from a consideration of the consumers' wants and needs (1).

The backbone of a customer orientation is consumer research. Formative research is used to gain a deeper understanding of a target audience's needs, aspirations, values, and everyday lives. Of special interest are consumers' perceptions of the products, benefits, costs, and other factors (e.g., perceived threat, self-efficacy, social influences) that motivate and deter them from adopting recommended behaviors. Research also provides information on distinct population subgroups and the social and cultural environments in which the people act on behavioral decisions. This information is used to make strategic marketing decisions about the audience segments to target, the benefits to offer, and the costs to lower, and about how to price, place, and promote products. Although consumer research need not be expensive or complex, it must be done. [For a discussion of inexpensive research methods, see Andreasen (3)].

The importance of evidence-based program planning and community-based approaches in public health has increased dramatically during the past two decades (30). As a result, social marketers are not alone in their reliance on research and careful consideration of consumers' needs when designing strategies to change behavior. Social marketing is distinctive, however, in its reliance on marketing's conceptual framework to guide the research process and the development of a strategic plan (i.e., based on the 4 Ps and an understanding of the competition). The VERB$_{TM}$ program, for instance, used existing data and consumer research to understand the behaviors, lifestyle, and mindsets of tweens, parents, and other key influencers. Research explored the cultural, ethnic, and economic dynamics that unify and differentiate the tween audience and provided insights into the competitive environment in which tweens make decisions about how to spend their time. Results were used to develop an integrated marketing plan based on the 4 Ps and communication guidelines that served as a blueprint for the national media campaign (56).

Ideally, the consumer orientation represents a commitment to provide consumers with satisfying exchanges that result in long-term, trusting relationships (15). If, for instance, health services are underutilized or dietary change recommendations are overlooked, program planners listen to consumers to find out what they can do to improve program offerings and make their recommendations more helpful. This willingness to change the product to meet consumer preferences is an essential feature of social marketing, one shared by total quality management or continuous improvement approaches but which is divergent from more traditional, expert-driven approaches in which public health professionals determine what consumers need to do.

CONTINUOUS MONITORING AND REVISION   Plans for evaluating and monitoring a social marketing intervention begin at the outset of the planning process. As program interventions are implemented, each is monitored to assess its effectiveness to determine if it is worthy of being sustained, and to identify activities that require midcourse revision. Although many public health programs conduct process and impact evaluations, marketing devotes considerable resources to this activity and practices it on a continuous basis. Social marketers are constantly checking with target audiences to gauge their responses to all aspects of an intervention, from the broad marketing strategy to specific messages and materials (7). The VERB$_{TM}$ program, for example, uses observation and intercept interviews at sponsored events to assess visitor demographics and interaction patterns of the tweens with the activities.

Comparing Marketing to Other Behavior Management Tools

Social marketing can also be understood by comparing it with other approaches to managing behavior change. Rothschild (47) developed a conceptual framework that contrasts marketing with education and law. In his view, education informs and persuades people to adopt healthy behaviors voluntarily by creating awareness of the benefits of changing. When health professionals educate people about the benefits of adopting healthy lifestyle behaviors, citizens have free choice in how they respond, and society accepts the costs when some people continue to practice undesirable behaviors. Education is most effective when the goals of society are consistent with those of the target audience, the benefits of behavior change are inherently attractive, immediate, and obvious, the costs of changing are low, and the skills and other resources needed to change are readily available [e.g., putting a baby to sleep on its back to prevent sudden infant death syndrome (SIDS)].

Law or policy development uses coercion or the threat of punishment to manage behavior. Legislation is the most effective tool for public health when society is not willing to pay the costs associated with continued practice of an unhealthy or risky behavior (e.g., drunk driving) yet citizens are unlikely to find it in their immediate self-interest to change.

In contrast, marketing influences behavior by offering alternative choices that invite voluntary exchange. Marketing alters the environment to make the recommended health behavior more advantageous than the unhealthy behavior it is designed to replace and then communicates the more favorable cost-benefit relationship to the target audience. Marketing is the most effective strategy when societal goals are not directly and immediately consistent with people's self-interest but citizens can be influenced to change by making the consequences more advantageous. Like education, marketing offers people freedom of choice; but unlike education, it alters the behavioral consequences rather than expects individuals to make a sacrifice on society's behalf. Education and policy changes are often components in a social marketing intervention; however, marketing also creates an environment more conducive for change by enhancing the attractiveness of the benefits offered and minimizing the costs.

Steps in the Social Marketing Process

The social marketing process is a continuous, iterative process that can be described as consisting of six major steps or tasks: initial planning; formative research; strategy development; program development and pretesting of material and nonmaterial interventions; implementation; and monitoring and evaluation. The initial planning stage involves gathering relevant information to help identify preliminary behavioral objectives, determine target markets, and recognize potential behavioral determinants and strategies. Formative research is then conducted to investigate factors identified during the initial planning phase to segment audiences and determine those factors that must be addressed to bring about behavior change. Strategy development involves the preparation of a realistic marketing plan comprised of specific, measurable objectives and a step-by-step work plan that will guide the development, implementation, and tracking of the project. The plan includes the overall goals of the program, a description of the target audience, specific behaviors that will be marketed toward them, and strategies for addressing the critical factors associated with the target behavior. The social marketing plan is organized around marketing's conceptual framework of the four Ps. Campaign strategies and materials are then developed, pretested, piloted, and revised prior to program implementation. Monitoring and evaluation activities continue throughout the program implementation to identify any necessary program revisions, as well as to understand program effectiveness and make midcourse corrections as needed.

CASE EXAMPLES OF SOCIAL MARKETING APPLICATIONS

Three case studies are provided to illustrate how social marketing can be used to develop new public health products (the Road Crew), improve service delivery and enhance program utilization (the Texas WIC Program), and promote healthy eating behaviors (the Food Trust).

The Road Crew

In the Road Crew project, social marketing was used to develop a new product to compete with a dangerous brand, "I can drive myself home, even though I've had too much to drink" (32). In an effort to curb alcohol-related automobile crashes, this program targets 21- to 34-year-old men who drive themselves home after an evening of drinking at taverns in rural Wisconsin. Formative research revealed that, although alternative forms of transportation were unavailable in these communities, even if offered a ride home, men were unwilling to leave their automobiles at the bars overnight. In response, program designers created a ride service that transported men from their homes to the bars, between bars, and back home again, allowing them to enjoy their evening without risk of driving while intoxicated. The program was not without controversy, as some critics argued that the ride service would lead to increased individual-level drinking. Nonetheless, three rural communities were given funds to establish ride services tailored to meet the unique opportunities and constraints in respective areas. Each community also developed a pricing scheme to cover costs. An advertising agency developed the program's name (Road Crew), slogan, and logo. At the end of the first year, and 19,575 rides later, evaluation results suggest that the program has decreased alcohol-related crashes by 17% and saved the state of Wisconsin $610,000 (32). Additionally, the evaluation found no evidence to support the criticism that the program increased individual-level drinking.

The Texas WIC Program

The second case study examines a social marketing program conducted to increase enrollment and improve customer and employee satisfaction with the Special Supplemental Nutrition Program for Women, Infants, and Children (WIC) in Texas. Participant observation, in-depth interviews, telephone interviews, focus groups, and surveys were used to understand the needs, preferences, and characteristics of four target audiences: families eligible but not participating in the program, program participants, program employees, and professionals who refer people to the program (9, 10). Research results were used to develop a comprehensive social marketing plan that included policy changes, service delivery improvements, staff and vendor training, internal promotion, public information and communications, client education, and community-based interventions. This plan worked to change families' perceptions of WIC as a welfare program that provided free food to poor people by emphasizing nutrition education, health checkups, immunizations, and referrals. It included recommendations for lowering costs by repositioning the program as a temporary assistance nutrition and health program—"WIC—Helping Families Help Themselves"—in which families can maintain their pride and self-esteem as they earn their WIC benefits and learn about nutrition and other ways to help their families. Because many women did not know they were eligible for the program and/or had trouble enrolling, the marketing plan also emphasized ways to help families understand eligibility guidelines, streamline the certification process, and make it easier for health and social service professionals to refer eligible women. Placement strategies recommended the location of WIC clinics outside of government assistance venues, and professional training programs were developed to enhance employees' skills in dealing with customers and teach grocery store cashiers to process WIC clients more efficiently and respectfully. Promotional efforts included a community outreach kit to reach referral sources as well as the use of mass media to reach eligible families. The Texas WIC Program was launched in the fall of 1995. Program data was used to monitor the number of families who called the toll-free number for more information after the program was launched and, more importantly, the number of people participating in Texas WIC. When results showed that increases in program enrollment were not sustained, midcourse revisions were made to improve program delivery. The program's caseload then grew from its baseline level of 582,819 in October 1993 to 778,558 in October 1998—an increase of almost 200,000 participants.

The Food Trust

The last case study examines the Food Trust, a nonprofit organization in Philadelphia, Pennsylvania, which aims to increase people's access to affordable and nutritious foods. The Food Trust's Corner Store Campaign seeks to reduce the incidence of diet-related disease and obesity by improving the snack food choices made by youth in local corner stores. The campaign uses social marketing to increase demand for healthy snacks, promote student participation in the school meals programs, and target the food industry to increase the availability of healthier choices in local stores. An initial budget of $10,000 (not including staff time) was allocated to develop the social marketing plan for the Corner Store Campaign. At the start of the planning process, Food Trust staff members interviewed 33 key informants on best practices in social marketing and also worked to identify other programs aimed at affecting youth snack choices nationwide. Survey research was conducted to understand the food choices available in the corner stores in five local communities and to provide a baseline for the development of strategies to increase the distribution of healthier snacks. Survey results found that healthy food choices were available only in limited quantities in most of these stores, e.g., only one store carried low-fat milk in single serving containers and none sold fresh fruit. Results of the assessment of the food environment were used to determine (a) which healthy snacks could be promoted in the short term and (b) how to facilitate food manufacturers and retailers distribution of healthier snacks. For example, the Food Trust developed partnerships with individual snack food companies to increase the distribution of healthier choices in neighborhood stores. Formative research was also conducted with youth ages 5–12 to understand their snacking behavior and how to best promote the currently available healthier snack choices. This formative research informed the development of a social marketing plan that was piloted in two local communities in the summer of 2004.

CHALLENGES AND MISCONCEPTIONS

Andreasen (4) has argued that social marketing is now moving into a period of early maturity with growing popularity among public health professionals. However, to continue developing, social marketing must overcome a variety of challenges. In public health, these challenges can be grouped into four categories: (a) misconceptions and other barriers to diffusion, (b) formative research and evaluation methodologies, (c) theoretical issues, and (d) ethical considerations.

Barriers to Diffusion

After initial resistance, the field of public health has readily embraced marketing's reliance on advertising and other promotional techniques and has begun to rely increasingly on consumer research to make evidence-based decisions (27). It has yet, however, to fully appreciate social marketing's "flexibility, range, and breadth of potential for addressing behavioral and social issues" (38). As previously noted, social marketing is often viewed as a method for designing communication campaigns rather than developing comprehensive interventions that integrate the full marketing mix of product, price, place, and promotion. In part, the diminished attention given to nonpromotional elements of the marketing mix reflects confusion surrounding the adaptation of these concepts to social marketing situations (a theoretical issue we discuss at greater length below). It also reflects difficulties social marketers have in modifying public health products (e.g., creating new and more attractive benefits for eating fruits and vegetables), lowering the costs associated with healthy behaviors (e.g., making fruits and vegetables cheaper to purchase or easier to prepare), and creating accessible action outlets (such as placing fruits and vegetables on fast-food restaurant menus). Finally, many of social marketing's earliest adopters were dazzled by advertising or came from the public relations and advertising fields and did not recognize the difference between marketing and health communication (51). Whatever the reason, the disproportionate amount of attention given to promotional activities has created the misconception that social marketing relies primarily on advertising to achieve its goals. To overcome this problem and realize social marketing's full potential, its practitioners must recognize the power that lies in the integration of all elements of the marketing mix rather than the magic of advertising messages.

Another criticism of social marketing is that it "blames the victim" by focusing on individual behavior rather than on the underlying environmental and social causes of the problems it addresses. Perhaps the most articulate of social marketing's critics is Wallack (52), who argues that social marketing, like many public health approaches, tries to rescue people from drowning "downstream," when the important work lies "upstream," combating the environmental and social structural factors that create the health problems. There is an element of truth in this criticism: Social marketers have been guilty of relying too heavily on strategies aimed at changing individual behavior and paying too little attention to environmental factors (15, 26). The field has benefited from this criticism, and today the importance of understanding the social environment and making it more conducive to individual healthy behavior is well established (25). For instance, Goldberg (20) describes how an intervention designed to persuade individual motorcyclists to wear helmets can be successful downstream in increasing individual helmet usage and succeed upstream by demonstrating health care savings that prompt policy makers to pass mandatory helmet laws. Nevertheless, although more cognizant of environmental factors, social marketing practitioners too infrequently target policy makers who can address the broader social determinants of health (e.g., social inequality, illiteracy, lack of community cohesiveness, poor housing, racism) (15, 26). [See Siegel & Doner (48) for a discussion of social marketing and policy development.]

Another long-standing complaint against social marketing is that it is manipulative. Some public health professionals in the developing world view social marketing as a colonial approach that implies disrespect by using language based on military metaphors (e.g., target markets) and commercialism (e.g., customers). As Wallack (52) points out, "even the term consumer evokes a metaphor of limited power that values people only for what they can purchase and not for how they can participate." Some public health professionals still reject social marketing because of its ties to Madison Avenue—style advertising, a field that has come under increased scrutiny and criticism (27). Yet, as Hastings & Saren (27) note, these criticisms ignore social marketing's consumer orientation and commitment to using research to understand and meet the wants and needs of consumers, an approach that "challenges the expert-driven hegemony in the health sector. . .." To successfully dispel the claim that marketing is manipulative, social marketers need to focus less on communication to inform people about public health products and place greater emphasis on developing affordable, accessible products that allow people to solve their problems and realize the aspirations that matter most in their lives and to modify the environment to make it easier and more enticing to adopt the healthy behavior. Efforts to involve consumers in goal-setting, participatory research and strategy development would also enable them to become true partners instead of targets of professionals' programs.

Social marketing's diffusion has also been affected by some public health professionals' reluctance to invest time and resources in consumer research. Fortunately, some funding agencies (e.g., the CDC, USDHHS, USDA, and the Robert Wood Johnson Foundation) now require a planning phase and allocate funds for community assessments, environmental scans, and consumer research for many of the grants they award. But many other federal, state, and nonprofit funding agencies still expect grantees to begin implementation before they have had ample time to understand their consumers and develop appropriate intervention strategies.

Whereas social marketing may be inappropriate when time and resources are not available to conduct formative research, in other cases, it may be possible to truncate planning time and minimize costs by relying more on existing information to develop a marketing plan. In addition to the published literature, local and state program data sets can provide important insights into service utilization rates, characteristics of current and previous program participants, and customer satisfaction ratings. Also, social marketers can now access unpublished reports of federally sponsored audience research on prevention topics from the Prevention Communication Research Database (PCRD) created by the U.S. Department of Health and Human Services (http://www.health.gov/communication/).

Another valuable way to save time and scarce financial resources is to build on existing program strategies and interventions. Many large-scale social marketing programs such as VERB$_{TM}$ or 5 A Day programs produce interventions, including educational, promotional, and/or training materials, that can be used at the state and local community level. These interventions make it possible to capitalize on extensive formative research and sophisticated creative development that local public health professionals can rarely afford. In some cases, careful pretesting and pilot testing of existing materials and program strategies may be needed to adapt existing program approaches to fit unique community characteristics and provide a local face for national programs. In other cases, this may not be necessary because the national program materials address issues that cut across state and regional boundaries. In either case, practitioners at the local level are wise to build on the brand equity created by national media coverage rather than replicate or compete with national initiatives.

Formative Research and Evaluation

The application of social marketing in public health would also benefit from improved research methodologies—a greater reliance on mixed methods, more creative audience segmentation, and improved evaluation studies.

Each year, the University of South Florida Social Marketing and Public Health conference issues a call for abstracts. And each year, the majority of respondents submit projects that have relied exclusively on focus groups to design a program intervention. Rarely is their marketing plan based on a solid foundation of secondary data and/or a mixture of qualitative and quantitative methods. The overreliance on focus groups in marketing research is problematic for at least two reasons. First, focus group interviews can be misleading: The issues that people discuss in a group setting are not always those that have the greatest impact on their behavioral decisions. Second, quantitative data is needed to segment populations into more distinct subgroups. Conversely, survey data alone can miss important insights into a consumer's "... everyday life and how either adopting or stopping certain types of behaviors impacts it" (35). For these reasons, social marketers would benefit from using mixed methodologies to develop effective marketing plans.

Audience segmentation in public health also is limited by an overreliance on ethnicity and other demographic variables and the Stages of Change theoretical framework (46). Many public health practitioners of social marketing have yet to heed the advice Walsh and her associates (53) gave more than a decade ago:

> Health programs could benefit from more diversified and customized segmentation strategies, taking account of variables—such as life stage, propensity for sensation seeking, interest in changing lifestyle, and entertainment and leisure-time activities—that may be especially germane to health.

The CDC employs two data sets that make it possible to link this type of psychographic data with health information on U.S. populations: Healthstyles and the merging of the PRIZM database with health data such as cancer screening rates and medically underserved status. The Healthstyles segmentation system, developed by Porter Novelli, integrates information on health beliefs and behaviors (e.g., physical activity and nutrition, smoking, alcohol consumption, weight control, and breastfeeding), lifestyle factors, and demographics (34). The PRIZM system, developed by Claritas, Inc., divides the U.S. population into 64 segments on the basis of demographic and lifestyle variables. CDC produces summary reports and maps based on the PRIZM data set, which provide insights into the media preferences, purchasing behavior, lifestyle activities and demographics of residents living in census tracts, ZIP codes, or other geographic units (5).

Program evaluation poses yet another challenge. The field still lacks convincing evidence that social marketing programs are more effective than those planned using traditional, top-down approaches (35). Many social marketing programs are evaluated poorly or not at all. Because social marketing interventions often vary continuously over long periods of time and attempt to reach large population units (e.g., U.S. tweens) they do not lend themselves to the gold standard randomized clinical trial or other experimental designs (29). However, other evaluation and monitoring designs can generate strong inferences about a program's impact and "satisfy critics that there is no other equally plausible or compelling reason change might have occurred even if absolute cause and effect cannot be demonstrated" (14). Alternative evaluation designs also can provide important insights into other aspects of the program's process and performance, e.g., by determining if the program is implemented as planned, identifying consumers the program has failed to reach, determining if consumers recognize the program's brand and can recall key messages, and recommending ways to improve the program (29). [For a discussion of less well-known designs that may be appropriate for evaluating social marketing programs see Hornik (29).]

McDermott (39) reminds us that evaluators should begin by asking a series of questions: Why are you going to be evaluating? Whom are you going to be evaluating? What are you going to be evaluating? Where are you going to be evaluating? When are you going to be evaluating? How are you going to be evaluating? and Who is going to be doing the evaluating? By answering these questions in advance we can avoid some of the common problems that compromise evaluations of social marketing interventions, such as

- measuring outcomes too early, before change can occur
- failing to measure exposure and expecting too much from a limited intervention "dose,"
- measuring the wrong outcomes (e.g., individual behavior change instead of policy changes), and
- using the wrong units of analysis when measuring effects (e.g., individuals instead of communities).

Theoretical Underpinnings

Over the past two decades, social marketers have looked largely to commercial marketing for theoretical grounding and attempted to make its principles and concepts fit social marketing situations. There has been considerable discussion on the Social Marketing List Serve, for instance, about how to apply the concept of product to the promotion of health behavior (44).

More recently, however, Peattie & Peattie (44) have warned that "[t]here is. . .a danger that an overemphasis on the direct translation of mainstream marketing principles and practices into social contexts may create practical problems and also confusion regarding the theoretical basis of social marketing." Some scholars (19), for instance, have questioned the usefulness of exchange theory for social marketing programs. Peattie & Peattie (44) also recommend that the 4 Ps be renamed and conceptualized as the social proposition (product), costs (price), accessibility (place), and communication (promotion). Other recent debates among social marketers have concerned the degree to which relationship marketing (24), branding (40), and an analysis of competition are useful in marketing public health products (23).

If careful not to throw the baby out with the bath water, the field could benefit by expanding its vocabulary and broadening its theoretical underpinnings (19, 35, 44, 51). Because no single theory or discipline is likely to provide all the guidance needed to direct social change, the following are some "next steps" to consider:

- explore other ways to conceptualize the exchange process that more appropriately account for the complex, social nature of health behavior change (19);
- look to marketing's subdisciplines (relationship marketing, service marketing, political marketing, nonprofit marketing) for additional insights into consumer behavior that are appropriate for social marketing situations (44);
- investigate a wide array of potential behavior change determinants (e.g., emotions and motivation), recognizing that the most important factors are unlikely to be the same for all health behaviors (35); and
- explore other theoretical frameworks for understanding change processes and other models for directing change (35, 51). In addition to public health's standard health behavior theories, social marketing could be blended with elements from community organization (41), media advocacy (52), and behavior analysis (18). Social marketers could learn also from risk compensation theory, the emotional contagion model, political risk compensation theory, risk homeostatis theory, and social capital (19, 35).

The intent of these explorations should not be to break social marketing's ties with its commercial counterpart, but rather to develop a better understanding of the factors that influence health behavior and improve social marketing's tools for modifying the social-structural, environmental, and individual-level determinants of social change. As social marketers adopt other theories and vocabularies, the field is likely to move away from its marketing roots. This raises important questions: Will it stop being social marketing and morph into a new model? And is it important to maintain distinct boundaries as social marketing as long as we become more effective in bringing about social change? One of our most influential social change agents Novelli (43) writes

> I realize that if you're going to have a discipline, you have to have some boundaries. But to me, that shouldn't interfere with the objective—to win. These are not programs for the faint of heart. There's not enough money, there's not enough time... I don't know how these definitional debates are going to turn out, but I hope they're not stymieing people from moving forward. (p. 45)

Ethical Considerations

Investigators increasingly are recognizing that if the field is to mature as a profession, its practitioners must pay careful attention to ethical standards and practices (2). The marketing of social products, services, and ideas is particularly prone to ethical dilemmas. Unlike most commercial marketing, social marketing involves some of our most deeply held beliefs and moral judgments (50). Recent work on ethics highlights unique issues about the moral justification of social marketing's aims (e.g., individual or social welfare versus individual satisfaction), procedures (e.g., how much disclosure is necessary in the promotion of a contraceptive about product side effects), and outcomes (e.g., moral changes in a community, especially when the social marketers are not members of that community) (2, 8, 50).

Many ethical criticisms of social marketing focus on power differentials that contribute to an unequal playing field between marketers and consumers. Some authors argue that incorporating consumers in the process, from the beginning of the social marketing design to its implementation and evaluation, would help counteract this issue (23). Hastings (24), for instance, notes that public health can learn as much from the consumer as it teaches them.

Given the ecological nature of most health conditions, efforts to change health behaviors can impact a variety of contextual factors; therefore, it also is important to anticipate any unintended effects social marketing activities may have on target audiences and others. Media messages, for instance, should not reinforce stereotypes or stigmatize population segments (21) [e.g., by presenting smokers as nasty or parents as unfit (50)] or divert program planners from addressing structural factors needed to facilitate change. For a more complete coverage of ethical issues see Andreasen (2).

THE NEXT STEPS: A VISION FOR THE FUTURE OF SOCIAL MARKETING IN PUBLIC HEALTH

For social marketing to become more widely accepted by public health professionals and carefully applied, several developments are necessary. Program administrators, health educators, and other program planners need to be trained in social marketing to enable them to imbue public health organizations with a marketing mindset. Currently, short training sessions are offered in the United States and elsewhere, and the University of South Florida offers certification in social marketing for public health professionals who hold graduate degrees. This program provides instruction in the basic skills required to manage social marketing programs. However, at this time, no schools of public health offer a concentration in social marketing, and most do not provide a complete course on the topic. Although it is debatable whether social marketing should develop into a distinct degree-granting discipline within public health, competency-based training is needed to prepare public health professionals to apply its principles correctly: specifically, to conduct rigorous formative research, develop integrated marketing plans, and evaluate social marketing programs.

Funding organizations need to provide training for their project officers and administrators to help them structure program grants in ways that optimize social marketing's impact. Grantees should be given sufficient time and resources to conduct formative research, develop evidence-based marketing strategies, pretest program interventions, and monitor program activities. Administrators should recognize the danger inherent in short funding cycles and limited budgets that prevent social marketing programs from achieving the intervention "dose" needed to bring about social change. Agencies that encourage grantees to use social marketing also need staff who can determine if social marketing principles are being applied correctly and provide technical assistance when necessary.

Evaluation of social marketing projects is critical to determine if social marketing programs are cost effective and to identify the conditions under which social marketing is the preferred program planning approach. Commercial marketers often rely on national databases to monitor their success in the marketplace. Similar data sets are needed that would allow social marketing's practitioners to monitor the health behavior of population segments in a timely fashion (14).

Public health practitioners now recognize the value of community-based approaches to social change. Ideally, social marketing practitioners will develop ways to incorporate consumers as partners into the planning process, allowing them to set agendas and directly participate in efforts to ameliorate the problems they decide to tackle. Community-based prevention marketing is one model that blends community mobilization, empowerment, and participatory research with marketing principles and processes in an attempt to balance the power differentials between public health professionals and consumers while benefiting from marketing's approach to social change (11). The prevention marketing initiative is another model in which social marketers work closely with community coalitions (33).

A final and admittedly idealistic goal is for public health to adopt social marketing's consumer orientation as a central value in its organizational culture. Rather than view marketing's orientation as just another program-planning tool or new type of intervention to prevent disease, public health organizations could benefit from viewing the consumer as the center of everything they do, inviting consumers to be true partners in determining how to best meet their health needs. We envision a public health field in which its practitioners, working at all levels, are committed to understanding and responding to the public's desires as well as their needs and routinely use consumer research to make strategic planning decisions about how best to help its consumers solve their problems and realize their aspirations. We believe the marketing mindset will optimize public health's ability to create trusting relationships with consumers and make their lives healthier and more fulfilling.

ACKNOWLEDGMENTS

Sonya Grier is a Robert Wood Johnson Foundation Health and Society Scholar at the University of Pennsylvania and an assistant professor of marketing (on leave) at the Stanford University Graduate School of Business.

The authors thank James Lindenberger for his thoughtful comments and editorial assistance with the manuscript. We also thank Alan Andreasen, Dominick Frosch, Shiriki Kumanyika, and Jose Pagan for their helpful comments on earlier drafts.

**The *Annual Review of Public Health* is online at
http://publhealth.annualreviews.org**

LITERATURE CITED

1. Andreasen AR. 1995. *Marketing Social Change: Changing Behavior to Promote Health, Social Development, and the Environment.* San Francisco, CA: Jossey-Bass

2. Andreasen AR. 2001. *Ethics in Social Marketing.* Washington, DC: Georgetown Univ. Press

3. Andreasen AR. 2002. *Marketing Research That Won't Break the Bank: A Practical Guide to Getting the Information You Need.* San Francisco: Jossey-Bass. 2nd ed.

4. Andreasen AR. 2003. The life trajectory of social marketing. *Mark. Theory* 3:293–303

5. Andreasen AR, Kotler P. 2003. *Strategic Marketing for Nonprofit Organizations.* Upper Saddle River, NJ: Prentice Hall

6. Bagozzi RP. 1978. Marketing as exchange: a theory of transactions in the marketplace. *Am. Behav. Sci.* 21:535–56

7. Balch GI, Sutton SM. 1997. Keep me posted: a plea for practical evaluation. In *Social Marketing: Theoretical and Practical Perspectives*, pp. 61–74. Mahwah, NJ: Erlbaum

8. Brenkert GG. 2001. The ethics of international social marketing. See Andreasen 2001, pp. 39–69

9. Bryant CA, Kent E, Brown C, Bustillo M, Blair C, et al. 1998. A social marketing approach to increase customer satisfaction with the Texas WIC Program. *Mark. Health Serv.* Winter: 5–17

10. Bryant CA, Lindenberger JH, Brown C, Kent E, Schreiber JM, et al. 2001. A social marketing approach to increasing enrollment in a public health program—Case

Study of the Texas WIC Program. *Hum. Org.* 60:234–46

11. Bryant CA, McCormack FM, Brown K, Landis D, McDermott RJ. 2000. Community-based prevention marketing: the next steps in disseminating behavior change. *Am. J. Health Behav.* 24:61–68

12. Coreil J, Bryant CA, Henderson JN. 2000. *Social and Behavioral Foundations of Public Health.* Thousand Oaks, CA: Sage

13. Courtney AH, Bryant CA, Peterson MF, Koonce D. 2004. *Kentucky youth nutrition and fitness project: progress report.* Tech. Rep. Div. Nutr. Health Educ., Lexington-Fayette County Health Dep., Lexington, Kentucky

14. Doner L. 2003. Approaches to evaluating social marketing programs. *Soc. Mark. Q.* IX: 18–26

15. Donovan RJ, Henley N. 2003. *Social Marketing: Principles and Practices.* Melbourne: IP Commun.

16. Farrelly MC, Healton CG, Davis KC, Messeri P, Hersey JC, Haviland ML. 2002. Getting to the truth: evaluating national tobacco countermarketing campaigns. *Am. J. Public Health* 92:901–7

17. Forthofer MS, Bryant CA. 2000. Using audience-segmentation techniques to tailor health behavior change strategies. *Am. J. Health Behav.* 24:36–43

18. Geller ES. 2002. The challenge of social change: a behavioral scientist's perspective. *Soc. Mark. Q.* VIII:15–24

19. Glenane-Antoniadis A, Whitwell GB. 2003. Extending the vision of social marketing through social capital theory:

marketing in the context of intricate exchange and market failure. *Mark. Theory* 3:323–43

20. Goldberg ME. 1995. Social marketing: Are we fiddling while Rome burns? *J. Consum. Psychol.* 4:347–70

21. Grier SA, Brumbaugh A. 1999. Noticing cultural differences: advertising meanings created by the target and non-target markets. *J. Advert.* 28:79–93

22. Harvey P. 1999. *Let Every Child Be Wanted: How Social Marketing Is Revolutionizing Contraceptive Use Around the World.* Westport, CT: Auburn House

23. Hastings G. 2003a. Competition in social marketing. *Soc. Mark. Q.* IX:6–10

24. Hastings G. 2003b. Relational paradigms in social marketing. *J. Macromark.* 23:6–15

25. Hastings G, Donovan RJ. 2002. International initiatives: introduction and overview. *Soc. Mark. Q.* 8:3–5

26. Hastings G, MacFadyen L, Anderson S. 2000. Whose behavior is it anyway? The broader potential of social marketing. *Soc. Mark. Q.* VI:46–58

27. Hastings G, Saren M. 2003. The critical contribution of social marketing: theory and application. *Mark. Theory* 3:305–22

28. Hill R. 2001. The marketing concept and health promotion: a survey and analysis of "recent health promotion" literature. *Soc. Mark. Q.* 2:29–53

29. Hornik RC. 2002. *Public Health Communication: Evidence for Behavior Change.* Mahwah, NJ: Erlbaum

30. Inst. Med. 2003. *The Future of the Public's Health in the 21st Century.* Washington, DC: Natl. Acad. Press

31. Jooste PL, Marks AS, van Erkom Schurink C. 1995. Factors influencing the availability of iodised salt in South Africa. *S. Afr. J. Food Sci. Nutr.* 7:49–52

32. Rothschild ML, Mastin B, Karsten C, Miller T. 2003. The Road Crew final report: a demonstration of the use of social marketing to reduce alcohol-impaired driving by individuals age 21 through 34. *Wis. Dep.* *Transp. Tech. Rep.*, Madison, Wis., http://www.dot.wisconsin.gov/library/publications/topic/safety/roadcrew.pdf

33. Kennedy MG, Mizuno Y, Seals BF, Myllyluoma J, Weeks-Norton K. 2000. Increasing condom use among adolescents with coalition-based social marketing. *AIDS* 14:1809–18

34. Kotler P, Roberto N, Lee N. 2002. *Social Marketing: Improving the Quality of Life.* Thousand Oaks, CA: Sage

35. Lefebvre C, Bryant CA. 2004. An interview with R. Craig Lefebvre. *Soc. Mark. Q.* 10:17–30

36. Maibach EW, Rothschild M, Novelli W. 2002. Social marketing. In *Health Behavior and Health Education: Theory, Research, and Practice*, ed. K Glanz, B Rimer, FM Lewis, pp. 437—61. Indianapolis, IN: Jossey-Bass

37. Marks AS, Greathead D. 1994. *The application of social marketing to the design of a programme aimed at fostering TB compliance.* Presented at Tuberculosis–Towards 2000 Int. Conf., Pretoria, South Africa

38. McDermott RJ. 2000. Social marketing: a tool for health education. *Am. J. Health Behav.* 24:6–10

39. McDermott RJ. 2003. Essentials of evaluating social marketing campaigns for health behavior change. *Health Educ. Monogr. Ser.* 20:31–38

40. McDivitt J. 2003. Is there a role for branding in social marketing. *Soc. Mark. Q.* IX:11–17

41. Minkler M, Wallerstein NB. 2002. Improving health through community organization and community building. In *Health Behavior and Health Education: Theory, Research, and Practice*, ed. BRK Glanz, FM Lewis, pp. 279–311. San Francisco, CA: Jossey-Bass

42. Mong Y, Kaiser R, Ibrahim D, Rasoatiana Razifimbololona L, Quick RE. 2001. Impact of the safe water system on water quality in cyclone-affected communities in Madagascar. *Am. J. Public Health* 91:1577–79

43. Novelli W. 1996. SMQ centerpiece: an interview with William D. Novelli. *Social Mark. Q* III:27–50

44. Peattie S, Peattie K. 2003. Ready to fly solo? Reducing social marketing's dependence on commercial marketing theory. *Mark. Theory* 3:365–85

45. Potter LD, Duke JC, Nolin MJ, Judkins D, Huhman M. 2004. Evaluation of the CDC VERB campaign: findings from the Youth Media Campaign Longitudinal Survey, 2002–2003. Rep. Contr. Number 200199900020, Rep. for U.S. Cent. Dis. Control Prev.

46. Prochaska JO, DiClemente CC. 1984. *The Transtheoretical Approach: Crossing the Traditional Boundaries of Therapy.* Homewood, IL: Dow Jones-Irwin

47. Rothschild ML. 1999. Carrots, sticks, and promises. *J. Mark.* 63:24–27

48. Siegel M, Doner L. 1998. *Marketing Public Health: Strategies to Promote Social Change.* Gaithersburg, MD: Aspen

49. Smith WA. 2000. Social marketing: an evolving definition. *Am. J. Health Behav.* 24:11–17

50. Smith WA. 2001. Ethics and the social marketer: a framework for practitioners. In *Ethics in Social Marketing*, ed. AR Andreasen, pp. 1–16. Washington, DC: Georgetown Univ. Press

51. Smith WA. 2002. Social marketing and its contribution to a modern synthesis of social change. *Soc. Mark. Q.* VIII:46–50

52. Wallack L. 2002. Public health, social change, and media advocacy. *Soc. Mark. Q.* VIII:25–31

53. Walsh DC, Rudd RE, Moeykens BA, Moloney TW. 1993. Social marketing for public health. *Health Aff.* Summer:104–19

54. Williams JD, Kumanyika S. 2002. Is Social Marketing an Effective Tool to Reduce Health Disparities? *Soc. Mark. Q.* 3:14–31

55. Williams PG. 1999. Social marketing to eliminate leprosy in Sri Lanka. *Soc. Mark. Q.* 4:27–31

56. Wong F, Huhman M, Heitzler C, Asbury L, Bretthauer-Mueller R, et al. 2003. VERB$_{TM}$—a social marketing campaign to increase physical activity among youth. *Prev. Chron. Dis.* 1:http://www.cdc.gov/pcd/

Annu. Rev. Public Health 2005. 26:341–65
doi: 10.1146/annurev.publhealth.26.021304.144708
Copyright © 2005 by Annual Reviews. All rights reserved
First published online as a Review in Advance on August 18, 2004

URBAN HEALTH: Evidence, Challenges, and Directions

Sandro Galea and David Vlahov

*Center for Urban Epidemiologic Studies, New York Academy of Medicine, and
Department of Epidemiology, Joseph T. Mailman School of Public Health, Columbia
University, New York, NY 10029; email: sgalea@nyam.org; dvlahov@nyam.org*

Key Words multilevel, methods, social epidemiology, cities, mechanisms

■ **Abstract** Urbanization is one of the most important demographic shifts world-wide during the past century and represents a substantial change from how most of the world's population has lived for the past several thousand years. The study of urban health considers how characteristics of the urban environment may affect population health. This paper reviews the empirical research assessing urban living's impact on population health and our rationale for considering the study of urban health as a distinct field of inquiry. The key factors affecting health in cities can be considered within three broad themes: the physical environment, the social environment, and access to health and social services. The methodologic and conceptual challenges facing the study of urban health, arising both from the limitations of the research to date and from the complexities inherent in assessing the relations among complex urban systems, disease causation, and health are discussed.

INTRODUCTION

Urbanization is likely the single most important demographic shift worldwide during the past century and in the new century, and it represents a sentinel change from how most of the world's population has lived for the past several thousand years (83). Current estimates suggest that the trend toward an urbanizing world will continue well into the twenty-first century (15). At the beginning of the nineteenth century only 5% of the world's population was living in urban areas. By the end of the century, about 46% of the world's population was living in urban areas (15, 49). There are ~50,000 urban areas in the world today and almost 400 cities containing a population of one million people or more (110). Around 1940, the New York metropolitan area became the first urban area to become a megacity containing more than 10 million inhabitants. Today there are more than 15 megacities worldwide (109, 110). Overall global population growth in the next 30 years will be primarily in cities. Current projections suggest that more than half the world's population will be living in urban areas by 2007 and that nearly two thirds of the world's population will live in urban areas within the next 30 years. By 2010, approximately 4000 million people will live in urban centers worldwide (49).

We might expect such a shift in how the majority of the world's population lives to have health implications. Indeed, researchers, both in the popular press and in the academic literature, have long been interested in cities and how they may affect the public's health. Writers from several eras in western European history considered cities as places that were detrimental to health, and in many ways, for much of history, cities were, in fact, characterized by features that were unquestionably linked to poor health. Charles Dickens's novels detail and offer insights into the difficulties of city life in the nineteenth century (22). As cities assumed a greater role in the life of European countries, population density, numbers of marginalized populations, pollution, and crime frequently increased, resulting, in many countries, in worse health in cities than outside of cities (76, 115). Multiple writers, commentators, and social theorists observed the problems endemic to these growing cities and suggested that the cities themselves had a role in shaping individual well-being (25, 26, 28, 80).

However, whereas writers in the eighteenth and nineteenth centuries overwhelmingly noted a connection between the urban context and poor health, the urban environment in many Western cities improved dramatically at the turn of the twentieth century, and coincident with this sanitary awakening, the health of urban populations improved. One historical analysis showed that, although for much of the nineteenth century infant mortality rates in Imperial Germany were higher in urban areas than they were in nonurban areas, there was a dramatic improvement in infant mortality rates in urban areas starting in the 1870s, which preceded a comparable decline in mortality in the rest of the country (126). This analysis suggested that improvements in the urban environment were responsible for this rapid improvement in infant health in Imperial Germany and that this pattern was typical of the pattern observed at around the same time in many European industrialized societies (112). Today, in many countries, including the United States, aggregate health, as measured by life expectancy, all-cause mortality, and many other health indicators, is actually better in many urban areas than it is in nonurban areas (102).

What then is urban health, and why should we concern ourselves with urban health as a specific subject of inquiry? As urban living becomes the predominant social context for most of the world's population, the very ubiquity of urban living promises both to shape health directly and indirectly to affect what we typically consider risk factors or determinants of population health. Therefore, despite the truism that the urban context inherently shapes population health in cities, not all public health is urban health. We consider urban health research to be the explicit investigation of the relation between the urban context and population distribution of health and disease. Urban health, then, concerns itself with the determinants of health and diseases in urban areas and with the urban context itself as the exposure of interest. As such, defining the evidence and research direction for urban health requires that researchers and public health professionals pay attention to theories and mechanisms that may explain how the urban context may affect health and to methods that can better illustrate the relation between the urban context and health. To that end, in this review we first discuss what we mean when considering urban areas; then we address potential mechanisms that can explain the relation between the urban context and health. We discuss particular challenges in the study of urban health and conclude with directions for potential research and practice.

CITIES AND THEIR ROLE IN THE WORLD

As we discuss urban health, we are implicitly assuming that readers share an image of cities and urban areas. However, our personal experiences likely have shaped what we think of when we discuss "cities" and "urban areas." Saul Bellow, the novelist and Nobel Prize laureate, in discussing how Americans think of New York City, suggested, "That is perhaps like asking how Scotsmen feel about the Loch Ness monster. It is our legendary phenomenon, our great thing, our world-famous impossibility. . . .New York is stirring, insupportable, agitated, ungovernable, demonic. No single individual can judge it adequately" (11a). In academic discourse investigators have long disputed the definition of "urban" (45). Cities are not static, and the very density and diversity that characterize most cities make generalizations about defining cities difficult. We discuss below the implications of these definitional challenges for the empirical study of urban health. Meanwhile we can consider different types of cities using an example that all readers are likely familiar with.

Cities can be sprawling, diffuse, and automobile-dependent metropolitan areas. This has led to recent substantial academic discourse about urban sprawl (37). For example, in Atlanta, Georgia, the average person travels by car more than 34 miles each day, which is more than twice as many miles as people in Philadelphia, Pennsylvania, drive (121). Conversely cities can be small and compact, as are many old European cities like Venice. Cities can be unique, cosmopolitan places (e.g., Paris, Casablanca), but also they can look tremendously alike, as do any number of midsized North American cities (e.g., Kansas City, Denver). Cities frequently include both sophisticated and wealthy areas, featuring commercial and entertainment interests that are among the best in their country, as well as areas of extreme poverty and deprivation. For example, Rio de Janeiro has among the world's most expensive tourist resorts abutting on extremely poor favelas; in New York City, the Upper East Side and Harlem are adjacent neighborhoods that are among the richest and poorest neighborhoods respectively in the United States. Cities are generally the centers of commerce and culture in their countries and geographic regions. However, proximity to other cities frequently defines the range of opportunities available in a particular city. For example, a regional capital in a large, sparsely populated area, such as Whitehorse in Canada's Yukon territory, is likely to have more diverse cultural offerings and a greater range of health services available than would a comparable-sized city close to other, far larger, urban areas. Therefore, cities can represent diverse conditions within which people live and can represent a range of human experiences. Throughout the rest of this review we discuss how these diverse places may affect health and how the systematic study of urban health may afford opportunities to improve population health.

MECHANISMS OF DISEASE: WHY CITIES MAY SHAPE POPULATION HEALTH

How does the urban context affect health? In particular, what are the mechanisms by which cities can affect health? Before answering this question, a couple of considerations are in order. First, there is no one way in which the urban context may affect health. Although, for the sake of explication, we generally discuss mechanisms and health in general, frequently different mechanisms are important potential explanations for the relations between the urban context and different diseases. As we discuss potential mechanisms, we consider health as one construct but make reference to specific theoretical distinctions and empirical examples that suggest how various factors may be important in different ways for diverse conditions. Second, as we highlight in the preceding section, cities ultimately are geographic places. Although cities are not static, and in fact cities' dynamism is one of their defining features, considering health in cities is fundamentally the study of how a particular type of place may affect health. Explanations for these potential effects then rest primarily on how characteristics of places, in this case cities, may be important health determinants. Several characteristics of cities may be important health determinants, each having multiple implications for urban dwellers. Academic interest in urban health has waxed and waned over the past century; several authors at different time points have proposed frameworks for considering the relation between city living and health, and they have identified features of the urban context that may be particularly important for specific diseases (42, 73, 91, 124). Many of these frameworks build on work that discusses the social and economic determinants of better population health (31, 52, 61). We find it useful to think of three broad categories of theories and mechanisms that may explain how city living can affect health: the physical environment, the social environment, and the availability of and access to health and social services.

The Urban Physical Environment

The urban physical environment includes the built environment: the air city dwellers breathe, the water they drink, the indoor and outdoor noise they hear, the park land inside and surrounding the city, and the geological and climate conditions of the site where the city is located. McNeill has suggested that primarily what distinguished the twentieth century from previous ones, and cities from nonurban areas, is the degree to which humans have become the primary influence on the physical environment (84). Although the literature on the relation between features of the physical environment and health is vast, we consider here some of the primary evidence linking key features of the physical environment to health.

THE BUILT ENVIRONMENT   The human built environment can influence both physical and mental health; empirical evidence about the relation between the built environment and health conditions includes, among others, asthma and other respiratory conditions, injuries, psychological distress, and child development (30, 71, 92). As an example, Weich and colleagues in 2002 (129) demonstrated higher levels of resident depression in areas that had less desirable built environments. In a study of New Orleans neighborhoods, Cohen (20) found that the prevalence of gonorrhea infection was higher in neighborhoods with deteriorating built environments. Different aspects of the built environment have been linked to specific health outcomes. For example, specific features of the built environment, including density of development, mixed land uses, scale of streets, aesthetic qualities of place, and connectivity of street networks, may affect physical activity (54). In turn, low levels of physical activity are a well-established risk factor for cardiovascular disease and all-cause mortality in urban areas (23, 97). A substantial literature addresses the relation between housing and health (68, 122). Recent work has begun to differentiate the roles of the external and the internal built environment in shaping health (56). Urban design may also affect health behaviors, crime, and violence rates (12, 89, 108), suggesting close interactions among urban physical and social environments.

URBAN INFRASTRUCTURE, WATER, AND SANITATION   The urban infrastructure is a critical part of the physical environment and determines how a city provides water, disposes of garbage, and provides energy (85). Water scarcity and water pollution are serious urban problems, particularly in less-wealthy countries. Nearly 1.5 billion people lack safe drinking water, and at least 5 million deaths per year can be attributed to waterborne diseases (70). The relation between the urban infrastructure and health is shaped by different forces in established urban areas and in rapidly growing urban areas. In longstanding urban areas, the decline of an aging infrastructure, coupled with frequently declining municipal resources, may challenge cities' ability to continue to provide safe water and sanitation for urban residents. Breakdowns may increase, causing health problems related to water, sewage, or disposal of solid waste (44). In rapidly urbanizing areas, frequently in less wealthy countries, cities are often challenged to maintain an adequate fresh water supply to growing numbers of urban residents and to transport accumulating sewage and other waste. The World Health Organization (WHO) estimates that most urban populations in developing countries do not have access to proper sanitation (136). Inadequate provision for solid waste collection frequently results in contamination of water bodies, which, coupled with the population density inherent to cities, presents a substantial risk for spreading epidemics rapidly (6, 18, 109).

POLLUTION   In the first half of the twentieth century, air pollution in the United States increased steadily as industrialization progressed, industries and homes used coal for power and heat, and cars proliferated. Cities had worse pollution than did nonurban areas (84). In the second half of the century, however, and especially in the past 25 years, many forms of pollution decreased as coal was phased out, manufacturing plants moved to the suburbs or abroad, lead was banned from gasoline, and the automobile industry was forced to build cleaner cars. However, cities still generate close to 80% of global carbon dioxide emissions and account for three quarters of industrial wood use worldwide (93). As late as the mid-1990s, investigators estimate that air pollution contributed to 30,000–60,000 deaths per year in the United States (24, 106). Indoor and outdoor air pollution are thought to contribute to 3 million deaths globally a year, with 90% of these deaths being in less wealthy countries (136). Worldwide, atmospheric pollution is thought to affect more than a billion people, mostly in cities (29, 104).

ACCESS TO GREEN SPACE   Some of the earliest studies that considered the relation between the urban context and health emphasized the role of access to parks and green space, or lack thereof, in shaping the health of urban populations. Griscom's report about housing in New York City in 1845 suggested that a lifestyle filled with "animal and vegetable exhalations" in the countryside provided "prima facie proofs" of the superiority of living in the countryside (45, 46). Although it remains generally recognized that public green spaces make for a more pleasant living environment (73), the empirical literature evaluating the relation between green space and health remains limited. Recent work has shown that living in areas with walkable green spaces, as opposed to living in areas without walkable green spaces, was associated with greater likelihood of physical activity (14), higher functional status (50), lower cardiovascular disease risk (74), and longevity among the elderly, independent of personal characteristics (119, 120). As more multidisciplinary work in urban health develops, more experimental and observational studies likely will assess the role of green space and urban planning in promoting health.

URBAN CLIMATE   Highways and streets can pollute water through runoff, destroy green space, influence motor vehicle use and accident rates, and contribute to the urban heat sink, absorption of heat that can increase by several degrees the temperature in cities. On warm days, urban areas can be more than 5°F warmer than surrounding areas, an effect known as the urban heat island effect (37). This effect is primarily due to dark surfaces absorbing heat and the limited ability of urban areas (with relatively few trees) to cool the air through transpiration. Global climate change may exacerbate this effect. Heat is a concern in urban areas in several ways, and ambient air temperature has been associated with a large number of hospitalizations and deaths yearly (10, 78). Heat exposure may result in direct health effects, including syncope or heat exhaustion, or exacerbate existing health disorders. Excess heat in urban areas can also exacerbate pollution, as cooling equipment (e.g., air conditioners) is put into heavier use to compensate for rising urban temperatures (60). Particular groups may be most at risk of the effects of heat in urban areas. Epidemic heat-related deaths have been particularly pronounced among socioeconomically disadvantaged and socially isolated elderly persons (67, 113).

OTHER FEATURES OF THE URBAN PHYSICAL ENVIRONMENT   Several other aspects of the urban physical environment may have specific relations to human health, and a full review of all relevant features of the physical environment is beyond the scope of this chapter. However, we note that city structures like bridges and skyscrapers may be vulnerable to natural or manmade disasters, as recent earthquakes in Japan and Iran and the September 11, 2001 terrorist attacks on New York City demonstrate, respectively. Features of the urban social environment, such as population density and social contagion, coupled with these vulnerable urban structures, can result in substantial health consequences after disasters in urban areas (39, 111). Other threats to health in cities include hazardous waste landfills, often located in or near urban areas, which may be associated with risks of low birth weight, birth defects, and cancers (127). Noise exposure, a common urban problem, may contribute to hearing impairment, hypertension, and ischemic heart disease (96).

The Urban Social Environment

The social environment has been broadly defined to include ". . .occupational structure, labor markets, social and economic processes, wealth, social, human, and health services, power relations, government, race relations, social inequality, cultural practices, the arts, religious institutions and practices, and beliefs about place and community" (9). This definition, by its very complexity, suggests that there are multiple ways in which the urban social environment may affect health. Building on the extant theoretical and empirical literature we consider here five features of the urban social environment that may be particularly important determinants of health in cities. Although these concepts have, in large part, arisen from sociological theory, many of them have been increasingly integrated into public health thinking that explores the relation between contextual characteristics and health.

SOCIAL DISORGANIZATION/STRAIN   Social disorganization theory was first developed in studies of urban crime by sociologists in Chicago in the 1920s and 1930s. In brief, social order, stability, and integration are conducive to conformity, whereas disorder is conducive to crime and poor integration into social structures (114). A parallel theory, frequently referred to as anomie/strain theory, suggests similar explanations for the relations between social structure and behavior. Drawing on the work of Durkheim (26), Merton suggested that anomie is the lack of societal integration, which arises from the tension between aspirations of industrialized persons and the means available to them to achieve those aspirations (86). In the urban context in particular, the exposure of persons of all social classes to high aspirations that are practically unachievable produces strain or pressure on these groups to take advantage of whatever effective means to income and success they can find, even if these means are illegitimate or illegal. Hence, Merton argued that social strain can be associated with crime. Contemporary anomie/strain theories suggest that other sources of strain in modern living, including confrontation with unpleasant stimuli, may be associated both with deviant behavior and with poor health (5, 19). A substantial body of research has established a relation between stress and social strain and mental and physical health (e.g., 27, 72, 98), and newer work has posited that features of the urban neighborhood context are associated with social strain and adverse health behaviors (13, 40).

SOCIAL RESOURCES   Separate from social strain, individual social experiences also may be important determinants of health in cities. For example, limited social support may predispose persons to poorer coping and adverse health (63, 82). Scant evidence exists that social connectedness in cities is better or worse than in nonurban areas. Informal social ties are an important feature of city living that ultimately affect social support, network, and cohesion (38). Social capital effects, including manifestations at the contextual level (e.g., at the level of the whole city or of urban neighborhoods) and at the social network level, are thought to offer both general economic and social support on an ongoing basis and also make specific resources available at times of stress (63). Social capital is often defined in terms of features of social organization and is associated with lower all-cause mortality (65, 116), reduced violent crime (66), and self-reported health (118) among other health outcomes. In the context of cities, the greater spatial proximity of one's immediate network may well accentuate the role of networks in shaping health. Social networks are associated, importantly, with a range of health behaviors (58, 79).

SOCIAL CONTAGION   Social learning theory emphasizes the importance of observing and modeling the behaviors and attitudes of others (8). This is particularly the case in densely populated areas where there are several persons on whom behavior can be modeled to determine behavior. In diverse urban settings, social learning can set both social norms and norms for social network behaviors. Similarly, theories of collective socialization emphasize the influence of the group on the individual (21, 134). These theories suggest that persons who are in positions of authority or influence in specific areas can affect norms and behavior of others in direct and indirect ways. One of the concepts that is linked to social learning that may have substantial implications for public health is contagiousness. Models of biological contagion, particularly in the context of infectious disease, are well established. For example, in recent years, group practices and social norms have been considered particularly important in transmission of sexually transmitted diseases and the transmission of human immunodeficiency virus (HIV) (101, 130). Newer theories include the possibility of contagiousness of ideas and social examples. In epidemiology it is understood that all things being equal, urban populations, characterized by high population density are at higher risk of transmission of biological organisms. Also, because concentrated urban populations share common resources (e.g., water) the practices of one group can affect the health of others. These observations may be extended to behavior and to health. For example, media representations of suicide may have some influence on the suicide of those exposed to them such that suicide becomes more likely (100). Several studies have provided both theoretical and empirical reasons to suggest that media representations of suicide could have some influence on a person's suicidality (35). In the urban context, the concentrated proximity of persons and sources of information may be a crucible for the exacerbation of this effect.

SPATIAL SEGREGATION   Spatial segregation of different racial/ethnic and socioeconomic groups also may be an important determinant of health in cities. Many cities worldwide are highly segregated with multiple historical, logistical, and practical barriers to mixing social groups. In their seminal work of mental disorder in urban areas, Faris & Dunham (32) describe a Chicago that had concentric circles wherein dwelled distinct groups whose social status was relatively unchanged even with migration of populations over time. Spatial segregation can have multiple effects, including the enforcement of homogeneity in resources and social network ties, suppressing diversity that may benefit persons of lower socioeconomic status. Persons who live in segregated communities may have disproportionate exposure, susceptibility, and response to economic and social deprivation, toxic substances, and hazardous conditions (132). One study of infectious disease transmission suggested that residential segregation contributes to the transmission of tuberculosis through concentrated poverty. Urban characteristics such as dilapidated housing and inadequate access to health care in turn are associated with concentrated poverty in cities (1). Racial segregation also may affect health through its influence on access to health care services. Segregated communities frequently face shortages of health care providers and disproportionately low rates of health insurance; both factors are among the most important predictors of differential access to medical care (81). More segregated communities may have lower levels of social capital, which, as discussed above, has been associated with poor health (64). Also, spatial heterogeneity permits persons of higher socioeconomic status to appreciate the issues faced by others and to use their power, money, and prestige to influence the development of better distributed salutary resources. Conversely, it is worth noting that spatial segregation, by virtue of keeping persons who are different apart from one another, may serve to minimize social strain (107).

INEQUALITY   Although it is related to many of the other features of the urban social environment discussed here, the particular role of inequality as a potential determinant of health in urban areas is worth noting briefly. Although there is ample evidence for the relation between poor individual and group socioeconomic status and health (4), in the urban context, rich and poor populations live in physically proximate neighborhoods. We do not consider disadvantage per se a hallmark of urban areas because in many instances aggregate wealth in cities is greater than it is in nonurban areas, but rather it is the relative proximity of rich and poor that is a common characteristic of cities worldwide. Empirical and theoretical work suggests that this inequality in the distribution of income and other resources may, in and of itself, shape health through multiple mechanisms. Ecologic evidence has long suggested that countries with more egalitarian distribution of income have lower mortality rates (103). In the early 1990s, a series of publications spurred further interest in the role of income distribution as an area-level determinant of health (131). Recent empirical evidence, although controversial, suggests that inequalities in income distribution contribute to health differentials between states and cities (62, 77, 105). The principal proponents of the hypothesized relation between income distribution and health suggest that perceived and actual inequity, caused by the discrepancies in income distribution, erode social trust and diminish the social capital that shapes societal well-being and individual health (65). Therefore, inequalities in urban areas may be important modifiers of the role of several other features of the social environment discussed here.

Health and Social Services

The relation between provision of health and social services and urban living is complicated and varies between cities and countries. In wealthy countries, cities are characterized by a rich array of health and social services (17, 33). Even the poorest urban neighborhood often has dozens of social agencies, each having a distinct mission and providing different services. Many of the health successes in urban areas in the past two decades, including reductions in HIV transmission, teen pregnancy rates, tuberculosis control, and new cases of childhood lead poisoning, have depended in part on the efforts of these groups (36). In addition, many urban areas serve as referral centers for surrounding communities, and as such there is often greater availability of health and social services in urban areas. In general there are far fewer physicians and hospitals in nonurban areas, and the travel time to health care providers is greater than in nonurban areas (94).

However, as previously discussed, many cities are characterized by sharp disparities in wealth between relatively proximate neighborhoods (131). These disparities are often associated with disparities in the availability and quality of care (7, 128). The presence of well-equipped, lucrative practice opportunities in the same city decreases the likelihood that service providers will work in lower-paid, public service clinics, particularly when these latter services face limited resources and wavering political commitment (34). Also, low-income urban residents continue to face significant obstacles in finding health care both in wealthy and less-wealthy countries (57). In the U.S. context, persons with lower socioeconomic status are more likely to lack health insurance coverage (48, 133). In turn, uninsured persons face barriers to care, receive poor quality care, and are more likely than are insured persons to use emergency systems (87). Recent immigrants, homeless people, inmates released from jail or prison, all disproportionately represented in urban areas, also face specific obstacles in obtaining health care (3, 51, 53, 59). In turn, these populations put a burden on health systems not adequately funded or prepared to care for them. Social services for disadvantaged or marginalized populations are often susceptible to changing municipal fiscal realities with the resultant decrease in service frequently coinciding with times of greater need in the urban population (33). In the past few years, for example, the decline in the national economy and tax revenues has forced many cities and states to reduce services at the very time unemployment, homelessness, and hunger are increasing (95). Internationally, several studies have highlighted the potential inadequacies of health systems in preventing and treating conditions such as malaria, dengue, and tuberculosis, spread of which is facilitated by high-density living characteristic of cities (69, 88, 117).

In summary, multiple mechanisms may explain how cities affect mental health, with different mechanisms being potentially important for different morbidities. Indeed, a big picture perspective on the relation between the urban context and health would suggest that these relations are undoubtedly complicated and that any single analysis that isolates a feature of urban living and health is just scratching the surface. Whereas specific features of cities may affect specific diseases adversely, other features may offer protection. Interrelationships between features of the urban environment further make generalization difficult. For example, further refinements on social strain theory in urban areas include an appreciation of the fact that in urban areas persons with different socioeconomic statuses may be differentially faced with stressors and have varying levels of access to resources that may help them cope with stressors. In particular, in urban areas, formal local resources can complement or substitute for individual or family resources for transient urban populations. Therefore, the relation between urban stressors and health is likely buffered by salutary resources (e.g., health care, social services) that are oftentimes more prevalent in urban compared with nonurban areas (41). Although these resources may be available to urban residents, socioeconomic disparities in cities are linked to differential access to these resources, which suggests that persons at different ends of the socioeconomic spectrum may have different opportunities to benefit from the resources available in cities.

INTERNATIONAL CONSIDERATIONS

In considering the mechanisms that may explain the relations between the urban context and health, we refer to potential differences in the role of certain mechanisms cross-nationally. This point is worth emphasizing, particularly in light of the varying pace of urbanization worldwide. The pace of urbanization is projected to differ by region of the world and by initial city size. In particular, most global population growth in the coming decades will occur in less wealthy regions of the world, with the most rapid pace of growth expected to occur in Asia and Africa (49). Although North America and Europe are currently the most urbanized regions, the number of urban dwellers in the least urbanized region, Asia, in 2000 was already greater than the urban population in North America and Europe combined. The proportion of people living in megacities is expected to rise from 4.3% of the global population in 2000 to 5.2% in 2015 (123). The growth rate of megacities in the developing world will be much higher. For example the anticipated growth rate for Calcutta, India, between 2000 and 2015 is 1.9%, compared with an anticipated growth rate of 0.4% for New York City, United States (15, 123). However, whereas the growth of large cities in developing countries will account for approximately one fifth of the increase in the world's population, small cities will account for almost half of this increase (109). A growing number of relatively small cities throughout the world will contain most of the world's population in the twenty-first century, and most of the growth in cities will take place in less wealthy countries.

Therefore, the relative importance of characteristics of the urban environment that may affect health may vary substantially in different cities and in different parts of the world. For example, in many rapidly growing urban areas in the developing world, lack of safe water and poor sanitation are likely to account for a greater proportion of the morbidity and mortality in a specific city than are all other factors identified here. As cities become more established, an aging infrastructure can threaten health and growing inequalities, and social strains can influence both health behaviors and access to resources. In addition, the course of urbanization in different cities worldwide may have different implications for health. A newly urbanizing city is likely to be under different and probably more substantial strains than is a long-established urban area. Therefore, when considering how cities may affect health it is important for the public health researcher or practitioner to consider both place, i.e., the particulars of a given city, and time, i.e., the trajectory of urbanization in a particular city. There are no simple solutions summarizing the relations between the different factors that can affect health in various countries. Rather, specific investigations and interventions would do well to bear in mind the relevant local and temporal context that may guide an appreciation of relevant and salient risk determination in a given urban area.

CHALLENGES IN THE STUDY OF URBAN HEALTH

Defining Cities and Urbanization

Given the growing preponderance of cities and the increasing contribution of urban populations to the world's total population, one might expect that our enumeration of "urban dwelling" populations is based on a universally agreed upon definition of "urbanization" and "urban." However, and perhaps unfortunately for the current science, there are multiple and inconsistent definitions of both urbanization and urban. An appreciation of this complication is essential to understanding how urbanization may affect human health. It is generally accepted that urbanization is the process of becoming urban, and it reflects aggregate population growth in cities, be it through natural population increase or migration. By contrast, different authors have used terms such as urbanism or urbanicity to refer to the inhabitation of human populations in concentrated areas at a given point in time.

Wirth (135), in his seminal essay "Urbanism as a way of life," suggested three distinct characteristics of urban areas: size, density, and heterogeneity of populations. Although this definition may be intuitive, and indeed most authors would consider this definition valid, there are multiple practical barriers to the quantification of what an urban area is that can then be applied to research or practice. The fundamental problem is that no definition of urban places has been universally adopted by national governments, and as such, multiple, inconsistent definitions of urban are used by different countries.

The U.S. Bureau of the Census (16) defines an urbanized area in the following way: "An urbanized area comprises a place and the adjacent densely settled surrounding territory that together comprise a minimum population of 50,000 people. . . . The 'densely settled surrounding territory' adjacent to the place consists of territory made up of one or more contiguous blocks having a population density of at least 1000 people per square mile." However, this definition raises a number of questions and is substantially different from the definition employed in other countries. Among 228 countries on which the United Nations has data, about half use administrative definitions of urban (e.g., living in the capital city), 51 use size and density, 39 use functional characteristics (e.g., economic activity), 22 have no definition of urban, and 8 define all (e.g., Singapore) or none (e.g., Polynesian countries) of their population as urban (15). These official statistics (i.e., all the statistics above) rely on country-specific designations and do not use a uniform definition of urban. In specific instances, definitions of urban in adjacent countries vary tremendously. For example, the Bolivian definition of urban includes localities containing 2000 or more inhabitants. In neighboring Peru, populated centers with 100 or more dwellings grouped contiguously and administrative centers of districts are considered urban. Therefore, global statistics on urbanization depend on international definitional differences that may be a function of statistical or historical precedent and, in some cases, political expedience. Ultimately, compounding these difficulties, definitions of urban have changed over time in different countries, and these different definitions are frequently embedded in calculations about changing urban proportions.

In addition to challenges in defining an urban area, the definition of urbanization also is complicated by multiple considerations in how to assess "population growth in cities." Urbanization, at its simplest level, may be calculated as the change in the proportion of the national population that is urban. However, this change in proportion is dependent both on the urban population growth and on the relative growth of the rest of the country. There are different implications for countries and cities where urbanization is driven by rural-urban migration or international migration compared with other countries where urbanization is driven largely by natural growth of cities. Together with changing urban proportions, changes in the absolute number of urban residents are also meaningful. Thus, although countries of vastly different sizes can share urbanization rates, these urbanization rates can represent vastly different absolute numbers of urban residents. Also, the percent of national growth influenced by growth in urban areas ultimately is reliant on the change of the overall national population. Thus, net urban growth is again differently meaningful in the context of larger and smaller countries.

Specification of the Research Question in Urban Health

Clear specification of a research question is the necessary first step in all etiologic research and is often one of the hardest steps. One of the greatest challenges in the study of urban health is in adequate specification of research questions that address how and why the urban context may affect health. Three primary reasons exemplify why the specification of a research question may be particularly challenging in urban health. First, much of what may be considered urban health research in the literature thus far has arisen from different disciplines, using different theoretical frameworks and applying disciplinary orientations and terminologies. For example, in demography and epidemiology, research into the role of urbanization in shaping health may focus on how population change in cities, resulting from migration and population growth, may influence the distribution of diseases (e.g., 99, 137). In contrast, the study of urbanization in sociology may focus on social activities and social organization in cities and their association with changing behaviors and consequences thereof. In considering how urban living may affect health, the study of changing urban population size and how individuals acquire different urban lifestyles is important. Although both arguably are features associated with changing cities, they may lend distinct understandings to health and health behavior. Second, many questions in urban health research do not meaningfully exist in isolation. Understanding how the urban context affects health requires consideration of multiple, often competing, influences. Continuing to consider the example of urbanization, different disciplines might study various aspects of urbanization that potentially exert varying effects on population health. This interdependence of research questions complicates the empirical task of assessing how cities may affect health. Specification of relevant research questions must at least acknowledge, if not take into account, the interrelated processes that ultimately determine health in cities. Third, as is the case with all research, clear specification of a research question rests, at least implicitly, on the acknowledgment of a theoretical framework that suggests how and why the characteristics of interest may affect health. The absence of such a framework in the study of urban health complicates the specification of research questions in the field, as well as the interpretation of research findings.

Complexity of Causation in the Urban Context

As discussed at various points in this chapter, cities are complex communities of heterogeneous individuals, and multiple factors may be important determinants of population health in cities. For example, understanding the role that racial/ethnic heterogeneity plays in shaping the health of urban populations requires an understanding of the role of segregation in restricting access to resources in urban neighborhoods (2) as well as the potential for greater tolerance of racial/ethnic differences in cities compared with nonurban areas. Assessing how the urban context may affect health raises challenges and introduces complexity that is often not easily addressed through the application of simple analytic methods.

In addition, cities are different from one another and may change over time. Empirical inquiry in health presupposes that identifiable factors influence health, and these factors can be identified (and potentially intervened upon). Typically, public health studies imply, for example, that we can generalize about how different foods will affect health across individuals, at least within the confines of effect modification across groups (e.g., age groups) or under different circumstances (e.g., at different levels of caloric intake). However, cities are characterized by multiple factors (e.g., population density, heterogeneity) that in many ways make each city unique. The complexity of cities and of city living may mean that urban characteristics important in one city may not be important in other cities, limiting the generalizations that can be drawn about how urban living influences health. Further complicating this task is the fact that cities change over time, and this change has implications for the relative contribution of different factors in determining health in cities. For example, municipal taxation of alcohol and cigarettes may control alcohol and cigarette consumption in a particular city at one point in time (47). However, changing social norms around smoking and alcohol use may either obviate or reinforce the influence of taxation. As such, in considering urban characteristics that affect health it may be important to note both the prevailing context within which such characteristics operate and that the role of these characteristics may change over time.

Choice of Appropriate Study Design

A broad array of methods in multiple disciplines have been used to address questions that pertain to urban health. In general, three types of published studies attempt to address somewhat different questions relevant to urban health: studies comparing rural and urban communities, studies comparing cities within countries or across countries, and studies examining intraurban variations in health.

Studies comparing rates and prevalence of morbidity and mortality in urban and rural areas are likely the most common, although they have become less common in recent years. These studies typically contrast several urban areas with rural areas in the same country or consider morbidity and mortality in urban versus nonurban areas; investigators frequently define the latter as all areas that do not meet urban criteria. Such urban-rural or urban-nonurban comparisons are useful to draw attention to particular features of urban areas that may be associated with health and that merit investigation. However, these studies are limited in their ability to shed light on what these features may be and on how urban areas may affect residents' health. That different urban-rural comparisons have provided conflicting evidence about the relative burden of disease in urban and nonurban areas is not surprising. Changing conditions within cities over time and differences in living conditions between cities suggest that these studies provide, at best, a crude snapshot of how the mass of urban living conditions at one point in time may affect population health.

The second type of study that attempts to address how cities affect health involves comparisons of health between cities, either within a country or between countries. Using the city itself as the key unit of analysis, these studies compare different cities to reach conclusions about urban characteristics associated with health. In comparing health between cities, these studies contribute to investigators' ability to discern features of cities that may promote or negatively affect population health. This research may suggest city-level practices that are amenable to intervention that could improve population health. Most saliently, these studies serve to highlight urban characteristics that, at least at the macro level, may be important determinants of urban health. However, by considering the city as the unit of analytic interest, these studies implicitly assume that aggregate behaviors or characteristics at the city level are equally important for all residents of those cities. This view limits to an analysis of city-wide characteristics that may or may not affect all urban residents equally the consideration of how cities may affect the health of urban residents.

The third group of studies that has contributed to our understanding of how city living may affect health is not frequently conceived of by researchers as studies of urban health per se. This group of studies has become more common in the past decade and often has included studies of how living in particular urban communities may be associated with health. Most commonly, these studies focus on spatial groupings of individuals (typically conceived of as neighborhoods, although several studies assess the contribution of administrative groupings that are not necessarily meaningful to residents as neighborhoods) and typically consider the impact of one's community of residence within an urban area on an individual's health. Relatively fewer studies have considered how membership in other urban communities, particularly social networks, may be associated with behavior and health (e.g., 72). Although these studies contribute important insights into urban conditions and their implications for health, they may be difficult to generalize to other cities or, more broadly, to urban areas. That is, the observation in one study that the quality of neighborhood sidewalks is associated with the likelihood of physical activity among urban residents may not necessarily be relevant in another urban context in which fear of assault is an important determinant of outdoor activity.

Therefore, different study designs can fruitfully address different questions that may be important to urban health. Unfortunately, results from these studies are frequently conflated, and the appreciable but nuanced differences in conclusions that can be drawn from different studies are not used to guide hypothesis generation to further urban health inquiry. Clear specification of the research question, coupled with appropriately choosing a study design, can point to inquiry and intervention in urban health.

A Common Language for Urban Health

The complexity of causation and the diversity of mechanisms that may explain how characteristics of the urban environment may affect the health of urban populations suggest that cross-disciplinary work is needed to improve our understanding, both general and specific, of the role urban context plays in shaping population health. Theoretically informed efforts that combine the perspectives of different traditions or disciplines, that use quantitative and qualitative methods when appropriate, and that apply theoretically driven sampling strategies are more likely to provide answers to questions about both how and why characteristics of urban living may affect health. Quantitative and qualitative methods may inform each other and help minimize the extent to which a priori decisions about conceptual frameworks may shape both the hypothesis being tested and the answers obtained from such inquiries. However, the isolation of academic disciplines from one another often means that there is little shared vocabulary between disciplines and that researchers and practitioners schooled in different academic traditions face considerable challenges when working together.

We suggested previously that the study of urban health may benefit from being constituted as a discipline by bringing together expertise and interests from academics and practitioners with complementary skills (125). Absent such a radical solution, many encouraging signs show that interest is growing in urban health as a cogent field of inquiry. Papers offering frameworks for the study of urban health have recently increased (42, 91, 124), as has the formation of cross-disciplinary meetings dedicated to urban health (11, 43). Also, public health practitioners and researchers have developed specific training programs and institutes aimed at teaching students skills from multiple disciplines (e.g., urban planning, epidemiology) that are relevant to the study of urban health. Meanwhile, international projects, particularly the Healthy Cities movement sponsored by the WHO, are working directly with local governments to promote health in cities. Most of the work of the Healthy Cities movement thus far has been in high-income countries, although more recently, the WHO supported Healthy City projects in low-income countries. In the first evaluation of these projects, evidence showed that key stakeholders had an improved understanding of the role of the urban environment in shaping health but had limited political will to act on this awareness (55). Although success of the Healthy Cities movement remains difficult to assess, it represents a worldwide effort to raise awareness among key decision makers about the role of cities in shaping health, potentially setting the stage for local interventions. All these efforts will be necessary eventually to guide public health training, research, and efforts to improve health in complex urban areas.

DIRECTIONS FOR URBAN HEALTH RESEARCH
AND PRACTICE

Throughout this review we consider the study of urban health inquiry into how features of the urban context may affect the health of populations. We also identify substantial challenges that may complicate urban health inquiry and practice. Moreover, we argue that the study of urban health lends itself to the creative application of methods from multiple disciplines and the nuanced appreciation of the role of multiple factors that may determine population health in cities. Despite this complexity, key factors can explicitly distinguish and guide the study and practice of urban health.

First, we need to consider whether there are specific features of the urban context that are causally related to health. Appropriate specification of the research question of interest is critical. For example, understanding how living in a city as a whole may affect smoking behavior requires a different set of tools than do questions about how intraurban differences in pollution affect variability in neighborhood prevalence of asthma. Similarly, understanding the quantitative relation between social capital in urban communities and resident well-being requires different tools than do questions about why social capital may have different implications for health in different communities or how social capital is produced or eroded in urban contexts.

Second, it is important to consider if these features are differentially distributed between urban and nonurban areas and within urban areas (e.g., between urban neighborhoods). As a corollary to this consideration, it becomes essential to consider the extent to which these features are unique to a particular city or differ between cities and, as such, to learn whether salutary features of the urban environment are adaptable in different contexts. For example, undoubtedly, much can be learned from well-studied urban areas in wealthy countries that can be applied to public health practice in less wealthy countries.

Third, identifying which characteristics of the urban context, and under which circumstances, are modifiable, is an important theoretical, empirical, public health question. In many ways the choice of an appropriate urban health framework may dictate, at least implicitly, the choice of both the question asked and the methods used in addressing the question. For example, a comprehensive framework that includes national-level policies that shape municipal financing may suggest that inquiry into and intervention on national policies may be of primary importance to urban health. In contrast, a framework that considers primarily physical characteristics of cities will address how features of the built environment at the local level can affect residents' health. Thus far, relatively little has been written about the processes through which the urban context may affect health and about further elucidation of these processes. A comprehensive appreciation of the processes that influence urban health can and should guide research and practice.

In conclusion, we note that although in this review we highlighted challenges inherent to the study of urban health, this work is informed by an appreciation for the potential of urban health inquiry. Although the study of urban health embeds substantial complexity, research with clearly specified research questions and appropriate study designs can help focus our appreciation of the relation between specific features of the urban context and health, both in specific cities and as generalizable to cities in national and international contexts. Recent methodologic advances, particularly the widespread acceptance of multilevel methods in public health research, have made it possible to test hypotheses about urban characteristics and their relation to specific health outcomes. Newer methods may eventually contribute to an improved understanding of the competing influences on the health of urban populations over time (75). Such research can inform local intervention and policies across urban areas. We hope that efforts such as this review, aimed to structure our thinking about cities and health, are helpful in stimulating both empirical and theoretical developments that can lead to improved health in cities worldwide.

ACKNOWLEDGMENTS

The authors thank Emily Gibble for editorial assistance. Funded in part by grant R01 DA 017642-01 from the National Institutes of Health and by grant U48/CCU 209663 from the Centers for Disease Control and Prevention.

The *Annual Review of Public Health* is online at
http://publhealth.annualreviews.org

LITERATURE CITED

1. Acevedo-Garcia D. 2000. Residential segregation and the epidemiology of infectious disease. *Soc. Sci. Med.* 51:1143–61

2. Acevedo-Garcia D, Lochner KA, Osypuk TL, Subramanian SV. 2003. Future directions in residential segregation and health research: a multilevel approach. *Am. J. Public Health* 93(2):215–21

3. Acosta O, Toro PA. 2000. Let's ask the homeless people themselves: a needs assessment based on a probability sample of adults. *Am. J. Community Psychol.* 28(3):343–66

4. Adler N, Newman K. 2002. Socioeconomic disparities in health: pathways and policies. Inequality in education, income, and occupation exacerbates the gaps between the health "haves" and "have-nots." *Health Aff.* 21(2):60–76

5. Agnew R. 1992. Foundation for a general strain theory of crime and delinquency. *Criminology* 30(1):47–87

6. Alexander SE, Ehrlich PR. 2000. Population and the environment. In *Earth Systems: Processes and Issues*, ed. WG Ernst, p. 341. Cambridge, UK: Cambridge Univ. Press

7. Andrulis DP. 2000. Community, service, and policy strategies to improve health care access in the changing urban environment. *Am. J. Public Health* 90:858–62

8. Bandura A. 1986. *Social Foundations of Thought and Action: A Social Cognitive Theory.* Engelwood Hills, NJ: Prentice-Hall

9. Barnett E, Casper M. 2001. A definition of "social environment." *Am. J. Public Health* 91(3):465

10. Basu R, Samet JM. 2002. Relation

between elevated ambient temperature and mortality: a review of the epidemiologic evidence. *Epidemiol. Rev.* 24:190–202

11. Bayoumi A, Hwang S. 2002. Methodological, practical, and ethical challenges to inner-city health research. *J. Urban Health* 79:S35–42

11a. Bellow S. 1970. World Famous Impossibility. *New York Times* Dec. 6:115

12. Berrigan D, Troiano RP. The association between urban form and physical activity in US adults. *Am. J. Prev. Med.* 23(2S):74–79

13. Boardman JD, Finch BK, Ellison CG, Williams DR, Jackson JS. 2001. Neighborhood disadvantage, stress, and drug use among adults. *J. Health Soc. Behav.* 42(2):151–65

14. Booth ML, Owen N, Bauman A, Clavisi O, Leslie E. 2000. Social-cognitive and perceived environment influences associated with physical activity in older Australians. *Prev. Med.* 31:15–22

15. Brockerhoff MP. 2000. An urbanizing world. *Popul. Bull.* 55(3):3–4

16. Bur. Census. 2002. *Qualifying urban areas for census 2000. Federal Register Part VII Department of Commerce.* http://www.census.gov/geo/www/ua/fdrgua2k.pdf

17. Casey MM, Thiede Call K, Klingner JM. 2001. Are rural residents less likely to obtain recommended preventive healthcare services? *Am. J. Prev. Med.* 21(3):182–88

18. Chanthikul S, Qasim SR, Mukhopadhyay B, Chiang WW. 2004. Computer simulation of leachate quality by recirculation in a sanitary landfill bioreactor. *Environ. Sci. Health Part A Tox. Hazard Subst. Environ. Eng.* 39(2):493–505

19. Cohen DA, Farley TA, Mason K. 2003. Why is poverty unhealthy? Social and physical mediators. *Soc. Sci. Med.* 57(9):1631–41

20. Cohen DA, Spear S, Scribner R, Kissinger P, Mason K, Wildgen J. 2000. Broken windows and the risk of gonorrhea. *Am. J. Public Health* 90(2):230–36

21. Coleman JS. 1988. Social capital in the creation of human capital. *Am. J. Sociol.* 94(Suppl.):S95–120

22. Dickens C. 1850. *The Personal History and Experience of David Copperfield the Younger.* New York: Collier

23. Diez-Roux AV. 2003. Residential environments and cardiovascular risk. *J. Urban Health* 80(4):569–89

24. Dockery DW, Pope CA 3rd, Xu X, Spengler JD, Ware JH, et al. 1993. An association between air pollution and mortality in six U.S. cities. *N. Engl. J. Med.* 9:329(24):1753–59

25. Durant W, Durant A. 1967. *The Story of Civilization.* Vol. 10—*The Age of Rousseau.* New York: Simon and Schuster

26. Durkheim E. 1951. *Suicide; 1897.* Glencoe, IL: Free Press

27. Elliott M. 2000. The stress process in neighborhood context. *Health Place* 6:287–99

28. Engels F. 1887. *The Condition of the Working Class in England.* New York: Lovell

29. Environ. Software Serv. GmbH AUSTRIA. 2002. *Energy impact assessment.* http://www.ess.co.at/AIR-EIA/LECTURES/L001.html

30. Evans GW, Wells NM, Chan HY, Saltzman H. 2000. Housing quality and mental health. *J. Consult. Clin. Psychol.* 68(3):526–30

31. Evans RG, Stoddart GL. 1990. Producing health, consuming health care. *Soc. Sci. Med.* 31:1347–63

32. Faris REL, Dunham HW. 1939. *Mental Disorders in Urban Areas: An Ecological Study of Schizophrenia and Other Psychoses.* Chicago, IL: Univ. Chicago Press

33. Felt-Lisk S, McHugh M, Howell E. 2002. Monitoring local safety-net providers: Do they have adequate capacity? *Health Aff. (Millwood)* 21(5):277–83

34. Franks P, Fiscella K 2002. Effect of patient socioeconomic status on physician

profiles for prevention, disease management, and diagnostic testing costs. *Med. Care* 40(8):717–24

35. Frei A, Schenker T, Finzen A, Dittmann V, Kraeuchi K, et al. 2003. The Werther effect and assisted suicide. *Suicide Life Threat. Behav.* 33(2):192–200

36. Freudenberg N, Silver D, Carmona JM, Kass D, Lancaster B, et al. 2000. Health promotion in the city: a structured review of the literature on interventions to prevent heart disease, substance abuse, violence and HIV infection in US metropolitan areas, 1980–1995. *J. Urban Health* 77(3):443–57

37. Frumkin H. 2002. Urban sprawl and public health. *Public Health Rep.* 117:201–17

38. Fullilove MT. 1998. Promoting social cohesion to improve health. *J. Am. Med. Womens Assoc.* 53(2):72–76

39. Galea S, Ahern J, Resnick H, Kilpatrick D, Bucuvalas M, et al. 2002. Psychological sequelae of the September 11th attacks in Manhattan, New York City. *N. Engl. J. Med.* 346:982–87

40. Galea S, Ahern J, Vlahov D, Coffin PO, Fuller C, et al. 2003. Income distribution and risk of fatal drug overdose in New York City neighborhoods. *Drug Alcohol. Depend.* 70(2):139–48

41. Galea S, Factor SH, Bonner S, Foley M, Freudenberg N, et al. 2002. Collaboration among community members, local health service providers, and researchers in an urban research center in Harlem, New York. *Public Health Rep.* 116(6):530–39

42. Galea S, Freudenberg N, Vlahov D. 2005. Cities and population health. *Soc. Sci. Med.* In press

43. Galea S, Vlahov D, Sisco S. 2003. The second annual international conference on urban health. October 15–18, 2003. *J. Urban Health* 80(3)(Suppl. 1):II1–2

44. Garrett L. 2001. *Betrayal of Trust the Collapse of Global Public Health*. New York: Oxford Univ. Press

45. Glaab CN, Brown AT. 1976. *A History of Urban America*. Toronto, Canada: Macmillan

46. Griscom J. 1845. *Sanitary Condition of the Laboring Poplation of New York*. New York: Harper

47. Grossman M. 1989. Health benefits of increases in alcohol and cigarette taxes. *Br. J. Addict.* 84:1193–204

48. Grumbach K, Vranizan K, Bindman AB. 1997. Physician supply and access to care in urban communities. *Health Aff.* 16(1):71–86

49. Guidotti TL, de Kok T, Kjellstrom T, Yassi A. 2001. *Basic Environmental Health*. New York: Oxford Univ. Press

50. Guralnik JM, Seeman TE, Tinetti ME, Nevitt MC, Berkman LF. 1994. Validation and use of performance measures of functioning in a non-disabled older urban population: MacArthur studies of successful aging. *Aging* 6:410–19

51. Guttmacher S. 1984. Immigrant workers: health, law, and public policy. *J. Health Polit. Policy Law* 9(3):503–14

52. Hamilton N, Bhatti T. 1996. *Population Health Promotion: An Integrated Model of Population Health and Health Promotion*. Ottawa, Ontario, Canada: Health Promot. Dev. Div., Health Canada

53. Hammett TM, Gaiter JL, Crawford C. 1998. Reaching seriously at-risk populations: health interventions in criminal justice settings. *Health Educ. Behav.* 25(1):99–120

54. Handy SL, Boarnet MG, Ewing R, Killingsworth RE. 2002. How the built environment affects physical activity: views from urban planning. *Am. J. Prev. Med.* 23(2S):64–73

55. Harpham T, Burton S, Blue I. 2001. Healthy city projects in developing countries: the first evaluation. *Health Promot. Int.* 16(2):111–25

56. Hembree C, Galea S, Ahern J, Tracy M, Markham Piper T, et al. 2004. The built environment and overdose mortality in New York City neighborhoods. *Health & Place.* In Press

57. Hoffman M, Pick WM, Cooper D, Myers JE. 1997. Women's health status and use of health services in a rapidly growing peri-urban area of South Africa. *Soc. Sci. Med.* 45(1):149–57

58. Kafka RR, London P. 1991. Communication in relationships and adolescent substance use: the influence of parents and friends. *Adolescence* 26:587–98

59. Kalet A, Gany F, Senter L. 2002. Working with interpreters: an interactive Web-based learning module. *Acad. Med.* 77(9):927

60. Kalkstein LS. 1993. Direct impacts in cities. *Lancet* 342:1397–98

61. Kaplan GA. 1999. What is the role of the social environment in understanding inequalities in health? *Ann. N.Y. Acad. Sci.* 896:116–19

62. Kaplan GA, Pamuk ER, Lynch JW, Cohen RD, Balfour JL. 1996. Inequality in income and mortality in the United States: analysis of mortality and potential pathways. *Br. Med. J.* 312:999–1003

63. Kawachi I, Berkman LF. 2001. Social ties and mental health. *J. Urban Health* 78(3):458–67

64. Kawachi I, Kennedy BP, Glass R. 1999. Social capital and self-rated health: a contextual analysis. *Am. J. Public Health* 89(8):1187–93

65. Kawachi I, Kennedy BP, Lochner K, Prothrow-Stith D. 1997. Social capital, income inequality and mortality. *Am. J. Public Health* 87:1491–98

66. Kennedy BP, Kawachi I, Prothrow-Stith D, Lochner K, Gupta V. 1998. Social capital, income inequality, and firearm violent crime. *Soc. Sci. Med.* 47(1):7–17. Erratum. *Soc. Sci. Med.* 47(10):1637

67. Kilbourne EM, Choi K, Jones TS, Thacker SB. 1982. Risk factors for heatstroke. A case-control study. *JAMA* 25(247)(24):3332–36

68. Kingsley GT. 2003. Housing, health, and the neighborhood context. *Am. J. Prev. Med.* 24(3S):6–7

69. Knudsen AB, Slooff R. 1992. Vector-borne disease problems in rapid urbanization: new approaches in vector control. *Bull. World Health Organ.* 70(1):1–6

70. Krants D, Kifferstein B. 1998. *Water pollution and society.* http://www.umich.edu/~gs265/society/waterpollution.htm

71. Krieger J, Higgins DL. 2002. Housing and health: time again for public health action. *Am. J. Public Health* 92:758–68

72. Latkin CA, Curry AD. 2003. Stressful neighborhoods and depression: a prospective study of the impact of neighborhood disorder. *J. Health Soc. Behav.* 44(1):34–44

73. Lawrence RJ. 1999. Urban health: an ecological perspective. *Rev. Environ. Health* 14(1):1–10

74. Lee IM, Rexrode KM, Cook NR, Manson JE, Buring JE. 2001. Physical activity and coronary heart disease in women: Is "no pain, no gain" passé? *JAMA* 285:1447–54

75. Levins R, Lopez C. 1999. Toward an ecosocial view of health. *Int. J. Health Serv.* 29:261–93

76. Lund VK. 1999. The Healthy Communities Movement: Bridging the Gap Between Urban Planning and Public Health. http://www.asu.edu/caed/proceedings99/LUND/LUND.HTM

77. Lynch J, Smith GD, Hillemeier M, Shaw M, Raghunathan T, et al. 2001. Income inequality, the psychosocial environment and health: comparisons of wealthy nations. *Lancet* 358:1285–87

78. Mackenbach JP, Borst V, Schols JM. 1997. Heat-related mortality among nursing-home patients. *Lancet* 349:1297–98

79. Madianos MG, Gefou-Madianou D, Richardson C, Stefanis CN. 1995. Factors affecting illicit and licit drug use among adolescents and young adults in Greece. *Acta. Psychiatr. Scand.* 4:258–64

80. Marsella AJ. 1995. Urbanization, mental health and psychosocial well-being: some historical perspectives and considerations. In *Urbanization and Mental Health in Developing Countries*, ed. T

Harpham, I Blue, pp. 3–14. Aldershot, UK: Avebury

81. Mayberry RM, Mili F, Ofili E. 2000. Racial and ethnic differences in access to medical care. *Med. Care Res. Rev.* 57(1):108–45

82. McLeod L, Kessler R. 1990. Socioeconomic status differences in vulnerability to undesirable life events. *J. Health Soc. Behav.* 31:162–72

83. McMichael AJ. 1999. Urbanization and urbanism in industrialized nations, 1850–present: implications for health. In *Urbanism, Health, and Human Biology in Unindustrialized Countries*, ed. LM Schell, pp. 22–26. Cambridge, UK: Cambridge Univ. Press

84. McNeill JR. 2000. *Something New Under the Sun: An Environmental History of the Twentieth Century.* New York: Norton

85. Melosi M. 2000. *The Sanitary City: Urban Infrastructure in America from Colonial Times to the Present.* Baltimore: Johns Hopkins Press

86. Merton RK. 1938. Social structure and anomie. *Am. Sociol. Rev.* 3:672–82

87. Merzel C. 2000. Gender differences in health care access indicators in an urban, low-income community. *Am. J. Public Health* 90(6):909–16

88. Molbak K, Aaby P, Ingholt N, Hojyling N, Gottschau A, et al. 1992. Persistent and acute diarrhea as the leading cause of child mortality in Urban Guinea Bissau. *Trans. R. Soc. Trop. Med.* 86(2):216–20

89. Newman O. 1986. *Defensible Space: Crime Prevention Through Urban Design.* New York: McMillan

90. Deleted in proof

91. Northridge ME, Sclar E. 2003. A joint urban planning and public health framework: contributions to health impact assessment. *Am. J. Public Health* 93(1): 118–21

92. Northridge ME, Sclar E, Biswas P. 2003. Sorting out the connections between the built environment and health: a conceptual framework for navigating pathways and planning healthy cities. *J. Urban Health* 80(4):556–68

93. O'Meara M. 1999. *Reinventing Cities for People and the Planet.* Washington DC: Worldwatch Inst.

94. Ormond BA, Zuckerman S, Lhila A. 2000. *Rural/Urban Differences in Health Care Are Not Uniform Across States.* Washington, DC: Urban Inst.

95. Pagano MA, Hoene CW. *National League of Cities. 2003. City fiscal conditions in 2003.* http://www.nlc.org/nlc_org/site/files/reports/fbrief03.pdf

96. Passchier-Vermeer W, Passchier WF. 2000. Noise exposure and public health. *Environ. Health Perspect.* 108(Suppl. 1): 123–31

97. Pate RR, Pratt M, Blair SN, Haskell WL, Macera CA, et al. 1995. Physical activity and public health: a recommendation from the Centers for Disease Control and Prevention and the American College of Sports Medicine. *JAMA* 273: 402–7

98. Pearlin L, Lieberman M, Menaghan E, Mullan J. 1981. The stress process. *J. Health Soc. Behav.* 22:337–56

99. Peters J. 1999. Urbanism and health in industrialized Asia. In *Urbanism, Health and Human Biology in Industrialised Countries*, ed. LM Schell, SJ Ulijaszek, pp. 159–64. Cambridge, UK: Cambridge Univ. Press

100. Phillips DP. 1974. The influence of suggestion on suicide: substantive and theoretical implications of the Werther effect. *Am. Sociol. Rev.* 39(3):340–54

101. Pick WM, Obermeyer CM. 1996. Urbanisation, household composition, and the reproductive health of women in a South African City. *Soc. Sci. Med.* 43(1):1431–41

102. Popul. Ref. Bur. 2004. *March 2004. The population bulletin Vol. 59, No. 1.* http://www.prb.org/Template.cfm?Section=PRB&template=/ContentManagement/ContntDisplay.cfm&ContentID=10110

103. Rodgers GB. 1979. Income and inequality as determinants of mortality: an international cross section analysis. *Int. J. Epidemiol.* 31:182–91

104. Roodman D. 1998. *The Natural Wealth of Nations: Harnessing the Market for the Environment.* New York: Norton

105. Ross NA, Wolfson MC, Dunn JR, Berthelot JM, Kaplan GA, et al. 2000. Relation between income inequality and mortality in Canada and in the United States: cross sectional assessment using census data and vital statistics. *BMJ* 1(30)(7239):898–902

106. Samet JM, Dominici F, Curreriro FC, Coursac I, Zeger SL. 2000. Fine particulate air pollution and mortality in 20 US cities, 1987–1994. *N. Engl. J. Med.* 343:1742–49

107. Sampson RJ. 2003. Neighborhood-level context and health: lessons from sociology. In *Neighborhoods and Health*, ed. I Kawachi, LF Berkman, p. 193. New York: Oxford Univ. Press

108. Sampson RJ, Raudenbush SW, Earls F. 1997. Neighborhoods and violent crime: a multilevel study of collective efficacy. *Science* 277:918–24

109. Satterthwaite D. 2000. Will most people live in cities? *BMJ* 321:1143–45

110. Satterthwaite D. 2002. *Coping with rapid urban growth. RICS Leading Edge Series.* http://www.rics.org/downloads/research_reports/urban_growth.pdf

111. Schlenger WE, Caddell JM, Ebert L, Jordan BK, Rourke KM, et al. 2002. Psychological reactions to terrorist attacks: findings from the National Study of Americans' Reactions to September 11. *JAMA* 288(5):581–88

112. Schofield R, Reher D, Bideau A. 1991. *Decline of mortality in Europe.* http://www.oup.co.uk/isbn/0–19–828328–8

113. Semenza JC, McCullough JE, Flanders WD, McGeehin MA, Lumpkin JR. 1999. Excess hospital admissions during the July 1995 heat wave in Chicago. *Am. J. Prev. Med.* 16(4):269–77

114. Shaw CR, McKay HD. 1969. *Juvenile Delinquency and Urban Areas.* Chicago, IL: Univ. Chicago Press

115. Sheard S, Power H. 2000. *Body and City: Histories of Urban Public Health.* Aldershot, UK: Ashgate

116. Skrabski A, Kobb M, Kawachi I. 2004. Social capital and collective efficacy in Hungary: cross sectional associations with middle aged female and male mortality rates. *J. Epidemiol. Community Health* 58(4):340–45

117. Sodermann M, Jakobsen MS, Molbak K, Aaby ICA, Aaaby P. 1997. High mortality despite good care-seeking behavior: a community study of childhood deaths in Guinea-Bissau. *Bull. World Health Organ.* 75(3):205–12

118. Subramanian SV, Kim DJ, Kawachi I. 2002. Social trust and self-rated health in US communities: a multilevel analysis. *J. Urban Health* 79(4 Suppl. 1):S21–34

119. Takano T, Nakamura K, Watanabe M. 2002. Urban residential environments and senior citizens' longevity in megacity areas: the importance of walkable greenspaces. *J. Epidemiol. Community Health* 56:913–18

120. Tanaka A, Takano T, Nakamura K, Takeuchi S. 1996. Health levels influenced by urban residential conditions in a megacity—Tokyo. *Urban Stud.* 33(6):879–94

121. Tex. Transp. Inst. *2002 annual urban mobility study.* http://tti.tamu.edu/researcher/v38n2/annual%5Fmobility%5Fstudy.stm

122. Thomson H, Pettricrew M, Douglas M. 2003. Health impact assessment of housing improvement: incorporating research evidence. *J. Epidemiol. Community Health* 57:11–16

123. United Nations. 1999. *World urbanization prospects: the 1999 revision.* http://www.un.org/esa/population/pubsarchive/urbanization/urbanization.pdf

124. Vlahov D, Galea S. 2002. Urbanization,

urbanicity, and health. *J. Urban Health* 79(Suppl. 1):S1–12

125. Vlahov D, Galea S. 2003. Urban health: a new discipline. *Lancet* 362(9390):1091–92

126. Vogele JP. 1994. Urban infant mortality in Imperial Germany. *Soc. Hist. Med.* 7(3):401–25

127. Vrijheid M. 2000. Health effects of residence near hazardous waste landfill sites: a review of the epidemiologic literature. *Environ. Health. Perspect.* 108(Suppl. 1): 101–12

128. Wan TTH, Gray LC. 1978. Differential access to preventive services for young children in low-income urban areas. *J. Health. Soc. Behav.* 19:312–24

129. Weich S, Blanchard M, Prince M, Burton E, Erens B, et al. 2002. Mental health and the built environment: cross-sectional survey of individual and contextual risk factors for depression. *Br. J. Psychiatry* 180:428–33

130. Wellington M, Ndowa F, Mbengeranwa L. 1997. Risk factors for sexually transmitted disease in Harare: a case-control study. *Sex. Transm. Dis.* 24(9):528–32

131. Wilkinson RG. 1992. Income distribution and life expectancy. *BMJ* 304:165–68

132. Williams DR, Collins C. 2002. Racial residential segregation: a fundamental cause of racial disparities in health. In *Race, Ethnicity and Health: A Public Health Reader*, ed. TA Laveiest, pp. 369–90. San Francisco: Jossey Bass

133. Williams DR, Rucker TD. 2000. Understanding and addressing racial disparities in health care. *Health Care Financ. Rev.* 21(4):75–90

134. Wilson WJ. 1987. *The Truly Disadvantaged: The Inner City, The Underclass and Public Policy.* Chicago, IL: Univ. Chicago Press

135. Wirth L. 1938. Urbanism as a way of life. *Am. J. Soc.* 44:1–24

136. World Health Organ. 1997. *Health and the Environment in Sustainable Development: Five years After the Earth Summit.* Geneva, Switz.: WHO

137. Yusuf S, Reddy S, Ounpuu S, Anand S. 2001. Global burden of cardiovascular diseases: part I: general considerations, the epidemiologic transition, risk factors, and impact of urbanization. *Circulation* 104(22):2746–53

Annu. Rev. Public Health 2005. 26:367–97
doi: 10.1146/annurev.publhealth.26.021304.144615

Acculturation and Latino Health in the United States: A Review of the Literature and its Sociopolitical Context

Marielena Lara,[1,2] Cristina Gamboa,[3] M. Iya Kahramanian,[3] Leo S. Morales,[4] and David E. Hayes Bautista[3]

[1]*UCLA/RAND Program on Latino Children with Asthma, RAND Health, Santa Monica, California, 90407; email: lara@rand.org*
[2]*Department of Pediatrics,* [3]*Center for Study of Latino Health and Culture,* [4]*Department of Medicine, David Geffen School of Medicine, University of California, Los Angeles, California, 90024; email: cgamboa@ucla.edu, mariamK@ucla.edu, leo_morales@rand.org, dhayesb@ucla.edu*

Key Words health outcomes, Hispanic, assimilation, health behaviors, health care use

■ **Abstract** This chapter provides an overview of the concept of acculturation and reviews existing evidence about the possible relationships between acculturation and selected health and behavioral outcomes among Latinos. The effect of acculturation on Latino health is complex and not well understood. In certain areas—substance abuse, dietary practices, and birth outcomes—there is evidence that acculturation has a negative effect and that it is associated with worse health outcomes, behaviors, or perceptions. In others—health care use and self-perceptions of health—the effect is mostly in the positive direction. Although the literature, to date, on acculturation lacks some breadth and methodological rigor, the public health significance of findings in areas in which there is enough evidence justifies public health action. We conclude with a set of general recommendations in two areas—public health practice and research—targeted to public health personnel in academia, community-based settings, and government agencies.

INTRODUCTION

Health outcomes for Latinos are generally favorable when compared with other racial and ethnic groups in the United States. Two commonly used measures of population health include rates of adult and infant mortality. Mortality statistics for adults show that Latinos in the United States have lower mortality rates than do non-Latino whites and blacks. For example, in 2001 the age-adjusted mortality rate for Latinos was 22% lower than was the age-adjusted mortality rate among

0163-7525/05/0421-0367$20.00

non-Latino whites and 41% lower than was the age-adjusted mortality rate for non-Latino blacks (6). Similarly, birth outcomes statistics for 2001 show that infant mortality among Latinos was similar to that of non-Latino whites, and it was 58% lower than that of non-Latino blacks (6).

Yet the health outcomes of U.S. Latinos present a pattern of substantial heterogeneity in several dimensions. First, important indicators of population health vary among Latinos of Mexican, Puerto Rican, Cuban, and other Latino origin or cultural heritage. For instance, mortality and prevalence rates of chronic illness vary among both Latino children and adults of these different subgroups (33, 53, 55, 98, 102). Second, wide ranges of factors have been explored to explain this heterogeneity. These factors include more traditionally studied attributes such as socioeconomic status, educational level, and age, as well as other, less studied, contextual factors such as language fluency and immigration status, including time and number of generations living in the United States. These factors often are described as part of the phenomenon of acculturation to U.S. mainstream culture.

The focus of this chapter is to provide public health practitioners with an understanding of the concept of acculturation as one of many factors influencing the health of Latinos in the United States. We begin with a brief historical review of the concept, followed by a synopsis of how the term acculturation has been defined and used in the public health literature to date. We then present a critical review of existing evidence about the possible relationships between acculturation and selected health and behavioral outcomes among U.S. Latinos. On the basis of this review of existing evidence, we conclude with a summary of the relevance of acculturation to the design, planning, and implementation of public health programs for the Latino population; and we present recommendations for public health personnel in community, academic, and government settings.

ACCULTURATION AND ASSIMILATION: A HISTORY OF THE CONCEPTS

Milton Gordon (61) summarized thinking on the experience of European immigrant ethnic groups in America during the late nineteenth and early twentieth centuries in his 1964 book *Assimilation in American Life*, in which assimilation and acculturation were presented as unidirectional and inevitable. To become assimilated into the host society, the immigrant ethnic group had to make the major accommodation and develop, in the words of Gordon's mentor, Robert E. Park, "the memories, sentiments and attitudes of other persons and groups and, by sharing their experience and history. . .[become] incorporated with them in a common cultural life" (113). Those memories, sentiments, and attitudes the immigrants had to adopt were, of course, the "middle-class cultural patterns of largely white Protestant, Anglo-Saxon origins," often referred to as the "core culture" (61). When immigrants had expunged their own ethnicity, the host society then would allow the "cleansed" ethnic group entry into "the social cliques, clubs and institutions of the core society," that is, into their inner-circle institutions (61). The most intimate entry, and the endpoint of the assimilation process, was intermarriage, upon which the minority groups' separate identity, having lost all value, would cease to be even a memory.

Acculturation, the acquisition of the cultural elements of the dominant society—language, food choice, dress, music, sports, etc.—was the process by which assimilation was to be achieved. Warner & Srole (151) described the acculturation process as one in which ethnic groups unlearned their inferior culturally based behaviors. The primary investigator of a maternal and child health project in Riverside County, California, sighed about the difficulty of getting Mexican immigrants to expunge their health-harming culture when she wrote, "So steeped are these people in their traditional ways and so accustomed are they to ill health and the constant presence of death, and so stupid are they in their ignorance, illiteracy and wasting diseases that lifting them out of this abyss is a real job" (84). In these views, acculturation to white, Anglo-Saxon norms would be the best thing to happen to ethnic groups, and the quicker the better.

Then, only months after Gordon published his state-of-the-art monograph, the Watts area of Los Angeles exploded in the first of the "long hot summers" that racked urban America, and changes in immigration law allowed the entry of a significant number of immigrants for the first time in nearly 40 years, only this time largely from Mexico, other Latin American countries, and Asia. Initially, experts assumed that the acculturation and assimilation models of the past would guide the fortunes of these new immigrant groups. But the unilinear, unidirectional, and inevitable assimilation of the earlier groups seemed suddenly to become an elusive goal. Some theorists tried to rework the old models, adding new elements that had been overlooked. Perlman & Waldinger (116), for example, pointed out that earlier European immigrant mobility had not been the result of individual choice and gumption alone; entry to inner-circle institutions came only after organized ethnic communities exerted economic, political, and legal pressure to force those institutions to accept individuals from ethnic communities.

Other theorists began to see some structural differences between earlier and current waves of immigrants. Alba (2) noticed a bimodal pattern of immigration. "Human capital immigrants," largely from Asia, who arrived with higher educational and occupational levels than those achieved on average by U.S.-born non-Latino whites, seemed to be succeeding quickly, in spite of racial distinctiveness. "Labor immigrants," largely from Mexico and Central America, with lower educational and occupational levels, made much slower progress. Portes & Rumbaut (119) noted in their study of second-generation children of immigrants that assimilation outcomes varied across immigrant minorities, and that archetypical rapid acceptance and integration into the American mainstream represented just one possible outcome. They offered a model of segmented assimilation, in which different groups could wind up in vastly different relationships to mainstream American society, depending on three different variables: the human capital possessed by the immigrant group (education, wealth, occupational skills, and English ability), the policies of governmental institutions and the attitudes of native populations, and the structure and resources of the immigrants' families and communities. Groups with high human capital, whose presence is welcomed by policies generated by native populations, are likely to experience a smooth transition akin to that perceived of the older, European immigrant groups. Groups with low human capital, however, whose presence is resented or even rejected by the policies of the native population, are likely to wind up in a subordinate, permanent multi-ethnic underclass. In between would be a group whose individual members might have low human capital but whose community resources and networks provide access to social and economic mobility; even if the group's presence is resented by the native population, its very ethnicity provides a source of strength.

In Portes & Rumbaut's model, the process of acculturation can vary, ranging from dissonant acculturation, in which the child acquires cultural capital before the parent does, thereby upsetting parental roles; to consonant acculturation, in which parent and child acquire cultural elements at the same speed, preserving parental authority; to selective acculturation, in which a functioning ethnic community mediates between parent and child.

DEFINITIONS OF ACCULTURATION USED IN THE PUBLIC HEALTH LITERATURE

Unidimensional and Bidimensional Acculturation Models

Influenced by this previous historical context, the use and application of the concept of acculturation in the public health literature to date has included both unidimensional and bidimensional models. Unidimensional definitions, sometimes referred to as a "zero-sum game" (17, 36, 37, 124), assume that the acculturation experience occurs along a linear continuum from not acculturated (total immersion in the culture of origin) to completely acculturated (total immersion in the dominant or host culture); as the individual acculturates into the dominant culture, he or she loses his or her original cultural paradigms (17, 36, 37, 86). Unidimensional models probably best describe the experience of assimilation by which individuals "become part of the new group, and 'fold in' with members of the new culture" (11, 86).

Bidimensional models, questioning the validity of these assumptions, propose that acquiring or adhering to a new dominant culture is independent of maintaining the original culture (11, 17, 85, 87, 124, 125). Cultural maintenance is the degree to which an individual continues to value and adhere to the norms of the culture of origin. The level of participation and contact the individual has with the new dominant culture also can vary. Both domains theoretically range from full participation to full rejection of either culture's values, behaviors, and attitudes (11, 17).

Bidimensional models emphasize integration or biculturalism, in that they aim to characterize the experience by which individuals "feel equally comfortable in both cultures, hold the values and respect for norms of both cultures, and retain a dual cultural identity" (86).

In bidimensional acculturation models, different subcategories or states are possible: (*a*) assimilation—complete acquisition of the new culture, from the lack of desire to maintain the culture of origin or for other reasons; (*b*) separation—maintenance of the culture of origin through rejection or avoidance of the new culture; (*c*) integration—embracing and valuing both cultures; and (*d*) marginalization—exclusion (voluntarily or not) by both cultures (17). A similar, somewhat parallel categorization for the possible states within the bidimensional model has been articulated by Mendoza: (*a*) cultural shift—substituting new alternate cultural norms for original customs; (*b*) cultural resistance—resisting acquiring new alternate cultural norms while maintaining original customs; (*c*) cultural incorporation—adapting customs from both original and new alternate customs; and (*d*) cultural transmutation—alternating between original and new alternate cultural practices, thus creating a unique subcultural entity (100).

Transition into one of these categories or states assumes that an individual has control over these domains (11). This is not necessarily the case. Separation or marginalization, as described previously, can result from societal circumstances—such as prejudice, institutional racism, and segregational rules or laws—or historical circumstances, such as when a territory is invaded or annexed by another country (86).

In conceptualizing the process of acculturation, Marin postulates that the "culture learning" that is part of the acculturation process can be described on three levels. (*a*) First is a mostly superficial level including "the learning (and forgetting) of the facts that are part of one's cultural history or tradition" and "changes in the consumption of food and in the uses of the media" (86). Perhaps the reason these are considered superficial is that the adoption of things like food and media depends on the relative availability of these versus the ones from the culture of origin. (*b*) Next is an intermediate level including behaviors that are central to a person's social life, such as language preference and use, and preference for the ethnicity of friends, neighbors, spouse, and media in a multicultural environment. (*c*) Last is a more significant level and perhaps more permanent cultural learning, or adoption, of values and norms, including both maintenance of original cultural norms (e.g., familism in Latinos) and nonlinear adoption of new values. For example, Sabogal et al. (126) have shown that although certain aspects of familism—a sense of obligation and the power of the family as a behavioral referent—change as an individual becomes more acculturated, others (e.g., support received and expected from relatives) remain important to highly acculturated Latinos as well as to the less acculturated (126).

Magaña, who found that biculturalism does not equate to the equal embrace of both cultures, has further highlighted the nonlinear nature of the acculturation process. For example, bicultural individuals may speak Spanish predominantly within the family, while maintaining social affiliations with individuals from both Latino and non-Latino cultural groups. In contrast, individuals who shift away from Latino to non-Latino culture speak English primarily within the home, yet at the same time they socialize predominantly with others of Latino descent (85).

Acculturation Measures and Scales

Public health researchers have used different proxy measures, including summary acculturation scales, to describe and understand the complex phenomenon of acculturation. Several unidimensional and bidimensional acculturation scales have been developed and published to date (9, 31, 32, 36, 37, 41, 54, 72, 87, 90, 100, 121, 134, 150, 159). Other than the key distinction of uni- versus bi-dimensionality, scales differ in the subconstructs of acculturation they intend to measure, including (a) engaging in culturally specific behaviors, such as music, diet, and media; (b) proficiency in, use of, and preference for the Spanish or English language; (c) knowledge of culture-specific history and current events; (d) a sense of cultural identity; and (e) adoption of and belief in culture-specific values. These scales have been used and validated to different degrees. All scales include language as a subconstruct. Some scales exclude the behavioral component because engaging in these behaviors reflects, to a certain extent, the availability and accessibility of culture-specific items such as music and food, not an individual's preference per se (86, 159). Also, values and norms are more difficult to measure than are language preferences and patterns in food consumption, and therefore they are not included in many of the scales (86).

The heavy dependence of acculturation measures and scales on language has pros and cons. Supporters argue that psychometric analyses show that language items, compared with other constructs, explain most of the variance of acculturation scales (86). Also, although language is a complex construct—involving differential capacities to read, speak, and think, as well as levels of use based on preferences or opportunity for use (87, 159)—it is among the easiest acculturation constructs to measure. In his Behavioral Acculturation Scale (BAS) scale, for instance, Marin (87) makes distinctions between language use, proficiency, and media exposure.

Critics, in contrast, argue that the language measures do not capture the complexity of language use among bicultural individuals. Marin (86) states that "among Latinos/as it is to easy to find people who are primarily English or Spanish speaking, regardless of either their place of birth or their length of residence in the U.S., as well as individuals who are fully bilingual." Furthermore, acquisition of the English language does not necessarily mean sustenance of the Spanish language, or vice versa. An initially monolingual person can become either bilingual in the native and host languages or monolingual in the host language (86).

Critics of acculturation scales outline other weaknesses aside from this potential overemphasis on language. These can include the lack of appropriate psychometric testing, such as in the informal adaptation of previously validated scales, and the inclusion of sociodemographic characteristics (e.g., generation of respondents) as measures instead of as correlates of acculturation (criterion variables). For instance, the large-scale Hispanic Health and Nutrition Examination Survey (HHANES) uses a mixture of criterion and measurement variables in identifying the level of acculturation. Critics argue that the inconsistent relationships observed between the effects of acculturation in different Latino health outcomes are, in fact, due in large part to these differences in measurement (86).

In addition to summary scales, researchers also have used some of the same individual constructs to measure by proxy the acculturation phenomenon. Other than language, some of these proxy measures—including generational status (first, second, or third U.S. generation), age at immigration, place of birth (United States versus foreign), and place of education—assume that acculturation can be approximated by the amount of exposure individuals have to the dominant culture (17, 105, 125).

Significant variability may exist in the effects and manifestations of acculturation at the individual level, and acculturation scales aim at capturing that variability. Groups may behave differently than do individuals, e.g., Mexican Americans may, as a group, show certain effects of acculturation, but an individual Mexican American might have different shades of use/effect of language, income, etc. (11, 17).

Understanding and measuring acculturation are complex and difficult undertakings. Ideally, they would involve describing not only proxy measures for the construct, but also important contextual factors likely to be important mediators of the process. Contextual factors influencing the process of acculturation have been summarized by Cabassa (17). These include context prior to immigration (society of origin factors and individual factors), immigration context, and settlement context (society of settlement factors and individual factors). Another important modifier is the variability among individuals in the degree of stress experienced, the coping capacity of individuals, and the actual outcome of the acculturation process (11, 17).

In summary, although Redfield's original definition of acculturation implies bidirectional influence (17, 86), most theories and measures to date have captured "the changes that occur in the group and individuals that are being acculturated to a dominant culture" and the "psychological and social changes that groups and individuals experience when they enter a new and different cultural context" (11, 17). Acculturation is a "rather fluid process that implies movement at different speeds across different dimensions (e.g., behaviors, attitudes, norms, and values) and planes. . .[and] that does not typically follow a deficit mode, but rather implies growth across a variety of continua" (86).

CURRENT EVIDENCE REGARDING THE EFFECTS OF ACCULTURATION ON LATINO HEALTH OUTCOMES

Literature Review Methods

Prior to conducting our review, we identified a list of areas on which to focus our literature search. Our process of selection and review of the scientific literature was as follows. In each area two of the investigators reviewed article and book titles for inclusion. The abstracts of those titles agreed on by two individuals were reviewed using a structured form for easy screening for relevance and summary of the key findings. A summary of findings in each area and resulting recommendations were discussed and approved by the coauthors. We supplemented our literature search with other key review articles familiar to the coauthors or referred to them by other experts in the field.

Overview of Findings

Table 1 presents a summary of the studies in the literature areas we reviewed: health behaviors, health care use and access, self-assessed health perceptions, birth outcomes, chronic diseases, and mental health outcomes. In evaluating the effect of acculturation we determined if the evidence from each study supported (*a*) a negative effect (acculturation is associated with worse health outcomes, behaviors, or perceptions), (*b*) a positive effect (acculturation is associated with better health outcomes, behaviors, or perceptions), or (*c*) a mixed or no effect. A mixed effect might be, for example, a study showing that acculturation had opposite effects by gender, or alternately a positive effect according to one measure of acculturation, e.g., foreign place of birth, but a negative or no effect according to another, e.g., language. In this section we provide an overview of the major findings of our review, followed by a more specific description by area of the findings of key studies.

Our most important overall finding is that the effect of acculturation, or more accurately, assimilation to mainstream U.S. culture, on Latino behaviors and health outcomes is very complex and not well understood. Although we can identify certain major positive or negative trends in the subject areas reviewed, the effects are not always in the same direction, and many times the effects are mixed. Thus, depending on the subject area, the measure of acculturation used, and factors such as age, gender, or other measured or unmeasured constructs, acculturation may have a negative, positive, or no effect on the health of Latinos.

Although not absolute, the strongest evidence points toward a negative effect of acculturation on health behaviors overall—substance abuse, diet, and birth outcomes (low birthweight and prematurity)—among Latinos living in the United States. More acculturated Latinos (those who are highly acculturated) are more likely to engage in substance abuse and undesirable dietary behaviors and experience worse birth outcomes compared with their less acculturated counterparts. Furthermore, the negative effect of acculturation on substance abuse, although not completely uniform across areas, appears to have a stronger relative effect on women than on men (144, 148).

However, evidence suggests that the acculturation process has a positive effect on health care use and self-perceptions of health. Some studies have found that more acculturated Latinos are more likely to use preventive services (75, 96) (e.g., cancer screening) and have a better self-perception of health than do the less

TABLE 1   Referenced studies examining the relationship between acculturation and selected behaviors, health care use measures, and health outcomes among U.S. Latinos[1]

Area	Negative effect[a]	Mixed or no effect	Positive effect[b]
Health Behaviors			
Nutrition	10, 42, 62, 64, 96, 106, 109	97	
Exercise	49, 62, 135	20	34
Substance abuse			
General drug use	14, 23, 57, 58, 108, 141, 147, 148	48	
Cocaine	3, 23, 144	128, 149	
Marijuana	3, 23, 144	141	
Alcohol	12, 23, 89, 96, 109, 117, 145, 147	20, 92, 95, 141	
Smoking	28, 30, 47, 58, 62, 78, 109, 145	20, 43, 88, 91, 127, 142	
In pregnancy			
Breastfeeding		15	
Smoking	1, 27, 73	156	
Diet and other behaviors	27, 158		
General substance abuse	29, 73, 158		
Health care use and access			
General health care use		94	24
Use of preventive services		134	26, 75, 96
Have a regular source of care			63
Insurance			63, 75, 140
Continuous Medicaid insurance		67	
Decreased barriers to care			26, 153
Satisfaction with care			75
Immunizations	4, 120	52, 101	
Cervical cancer screening		137, 157	44, 59, 68, 96, 133
Breast cancer screening		122, 137, 157	13, 44, 59, 68, 107, 114, 115, 133
Health perceptions and outcomes			
Self health assessed reported health			5, 51, 98, 131
Birth outcomes			
Low birthweight	17, 22, 27, 45, 77, 129, 132	7, 46, 123, 156, 158	

(*Continued*)

TABLE 1   (*Continued*)

Area	Negative effect[a]	Mixed or no effect	Positive effect[b]
Prematurity	22, 35	156, 158	
Teenage pregnancy	29		
Caesarean birth/postpartum complications		73, 123	
Neonatal and Post-neonatal mortality	132	45, 82	
Childhood illness at 8–16 months	65		
Chronic conditions			
Childhood asthma	81, 99	83	
Diabetes	29, 135, 155	69, 80	72
Hypertension	50	93	
Coronary artery disease mortality		139	
Obesity—adolescent	62, 118	20, 79, 138	
Mental health	1, 108, 147	14	
Depression—adolescents	74, 103	38, 76, 141	60

[a] Acculturation associated with worse/detrimental outcomes or behaviors; [b] Acculturation associated with better/beneficial outcomes or behaviors.

[1] Shaded boxes indicate overall tendency of acculturation effect on shown outcomes: negative effect, mixed or no effect, or positive effect.

acculturated (51). There are important exceptions, however, in which the evidence is not as clear: for example, the effect of acculturation on immunization rates, where studies have shown both a negative and no effect (4, 52, 101, 120).

When reviewing the literature, we found that, across the board, past research studies have not been consistent in their measurement of acculturation or in their adjustments for possible confounding factors. This inconsistency is very important to consider in the overall interpretation of the findings. In some cases, the acculturation effect on health outcomes can be related to whether language, country of origin, or an acculturation scale was used to measure acculturation. For example, English (46) found that Mexican maternal nativity, and not necessarily speaking Spanish, was associated with better birth outcomes. In other cases, when studies have controlled for factors such as age, educational attainment, income, insurance, and other predisposing, enabling, or need factors, the effects of acculturation diminish or disappear (67, 157, 158). For example, in some studies, the "protective" or positive effect of acculturation on some health care use behaviors (e.g., cancer screening) has been accounted for by higher educational and income levels among the more acculturated (157). Solis and colleagues (134) found that socioeconomic status (SES) characteristics, and an access "score," predicted health care use more strongly than did acculturation. Of the acculturation variables, language but not ethnic identification predicted use. From these findings Solis and colleagues (134) concluded that "the effect of language on screening practices should not be interpreted as a cultural factor, but as an access factor."

Finally, almost all research on the effects of acculturation on Latinos in the United States has been done on persons of Mexican origin. The very few studies that have compared the effect of acculturation across Latino subgroups suggest that the experience of acculturation and its effects on health outcomes may be different for Mexicans and Puerto Ricans. The prevalence of childhood asthma and related risk factors is associated with different effects in Mexicans and Puerto Ricans according to place of birth. Island-born Puerto Ricans—presumed to be less acculturated—have a higher prevalence of asthma than do those born in the 50 U.S. states and the District of Columbia. On the contrary, less acculturated (foreign-born) Mexican American children have a lower prevalence of asthma and related risk factors than do their more acculturated (U.S.-born) counterparts (81, 83). Likewise, diabetes in pregnancy is more prevalent among Island-born Puerto Ricans but not in foreign-born Mexicans (80). Investigators have shown some small differences in illness-related beliefs for asthma and diabetes among individuals of different Latino subgroups (110–112, 152). It is unlikely, however, that these small differences account for the large differences in prevalence. Another possibility is varying patterns in disease recognition, diagnosis, and actual predisposition to disease. The degree to which possible differences in the acculturation experiences between Mexicans and Puerto Ricans account for this effect is a question for future research. The relevance of the concept of acculturation to Puerto Ricans—given that they are U.S. citizens and, thus, exposed to U.S. mainstream culture from birth—also should be examined.

ACCULTURATION IS ASSOCIATED WITH SEVERAL NEGATIVE HEALTH-RELATED BEHAVIORS AND HEALTH OUTCOMES IN LATINOS   Most studies evaluating the relationship between acculturation and substance abuse have found a negative effect of acculturation on substance abuse behaviors, both in general and specifically in pregnancy, including use of illicit drugs, alcohol, and smoking. Negative effects of acculturation also have been demonstrated regarding dietary practices and birth outcomes.

1. *Illicit drug use*   The negative effect of acculturation on drug use, including marijuana, cocaine, and other illicit drugs, has been demonstrated in adults, pregnant women, and adolescents (3, 57, 58, 144, 146). Some of these studies have shown a stronger negative effect in females than in males (144, 148). Although most studies have been conducted in Mexican American populations, some have included other Latino subgroups. Turner (141) found a negative effect of acculturation among U.S.-born Cubans and other U.S.-born Caribbean-origin Latinos in southern Florida, and Velez (148) showed that, among Puerto Rican female adolescents, the effect of acculturation on drug use was more pronounced and was related to length of time lived in New York City. Some of these studies evaluated possible confounders and

interactions. For example, Amaro (3) found that among Mexican Americans and Puerto Ricans of lower educational attainment, illicit drug use was linked more strongly with predominant use of English than it was among those of higher educational attainment. The relation between acculturation, as measured by language, and drug use also varied by sex, marital status, and place of birth. From these findings, Amaro concluded that the experience of acculturation is associated with socioeconomic context. Velez (148) found that lower socioeconomic status was associated with drug involvement by adolescents in New York City, but not among Puerto Ricans on the Island.

2. *Drinking* The detrimental effect of acculturation on patterns of alcohol use is clearest in women; the effect is more ambiguous among men (12, 92, 95, 96, 109, 117). Men have a higher prevalence of alcohol consumption to begin with, so the acculturation effect reflects a closing of the gap between men and women (89, 96, 154). Gender differences observed in the data from the HHANES analyzed by Marks et al. (96) illustrate that, on average, Mexican American, Cuban American, and Puerto Rican men are more than two times as likely to be alcohol users, compared with women (e.g., 77.4% for Mexican American men compared with 34.7% for Mexican American women). The correlation of acculturation and drinking was close to three times greater for Mexican American and Cuban American women than for men (0.30 versus 0.11, 0.36 versus 0.13, respectively) and six times greater for Puerto Rican women than for men (0.26 versus 0.04). The strong influence of non-Latino norms results in the adoption of practices similar to those of non-Latina women as Latinas acculturate. This effect is not observed in men because Latino and non-Latino men exhibit similar drinking behaviors to begin with.

The effect of acculturation on drinking is complicated and related to both frequency and volume of drinking. The relationship of consumption frequency, i.e., the number of days a person consumed any alcoholic beverage, and acculturation observed by Marín & Posner (89) showed that increased drinking is related to an increase in acculturation. Less acculturated Mexican Americans and Central Americans drank less often than did the more acculturated (6.3 days versus 8.3 and 3.9 days versus 5.9, respectively). A reverse effect, however, was noticed with respect to volume, or the mean number of drinks per day. Less acculturated Latinos drank in greater volume, compared with the more acculturated—on average 3.1 drinks versus 2.8 drinks in Mexican Americans and 2.9 drinks versus 2.7 drinks in Central Americans. Furthermore, the pattern of frequency and volume of alcohol consumption is heightened in men. There does not seem to be an age effect, however, in the relationship between acculturation and drinking patterns (18, 89).

3. *Smoking* Acculturation also has an overall negative health effect on smoking in both men and women, but the effect is not as strong as on drinking (28, 30, 96). According to Marks et al., (96) the correlation of drinking and

acculturation in Mexican American women (0.30) is three times greater than that of smoking and acculturation (0.09). There is also a gender pattern in the relationship between acculturation and smoking. Although the prevalence of smoking is shown to be greater in men (32.4%) than in women (16.8%), acculturation in women is associated with more smoking, including smoking during pregnancy (109). For example, the analysis of a phone survey conducted by Marín et al. (88) found age-adjusted smoking rates to be greater among more acculturated women (22.3%) versus less acculturated women (13.6%). In men, the pattern was not as clear.

4. *Nutrition and dietary patterns*   Diets can be more nutritious among the less acculturated. Several studies have found that less acculturated Latinos consume healthier diets than do their more acculturated counterparts. Less acculturated Mexican American women consume less fat and more fiber. They have a higher intake of protein; vitamins A, C, E, and B_6; and folate, calcium, potassium, and magnesium than do their more acculturated counterparts (42, 64). Although Latino elders overall consume significantly less saturated fats and simple sugars and more complex carbohydrates than do non-Latino whites, Latino elderly who have resided in the United States for a longer time have macronutrient profiles and eating patterns more similar to those of non-Latino whites (10). Latinos, on average, consume one or more servings of fruits and vegetables more per day than do non-Latino whites. However, highly acculturated Latinos eat half the servings of fruits and vegetables less than do the less acculturated (106). Another study (97), however, on the basis of the National Health and Nutrition Examination Survey, found that lower levels of acculturation only partially ameliorated the negative association between poverty and undesirable dietary patterns in Latino youth.

5. *Birth outcomes*   Among the negative effects of acculturation on health outcomes, the effect on birth outcomes stands out. An extensive literature documents that a higher acculturation level is associated with worse birth and perinatal outcomes [prematurity, low birthweight (LBW), teen pregnancy, neonatal mortality], as well as with undesirable prenatal and postnatal behaviors (smoking and drug use during pregnancy, decreased number of breast-feeding mothers). The effect is the "cleanest" in Mexican American women. Among Mexican American women, acculturation is associated with lower birth weight (19, 22, 27, 56, 129, 132, 156), prematurity (22, 35, 156), and teenage (<17 years) births (29). Cobas found that acculturation appears to affect LBW status indirectly through smoking and dietary intake (27). Wolff (156) found that more acculturated pregnant women smoke more. Acculturation is associated with more smoking, alcohol, and street drug use during pregnancy (29, 73, 156, 158). Coonrad et al. (29) found that highly acculturated Latina women were four to seven times more likely to acknowledge substance abuse during pregnancy. Frequency of tobacco use in highly

acculturated pregnant Latina women was 13.8%, compared with 3.4% in the less acculturated. Likewise, alcohol use and drug use in highly acculturated and less acculturated pregnant women was 7.8% versus 1.8% and 14.5% versus 2.0%, respectively (29).

For Puerto Rican women and their babies, the effects of acculturation are similar to those on Mexican Americans, except for neonatal mortality; Island-born babies have a higher birthweight-specific neonatal mortality rate than do mainland-born Puerto Rican babies (7.8 versus 6.8). Infants of island-born Puerto Rican mothers, however, had lower birthweight-specific postneonatal mortality rates than did babies of Mainland-born Puerto Rican mothers, a rate of 3.5 compared with 4.4 (45).

Yet some literature also suggests mixed or no effects on birth outcomes. This is related to the fact that acculturation is a complex phenomenon: Language, place of birth, and length of stay in the United States contribute to different effects. For instance, Zambrana (158) found that although higher acculturation was significantly associated with more undesirable prenatal behaviors and risk factors in Mexican American women, there were no direct effects of acculturation on infant gestational age or birthweight. In a study of related birth outcomes, Acevedo (1) found that Mexican American mothers were at lower risk for cigarette smoking during pregnancy but at higher risk for adverse parenting beliefs, such as lack of empathy, physical punishment, unrealistic expectations, and role reversals, than were European American women of the same low-income background. Among Mexican American women, Spanish speakers were at lower risk for cigarette smoking and mental health problems during pregnancy, but were at a higher risk for adverse parenting beliefs, than were bilingual and English-only speakers. Reynoso (123) compared Mexican American pregnant teenagers who were more acculturated with those who were less so. More acculturated teenagers were younger on first instance of sexual intercourse, were more educated, and sought earlier prenatal care, but no differences in birthweight between groups were observed. Landale (82) compared Mainland-born Puerto Ricans, Island-born Puerto Ricans in Puerto Rico, and Island-born recent immigrants to the United States. Controlling for age, income, marital status, social support, previous history of LBW, substance abuse during pregnancy, prenatal care, and WIC participation, he found that Mainland-born and Island-born Puerto Ricans in Puerto Rico have similar rates of infant mortality, although these two groups had higher rates than did those of Island-born immigrants to the Mainland, when the study also controlled for LBW. Without controlling for LBW, however, children of Puerto Rican women in Puerto Rico had higher infant mortality.

Some studies have found that foreign place of birth and language have different, individual effects on birth outcomes. As stated previously, English et al. (46) found that the mother's birthplace was correlated more closely with low rates of LBW than to Spanish language preference. Heilemann (73) found that more acculturated Mexican American women had more prenatal complications, excessive maternal weight gain, cesarean births, postpartum complications, and a higher prevalence of sexually transmitted diseases and substance abuse than did less acculturated women. Yet these effects were predicted most consistently by place of birth, not language. Similarly, Wolff & Portis (156) found that Mexican American women with a moderate American orientation experienced significantly poorer birth outcome indicators (LBW and prematurity) and higher rates of smoking than did women with either a stronger American orientation or a Mexican orientation. Finally, although the overall direction of Balcazar's (7) findings was like that of most studies in the field, surprisingly, he found that length of U.S. residence had an opposite effect in predicting both birth outcome indicators, when compared with acculturation.

Evidence for the effect of acculturation on breastfeeding is more mixed than birth outcomes. Lower acculturation is associated with a more likely decision to breastfeed, yet more breastfeeding is observed among the more educated. Byrd et al. (15) found that lower levels of acculturation are associated with a history of breastfeeding and intention to breastfeed, with multipara women born in Mexico or primipara women who grew up and were educated in Mexico more likely to intend to breastfeed. Yet women with less education, women who were single, and women who did not receive any prenatal care were less likely to intend to breastfeed than were women with a college education, women with a partner, and women who received prenatal care.

Acculturation is Associated with Improved Access to Care and Use of Preventive Health Services Among Latinos

More acculturated Latinos have higher rates of insurance coverage and access to health care. Thamer et al. (140), using the 1989–1990 NHIS (National Health Interview Survey), found that foreign-born Latinos who had resided in the United States for fewer than 15 years were 2–5 times more likely to be uninsured than were non-Latino whites. Granados and colleagues (63) found, in a predominantly Latino sample in Wilmington, Los Angeles, that the proportion of insured children enrolled in public or private insurance at the time of study and those reporting a usual source of care increased, respectively, from both foreign-born parent-children dyads to mixed dyads to U.S.-born parent-children dyads. Hu & Covell (75) found, in a study of Latino adults in San Diego, that the primary use of English, as compared with two other groups—bilingual and primarily Spanish—was positively correlated with a higher frequency of general physical, vision, and dental check-ups; being more satisfied with health care; having insurance; having a self-perception of excellent health; and having ever been hospitalized. These relationships remained constant when controlled for income, age, sex, and having a regular source of care.

Other studies have shown mixed results. Markides et al. (94) undertook a path analysis to evaluate the contribution of factors in the Andersen model vis-à-vis acculturation in a three-generation study of Mexican Americans in San Antonio. When controlled for potential predisposing (age, sex, marital status), enabling (insurance, employment), and need (number of chronic diseases, physical symptom scale, self-rated health, worry about health) factors, acculturation was not directly associated with increased physician visits in the previous year among the more acculturated. Similarly, Halfon and colleagues (67) found that continuous Medicaid enrollment among Latino families in South Central and East Los Angeles was not associated with residency status, length of U.S. residency, or language preference. Moreover, he found that "insurance status and provider type were more consistently associated with access rather than residency and language preference" (p. 636). Finally, Solis et al. (134) used the HHANES to evaluate the relationship of use of preventive health services (physical, dental, and vision examinations) among Mexican Americans, Cuban Americans, and Puerto Rican adults to an "access score"—measured by a scale of insurance, having a regular place for care, type of facility used, having a regular provider, and travel time—and to an acculturation scale, eight subset items from the Cuellar scale. Solis found that socioeconomic status characteristics and the access score predicted health care use more strongly than did acculturation. Of the acculturation variables, language, but not ethnic identification, predicted use.

The more acculturated also have fewer barriers to care. Wells (153), even after controlling for poverty, transportation, and other barriers, found that the less acculturated have more barriers to mental heath care and that these barriers are associated with predisposing and enabling factors in this group. Chesney (24), while controlling for social class and social isolation, found in a largely Mexican American population living near the Texas-Mexico border that their predisposition to use of health care services was directly related to acculturation: The highly acculturated had twice the rates of utilization of the less acculturated. In an ethnographic study of Latina women in the Rocky Mountain West, Clark (26) found that immigrant or less acculturated Latina mothers described more barriers to care than did more acculturated mothers.

Finally, acculturation is associated with higher use of some preventive services by women, including screening for breast cancer and pap smears (13, 44, 59, 68, 96, 107, 114, 115, 133). Borrayo et al. (13) found that 58.2% of U.S.-born women of Mexican descent had received a mammogram in the past year, compared with 48.6% of Mexico-born women. Furthermore, 62% of the U.S.-born women reported a breast self-exam (BSE) in the past month, compared with 45% of Mexico-born women. Goel et al. reported that Latinas were less likely to undergo a pap smear (77%) than were non-Latina whites (86%). After controlling for sociodemographic and other covariates, foreign-born Latina women had 0.65 (95% C.I. 0.53–0.79) the odds of receiving a pap smear when compared with non-Latina whites. There were no differences in pap smear rates between U.S.-born Latinas and U.S.-born non-Latina whites (59).

In Other Areas, the Effects of Acculturation are not Clear to Date

Our review did not demonstrate a clear relationship between acculturation and the other conditions and areas studied. This lack of clear relationship resulted either from an insufficient number and/or quality of studies or from multiple studies that demonstrated opposite or no effects. This included studies related to the effect of acculturation on certain Latino behaviors (e.g., exercise), prevalence of chronic diseases (e.g., asthma, diabetes, hypertension, obesity), and mental health outcomes. The lack of clarity about the effects of acculturation on various mental health outcomes also has been documented by others (8).

RECOMMENDATIONS FOR PUBLIC HEALTH PRACTICE AND RESEARCH

On the basis of our review's findings, we present in this section general recommendations for public health personnel and scientists in two general areas: public health practice and research. Given the state of the literature on acculturation and health outcomes in Latinos, our desire is to outline both the major opportunities and the remaining challenges in this field.

Public Health Practice Recommendations

The literature on acculturation to date lacks sufficient breadth and methodological rigor to make comprehensive and definitive evidence-based recommendations about how to modify the acculturation effects of the U.S. social and physical environments on the health of Latino children and adults in all areas. Yet in some areas—substance abuse, dietary practices, birth outcomes, and health care utilization—there is enough evidence, to date, to justify public health action.

The following recommendations apply to public health practitioners in community, academic, and/or government settings.

INCREASE KNOWLEDGE AND AWARENESS OF THE ROLE OF ACCULTURATION IN LATINO BEHAVIORS, HEALTH OUTCOMES, AND HEALTH CARE USE Given evidence of the detrimental effects of acculturation on some health behaviors and outcomes among U.S. Latinos, planners and implementers of public health programs to promote healthy dietary practices, improve birth outcomes, decrease alcohol and illicit drug usage, and increase health care use among Latinos/as should take into account acculturation in the design and actual implementation of their programs. At the field level, for example, public health staff working in community settings could be educated about the general role of acculturation, its effects in key areas, and strategies to better target Latinos for services based on their acculturation levels. At the administrative level, awareness-promoting activities could target government public health officials administering, funding, and implementing programs. In an era of limited resources, this would facilitate selection of and favorable review of effective Latino public health programs that incorporate acculturation as part of their planning and implementation strategies. Finally, at the academic level, teaching and application of the concept of acculturation and its relevance to Latino health should be included in public health schools' curricula.

INCREASE USE OF ACCULTURATION MEASURES AMONG PUBLIC HEALTH PERSONNEL
Although language and nativity are imperfect proxy measures for acculturation,
they are the most practical measures that can be used in real-life public health
settings. It is better to use some measure of acculturation than none at all. At
a minimum, public health practioners should have information on the language
and nativity of all their Latino clients. They also should have information on
immigrants' length of residence in the United States and be able to differentiate between language of preference and that of use in evaluating acculturation
among Latino clients. Government public health officials also should promote
the inclusion of acculturation measures in all major government health
surveys.

PROMOTE THE MAINTENANCE OF HEALTHY BEHAVIORS AMONG THE LESS ACCUL-
TURATED AND PROMOTE THE REACQUISITION OF THESE BEHAVIORS AMONG THE
MORE ACCULTURATED   A key public health issue is avoiding the erosion of certain
healthy behaviors among less acculturated Latinos to the less desirable population
average of other groups. The goal would be to reinforce positive behaviors among
the least acculturated and inspire a return to good behaviors among those who are
becoming acculturated. Strategies might include educational programs to prevent
the acquisition of drinking, smoking, illicit drug use, and other unhealthy behaviors, and to encourage the maintenance of beneficial nutritional practices and other
desirable behaviors among the less acculturated. Social marketing and/or behavioral modification techniques could be tested, among other strategies, to provide
positive reinforcement and a sense of pride in individuals who, although less acculturated, undertake healthier behaviors (e.g., eating more nutritious meals even
if families are low-income).

Because of the considerable evidence of the negative effect of acculturation on
dietary practices among Mexican Americans, we also recommend testing novel
strategies that would encourage the use of recipes and staples of a healthy, less-
acculturated diet in existing educational and nutritional public health programs,
such as the WIC program. For example, financial incentives for healthy diet choices
among the least acculturated, such as more credit on WIC food coupons for these
foods, could be an effective strategy to promote continuation of good nutritional
practices.

In the specific case of substance abuse programs (including smoking, alcohol,
and illicit drugs), prevention, educational, and other treatment programs should be
tailored to the individual's level of acculturation and gender. Highly acculturated
Latinas are a group with significant potential for risk reduction, on the basis of the
stronger relative effects of acculturation on unhealthy behaviors and outcomes in
women as compared with men. Contrary to other areas, in which the evidence of
the effects of acculturation are mostly on persons of Mexican origin, in the area
of illicit drug use, there is a strong argument for targeting prevention and control
programs to the more acculturated youth of all Latino groups: Mexican American,
Puerto Rican, Cuban, and others.

PROMOTE THE USE OF BOTH GENERAL AND SPECIFIC HEALTH SERVICES AMONG LESS ACCULTURATED LATINOS   More research is necessary to confirm the positive effect of acculturation on health care use by Latinos: specifically, to study the degree to which decreased health care use among less acculturated Latinos is due to acculturation level per se, versus mediating factors associated with less acculturation, such as lack of insurance and greater language barriers to care. We understand, however, that there already exists enough evidence to justify public health action to improve access to health care among less acculturated Latinos living in this country, and that strategies to increase the proportion of unacculturated Latinos who have medical insurance should be explored and implemented. For example, implementation of the national standards for Culturally and Linguistically Appropriate Services in Health Care recommended by the Office of Minority Health of the U.S. Department of Health Services (143) would improve the cultural competency of services—including language accessibility—and improve health care access and use in the least acculturated groups.

We also recommend the implementation and evaluation of outreach programs for less acculturated Latinos who are at risk of worse health and behavioral outcomes. There is a strong argument for implementation of public health programs that would increase utilization of preventive health and dental care, as well as breast cancer and cervical cancer screening, among less acculturated Latinos. In the case of prenatal programs for more acculturated Latinas, evidence also supports a need for the early identification and treatment of risk behaviors, including smoking and illicit drug use, during pregnancy. Educational and other programs to promote the continuation of good prenatal behaviors among the less acculturated also would be beneficial.

Research Recommendations

In this section we outline general research recommendations to address important methodological limitations and knowledge gaps in the field, as well as current research questions in specific areas.

PROMOTE THE USE AND IMPROVEMENT OF ACCULTURATION MEASURES AND THEORETICAL MODELS IN PUBLIC HEALTH RESEARCH   A recent comprehensive review of acculturation theory, measurement, and applied research (25) summarizes general challenges in this area. The main measures used to measure acculturation (e.g., language, generation, self-reported ethnic identity) are at best proxy variables and do not fully capture the construct of acculturation. Also, unidimensional and unidirectional definitions of acculturation are used prevalently. These oversimplify a process that is at least bidimensional and more likely multidimensional.

Several research strategies could be used to address these gaps. There needs to be increased use of multidimensional statistical and other modeling techniques, such as path modeling and structural equations, that better comprehend the effects of acculturation and differentiate between direct and indirect, or mediation, effects. The relationship between acculturation and specific outcomes may not be straight-forward or unidirectional. For example, acculturation may shape how individuals gain access to care, whereas certain access-to-care characteristics (e.g., having insurance) may influence the overall effect of acculturation in health outcomes.

Public health researchers also should apply, and modify as necessary, existing theories to account for likely differences in the history, context, and prevalence of certain behaviors and illnesses among Latino subgroups as a possible way of exploring the impact of acculturation. Investigators should ask how much possible difference in the effects of acculturation experience across Latino subgroups—including Mexicans, Puerto Ricans, Cubans, and others—relates to individual char-acteristics of the respective subgroups, beyond the acculturation experience per se?

In addition, more research on the use, validity, and application of acculturation scales would be beneficial. For example, can the number of items in the most used and evaluated scales be decreased further without losing validity? What are the reliability and validity of currently available scales and future measures in non-Mexican Latino subgroups? What is the most effective and feasible way to operationalize nonlanguage domains of acculturation, such as values, attitudes, and behaviors?

FUND AND CONDUCT PUBLIC HEALTH RESEARCH TO ADDRESS AREA-SPECIFIC RE-SEARCH TO ANSWER EXISTING QUESTIONS ABOUT THE PHENOMENON AND EFFE-CTS OF ACCULTURATION AMONG LATINOS   The following are examples of current research questions in the areas we reviewed.

Nutrition   What are the relationships between acculturation and specific types of dietary intake by age group, in both Mexican-origin and non-Mexican Latino groups? Are such relationships linked to acculturation status and/or to dietary practices and behaviors (e.g., exercise) that promote physical health and prevent obesity? To what extent do favorable dietary patterns in the less acculturated ame-liorate the negative effects of poverty and lower educational attainment?

Substance abuse, including drinking, smoking, and drug use   Why are there gender differences in the acquiring of unhealthy behaviors as a result of acculturation? Are they related to gender-specific factors that also are associated with increased income and education, irrespective of ethnicity? Is there something specific about the context of immigrant Latina women's experiences in the United States? Is the phenomenon like the closing of the gap between women and men in other areas? If so, what are possible public health intervention points, both for prevention and for treatment?

Mental health   What aspects of the acculturation process appear, in some stud-ies, to lead to higher rates of depression among more acculturated Latinos? Do the apparent differences in prevalence and morbidity related to mental health disorders among Latino subgroups reflect differences in acculturation experience, for instance, between Mexicans, Puerto Ricans, and Cubans? There is a need to tease out the differences between processes of acculturative stress versus adaptation to acculturative experiences. What is a mental health problem, and what is merely part of the normal process of adaptation? What are the roles of acculturative stress, context of immigration, and other important factors in the expression of mental illness among Latino immigrants?

Birth outcomes   What is it about acculturation to U.S. norms among Latinas that leads to lower birthweights in their offspring, in spite of greater access to prenatal care? What are the relative contributions of smoking, illicit drug use, dietary changes, and other factors among more acculturated Latinas that lead to worse birth outcomes?

Effect of income and education   What is the relative contribution of increased education for highly acculturated women, in terms of improving health outcomes among the most acculturated? Is there a U-shaped curve relationship? In other words, is acculturation associated with some undesirable health and behavioral outcomes until the individual attains a certain level of acculturation, and the effect levels off or decreases with increased educational and socioeconomic status?

Paradox of increased health care use with worse behavioral outcomes   In reviewing the overall effects of acculturation on Latino outcomes, evidence to date, although not perfect, suggests that more acculturated Latinos have worse behavioral and birth outcomes but have more frequent health care use than do less acculturated Latinos. The reasons for this apparent paradox need to be understood. Does acculturation have a different effect on behaviors and health care use? In other words, do acculturated individuals have different attitudes and related behaviors about going to the doctor versus abusing alcohol, cigarettes, and illicit drugs? Alternatively, do unhealthy behaviors drive higher health care use among the more acculturated because these unhealthy behaviors lead to real disease, for which individuals then seek medical care? Or is acculturation associated with mixed effects? For example, language acquisition leads to higher SES through higher paying jobs; in this way acculturation is good for health. Yet there is also evidence that greater acculturation leads to worsening health behaviors and other risk factors, such as family disintegration, which may in turn be associated with unhealthy behaviors. A summary question might be, what is the net effect of acculturation on Latino health?

Perceptions of health   The literature suggests that more acculturated Latinos perceive themselves as being in better health than less acculturated Latinos, in spite of having a trend toward certain worse health outcomes (51). Some of this apparent inconsistency of effect may be due to lack of study controls for important SES and health care–related factors and to a lack of multidimensional, consistent measures of acculturation (104). Yet it may also indicate that acculturation has opposite effects with respect to access to care and health habits—including diet, exercise, and substance abuse—on the one hand, and with respect to actual disease burden, morbidity, and perception of health, on the other.

Related research questions include, is increased access to care among more acculturated Latino/as associated with more diagnosis of disease and more patient report of disease, and yet a sense of better health because medical care helps control symptoms? And/or does contact with a physician gives more acculturated patients a sense of more disease control, irrespective of real morbidity? Alternatively, does worse access to care by the less acculturated account for lower parent- or self-rated health because existing conditions are undertreated? In a recent study of socioeconomic status and health, Case and colleagues (21) showed that children with a health condition and higher SES had better parent-reported health status than did children with a health condition and lower SES. Higher socioeconomic status is presumed to provide more access to higher quality medical care. Or, is it possible that English and Spanish measures of parent- or self-rated health are not interpreted similarly by more and less acculturated individuals? Some research suggests that more and less acculturated persons respond to this measure differently for cultural or linguistic reasons (51, 71).

CONCLUSIONS

The phenomenon of acculturation in U.S.-residing Latinos is complex. Although more research in this area is clearly necessary, public health action based on the evidence that does exist would help promote the health of Latinos. For those areas where there is evidence that acculturation has a negative effect—substance abuse, dietary practices, and birth outcomes—a key public health issue is how to avoid the erosion of healthy behaviors among less acculturated Latinos to the population average of other groups. Alternatively, for those areas where the effect is mostly in the positive direction—health care use and self-perceptions of health—the questions are how to improve access to health care among less acculturated populations and how to understand the relationship between perceived health and actual health.

On the basis of our literature review, we presented specific recommendations in two general areas public health practice and research. The recommended public health and research actions depend on and supplement one another. Implementation and evaluation of public health interventions based on existing evidence would provide further direction to research aimed at understanding the complex and interrelated processes associated with acculturation and health among Latinos.

ACKNOWLEDGMENTS

This work was conducted while M.L. was a Mentored Clinical Scientist sponsored by the Agency for Healthcare Research and Quality (Grant K08 HS00008) and was supported by the Center for the Study of Latino Health and Culture. During the writing of this paper, L.M. was a Robert Wood Johnson Foundation Harold Amos Fellow and received partial support from the UCLA Center for Health Improvement in Minority Elders, National Institute of Aging (AG-02-004), and the UCLA/Drew Project EXPORT, National Center on Minority Health and Health Disparities (P20-MD00148-01). The authors thank Peter Gutiérrez and Dr. José Jalil Colomé for assistance with data analysis and the literature review; Cynthia L. Chamberlin for editorial support; and Linda Escalante and Louis Ramirez for other essential administrative support. Finally, M.L. thanks also her husband, Richard Greenberg, and their daughter, Serena Michelle Lara-Greenberg, for their unwavering support of this and other projects. This paper is dedicated to all Latinos in the United States regardless of their level of acculturation.

The *Annual Review of Public Health* is online at
http://publhealth.annualreviews.org

LITERATURE CITED

1. Acevedo MC. 2000. The role of acculturation in explaining ethnic differences in the prenatal health-risk behaviors, mental health, and parenting beliefs of Mexican American and European American at-risk women. *Child Abuse Negl.* 24(1):111–27

2. Alba R. 1997. Rethinking assimilation theory for a new era of immigration. *Int. Migr. Rev.* 31(4):826–74

3. Amaro H, Whitaker R, Coffman G, Heeren T. 1990. Acculturation and marijuana and cocaine use: findings from HHANES 1982–84. *Am. J. Public Health* 80(Suppl.):54–60

4. Anderson LM, Wood DL, Sherbourne CD. 1987. Maternal acculturation and childhood immunization levels among children in Latino families in Los Angeles. *Am. J. Public Health* 87(12):2018–21

5. Angel R, Guarnaccia PJ. 1989. Mind, body, and culture: somatization among Hispanics. *Soc. Sci. Med.* 28(12):1229–38

6. Arias E, Anderson RN, Kung HC, Murphy SL, Kochanek KD. 2003. Deaths, final report for 2001. *Natl. Vital Stat. Rep.* 52(3):1–48

7. Balcazar H, Krull JL. 1999. Determinants of birth-weight outcomes among Mexican-American women: examining conflicting results about acculturation. *Ethn. Dis.* 9(3):410–22

8. Balls Organista P, Organista KC, Kurasaki K. 2003. The relationship between acculturation and ethnic minority mental health. See Ref. 25, pp. 136–61

9. Barona A, Miller JA. 1994. Short acculturation scale for Hispanic Youth (SASH-Y): a preliminary report. *Hisp. J. Behav. Sci.* 16(2):155–62

10. Bermudez OI, Falcon LM, Tucker KL. 2000. Intake and food sources of macronutrients among older Hispanic adults: association with ethnicity, acculturation, and length of residence in the United States. *J. Am. Diet Assoc.* 100(6): 665–73

11. Berry JW. 2003. Conceptual approaches to acculturation. See Ref. 25, pp. 17–37

12. Black SA, Markides KS. 1993. Acculturation and alcohol consumption in Puerto Rican, Cuban-American, and Mexican-American women in the United States. *Am. J. Public Health* 83(6):890–93

13. Borrayo EA, Guarnaccia CA. 2000. Differences in Mexican-born and U.S.-born women of Mexican descent regarding factors related to breast cancer screening

behaviors. *Health Care Women Int.* 21(7):599–613

14. Burnam MA, Hough RL, Karno M, Escobar JI, Telles CA. 1987. Acculturation and lifetime prevalence of psychiatric disorders among Mexican Americans in Los Angeles. *J. Health Soc. Behav.* 28(1):89–102

15. Byrd TL, Balcazar H, Hummer RA. 2001. Acculturation and breast-feeding intention and practice in Hispanic women on the US-Mexico border. *Ethn. Dis.* 11(1):72–79

16. Byrd TL, Peterson SK, Chavez R, Heckert A. 2004. Cervical cancer screening beliefs among young Hispanic women. *Prev. Med.* 38:192–97

17. Cabassa LJ. 2003. Measuring acculturation: where we are and where we need to go. *Hisp. J. Behav. Sci.* 25(2):127–46

18. Caetano R. 1987. Acculturation, drinking and social settings among U.S. Hispanics. *Drug Alcohol Depend.* 19(3):215–26

19. Callister LC, Birkhead A. 2002. Acculturation and perinatal outcomes in Mexican immigrant childbearing women: an integrative review. *J. Perinat. Neonatal Nurs.* 16(3):22–38

20. Cantero PJ, Richardson JL, Baezconde-Garbanati L, Mark G. 1999. The association between acculturation and health practices among middle-aged and elderly Latinas. *Ethn. Dis.* 9(2):166–80

21. Case A, Lubotsky D, Paxson C. 2002. Economic status and health in childhood: the origins of the gradient. *Am. Econ. Rev.* 92(5):1308–34

22. Cervantes A, Keith L, Wyshak G. 1999. Adverse birth outcomes among native-born and immigrant women: replicating national evidence regarding Mexicans at the local level. *Matern. Child Health J.* 3(2):99–109

23. Cherpitel CJ, Borges G. 2002. Substance use among emergency room patients: an exploratory analysis by ethnicity and acculturation. *Am. J. Drug Alcohol Abuse* 28(2):287–305

24. Chesney AP, Chavira JA, Hall RP, Gary HE Jr. 1982. Barriers to medical care of Mexican-Americans: the role of social class, acculturation, and social isolation. *Med. Care* 20(9):883–91

25. Chun KM, Balls Organista P, Marín G, eds. 2003. *Acculturation: Advances in Theory, Measurement and Applied Research.* Washington, DC: Am. Psychol. Assoc.

26. Clark L. 2002. Mexican-origin mothers' experiences using children's health care services. *West. J. Nurs. Res.* 24(2):159–79

27. Cobas JA, Balcazar H, Benin MB, Keith VM, Chong Y. 1996. Acculturation and low-birthweight infants among Latino women: a reanalysis of HHANES data with structural equation models. *Am. J. Public Health* 86(3):394–96

28. Coonrod DV, Balcazar H, Brady J, Garci S, Van Tine M. 1995. Smoking, acculturation and family cohesion in Mexican-American women. *Ethn. Dis.* 9(3):434–40

29. Coonrod DV, Day RC, Balcazar H. 2004. Ethnicity, acculturation and obstetric outcomes: different risk factor profiles in low- and high-acculturation Hispanics and in white non-Hispanics. *J. Reprod. Med.* 49(1):17–22

30. Coreil J, Ray LA, Markides KS. 1991. Predictors of smoking among Mexican-American: findings from Hispanic HANES. *Prev. Med.* 20(4):508–17

31. Cortés DE, Deren S, Andía J, Colón H, Robles R, Kang SY. 2003. The use of the Puerto Rican Biculturality Scale with Puerto Rican drug users in New York and Puerto Rico. *J. Psychol. Drugs* 35(2):197–207

32. Cortés DE, Rogler LH. 1994. Biculturality among Puerto Rican adults in the United States. *Am. J. Community Psychol.* 22(5):707–21

33. Counc. Sci. Aff. 1991. Hispanic Health in the United States. *JAMA* 265:248–52

34. Crespo CJ, Smit E, Carter-Pokras O, Andersen R. 2001. Acculturation and

leisure-time physical inactivity in Mexican American adults: results from NHANES III, 1988–1994. *Am. J. Public Health* 91(8):1254–57

35. Crump C, Lipsky S, Mueller BA. 1999. Adverse birth outcomes among Mexican-Americans: Are US-born women at greater risk than Mexico-born women? *Ethn. Health* 4(1–2):29–34

36. Cuellar I, Arnold B, Maldonado R. 1995. Acculturation rating scale for Mexican Americans–II: a revision of the original ARSMA Scale. *Hisp. J. Behav. Sci.* 17(3):275–304

37. Cuellar I, Harris L, Jasso R. 1980. An acculturation scale for Mexican Americans, normal and clinical populations. *Hisp. J. Behav. Sci.* 2(3):199–217

38. Cuellar I, Roberts RE. 1997. Relations of depression, acculturation, and socioeconomic status in a Latino sample. *Hisp. J. Behav. Sci.* 19(2):230–38

39. Dawson DA. 1998. Beyond black, white and Hispanic: race, ethnic origin and drinking patterns in the United States. *J. Subst. Abuse* 10(4):321–39

40. De La Rosa M, Vega R, Radish MA. 2000. The role of acculturation in the substance abuse behavior of African-American and Latino adolescents: advances, issues and recommendations. *J. Psychoact. Drugs* 32(1):33–42

41. Deyo RA, Diehl AK, Hazuda H, Stern MP. 1985. A simple language-based acculturation scale for Mexican-Americans: validation and application to health care research. *Am. J. Public Health* 75(1):51–55

42. Dixon LB, Sundquist J, Winkleby M. 2000. Differences in energy, nutrient, and food intakes in a US sample of Mexican-American women and men: findings from the Third National Health and Nutrition Examination Survey, 1988–1994. *Am. J. Epidemiol.* 152(6):548–57

43. Dusenbery L, Epstein JA, Botvin GJ, Diaz T. 1994. The relationship between language spoken and smoking among Hispanic-Latino youth in New York City. *Public Health Rep.* 109(3):421–27

44. Elder JP, Castro FG, de Moor C, Mayer J, Candelaria JI, et al. 1991. Differences in cancer-risk-related behaviors in Latino and Anglo adults. *Prev. Med.* 20(6):751–63

45. Engel T, Alexander GR, Leland NL. 1995. Pregnancy outcomes of U.S.-born Puerto Ricans: the role of maternal nativity status. *Am. J. Prev. Med.* 11(1):34–39

46. English PB, Kharrazi M, Guendelman S. 1997. Pregnancy outcomes and risk factors in Mexican Americans: the effect of language use and mother's birthplace. *Ethn. Dis.* 7(3):229–40

47. Epstein JA, Botvin GJ, Diaz T. 1998. Linguistic acculturation and gender effects on smoking among Hispanic youth. *Prev. Med.* 27(4):583–89

48. Epstein JA, Doyle M, Botvin GJ. 2003. A mediational model of the relationship between linguistic acculturation and polydrug use among Hispanic adolescents. *Psychol. Rep.* 93:859–66

49. Esparza J, Harper IT, Bennett PH, Schultz LO, Valencia ME, Ravussin E. 2000. Daily energy expenditure in Mexican and USA Pima indians: low physical activity as a possible cause of obesity. *Int. J. Obes. Relat. Metab. Disord.* 24(1):55–59

50. Espino DV, Maldonado D. 1990. Hypertension and acculturation in elderly Mexican Americans: results from 1982–84 Hispanic HANES. *J. Gerontol.* 45(6): M209-13

51. Finch BK, Hummer RA, Reindl M, Vega WA. 2002. Validity of self-rated health among Latinos. *Am. J. Epidemiol.* 155(8): 755–59

52. Findley SE, Irigoyen M, Schulman A. 1999. Children on the move and vaccination coverage in a low-income, urban Latino population. *Am. J. Public Health* 89(11):1728–31

53. Flores G, Fuentes-Afflick E, Barbot O, Carter-Pokras O, Claudio L, et al. 2002. The health of Latino children: urgent

priorities, unanswered questions, and a research agenda. *JAMA* 288(1):82–90

54. Franco JN. 1983. An acculturation scale for Mexican-American children. *J. Gen. Psychol.* 108:175–81

55. Fuentes-Afflick E, Hessol NA, Perez-Stable EJ. 1999. Testing the epidemiologic paradox of low birth weight in Latinos. *Arch. Pediatr. Adolesc. Med.* 153:14–53

56. Fuentes-Afflick E, Lurie P. 1997. Low birth weight and Latino ethnicity, examining the epidemiologic paradox. *Arch. Pediatr. Adolesc. Med.* 151(7):665–74

57. Gfroerer J, De La Rosa M. 1993. Protective and risk factors associated with drug use among Hispanic youth. *J. Addict Dis.* 12(2):87–107

58. Gfroerer JC, Tan LL. 2003. Substance use among foreign-born youths in the United States: Does the length of residence matter? *Am. J. Public Health* 93(11):1892–95

59. Goel MS, Wee CC, McCarthy EP, Davis RB, Ngo-Metzger Q, Phillips RS. 2003. Racial and ethnic disparities in cancer screening: the importance of foreign birth as a barrier to care. *J. Gen. Intern. Med.* 18(12):1028–35

60. Gonzales HM, Haan MN, Hinton L. 2001. Acculturation and the prevalence of depression in older Mexican Americans: baseline results of the Sacramento area Latino study on aging. *J. Am. Geriatr. Soc.* 49(7):948–53

61. Gordon M. 1964. *Assimilation in American Life: The Role of Race, Religion and National Origins*. New York: Oxford Univ.

62. Gordon-Larsen P, Harris KM, Ward DS, Popkin BM. 2003. Acculturation and overweight-related behaviors among Hispanic immigrants to the US: the National Longitudinal Study of Adolescent Health. *Soc. Sci. Med.* 57:2023–34

63. Granados G, Puvvula J, Berman N, Dowling PT. 2001. Health care for Latino children: impact of child and parental birth-place on insurance status and access to health services. *Am. J. Public Health* 91(11):1806–7

64. Guendelman S, Abrams B. 1995. Dietary intake among Mexican-American women: generational differences and a comparison with white non-Hispanic women. *Am. J. Public Health* 85(1):20–25

65. Guendelman S, English P, Chavez G. 1995. Infants of Mexican immigrants: health status of an emerging population. *Med. Care* 33(1):41–52

66. Guzman B. 2001. *The Hispanic Population. Census 2000 Brief C2KBR/01–3*. U.S. Census Bur.

67. Halfon N, Wood DL, Valdez RB, Pereyra M, Duan N. 1997. Medicaid enrollment and health services access by Latino children in inner-city Los Angeles. *JAMA* 277(8):636–41

68. Harmon MP, Castro FG, Coe K. 1996. Acculturation and cervical cancer: knowledge, beliefs, and behaviors of Hispanic women. *Women Health* 24(3):37–57

69. Harris MI. 1991. Epidemiological correlates of NIDDM in Hispanics, Whites and Blacks in the U.S. population. *Diabetes Care* 14(7):639–48

70. Harris-Reid MA. 1999. Coming to America: immigration, stress, and mental health. *Diss. Abstr. Int. A. Humanit. Soc. Sci.* 59(10-A):3975

71. Hayes RP, Baker DW. 1998. Methodological problems in comparing English-Speaking and Spanish-speaking patients' satisfaction with interpersonal aspects of care. *Med. Care* 36(2):230–36

72. Hazuda HP, Haffner SM, Stern MP, Eifler CW. 1988. Effects of acculturation and socioeconomic status on obesity and diabetes in Mexican Americans. *Am. J. Epidemiol.* 128(6):1289–301

73. Heilemann MV, Lee KA, Stinson J, Koshar JH, Gross G. 2000. Acculturation and perinatal health outcomes among rural women of Mexican descent. *Res. Nurs. Health* 23(2):118–25

74. Hovey JD. 2000. Acculturative stress, depression and suicidal ideation in Mexican immigrants. *Cult. Divers. Ethn. Minor. Psychol.* 6(2):134–51

75. Hu DJ, Covell RM. 1986. Health care usage by Hispanic outpatients as function of primary language. *West. J. Med.* 144(4):490–93

76. Kaplan MS, Marks G. 1990. Adverse effects of acculturation psychological distress among Mexican American young adults. *Soc. Sci. Med.* 31(12):1313–19

77. Kelaher M, Jessop DJ. 2002. Differences in low-birth weight among documented and undocumented foreign-born and US-born Latinas. *Soc. Sci. Med.* 55:2171–75

78. Kerner JF, Breen N, Tefft MC, Silsby J. 1998. Tobacco use among multi-ethnic Latino populations. *Ethn. Dis.* 8(2):167–83

79. Khan LK, Sobal J, Martorell R. 1997. Acculturation, socioeconomic status, and obesity in Mexican Americans, Cuban Americans, and Puerto Ricans. *Int. J. Obes.* 21(2):91–96

80. Kieffer EC, Martin JA, Herman WH. 1999. Impact of maternal nativity on the prevalence of diabetes during pregnancy among U.S. ethnic groups. *Diabetes Care* 22(5):729–35

81. Klinnert MD, Price MR, Liu AH, Robinson JL. 2002. Unraveling the ecology of risks for early childhood asthma among ethnically diverse families in the southwest. *Am. J. Public Health* 92(5):792–98

82. Landale NS, Oropesa RS, Gorman BK. 2000. Migration and infant death: assimilation or selective migration among Puerto Ricans? *Am. Sociol. Rev.* 65(6):888–909

83. Lara M, Akinbami L, Flores G, Morgenstern H. 2004. Heterogeneity of childhood asthma among Hispanics: Puerto Ricans bear a disproportionate burden. *Pediatrics*. In press

84. MacCoy EL. 1938. *Maternal and Child Health Among the Mexican Groups in San Bernardino and Imperial Counties: A Study and Comparison.* Calif. State Dep. Public Health Bur. Child Hyg.

85. Magaña JR, de la Rocha O, Amsel J, Magaña HA, Fernandez MI, Rulnick S. 1996. Revisting the dimensions of acculturation: cultural theory and psychometric practice. *Hisp. J. Behav. Sci.* 18(4):444–68

86. Marín G. 1992. Issues in the measurement of acculturation among Hispanics. In *Psychological Testing of Hispanics*, ed. KF Geisinger, pp. 23–51. Washington, DC: Am. Psychol. Assoc.

87. Marín G, Gamba RJ. 1996. A new measure of acculturation for Hispanics: The Bidimensional Scale for Hispanics (BAS). *Hisp. J. Behav. Sci.* 18(3):297–316

88. Marín G, Perez-Stable EJ, Marin BV. 1989. Cigarette smoking among San Francisco Hispanics: the role of acculturation and gender. *Am. J. Public Health* 79(2):196–98

89. Marín G, Posner SF. 1995. The role of gender and acculturation on determining the consumption of alcoholic beverages among Mexican-Americans and Central Americans in the United States. *Int. J. Addict.* 30(7):779–94

90. Marín G, Sabogal F, Marin BVO, Otero-Sabogal R, Perez-Stable EJ. 1987. Development of a short acculturation scale for Hispanics. *Hisp. J. Behav. Sci.* 9(2):183–205

91. Markides KS, Coreil J, Ray JA. 1987. Smoking among Mexican Americans: a three-generational study. *Am. J. Public Health* 77(6):708–11

92. Markides KS, Krause N, Mendes de Leon CF. 1988. Acculturation and alcohol consumption among Mexican Americans: a three-generation study. *Am. J. Public Health* 78(9):1178–81

93. Markides KS, Lee DJ, Ray LA. 1993. Acculturation and hypertension in Mexican Americans. *Ethn. Dis.* 3:70–74

94. Markides KS, Levin JS, Ray LA. 1985. Determinants of physician utilization

among Mexican-Americans. A three-generations study. *Med. Care* 23(3):236–46

95. Markides KS, Ray LA, Stroup-Benham CA, Trevino F. 1990. Acculturation and alcohol consumption in the Mexican-American population of the southwestern United States: findings from HHANES 1982–84. *Am. J. Public Health* 80(Suppl.):42–46

96. Marks G, Garcia M, Solis JM. 1990. Health risk behaviors of Hispanics in the United States: findings from HHANES, 1982–84. *Am. J. Public Health* 80(Suppl.):20–26

97. Mazur RE, Marquis GS, Jensen HH. 2003. Diet and food insufficiency among Hispanic youths: acculturation and socioeconomic factors in the third National Health and Nutrition Examination Survey. *Am. J. Clin. Nutr.* 78(6):1120–27

98. Mendoza FS. 1994. The health of Latino children in the United States. *Crit. Health Issues Child Youth* 4(3):43–72

99. Mendoza FS. 2000. Health risk profiles and race, culture and socioeconomic status. In *Child Health in the Multicutural Environment. Report of the Thirty-First Ross Roundtable on Critical Approaches to Common Pediatric Problems*, ed. LM Pachter, pp. 5–18. Columbus, OH: Ross Products Div., Abbott Labs.

100. Mendoza RH. 1989. An empirical scale to measure type and degree of acculturation in Mexican-American adolescents and adults. *J. Cross-Cult. Psychol.* 20(4):372–85

101. Moore P, Fenlon N, Hepworth JT. 1996. Indicators of differences in immunization rates of Mexican Americans and white non-Hispanic infants in a Medicaid managed care system. *Public Health Nurs.* 13(1):21–30

102. Morales LS, Lara M, Kington RS, Valdez RO, Escarse JJ. 2002. Socioeconomic, cultural, and behavioral factors affecting Hispanic health outcomes. *J. Health Care Poor Underserv.* 13(4):477–502

103. Moscicki EK, Locke BZ, Rae DS, Boyd JH. 1989. Depressive symptoms among Mexican Americans: the Hispanic Health and Nutrition Examination Survey. *Am. J. Epidemiol.* 130(2):348–60

104. Negy C, Woods DJ. 1992. A note on the relationship between acculturation and socioeconomic status. *Hisp. J. Behav. Sci.* 14(2):248–51

105. Negy C, Woods DJ. 1992. The importance of acculturation in understanding research with Hispanic-Americans. *Hisp. J. Behav. Sci.* 14(2):224–47

106. Neuhouser ML, Thompson B, Coronado GD, Solomon CC. 2004. Higher fat intake and lower fruit and vegetables intakes are associated with greater acculturation among Mexicans living in Washington State. *J. Am. Diet Assoc.* 104(1):51–57

107. O'Malley AS, Kerner J, Johnson AE, Mandelblatt J. 1999. Acculturation and breast cancer screening among Hispanic women in New York City. *Am. J. Public Health* 89(2):219–27

108. Ortega AN, Rosenheck R, Alegria M, Desai RA. 2000. Acculturation and the lifetime risk of psychiatric and substance use disorders among Hispanics. *J. Nerv. Ment. Dis.* 188(11):728–35

109. Otero-Sabogal R, Sabogal F, Perez-Stable EJ, Hiatt RA. 1995. Dietary practices, alcohol consumption, and smoking behavior: ethnic, sex and acculturation differences. *J. Natl. Cancer Inst. Monogr.* (18):73–82

110. Pachter LM, Cloutier MM, Bernstein BA. 1995. Ethnomedical (folk) remedies for childhood asthma in a mainland Puerto Rican community. *Arch. Pediatr. Adolesc. Med.* 149:982–88

111. Pachter LM, Weller SC. 1993. Acculturation and compliance with medical therapy. *J. Dev. Behav. Pediatr.* 14(3):163–68

112. Pachter LM, Weller SC, Baer RD, de Alba Garcia JE, Trotter RT, et al. 2002. Variation in asthma beliefs and practices among mainland Puerto Ricans,

Mexican-Americans, Mexicans and Guatemalans. *J. Asthma* 39(2):119–34

113. Park RE, Burgess EW. 1969. *Introduction to the Science of Sociology*. Chicago: Univ. Chicago Press

114. Peragallo NP, Fox PG, Alba ML. 1998. Breast care among Latino immigrant women in the U.S. *Health Care Women Int.* 19(2):165–72

115. Peragallo NP, Fox PG, Alba ML. 2000. Acculturation and breast self-examination among immigrant Latina women in the USA. *Int. Nurs. Rev.* 47(1):38–45

116. Perlman J, Waldinger R. 1997. Second generation decline? Children of immigrants, past and present—a reconsideration. *Int. Migr. Rev.* 31(4):893–922

117. Polednak AP. 1997. Gender and acculturation in relation to alcohol use among Hispanic (Latino) adults in two areas of the northeastern United States. *Subst. Use Misuse* 32(11):1513–24

118. Popkin BM, Udry JR. 1998. Adolescent obesity increases significantly in second and third generation U.S. immigrants: the National Longitudinal Study of Adolescent Health. *J. Nutr.* 128(4):701–6

119. Portes A, Rumbaut RG. 2001. *Legacies: The Story of the Immigrant Second Generation*. Berkeley: Univ. Calif. Press

120. Prislin R, Suarez L, Simpson DM, Dyer JA. 1998. When acculturation hurts: the case of immunization. *Soc. Sci. Med.* 47(12):1947–56

121. Ramirez A, Cousins JH, Santos Y, Supik JD. 1986. A media-based acculturation scale for Mexican-Americans: application to public health education programs. *Fam. Community Health* 9(3):63–71

122. Randolph WM, Freeman DH Jr, Freeman JL. 2002. Pap smear use in a population of older Mexican-American women. *Women Health* 36(1):21–31

123. Reynoso TC, Felice ME, Shragg GP. 1993. Does American acculturation affect outcome of Mexican-American teenage pregnancy? *J. Adolesc. Health* 14(4):257–61

124. Rogler LH, Cortes DE, Malgady RG. 1991. Acculturation and mental health status among Hispanics. *Am. Psychol.* 46(6):585–97

125. Ryder AG, Alden LE, Paulhus DL. 2000. Is acculturation unidimensional or bidimensional? A head-to-head comparison in the prediction of personality, self-identity, and adjustment. *J. Personal. Soc. Psychol.* 79(1):49–65

126. Sabogal F, Marín G, Otero-Sabogal R. 1987. Hispanic familism and acculturation: What changes and what doesn't? *Hisp. J. Behav. Sci.* 9(4):397–412

127. Samat JM, Howard CA, Coultas DB, Skipper BJ. 1992. Acculturation, education, and income as determinants of cigarette smoking in New Mexico Hispanics. *Cancer Epidemiol. Biomark. Prev.* 1(3):235–40

128. Schutz CG, Chilcoat HD, Anthony JC. 1994. Degree of acculturation and the risk of crack cocaine smoking among Hispanic Americans. *Am. J. Public Health* 84(11):1825–27

129. Scribner R, Dwyer JH. 1989. Acculturation and low birthweight among Latinos in the Hispanic HANES. *Am. J. Public Health* 79(9):1263–67

130. Serrano E, Anderson J. 2003. Assessment of a refined short acculturation scale for Latino preteens in rural Colorado. *Hisp. J. Behav. Sci.* 25(2):240–53

131. Shetterly SM, Baxter J, Mason LD, Hamman RF. 1996. Self-rated health among Hispanic vs. non-Hispanic white adults: the San Luis Valley Health and Aging Study. *Am. J. Public Health* 86(12):1798–801

132. Singh GK, Yu SM. 1996. Adverse pregnancy outcomes: differences between US and foreign-born women in major US racial and ethnic groups. *Am. J. Public Health* 86(6):837–43

133. Skaer TL, Robison LM, Sclar DA, Harding GH. 1996. Cancer-screening determinants among Hispanic women using

migrant health clinics. *J. Health Care Poor Underserv.* 7(4):338–54

134. Solis JM, Marks G, Garcia M, Shelton D. 1990. Acculturation, access to care, and use of preventive services by Hispanics: findings from HHANES 1982–84. *Am. J. Public Health* 80(Suppl.):11–19

135. Stern MP, Gonzalez C, Mitchell BD, Villalpando E, Haffner SM, Hazud HP. 1992. Genetic and environmental determinants of type II diabetes in Mexico City and San Antonio. *Diabetes* 41(4):484–92

136. Stern MP, Knapp JA, Hazuda HP, Haffner SM, Patterson JK, Mitchell BD. 1991. Genetic and environmental determinants of Type II diabetes in Mexican Americans: Is there a "descending limb" to the modernization/diabetes relationship? *Diabetes Care* 14(7):649–54

137. Suarez L. 1994. Pap smear and mammogram screening in Mexican American women: the effects of acculturation. *Am. J. Public Health* 84(5):742–46

138. Sundquist J, Winkleby M. 2000. Country of birth, acculturation status and abdominal obesity in a national sample of Mexican-American women and men. *Int. J. Epidemiol.* 29(3):470–77

139. Sundquist J, Winkleby MA. 1999. Cardiovascular risk factors in Mexican American adults: a transcultural analysis of NHANES III, 1988–1994. *Am. J. Public Health* 89(5):723–30

140. Thamer M, Richard C, Casebeer AW, Ray NF. 1997. Health insurance coverage among foreign-born US residents: the impact of race, ethnicity, and length of residence. *Am. J. Public Health* 87(1):96–102

141. Turner RJ, Gil AG. 2002. Psychiatric and substance use disorders in South Florida: racial/ethnic and gender contrasts in a young adult cohort. *Arch. Gen. Psychiatry* 59(1):43–50

142. Unger JB, Cruz TB, Rohrbach LA, Ribiski KM, Baezconde-Garbanati L, et al. 2000. English language use as a risk factor for smoking initiation among Hispanic and Asian American adolescents: evidence for

mediation by tobacco-related beliefs and social norms. *Health Psychol.* 19(5):403–10

143. U.S. Dep. Health Hum. Serv., Off. Minor. Health. 2001. *National Standards for Culturally and Linguistically Appropriate Services in Health Care: Final Rep.* Washington, DC. http://www.omhrc.gov/omh/programs/2pgprograms/finalreport.pdf

144. Vega WA, Alderete E, Kolody B, Aguilar-Gaxiola S. 1998. Illicit drug use among Mexicans and Mexican Americans in California: the effects of gender and acculturation. *Addiction* 93(12):1839–50

145. Vega WA, Gil AG, Zimmerman RS. 1993. Patterns of drug use among Cuban-American, African-American, and White non-Hispanic boys. *Am. J. Public Health* 83(2):257–59

146. Vega WA, Kolody B, Hwang J, Noble A, Porter PA. 1997. Perinatal drug use among immigrant and native-born Latinas. *Subst. Use Misuse* 32(1):43–62

147. Vega WA, Scribney WM, Achara-Abrahams I. 2003. Co-occurring alcohol, drug and other psychiatric disorders among Mexican-origin people in the United States. *Am. J. Public Health* 93(7):1057–64

148. Velez CN, Ungemack JA. 1989. Drug use among Puerto Rican youth: an exploration of generational status differences. *Soc. Sci. Med.* 29(6):779–89

149. Wagner-Echeagaray FA, Schütz CG, Chilcoat HD, Anthony JC. 1994. Degree of acculturation and the risk of crack cocaine smoking among Hispanic Americans. *Am. J. Public Health* 84(11):1825–27

150. Wallen GR, Feldman RH, Anliker J. 2002. Measuring acculturation among Central American Women with the use of a Brief Language Scale. *J. Immigr. Health* 4(2):95–102

151. Warner WL, Srole L. 1945. *The Social Systems of American Ethnic Groups.* New Haven, CT: Yale Univ. Press

152. Weller SC, Baer RD, Pachter LM, Trotter RT, Glazer M, et al. 1999. Latino beliefs about diabetes. *Diabetes Care* 22(5):722–28

153. Wells KB, Golding JM, Hough RL, Burnam MA, Karno M. 1989. Acculturation and the probability of use of health services by Mexican Americans. *Health Serv. Res.* 24(2):237–57

154. Welte JW, Barnes GM. 1995. Alcohol and other drug use among Hispanics in New York State. *Alcohol. Clin. Exp. Res.* 19(4):1061–66

155. West SK, Muñoz B, Klein R, Broman AT, Sanchez R, et al. 2002. Risk factors for Type II diabetes and diabetic retinopathy in a Mexican-American population: Proyecto VER. *Am. J. Ophthalmol.* 134(3):390–98

156. Wolff CB, Portis M. 1996. Smoking, acculturation, and pregnancy outcome among Mexican Americans. *Health Care Women Int.* 17(6):563–73

157. Zambrana RE, Breen N, Fox SA, Gutierrez-Mohamed ML. 1999. Use of cancer screening practices by Hispanic women: analyses by subgroup. *Prev. Med.* 29:466–77

158. Zambrana RE, Scrimshaw SC, Collins N, Dunkel-Schetter C. 1997. Prenatal health behaviors and psychosocial risk factors in pregnant women of Mexican origin: the role of acculturation. *Am. J. Public Health* 87(6):1022–26

159. Zea MC, Asner-Self KK, Birman D, Buki LP. 2003. The abbreviated multidimensional acculturation scale: empirical validation with two Latino/Latina samples. *Cult. Divers. Ethn. Minor. Psychol.* 9(2):107–26

Annu. Rev. Public Health 2005. 26:399–419
doi: 10.1146/annurev.publhealth.26.021304.144357
First published online as a Review in Advance on October 26, 2004

ADOLESCENT RESILIENCE: A Framework for Understanding Healthy Development in the Face of Risk

Stevenson Fergus and Marc A. Zimmerman

*Department of Health Behavior and Health Education, School of Public Health,
University of Michigan, Ann Arbor, Michigan 48109; email: ferguss@umich.edu,
marcz@umich.edu*

Key Words   positive development, protective factors, alcohol, tobacco, illegal
drugs, sexual behavior, violent behavior

■ **Abstract**   Adolescent resilience research differs from risk research by focusing on
the assets and resources that enable some adolescents to overcome the negative effects
of risk exposure. We discuss three models of resilience—the compensatory, protective,
and challenge models—and describe how resilience differs from related concepts. We
describe issues and limitations related to resilience and provide an overview of recent
resilience research related to adolescent substance use, violent behavior, and sexual
risk behavior. We then discuss implications that resilience research has for intervention
and describe some resilience-based interventions.

INTRODUCTION

Resilience refers to the process of overcoming the negative effects of risk exposure, coping successfully with traumatic experiences, and avoiding the negative
trajectories associated with risks (43, 65, 72, 84, 106). A key requirement of resilience is the presence of both risks and promotive factors that either help bring
about a positive outcome or reduce or avoid a negative outcome. Resilience theory, though it is concerned with risk exposure among adolescents, is focused on
strengths rather than deficits. It focuses on understanding healthy development in
spite of risk exposure.

The promotive factors that can help youth avoid the negative effects of risks may
be either assets or resources (6). Assets are the positive factors that reside within
the individual, such as competence, coping skills, and self-efficacy. Resources
are also positive factors that help youth overcome risk, but they are external to
the individual. Resources include parental support, adult mentoring, or community organizations that promote positive youth development. The term resources
emphasizes the social environmental influences on adolescent health and development, helps place resilience theory in a more ecological context, and moves

399

away from conceptualizations of resilience as a static, individual trait (87). It also stresses that external resources can be a focus of change to help adolescents face risks and prevent negative outcomes.

Adolescents growing up in poverty, for example, are at risk of a number of negative outcomes, including poor academic achievement (2, 96) and violent behavior (34, 37). One approach to understanding why poverty results in negative outcomes is to focus on other deficits to which poverty may be related, such as limited community resources or a lack of parental monitoring. Researchers and practitioners working within a resilience framework recognize that, despite these risks, many adolescents growing up in poverty exhibit positive outcomes. These adolescents may possess any number of promotive factors, such as high levels of self-esteem (21) or the presence of an adult mentor (114), which help them avoid the negative outcomes associated with poverty. Using assets or resources to overcome risks demonstrates resilience as a process. Researchers have also described resilience as an outcome when they identify as resilient an adolescent who has successfully overcome exposure to a risk.

Researchers have suggested that resilience and vulnerability are opposite poles on the same continuum (40), but this may not always be the case. Vulnerability refers to increased likelihood of a negative outcome, typically as a result of exposure to risk. Resilience refers to avoiding the problems associated with being vulnerable. The relationship and distinction between resilience and vulnerability can be depicted in a two-by-two table (104). Table 1 represents four possible combinations of a risk and an outcome. Cell A represents adolescents who are exposed to low levels of a risk factor and who achieve positive outcomes. These adolescents follow trajectories typically considered normative development and are generally not the focus of resilience research. Cell B represents adolescents who are exposed to high levels of risk but who nonetheless achieve positive outcomes. Such adolescents are said to have followed a resilient trajectory. Adolescents in cell C are exposed to low levels of the risk factor and achieve negative outcomes. The adolescents in this cell exhibit an unexpected trajectory. It is likely that these adolescents have been exposed to some risk factor that was either poorly assessed or not measured. Finally, cell D represents adolescents with the expected outcome in risk models because they are exposed to high levels of the risk factor, which results in negative outcomes.

A factor can be considered a risk exposure, or an asset or resource, depending on the nature of the factor and the level of exposure to it. For some constructs, one

TABLE 1 Depiction of a population of adolescents

	Low risk	High risk
Positive outcome	A (normative development)	B (resilience theory)
Negative outcome	C (inadequate risk assessment)	D (risk models)

Note: Adapted from Reference 104.

extreme may be a risk factor, whereas the other extreme may be promotive. Having low self-esteem, for example, may place an adolescent at risk for developing a number of undesirable outcomes. Having high self-esteem, in contrast, may be an asset that can protect youth from negative outcomes associated with risk exposure. For other constructs, opposite poles may simply mean more or less of the construct. The opposite of positive friend influence is not necessarily bad influence of friends. Rather it may just be limited positive influence of friends. Similarly, involvement in extracurricular or community activities may be related to positive outcomes among adolescents, but this outcome does not mean that not participating in such activities should necessarily be considered a risk.

Resilience is sometimes confused with positive adjustment, coping, or competence. Although each of these constructs is related to resilience, they are also distinct. Positive adjustment refers to an outcome of resilience. When youth overcome a risky situation (e.g., the transition to middle school) as evidenced by healthy development (e.g., academic achievement) they have adjusted to their new context. In this case, positive adjustment is a resilient outcome, but the process of overcoming the risk is resilience. Youth may also be considered positively adjusted, however, even though they may not have been exposed to a risk. Resilience processes can have other outcomes as well, such as avoiding a negative outcome or coping successfully with a traumatic event (e.g., the death of a loved one). Resilience is also distinguished from competence. Competence is an asset (i.e., an individual-level promotive factor) that can be a vital component in a resilience process. Competent youth are expected to be more likely to overcome the negative effects of a risk. Competence, however, is only one of many assets that help adolescents overcome adversity. Because resilience models stress the importance of ecological context, external factors in addition to competence may help youth avoid the negative effects of risks.

Models of Resilience

Researchers have identified three models of resilience—compensatory, protective, and challenge—that explain how promotive factors operate to alter the trajectory from risk exposure to negative outcome (43, 84, 113). A compensatory model is defined when a promotive factor counteracts or operates in an opposite direction of a risk factor. A compensatory model therefore involves a direct effect of a promotive factor on an outcome. This effect is independent of the effect of a risk factor (113). Model 1 in Figure 1 depicts how compensatory factors operate to influence outcomes. Youth living in poverty, for example, are more likely to commit violent behavior than are youth not living in poverty (37), but adult monitoring of behavior may help compensate for the negative effects of poverty. This model can be examined using a number of statistical and methodological approaches but is typically tested by examining unique, direct effects in a multiple regression analysis or with structural equation modeling.

Another model of resilience is the protective factor model. In this model, assets or resources moderate or reduce the effects of a risk on a negative outcome.

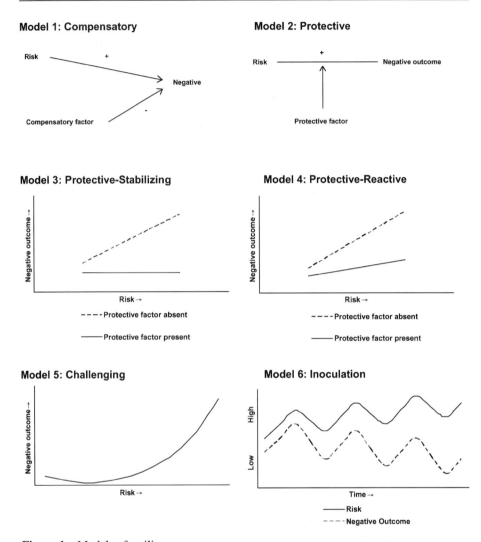

Figure 1 Models of resilience.

A protective model exists if, for example, the relationship between poverty and violent behavior is reduced for youth with high levels of parental support. In this example, parental support operates as a protective factor because it moderates the effects of poverty on violent behavior. Model 2 in Figure 1 shows how a protective factor may influence the relationship between a risk and an outcome. This model can be examined a number of different ways yet is typically tested with an interaction term in multiple regression or with group comparisons in structural equation modeling.

Protective factors may operate in several ways to influence outcomes. Luthar and colleagues (65), for example, define protective-stabilizing and protective-reactive models. A protective-stabilizing model, depicted in Model 3 in Figure 1, refers to instances when a protective factor helps to neutralize the effects of risks. Thus, higher levels of risk are associated with higher levels of a negative outcome when the protective factor is absent, but there is no relationship between the risk and the outcome when the protective factor is present. Among youth whose parents do not provide adequate support or monitoring (risk factors), for example, those without an adult mentor (a protective resource) may exhibit delinquent behaviors (an outcome), whereas those with a nonparental adult mentor may not.

A protective-reactive model, depicted in Model 4 in Figure 1, refers to instances when a protective factor diminishes, but does not completely remove, the expected correlation between a risk and an outcome. Thus, the relationship between the risk and the outcome is stronger when the protective factor is absent. Adolescents who abuse drugs, for example, may be more likely to engage in sexual risk behavior. The relationship between drug abuse (a risk factor) and sexual risk behavior (an outcome), however, may be weaker among adolescents who are exposed to comprehensive sexuality education in their schools (a protective resource) than among adolescents who do not receive such education.

Brook and colleagues (17, 18) also posit a protective-protective model. In this model, a protective factor enhances the effect of another promotive factor in producing an outcome. Parental support, for example, may enhance the positive effect of academic competence for producing more positive academic outcomes than for either factor alone. Yet, resilience requires the presence of risk, so the protective-protective model may not be a resilience model, unless the two protective factors are studied in a population defined to be at risk for a particular negative outcome (115).

A third model of resilience is the challenge model (43), depicted in Model 5 of Figure 1. In this model, the association between a risk factor and an outcome is curvilinear. This suggests that exposure to low levels and high levels of a risk factor are associated with negative outcomes, but moderate levels of the risk are related to less negative (or positive) outcomes (66). The idea is that adolescents exposed to moderate levels of risk are confronted with enough of the risk factor to learn how to overcome it but are not exposed to so much of it that overcoming it is impossible. A vital point concerning the challenge model is that low levels of risk exposure may be beneficial because they provide youth with a chance to practice skills or employ resources. The risk exposure, however, must be challenging enough to elicit a coping response so the adolescent can learn from the process of overcoming the risk. In challenge models, the risk and promotive factors studied are the same variable—whether it is a risk or is promotive for an adolescent depends on the level of exposure. Too little family conflict, for example, may not prepare youth with an opportunity to learn how to cope with or solve interpersonal conflicts outside of the home. Yet, too much conflict may be debilitating and lead youth to feel hopeless and distressed. A moderate amount of conflict, however, may provide youth with enough exposure to learn from the development and resolution of the conflict. They essentially learn through modeling or vicarious experience. Challenge models of resilience are typically tested with polynomial terms in multiple regression (e.g., quadratic or cubic terms).

The challenge model of resilience can be considered inoculation or steeling (70, 85, 113) if it includes a developmental (i.e., longitudinal) focus. This model, depicted in Model 6 of Figure 1, suggests that continued or repeated exposure to low levels of a risk factor helps inoculate adolescents so they are prepared to overcome more significant risks in the future. The inoculation model is similar to the challenge model because a factor may be seen as risky when it leads to negative outcomes or promotive when it teaches adolescents to better handle stressors in the future. Yates et al. (112) have described this model of resilience as an ongoing developmental process, in which children learn to mobilize assets and resources as they are exposed to adversity. As youth successfully overcome low levels of risk, they become more prepared to face increasing risk. As people age and mature, and continue to be exposed to adversity, their capacity to thrive despite risks increases. Such models must be tested with longitudinal data. In this way, compensatory, protective, or challenge models can operate within a framework of inoculation, as repeated exposures to compensatory, protective, and/or challenge processes prepare adolescents for dealing with adversities in the future.

Issues and Limitations

A number of issues related to resilience research have created confusion within the field and fueled criticism of resilience theory. Unfortunately, as several researchers have pointed out (65), differing uses of terminology has seemed to slow down the development of the field, and we need to develop a common language to bring the field to the next level. Some researchers who have criticized resilience research have assumed that resilience is a trait (103). It is vital to note, however, that resilience is not a static trait (58). That is, resilience is not a quality of an adolescent that is always present in every situation. Rather, resilience is defined by the context, the population, the risk, the promotive factor, and the outcome. Thus, the measurement of resilience with a self-report assessment (76, 105) may not be consistent with resilience theory. Part of the confusion may be because some individual-level assets such as self-efficacy, competence, or coping skills may be involved in resilience processes. This should not be interpreted to mean, however, that resilience lies only within the individual or is a static, personal trait. An analytic approach that examines relationships among risk and promotive factors is necessary for understanding adolescent resilience (72, 113).

As a way of stressing that resilience is not a trait, some researchers have suggested that the term resilience be used in place of resiliency (65), a term favored by others in the field. Although this distinction may not be important as both words are synonymous nouns, it is vital to distinguish resilience from a trait-based conception. Further, Luthar & Zelazo (66) point out that the term resilient should not be used as an adjective describing a person but as a descriptor of profiles or trajectories. This distinction further assures that the construct of resilience is not taken to be an individual trait. The concern in treating or considering resilience as a trait is that it places blame on the adolescent for failing to overcome adversity or risk. It also raises questions about the usefulness of prevention efforts because individual trait-like characteristics may not be amenable to change. Finally, trait conceptions ignore contextual factors, but resilience theory incorporates social and environmental influences.

Another issue to consider is that resilience may be content- and context-specific (26). That is, an adolescent may be resilient in the face of one type of risk but may be unable to overcome other types of risk. Some adolescents, for example, may be resilient against certain negative effects of poverty because they have supportive families, but some of these same adolescents may be less successful overcoming the effects of attending underfunded schools. The risk of an underfunded school may take more than family support to overcome. Researchers have also found that different assets may be associated with different risk and outcome pairings (32, 49). This makes it difficult to identify universal promotive factors and raises concerns that asset lists (7, 60, 73) may be interpreted to operate in the same manner for all groups, all contexts, or all outcomes.

The process of resilience may also vary for different groups of adolescents (28). Resilience for urban and suburban youth, for example, may differ from resilience for rural youth. Similarly, resilience may differ for high- and low-socioeconomic-status youth, for males and females (41), for early adolescents and late adolescents, or for immigrant and nonimmigrant youth. Sameroff et al. (86), for example, describe how parental control may be beneficial in environments characterized by certain risk exposures such as street crime but may be detrimental in environments where such risks do not exist. Similarly, Gutman et al. (49) found among African American adolescents an interaction between number of risk factors and democratic decision making in the family for predicting grade point average and math achievement. Their results indicated that democratic decision making increased the effects of risk factors on the outcomes. This finding suggests that democratic decision making, often considered a resource, may be detrimental in high-risk-exposed environments. This is a critical issue because researchers and practitioners may need to be aware that findings from one context or population may not apply to their given context or population.

Another key point about resilience theory is that, by definition, resilience requires the presence of a risk factor (45). Some have attempted to study resilience among youth not faced with risk (33), but this type of study may be more appropriately defined as research on adolescent development and adjustment more generally. Positive outcomes alone are not sufficient for inferring resilience. Adolescents must have been exposed to some factor or factors (i.e., risks) that increase the likelihood of a poor outcome for promotive factors to be relevant in a study of resilience. Yet, longitudinal research that includes a sample selected on the basis of being at a high level of a risk factor (e.g., poverty) may be problematic because of the tendency for the sample to regress toward the mean. This phenomenon, and not the presence of a promotive factor, may explain why some youth with a risk factor show fewer negative outcomes over time. In other words, some vulnerable youth may improve simply because of a statistical artifact, regardless of the presence of a promotive factor. Resilience researchers who choose such an approach must be sure to apply designs that will help them eliminate regression to the mean as an explanation of their results.

Adversities facing youth can range from long-term chronic stressors to short-term acute stressors, or to traumatic stressful events (8, 83, 108). Some risk exposures may have immediate, acute effects on adolescents, but the effects may dissipate relatively quickly. Other exposures may not be as dramatic but may be chronic and linger over time. A youth who is HIV positive, for example, faces a number of risk exposures that can lead to poor outcomes. The consistent need to remember to take medications may be considered a long-term chronic stressor, disclosing one's HIV status to a significant other may be a short-term acute stressor, and being hospitalized for a serious opportunistic infection may be a traumatic stressful event. Each of these risk exposures may be responsive to different assets and resources and may be related to different adverse outcomes.

Another issue related to risk exposure is that experiences of the same adverse event or condition may differ across adolescents. For many youth, for example, the divorce of one's parents may be experienced as a negative event. For some youth, however, the same experience may be positive, if it removes family conflict from the home environment (53). Researchers may therefore not always want to assume that because an event is normatively considered negative (or, conversely, normatively considered positive) it is experienced as negative (or positive) by all youth. Researchers may wish to include assessments of how the youth experienced an event in their studies. Failure to consider such a possibility may attenuate research findings, as relationships expected by researchers may operate among some youth in a way that is opposite the hypothesized direction. Similarly, even when an exposure is universally experienced as a risk, the level of adversity may differ. One way to handle this problem is to include measures related to the level of risk exposure in studies. Buckner et al. (21), for example, controlled for variation in experiences of negative events and chronic strains in their study of youth living in poverty. They found that the number of negative events and chronic strains reported was associated with a composite measure of behavior problems, mental health symptoms, functioning and adaptation, and competence.

Resilience research is also somewhat limited because it typically includes single risks and a single promotive factor (111), but most youth are actually exposed to multiple risks, may possess multiple assets, and may have access to multiple resources (45, 86). Several researchers have found that risks (or promotive factors) do not necessarily operate independently in the lives of youth but rather mutually influence each other (49, 65, 74, 75, 86, 94). Masten (71) describes a cascading effect of risks and promotive factors where positive constructs can also be either outcomes or predictors, depending on the situation and when a youth is assessed

(66). A rich understanding of resilience processes therefore necessitates including cumulative risks, assets, and resources studied over time (27, 28, 86, 112).

A final key component of resilience research, though one that is often over-looked, is investigating explanations for how assets or resources interact with risk exposures to produce particular outcomes (65). If researchers find evidence, for example, that parental support (a resource) interacts with negative peer influence (a risk) to predict smoking (an outcome), the next step should be to understand why this is so. The type of parental support provided may be decisive. Parents may provide emotional support necessary to develop the emotional capacity to with-stand peer influences, or they may provide informational support related to the health consequences of smoking, increasing the perceived threat of the behavior. Research on the mechanisms by which resilience processes occur, or what Sandler et al. (87) call "small theories," could yield information to be applied in developing interventions. Qualitative studies, like those conducted by Werner and colleagues (106, 107), may also help to answer such questions.

SELECTED RESEARCH FINDINGS ON ADOLESCENT RESILIENCE

Research on resilience has grown exponentially in the past 10 years. A simple Med-line search using PubMed and the key words adolescence, adolescent, resilience, resiliency, and protective factors produced 49 citations from 1975 through 1984, 206 citations from 1985 through 1994, and 756 citations from 1995 through 2004. Consequently, we focus our review on recent articles investigating substance use (alcohol, tobacco, and other drugs), violent behavior, and sexual behavior. We chose these outcomes for several reasons. First, most research on adolescent re-silience focuses on psychopathology (75), rather than behavior. Second, these three behaviors pose considerable health risks to adolescents and play a significant role in adolescent development. Finally, these behaviors may be particularly amenable to public health intervention.

Substance Use

Researchers have found a number of assets and resources that may compensate for or protect against risks for substance use at the individual, peer, family, school, and community levels. Researchers have found adolescents to be protected from the substance use consequences of stressful or negative life events by assets such as self-esteem (22), internal locus of control (92), positive affect (92), and religiosity (110). Wills et al. (109) found among 1702 adolescents followed from age 12 to age 15 that positive affectivity, or feeling happy, interested, and relaxed, was protective against the risk of emotional distress for cigarette, alcohol, and marijuana use. Resources that have been found to compensate for the effects of emotional distress include family connectedness (42, 63) and parental involvement with school (42).

Similar promotive factors, including planning to attend college (19), and resources such as family connectedness (42, 63) and parental involvement with school (42) have been found to compensate for the effects of delinquent behavior on substance use. Scheier et al. (91) found three assets to compensate for the effects of risk-taking on alcohol use among adolescents: self-control, substance-use refusal skills, and academic achievement. Psychological well-being and social competence (47) compensated for the effects of prior cigarette, alcohol, and marijuana use for predicting current use among 1184 junior high school students in New York City. Academic achievement is a consistent protective factor for substance use. This asset helps protect against the risks of low academic motivation (20) and age-related increases in substance use (19). Parental support resources protect youth from the risks of acculturation (50) and low ethnic identification (16, 93) for substance use.

Individual-level assets and family-level resources are consistent promotive factors for substance-use risks associated with peer influences. Participation in extracurricular and community activities (31) have compensated for the negative influences of peer tobacco, alcohol, and illegal drug use. Decision-making skills (12) and positive orientation toward school (30) have also protected youth from the negative effects of peer substance use. Legitimization of parental authority (57), family connectedness (63), parental monitoring (81), and open communication with parents (100) are resources that appear to compensate for peer substance use. Parental support may also protect against the negative effects of peer substance use (39, 59), peer pressure (39), and age-related increases (90). Similarly, decision-making skills (12) protect against having peers with favorable attitudes toward substance use for alcohol and marijuana use.

Parental substance use is also a significant risk factor for adolescent substance use. Among personal assets, social competence helps compensate for the risk posed by parental use (44), and religiosity helps protect youth from the adverse effects of parental substance use on their own use (15). Family connectedness (63) and parental authority (57) are resources that protect youth from the negative influence of parental substance use. Decision-making skills (12) have also protected youth from the negative effects of parental permissiveness on alcohol and marijuana use.

Family connectedness compensated for the risk of low school connectedness on cigarette smoking in a nationally representative sample (63). Parental support protects against the community-level risk factors of drug availability and low community norms for family closeness (16) on marijuana use. Family income has also moderated the relationship between neighborhood problems and adolescent alcohol and marijuana use (35). Higher family income protected youth from adverse neighborhood effects.

Most studies include analysis of one risk and promotive factor at a time, but other approaches are to study multiple risks and promotive factors or to combine multiple risk and promotive factors to form cumulative measures. Researchers have studied cumulative risk measures and adolescent substance use, both with single assets or resources and with cumulative promotive measures. Scal et al. (89), for example, investigated the effects of different combinations of assets and resources for smoking in the presence of a number of risks at the individual, peer, and parental levels. They found that religiosity, academic achievement, family connectedness, and parental education expectations all compensated for the effects of the risks. Other researchers studied cumulative risk measures with cumulative promotive measures. Cumulative measures made up solely of resources (5) and made up of assets and resources (38, 79, 92, 102) have been protective against cumulative risk measures.

Violent Behavior

Empirical evidence also supports the compensatory and protective models for adolescent violent behavior. Assets that have compensated for individual-level risk factors include prosocial beliefs compensating for antisocial socialization (56), religiosity compensating for interest in gang involvement (4), and anger control skills compensating for risk-taking behavior (48). Two dimensions of racial identity, public regard and centrality, are assets that Caldwell et al. (23) found to protect against the effects of racial discrimination on violent behavior among 325 African American adolescents studied from ages 14 to 20. Maternal support has both compensated for and protected against the risk factor for violent behavior of getting in a fight, whereas paternal support has been protective (116). Finally, the resource parental monitoring has compensated for the effects of risk-taking behavior on violent behavior (48).

Peer behaviors and attitudes may also pose a risk for violent behavior that promotive factors may compensate for or protect against. Anger-control skills compensate for the effects of peer delinquent behavior for predicting adolescent violent behavior (48). Perceived social status was found to moderate (i.e., a protective factor) the relationship between peer delinquent behaviors and adolescent violent behavior (80). Parental monitoring was also a compensatory factor (48). Adolescents' religiosity also compensated for the risk of peer substance use (55) and exposure to violence for violent behavior (4). Parental factors are also consistent resources to help youth overcome risks for violent behavior. Maternal support protected youth from the negative influences of peer violent behavior (116). Parental monitoring and paternal support were found to compensate for peer violent behavior (55, 116). Parental monitoring also compensated for the risk of living in a risky neighborhood (48). Maternal and paternal support also compensated for and protected youth from the negative consequences of exposure to violence (116).

Researchers have also found assets and resources that compensate for cumulative risk factors for violent behavior. Borowsky et al. (9) found among 13,781 seventh- through twelfth-grade adolescents studied over two years that academic performance, parental presence, parent-family connectedness, and school connectedness, alone and in combination, compensated for the cumulative effects of prior violent behavior, violence victimization, substance use, and school problems on violent behavior. Other researchers have found that cumulative measures of assets and resources compensate for cumulative risk factors (79, 101).

Sexual Behavior

Sexual behavior among adolescents includes initiation of sex, level of sexual activity, and risky sexual behavior. Substance use is an individual-level risk factor for adolescent sexual behavior that is compensated for by personal assets such as self-esteem (78), participation in extracurricular activities (1), school achievement and attachment (62, 67, 78, 88), religiosity (62, 67), HIV and reproductive health knowledge (67), positive attitudes toward condoms (69), safer sex intentions (69), seeing sex as nonnormative (88), and self-efficacy to refuse drugs and use condoms (88). Resources that have compensated for substance use in predicting sexual behavior include father's education (1), teacher support (1), residence with both parents (1, 62), peer norms for sexual behavior (3), and family socioeconomic status.

Family socioeconomic status (68), parental monitoring (81), and open parental communication (100) have compensated for the risk of peer sexual behavior for adolescent sexual behavior. Paul et al. (78) reported for their 21-year longitudinal study of 1020 participants in New Zealand that school attachment and self-esteem helped compensate for the risk of sexual intercourse before age 16 associated with mothers having had a child before the age of 20. Participation in extracurricular activities and community organizations has also helped counteract the effects of neighborhood poverty on a composite measure of adolescent sexual risk behavior in a study of 370 urban African American adolescents (82).

Research Findings Summary

Across most risk factors for adolescent substance use, violent behavior, and sexual behavior, parental factors seem to be particularly vital in helping youth be resilient. The compensatory model appears to have more empirical support, but for substance use and violent behavior, several promotive factors are also protective. To date, researchers have not yet tested the challenge or inoculation models for these outcomes.

One limitation in the research literature on adolescent resilience is that most studies focus on individual assets and family-level resources. Research that examines adolescent resilience with the help of school and community-level resources would be useful. Another limitation of this literature is the almost complete reliance on cross-sectional research (1, 3–5, 12, 15, 16, 22, 38, 39, 48, 55, 57, 59, 62, 63, 67–69, 79–82, 92, 102, 116). The studies that are longitudinal typically include only two time points (9, 23, 42, 50, 88, 89). It is necessary to include many waves of observation over longer periods of time to understand more completely the developmental factors associated with resilience processes for adolescent substance use, violent behavior, and sexual behavior.

Although the research described provides empirical support for the resilience models described, the researchers did not necessarily use resilience theory to guide the analyses. Rather, they found that positive factors (what we have called promotive factors) counteract (compensate) or moderate (protect) against risks youth face. More research that specifically applies resilience theory and tests the models within it will help us further understand how resilience processes operate to help youth overcome the risks they face.

Notably, most research on resilience has focused on either nationally representative samples (9, 19, 35, 63, 89), predominantly white youth (42, 62), or predominantly African American samples (3, 20, 23, 39, 48, 55, 57, 81, 82, 88, 93, 100, 102, 116). Research that focuses on other ethnic groups, such as Latino, Native American, or Arab American youth, or on recent immigrants, would further our understanding of resilience among adolescents. In addition, there are virtually no studies of resilience for gay, lesbian, bisexual, or transgendered youth, leaving a significant void in the literature.

RESILIENCE-BASED INTERVENTIONS

The concept of resilience and its associated evidence suggest several implications for prevention. A key idea is that interventions may need to focus on developing assets and resources for adolescents exposed to risk (26, 64, 112) instead of the more traditional approach of focusing on risk amelioration. The educational and ecological assessment phase of the widely used health planning model PRECEDE/PROCEED (46), for example, calls for practitioners to catalog the predisposing, enabling, and reinforcing factors associated with the behavior targeted for change. The usual practice is to list deficits that predispose, enable, and reinforce some negative behavior. A resilience approach, however, emphasizes assets and resources as the focus for change. Internal assets that may be particularly critical to develop include social skills for relating to peers, self-efficacy for health-promoting behavior, academic skills, and participation in extracurricular and community activities.

Botvin and colleagues (11, 13, 14) have suggested that skill building for life in general, such as the development of generic social and problem-solving skills, can be just as important as building skills for risk avoidance. External resources that may be developed include opportunities for adult mentorship (51, 114), parenting skills (61), and provision of health-promoting settings for adolescents (36). Another key idea is that, because of the multidimensional nature of resilience, interventions that cut across behaviors may be most effective. Interventions that focus solely on substance use avoidance, for example, may be too narrowly focused to alter the entire context of influences in adolescents' lives. Yet, it may be critical for practitioners to focus attention on those assets and resources that have been found to promote healthy outcomes in their particular populations.

A number of interventions include development of assets and resources in adolescents' lives. Life Skills Training (10, 13) is a classroom-based program that focuses on general adolescent skill development and on developing skills for resisting social influences to use substances. The intervention includes a number of activities such as demonstration, role-playing, and behavioral homework assignments. This intervention's focus on cognitive-behavior skills related to building self-esteem, decreasing anxiety, communicating effectively, developing relationships with others, and asserting rights suggests a resilience approach because it focuses on vital individual assets for healthy and effective social interaction. These skills are assets that can counteract risks for a variety of outcomes. The Resourceful Adolescent Program (RAP) (95) is another individual-level intervention focused on enhancing adolescents' skills and social resources. It includes sessions on affirming participants' strengths, learning skills for handling stress, developing social support networks, and conducting interpersonal relationships with others, including family members.

Several interventions focus on families as a way to develop both assets and resources. The RAP (95), for example, includes three sessions for participants' parents, with a similar focus as in the adolescent sessions. The Multidimensional Family Prevention project (54) trains counselors to visit participating inner-city families in their homes and to work with the families to identify their existing assets and resources. The program helps the adolescent and parent develop new skills to communicate more effectively in general and with each other. It is also designed to help both parents and youth engage more effectively in their interactions in the community. The Preparing for the Drug Free Years (PDFY) and Iowa Strengthening Families (ISF) programs (97–99) similarly focus on parental skills and adolescent prosocial and peer-pressure resistance skills. PDFY is an intervention with parents of sixth graders; it teaches them how to enhance their relationships with their children, develop appropriate monitoring practices, and manage anger and conflict within the family. Children are included in one of the intervention's sessions. The ISF program includes both parents and children; the parenting content is similar to the PDFY program, and the adolescent content focuses on peer resistance and relationship skills. In some of the sessions, parents and children are brought together to practice the skills they have been learning about. These programs are examples of employing a resilience approach because they focus on building positive relationships as a way to prevent negative outcomes, and they stress the importance of family members as resources for healthy adolescent development. In contrast, a more traditional approach may focus on reducing or eliminating the negative factors in youths' lives.

Some family-based interventions focus on particular racial or ethnic groups so that the intervention stresses risks, assets, and resources unique to the group. The Flint Fathers and Sons program (24, 25) is a family-based intervention focused on strengthening father-son relationships among African American participants. It involves family members in activities to learn skills (e.g., communication skills), participate in community and school activities, and enhance cultural pride and racial/ethnic identity. The focus of the intervention is to prevent or reduce substance use, violent behavior, and sexual risk behavior among the fathers and sons. The Adolescent and Family Rites of Passage program (52) is a similar intervention for African American adolescent males in Washington, D.C., that includes after-school activities, family enhancement, and empowerment activities. The activities include elements of African culture and aim to foster self-esteem, positive peer relationships, and interpersonal skills among the adolescents. It also includes programs for parents to enhance parenting skills, parent-child bonds, and participation in school and the community. Finally, Familias Unidas is a family-centered intervention for immigrant Latino families in South Florida (29, 77). This program focuses on parents and begins with the development of small parental support networks, which then develop and plan the remaining activities, including family meetings, home visits, parent-child discussion sessions, activities with adolescents, activities with adolescents and peers, meetings with school counselors, and family therapy. These three programs are examples of connecting parents and children in constructive ways so they are both more prepared to address risks for which adolescents are inevitably exposed. Their focus on youths' assets and family resources suggests they use a resilience approach.

CONCLUSION

The goal of this review is to help provide a common language and understanding to conduct research and interventions that focus on assets and resources. Resilience models help us understand why some youth exposed to risks are able to overcome them and avoid negative outcomes. Although assets and resources that help youth overcome the adverse effects of risks may differ by outcome, context, and population studied, several common themes do emerge. Parental factors are consistent and critical resources for youth. These factors include support, monitoring, and communication skills. Youth who have self-confidence and social skills also are somewhat predisposed to being resilient regardless of the risk or outcome. Nevertheless, it is vital that public health interventions that use a resilience approach pay particular attention to the unique features of the population of interest and the context in which the approach is employed. Resilience theory provides researchers and practitioners with a conceptual model that can help them understand how youth overcome adversity and how we can use that knowledge to enhance strengths and build the positive aspects of their lives.

The *Annual Review of Public Health* is online at
http://publhealth.annualreviews.org

LITERATURE CITED

1. Anteghini M, Fonseca H, Ireland M, Blum RW. 2001. Health risk behaviors and associated risk and protective factors among Brazilian adolescents in Santos, Brazil. *J. Adolesc. Health* 28:295–302

2. Arnold DH, Doctoroff GL. 2003. The early education of socioeconomically dis-

advantaged children. *Annu. Rev. Psychol.* 54:517–45

3. Bachanas PJ, Morris MK, Lewis-Gess JK, Sarett-Cuasay EJ, Sirl K, et al. 2002. Predictors of risky sexual behavior in African American adolescent girls: implications for prevention interventions. *J. Pediatr. Psychol.* 27:519–30

4. Barkin S, Kreiter S, Durant RH. 2001. Exposure to violence and intentions to engage in moralistic violence during early adolescence. *J. Adolesc.* 24:777–89

5. Beam MR, Gil-Rivas V, Greenberger E, Chen CS. 2002. Adolescent problem behavior and depressed mood: risk and protection within and across social contexts. *J. Youth Adolesc.* 31:343–57

6. Beauvais F, Oetting ER. 1999. Drug use, resilience, and the myth of the golden child. See Ref. 44a, pp. 101–8

7. Benson PL, Leffert N. 2001. Childhood and adolescence: developmental assets. In *International Encyclopedia of the Social and Behavioral Sciences*, ed. NJ Smelser, PG Baltes, pp. 1690–97. Oxford: Pergamon

8. Bonanno GA. 2004. Loss, trauma, and human resilience: Have we underestimated the human capacity to thrive after extremely aversive events? *Am. Psychol.* 59:20–28

9. Borowsky IW, Ireland M, Resnick MD. 2002. Violence risk and protective factors among youth held back in school. *Ambul. Pediatr.* 2:475–84

10. Botvin GJ, Baker E, Dusenbury L, Botvin EM, Diaz T. 1995. Long-term follow-up results of a randomized drug abuse prevention trial in a white middle-class population. *JAMA* 273:1106–12

11. Botvin GJ, Griffin KW. 2002. Life skills training as a primary prevention approach for adolescent drug abuse and other problem behaviors. *Int. J. Emerg. Ment. Health* 4:41–47

12. Botvin GJ, Malgady RG, Griffin KW, Scheier LM, Epstein JA. 1998. Alcohol and marijuana use among rural youth: interaction of social and intrapersonal influences. *Addict. Behav.* 23:379–87

13. Botvin GJ, Schinke SP, Epstein JA, Diaz T. 1994. The effectiveness of culturally focused and generic skills training approaches to alcohol and drug abuse prevention among minority youths. *Psychol. Addict. Behav.* 8:116–27

14. Botvin GJ, Schinke SP, Epstein JA, Diaz T, Botvin EM. 1995. Effectiveness of culturally focused and generic skills training approaches to alcohol and drug-abuse prevention among minority adolescents—2-year follow-up results. *Psychol. Addict. Behav.* 9:183–94

15. Brook JS, Brook DW, De La Rosa M, Whiteman M, Johnson E, Montoya I. 2001. Adolescent illegal drug use: the impact of personality, family, and environmental factors. *J. Behav. Med.* 24:183–203

16. Brook JS, Brook DW, De La Rosa M, Whiteman M, Montoya ID. 1999. The role of parents in protecting Colombian adolescents from delinquency and marijuana use. *Arch. Pediatr. Adolesc. Med.* 153:457–64

17. Brook JS, Gordon AS, Whiteman M, Cohen P. 1986. Dynamics of childhood and adolescent personality traits and adolescent drug use. *Dev. Psychol.* 22:403–14

18. Brook JS, Whiteman M, Gordon AS, Cohen P. 1989. Changes in drug involvement: a longitudinal study of childhood and adolescent determinants. *Psychol. Rep.* 65:707–26

19. Bryant AL, Schulenberg JE, O'Malley PM, Bachman JG, Johnston LD. 2003. How academic achievement, attitudes, and behaviors relate to the course of substance use during adolescence: a 6-year, multiwave national longitudinal study. *J. Res. Adolesc.* 13:361–97

20. Bryant AL, Zimmerman MA. 2002. Examining the effects of academic beliefs and behaviors on changes in substance use among urban adolescents. *J. Educ. Psychol.* 94:621–37

21. Buckner JC, Mezzacappa E, Beardslee WR. 2003. Characteristics of resilient youths living in poverty: the role of self-regulatory processes. *Dev. Psychopathol.* 15:139–62

22. Byrne DG, Mazanov J. 2001. Self-esteem, stress and cigarette smoking in adolescents. *Stress Health* 17:105–10

23. Caldwell CH, Kohn-Wood LP, Schmeelk-Cone KH, Chavous TM, Zimmerman MA. 2004. Racial discrimination and racial identity as risk or protective factors for violent behaviors in African American young adults. *Am. J. Community Psychol.* 33:91–105

24. Caldwell CH, Wright JC, Zimmerman MA, Walsemann KM, Williams D, Isichei PAC. 2004. Enhancing adolescent health behaviors through strengthening non-resident father-son relationships: a model for intervention with African American families. *Health Educ. Res.* http://her.oupjournals.org/cgi/reprint/cyg078v1

25. Caldwell CH, Zimmerman MA, Isichei PA. 2001. Forging collaborative partnerships to enhance family health: an assessment of strengths and challenges in conducting community-based research. *J. Public Health Manag. Pract.* 7:1–9

26. Cauce AM, Stewart A, Rodriquez MD, Cochran B, Ginzler J. 2003. Overcoming the odds? Adolescent development in the context of urban poverty. See Ref. 63a, pp. 343–63

27. Cicchette D. 2003. Foreword. See Ref. 63a, pp. xix–xxvii

28. Cicchetti D, Rogosch FA. 2002. A developmental psychopathology perspective on adolescence. *J. Consult. Clin. Psychol.* 70:6–20

29. Coatsworth JD, Pantin H, Szapocznik J. 2002. Familias Unidas: A family-centered ecodevelopmental intervention to reduce risk for problem behavior among Hispanic adolescents. *Clin. Child Fam. Psychol. Rev.* 5:113–32

30. Costa FM, Jessor R, Turbin MS. 1999. Transition into adolescent problem drinking: the role of psychosocial risk and protective factors. *J. Stud. Alcohol* 60:480–90

31. Crosnoe R. 2002. Academic and health-related trajectories in adolescence: the intersection of gender and athletics. *J. Health Soc. Behav.* 43:317–35

32. Crosnoe R, Erickson KG, Dornbusch SM. 2002. Protective functions of family relationships and school factors on the deviant behavior of adolescent boys and girls—reducing the impact of risky friendships. *Youth Soc.* 33:515–44

33. Davey M, Eaker DG, Walters LH. 2003. Resilience processes in adolescents: personality profiles, self-worth, and coping. *J. Adolesc. Res.* 18:347–62

34. Dornbusch SM, Erickson KG, Laird J, Wong CA. 2001. The relation of family and school attachment to adolescent deviance in diverse groups and communities. *J. Adolesc. Res.* 16:396–422

35. Duncan SC, Duncan TE, Strycker LA. 2000. Risk and protective factors influencing adolescent problem behavior: a multivariate latent growth curve analysis. *Ann. Behav. Med.* 22:103–9

36. Eccles J, Gootman JA, eds. 2002. *Community Programs to Promote Youth Development.* Washington, DC: Natl. Acad. Press

37. Edari R, McManus P. 1998. Risk and resiliency factors for violence. *Pediatr. Clin. North Am.* 45:293–305

38. Epstein JA, Botvin GJ, Griffin KW, Diaz T. 2001. Protective factors buffer effects of risk factors on alcohol use among inner-city youth. *J. Child Adolesc. Subst. Abuse* 11:77–90

39. Farrell AD, White KS. 1998. Peer influences and drug use among urban adolescents: family structure and parent-adolescent relationship as protective factors. *J. Consult. Clin. Psychol.* 66:248–58

40. Fergusson DM, Beautrais AL, Horwood LJ. 2003. Vulnerability and resiliency to suicidal behaviours in young people. *Psychol. Med.* 33:61–73

41. Fergusson DM, Horwood LJ. 2003. Resilience to childhood adversity: results of a 21-year study. See Ref. 63a, pp. 130–55

42. Fleming CB, Kim H, Harachi TW, Catalano RF. 2002. Family processes for children in early elementary school as predictors of smoking initiation. *J. Adolesc. Health* 30:184–89

43. Garmezy N, Masten AS, Tellegen A. 1984. The study of stress and competence in children: a building block for developmental psychopathology. *Child Dev.* 55:97–111

44. Garnier HE, Stein JA. 2002. An 18-year model of family and peer effects on adolescent drug use and delinquency. *J. Youth Adolesc.* 31:45–56

44a. Glantz MD, Johnson JL, eds. 1999. *Resilience and Development: Positive Life Adaptations.* New York: Kluwer Acad./Plenum

45. Glantz MD, Sloboda Z. 1999. Analysis and reconceptualization of resilience. See Ref. 44a, pp. 109–28

46. Green LW, Kreuter MW. 1999. *Health Promotion Planning: An Educational and Ecological Approach.* Mountain View, CA: Mayfield

47. Griffin KW, Botvin GJ, Scheier LM, Epstein JA, Doyle MM. 2002. Personal competence skills, distress, and well-being as determinants of substance use in a predominantly minority urban adolescent sample. *Prev. Sci.* 3:23–33

48. Griffin KW, Scheier LM, Botvin GJ, Diaz T, Miller N. 1999. Interpersonal aggression in urban minority youth: mediators of perceived neighborhood, peer, and parental influences. *J. Community Psychol.* 27:281–98

49. Gutman LM, Sameroff AJ, Eccles JS. 2002. The academic achievement of African American students during early adolescence: an examination of multiple risk, promotive, and protective factors. *Am. J. Community Psychol.* 30:367–99

50. Hahm HC, Lahiff M, Guterman NB. 2003. Acculturation and parental attachment in Asian-American adolescents' alcohol use. *J. Adolesc. Health* 33:119–29

51. Hanlon TE, Bateman RW, Simon BD, O'Grady KE, Carswell SB. 2002. An early community-based intervention for the prevention of substance abuse and other delinquent behavior. *J. Youth Adolesc.* 31:459–71

52. Harvey AR, Hill RB. 2004. Africentric youth and family rites of passage program: promoting resilience among at-risk African American youths. *Soc. Work* 49:65–74

53. Hetherington EM, Stanley-Hagan M. 1999. The adjustment of children with divorced parents: a risk and resiliency perspective. *J. Child Psychol. Psychiatry* 40:129–40

54. Hogue A, Liddle HA, Becker D, Johnson-Leckrone J. 2002. Family-based prevention counseling for high-risk young adolescents: immediate outcomes. *J. Community Psychol.* 30:1–22

55. Howard D, Qiu Y, Boekeloo B. 2003. Personal and social contextual correlates of adolescent dating violence. *J. Adolesc. Health* 33:9–17

56. Huang B, Kosterman R, Catalano RF, Hawkins JD, Abbott RD. 2001. Modeling mediation in the etiology of violent behavior and adolescence: a test of the social development model. *Criminology* 39:75–107

57. Jackson C. 2002. Perceived legitimacy of parental authority and tobacco and alcohol use during early adolescence. *J. Adolesc. Health* 31:425–32

58. Kaplan HB. 1999. Toward an understanding of resilience: a critical review of definitions and models. See Ref. 44a, pp. 17–83

59. Kim IJ, Zane NWS, Hong S. 2002. Protective factor against substance use among Asian American youth: a test of the peer cluster theory. *J. Community Psychol.* 30:565–84

60. Kumpfer KL. 1999. Factors and processes contributing to resilience: the resilience framework. See Ref. 44a, pp. 179–224

61. Kumpfer KL, Alvarado R. 2003. Family-strengthening approaches for the prevention of youth problem behaviors. *Am. Psychol.* 58:457–65

62. Lammers C, Ireland M, Resnick M, Blum R. 2000. Influences on adolescents' decision to postpone onset of sexual

intercourse: a survival analysis of virginity among youths aged 13 to 18 years. *J. Adolesc. Health* 26:42–48

63. Lloyd-Richardson EE, Papandonatos G, Kazura A, Stanton C, Niaura R. 2002. Differentiating stages of smoking intensity among adolescents: stage-specific psychological and social influences. *J. Consult. Clin. Psychol.* 70:998–1009

63a. Luthar SS, ed. 2003. *Resilience and Vulnerability: Adaptation in the Context of Childhood Adversities*. New York: Cambridge Univ. Press

64. Luthar SS, Cicchetti D. 2000. The construct of resilience: implications for interventions and social policies. *Dev. Psychopathol.* 12:857–85

65. Luthar SS, Cicchetti D, Becker B. 2000. The construct of resilience: a critical evaluation and guidelines for future work. *Child Dev.* 71:543–62

66. Luthar SS, Zelazo LB. 2003. Research on resilience: an integrative review. See Ref. 63a, pp. 510–50

67. Magnani RJ, Karim AM, Weiss LA, Bond KC, Lemba M, Morgan GT. 2002. Reproductive health risk and protective factors among youth in Lusaka, Zambia. *J. Adolesc. Health* 30:76–86

68. Magnani RJ, Seiber EE, Gutierrez EZ, Vereau D. 2001. Correlates of sexual activity and condom use among secondary-school students in urban Peru. *Stud. Fam. Plann.* 32:53–66

69. Malow RM, Devieux JG, Jennings T, Lucenko BA, Kalichman SC. 2001. Substance-abusing adolescents at varying levels of HIV risk: psychosocial characteristics, drug use, and sexual behavior. *J. Subst. Abuse* 13:103–17

70. Masten AS. 1999. Resilience comes of age: reflections on the past and outlook for the next generation. See Ref. 44a, pp. 281–96

71. Masten AS. 2001. Ordinary magic—resilience processes in development. *Am. Psychol.* 56:227–38

72. Masten AS, Powell JL. 2003. A resilience framework for research, policy, and practice. See Ref. 63a, pp. 1–28

73. Murray C. 2003. Risk factors, protective factors, vulnerability, and resilience—a framework for understanding and supporting the adult transitions of youth with high-incidence disabilities. *Remedial Spec. Educ.* 24:16–26

74. Newcomb MD, Felix-Ortiz M. 1992. Multiple protective and risk factors for drug use and abuse—cross-sectional and prospective findings. *J. Pers. Soc. Psychol.* 63:280–96

75. Olsson CA, Bond L, Burns JM, Vella-Brodrick DA, Sawyer SM. 2003. Adolescent resilience: a concept analysis. *J. Adolesc.* 26:1–11

76. Oshio A, Kaneko H, Nagamine S, Nakaya M. 2003. Construct validity of the Adolescent Resilience Scale. *Psychol. Rep.* 93:1217–22

77. Pantin H, Coatsworth JD, Feaster DJ, Newman FL, Briones E, et al. 2003. Familias Unidas: the efficacy of an intervention to promote parental investment in Hispanic immigrant families. *Prev. Sci.* 4:189–201

78. Paul C, Fitzjohn J, Herbison P, Dickson N. 2000. The determinants of sexual intercourse before age 16. *J. Adolesc. Health* 27:136–47

79. Pollard JA, Hawkins JD, Arthur MW. 1999. Risk and protection: Are both necessary to understand diverse behavioral outcomes in adolescence? *Soc. Work Res.* 23:145–58

80. Prinstein MJ, Boergers J, Spirito A. 2001. Adolescents' and their friends' health-risk behavior: factors that alter or add to peer influence. *J. Pediatr. Psychol.* 26:287–98

81. Rai AA, Stanton B, Wu Y, Li XM, Galbraith J, et al. 2003. Relative influences of perceived parental monitoring and perceived peer involvement on adolescent risk behaviors: an analysis of six cross-sectional data sets. *J. Adolesc. Health* 33:108–18

82. Ramirez-Valles J, Zimmerman MA, Newcomb MD. 1998. Sexual risk behavior among youth: modeling the influence of prosocial activities and socioeconomic factors. *J. Health Soc. Behav.* 39:237–53

83. Rosenthal S, Feiring C, Taska L. 2003. Emotional support and adjustment over a year's time following sexual abuse discovery. *Child Abuse Negl.* 27:641–61

84. Rutter M. 1985. Resilience in the face of adversity. Protective factors and resistance to psychiatric disorder. *Br. J. Psychiatry* 147:598–611

85. Rutter M. 1987. Psychosocial resilience and protective mechanisms. *Am. J. Orthopsychiatry* 57:316–31

86. Sameroff A, Gutman LM, Peck SC. 2003. Adaptation among youth facing multiple risks: prospective research findings. See Ref. 63a, pp. 364–91

87. Sandler I, Wolchik S, Davis C, Haine R, Ayers T. 2003. Correlational and experimental study of resilience in children of divorce and parentally bereaved children. See Ref. 63a, pp. 213–43

88. Santelli JS, Kaiser J, Hirsch L, Radosh A, Simkin L, Middlestadt S. 2004. Initiation of sexual intercourse among middle school adolescents: the influence of psychosocial factors. *J. Adolesc. Health* 34:200–8

89. Scal P, Ireland M, Borowsky IW. 2003. Smoking among American adolescents: a risk and protective factor analysis. *J. Community Health* 28:79–97

90. Scaramella LV, Conger RD, Simons RL. 1999. Parental protective influences and gender-specific increases in adolescent internalizing and externalizing problems. *J. Res. Adolesc.* 9:111–41

91. Scheier LM, Botvin GJ, Griffin KW, Diaz T. 1999. Latent growth models of drug refusal skills and adolescent alcohol use. *J. Alcohol Drug Educ.* 44:21–48

92. Scheier LM, Botvin GJ, Miller NL. 1999. Life events, neighborhood stress, psychosocial functioning, and alcohol use among urban minority youth. *J. Child Adolesc. Subst. Abuse* 9:19–50

93. Sellers RM, Caldwell CH, Bernat DH, Zimmerman MA. 2001. *Racial identity and alcohol use in a sample of academically at-risk African American high school students.* Presented at biennial meeting of Soc. Res. Child Dev., Minneapolis, MN

94. Serbin LA, Karp J. 2004. The intergenerational transfer of psychosocial risk: mediators of vulnerability and resilience. *Annu. Rev. Psychol.* 55:333–63

95. Shochet IM, Dadds MR, Holland D, Whitefield K, Harnett PH, Osgarby SM. 2001. The efficacy of a universal school-based program to prevent adolescent depression. *J. Clin. Child Psychol.* 30:303–15

96. Shumow L, Vandell DL, Posner J. 1999. Risk and resilience in the urban neighborhood: predictors of academic performance among low-income elementary school children. *Merrill-Palmer Q.-J. Dev. Psychol.* 45:309–31

97. Spoth R, Lopez Reyes M, Redmond C, Shin C. 1999. Assessing a public health approach to delay onset and progression of adolescent substance use: latent transition and log-linear analyses of longitudinal family preventive intervention outcomes. *J. Consult. Clin. Psychol.* 67:619–30

98. Spoth RL, Redmond C, Shin C. 2001. Randomized trial of brief family interventions for general populations: adolescent substance use outcomes 4 years following baseline. *J. Consult. Clin. Psychol.* 69:627–42

99. Spoth RL, Redmond C, Trudeau L, Shin C. 2002. Longitudinal substance initiation outcomes for a universal preventive intervention combining family and school programs. *Psychol. Addict. Behav.* 16:129–34

100. Stanton B, Li X, Pack R, Cottrell L, Harris C, Burns JM. 2002. Longitudinal influence of perceptions of peer and

parental factors on African American adolescent risk involvement. *J. Urban Health* 79:536–48

101. Stouthamer-Loeber M, Loeber R, Wei E, Farrington DP, Wikstrom POH. 2002. Risk and promotive effects in the explanation of persistent serious delinquency in boys. *J. Consult. Clin. Psychol.* 70:111–23

102. Sullivan TN, Farrell AD. 1999. Identification and impact of risk and protective factors for drug use among urban African American adolescents. *J. Clin. Child Psychol.* 28:122–36

103. Tarter RE, Vanyukov M. 1999. Re-visiting the validity of the construct of resilience. See Ref. 44a, pp. 85–100

104. Tiet QQ, Huizinga D. 2002. Dimensions of the construct of resilience and adaptation among inner-city youth. *J. Adolesc. Res.* 17:260–76

105. Tugade MM, Fredrickson BL. 2004. Resilient individuals use positive emotions to bounce back from negative emotional experiences. *J. Pers. Soc. Psychol.* 86:320–33

106. Werner EE. 1992. The children of Kauai: resiliency and recovery in adolescence and adulthood. *J. Adolesc. Health* 13:262–68

107. Werner EE, Smith RS. 1992. *Overcoming the Odds: High Risk Children from Birth to Adulthood*. Ithaca/London: Cornell Univ. Press

108. Williams NR, Davey M, Klock-Powell K. 2003. Rising from the ashes: stories of recovery, adaptation and resiliency in burn survivors. *Soc. Work Health Care* 36:53–77

109. Wills TA, Sandy JM, Shinar O, Yaeger A. 1999. Contributions of positive and negative affect to adolescent substance use: test of a bidimensional model in a longitudinal study. *Psychol. Addict. Behav.* 13:327–38

110. Wills TA, Yaeger AM, Sandy JM. 2003. Buffering effect of religiosity for adolescent substance use. *Psychol. Addict. Behav.* 17:24–31

111. Wong CA, Eccles JS, Sameroff A. 2003. The influence of ethnic discrimination and ethnic identification on African American adolescents' school and socioemotional adjustment. *J. Pers.* 71:1197–232

112. Yates TM, Egeland B, Sroufe LA. 2003. Rethinking resilience: a developmental perspective. See Ref. 63a, pp. 243–66

113. Zimmerman MA, Arunkumar R. 1994. Resiliency research: implications for schools and policy. *Soc. Policy Rep.* 8:1–17

114. Zimmerman MA, Bingenheimer JB, Notaro PC. 2002. Natural mentors and adolescent resiliency: a study with urban youth. *Am. J. Community Psychol.* 30:221–43

115. Zimmerman MA, Ramirez J, Washienko KM, Walter B, Dyer S. 1995. Enculturation hypothesis: exploring direct and protective effects among Native American youth. In *Resiliency in Ethnic Minority Families: Native and Immigrant American Families*, ed. HI McCubbin, EA Thompson, AI Thompson, JE Fromer, pp. 199–220. Madison: Univ. Wis. Cent. Excell. Fam. Stud.

116. Zimmerman MA, Steinman KJ, Rowe KJ. 1998. Violence among urban African-American adolescents: the protective effects of parental support. In *Addressing Community Problems: Research and Intervention*, ed. S Oskamp, XB Arriaga, pp. 78–103. Newbury Park, CA: Sage

Annu. Rev. Public Health 2005. 26:421–43
doi: 10.1146/annurev.publhealth.26.021304.144437

DECLINING RATES OF PHYSICAL ACTIVITY IN THE UNITED STATES: What Are the Contributors?

Ross C. Brownson, Tegan K. Boehmer, and Douglas A. Luke
*Department of Community Health and Prevention Research Center, Saint Louis University
School of Public Health, St. Louis, Missouri 63104; email: brownson@slu.edu,
boehmert@slu.edu, dluke@slu.edu*

Key Words   community, environment, exercise, health surveys, physical activity, surveillance

■ **Abstract**   This review describes current patterns and long-term trends (up to 50 years when possible) related to (*a*) physical activity, (*b*) employment and occupation, (*c*) travel behavior, (*d*) land use, and (*e*) related behaviors (e.g., television watching). On the basis of available data, the following trends were observed according to type of physical activity: relatively stable or slightly increasing levels of leisure-time physical activity, declining work-related activity, declining transportation activity, declining activity in the home, and increasing sedentary activity. These result in an overall trend of declining total physical activity. Large differences were noted in the rates of walking for transportation across metropolitan statistical areas. A strong linear increase existed in vehicle miles traveled per person over the past half century, coupled with a strong and consistent trend toward Americans living in suburbs. Although it is difficult to precisely quantify owing to the lack of long-term data, it is apparent that a combination of changes to the built environment and increases in the proportion of the population engaging in sedentary activities put the majority of the American population at high risk of physical inactivity.

INTRODUCTION

Regular physical activity reduces the risk of premature death and disability from a variety of conditions including coronary heart disease, diabetes, colon cancer, osteoarthritis, and osteoporosis (51). In the United States, estimates of the annual cost in lives lost have ranged from 200,000 to 300,000 (17, 26–28, 32), and medical costs due to inactivity and its consequences are estimated at $76 billion in 2000 dollars (33). To reduce this large health burden, public health recommendations have evolved to emphasize a lifestyle approach to increasing activity that includes common behaviors such as brisk walking, climbing stairs, doing house and yard work, and engaging in active recreational pursuits (31, 51).

The terms physical activity and exercise have often been used interchangeably (5, 48). Physical activity is "bodily movement that is produced by the contraction of skeletal muscle and that substantially increases energy expenditure" (51). Although the terms are similar in that they involve any bodily movement that expends energy, exercise is a subset of physical activity that has been defined as "planned, structured, and repetitive bodily movement done to improve or maintain one or more components of physical fitness," and physical fitness is "a set of attributes that people have or achieve that relates to the ability to perform physical activity" (5). To learn about the impact of environmental influences on all domains of physical activity, researchers recently have begun to collect reliable data on the forms of physical activity in addition to leisure-time (or recreational) physical activity (3, 25). These newer surveys and surveillance systems collect data on five domains including leisure activity, household and yard work activity, occupational activity, self-powered transport, and sedentary activity (12). There is also growing recognition that a variety of disciplines outside of the traditional domains of public health need to be engaged in research and practice to increase rates of physical activity (19, 22). These disciplines include urban design, city planning, and transportation engineering.

Land use characteristics in the physical (or built) environment are important in providing cues and opportunities for activity (14, 16, 20) and are associated with rates of physical activity in population-based studies. Using empirical methods, researchers have examined the relation between community design variables and walking or cycling for transportation. A recent review shows that people walk and cycle more when their neighborhoods have higher residential density, a mixture of land uses (e.g., shops are within walking distance of homes), and connected streets (e.g., grid-like pattern instead of many cul-de-sacs) (38).

Dramatic changes have taken place in the urban landscape over the past 50 years. Muller (29) has described the period from 1945 to the present as the "Freeway Era," in which the automobile is no longer a luxury but has become essential for commuting, shopping, and socializing. This trend also contributed to the advent of the suburban ring and the accompanying freeway segments, which now girdle most central cities in the United States. The migration to suburban environments relates to the proliferation of zoning across the United States, characterized by segregation of residential land uses from other types of uses (39). The landmark Supreme Court case of Euclid vs. Ambler Realty (272 U.S. 365, 1926) affirmed the zoning authority of municipalities. This decision was carried into the suburbs in later decades, leading to increased adoption of zoning ordinances by towns and cities in the name of protecting residential uses from the perceived negative impact of mixed uses.

In the area of transportation, researchers are interested in defining the relationship between rates of physical activity and travel behavior, particularly use of the automobile. For example, traffic congestion has grown in urban areas over the past few decades—the average annual traffic delay per person was 7 hours in 1982 and 26 hours in 2001 (40). Travel behavior researchers measure "trips," defined as the movement from one street address to another (18). The trip metric is often defined according to various components including trip frequency, trip duration and length, and mode of travel (i.e., automobile, transit, walking, biking). Although these travel data have not been intentionally collected to inform public health efforts, some of the information from travel behavior research is beneficial in understanding patterns and trends in physical activity.

Although selected reports have described trends in leisure-time physical activity (6, 46, 51), there has been sparse examination of physical activity trends by domain, along with other important lifestyle and behavior trends. The main purpose of this paper is to describe current patterns and long-term trends (up to 50 years when possible) related to (*a*) physical activity, (*b*) employment and occupation, (*c*) travel behavior, (*d*) land use, and (*e*) related behaviors (e.g., television watching).

CURRENT PATTERNS AND TIME TRENDS

We describe data sets that provide relevant current data as well as historical data. Under each of the categories of interest (i.e., physical activity, employment and occupation, travel behavior, land use), a primary data set is identified. When possible, the strengths and limitations of these data are described. Also when possible, data are broken down by population subgroup (e.g., age, gender, ethnicity).

When examining time trend data, we followed the criteria proposed by Stephens (44): Data needed to have (*a*) a minimum of three time points; (*b*) for physical activity data, a conceptually adequate definition of "active"; (*c*) a national probability sample; and (*d*) consistent data collection procedures. In addition, we included only data sets for which at least 10 years worth of data were available.

For key variables, we calculated rates of absolute change and relative change (absolute change/baseline rate). We also calculated the annual compound percent change, which is a description of the annual growth accounting for the compounding of values from the previous year. The compound growth rate was calculated using the following formula:

$$\text{Annual compound change} = [(\text{current value/baseline value})^{1/n}] - 1,$$

where n = number of years. In addition, for trends that strongly fit a linear model, beta coefficients were calculated to estimate rates of linear change, and R-squared was reported to measure the amount of variability accounted for by the data.

Physical Activity in Adults

National data on adult physical activity patterns can be obtained from several sources including the Behavioral Risk Factor Surveillance System (BRFSS), the National Health Interview Survey (NHIS), and the National Health and Nutrition Examination Survey (NHANES). We primarily describe data from the BRFSS because it provides the largest number of yearly estimates of physical activity. In addition, national data are available from the Youth Risk Behavior Surveillance System (YRBSS), although historical data are limited in YRBSS.

OVERVIEW OF THE BRFSS AND ITS PHYSICAL ACTIVITY INDEXES   Begun in 1981 by the Centers for Disease Control and Prevention (CDC), the BRFSS provides a flexible, state health agency-based surveillance system to assist in planning, implementing, and evaluating health promotion and disease prevention programs (15, 35, 42). It involves monthly, year-round, telephone interviews with noninstitutionalized adults aged 18 years and older, using the two-stage, Waksberg technique (57), which is a standard random-digit dialing method. In 2000, 50 states, the District of Columbia, and Puerto Rico participated. The total sample size in 2000 was 205,140, and the response rate was 51.1%. The BRFSS is generally representative of the overall U.S. population, although it underrepresents non-Whites, persons with less than a high school education, and those with lower incomes. To provide national estimates, data from the BRFSS were weighted according to the age, sex, and racial distributions of the United States.

BRFSS questions on physical activity have been consistent since 1986. When examining trend data in this review, however, only even-yeared data from 1990 to 2000 are shown because these survey years sampled at least 43 states and the District of Columbia and are considered to be the most reliable of BRFSS data (S. Ham, personal communication).

Physical activity indices were based on a series of BRFSS questions, the first of which asks "During the past month, did you participate in any physical activities such as running, calisthenics, golf, gardening, or walking for exercise?" If a respondent answered "yes" he or she was asked to identify his or her two most common activities and to indicate the frequency of activity in the previous month and duration per occasion (4).

We used a standard index for physical activity analyses with BRFSS data. Recommended activity requires meeting the CDC and the American College of Sports Medicine 1993 Physical Activity Recommendation, which states "every U.S. adult should accumulate 30 min or more of moderate-intensity physical activity on most, preferably all, days of the week" (31). Recommended physical activity was defined as 30 min of moderate physical activity at least 5 times per week or 20 consecutive minutes of vigorous activity at least 3 times per week, acquired during recreational or leisure-time activities (i.e., not work-related).

The strengths of the BRFSS include its large and representative sample, its ability to estimate physical activity for subgroups (e.g., women, various ethnic groups), and the consistency of questions over time. Its weaknesses include reliance on self-reported data, restriction to collect only data on leisure-time physical activity, and lack of coverage for some population subgroups (e.g., lower-income individuals) who are less likely to have telephones.

CURRENT PATTERNS   On the basis of BRFSS data from 2000, 26.2% of U.S. adults engaged in recommended levels of physical activity during recreational pursuits. Men were slightly more likely to meet recommended levels than were women (27.1% versus 25.5%). Among ethnic groups, non-Hispanic Blacks (21.9%) and Hispanics (21.1%) were least likely to meet recommended levels of physical activity, and non-Hispanic Whites (27.5%) were most likely to meet recommendations. A gradient in likelihood to reach recommended levels of physical activity exists across education levels; among persons with fewer than 12 years of education, 14.5% met recommendations, compared with 34.2% among persons with a college education. Considerable geographic variation for meeting recommended levels of physical activity occurs within the United States. Rates are lowest in southern states such as Kentucky (17.7%), Louisiana (18.3%), and Mississippi (21.3%) and are highest in western states such as Hawaii (34.8%), Washington (32.4%), and Oregon (32.4%) (8). These findings are consistent with those from the NHIS (51).

TIME TRENDS   Trends in recommended physical activity show slight improvements for both men and women between 1990 and 2000 (Figure 1). Over the 10-year period men showed a relative improvement of 9.7% in recommended activity, compared with 5.8% in women (Table 1). Trend data for recommended physical activity by educational group show slightly diverging trends: Data over time show a relative decline of 7.6% for persons with fewer than 12 years of education, compared with a relative increase of 8.9% for persons with a college education. Data by race/ethnicity show slight improvements in rates of recommended physical activity for Whites and Blacks and yet show a slight decrease for Hispanic adults.

Physical Activity in Youth

OVERVIEW OF THE YRBSS AND ITS PHYSICAL ACTIVITY INDEXES   The YRBSS was developed in 1990 to monitor priority health risk behaviors that contribute markedly to the leading causes of death, disability, and social problems among youth and adults in the United States; these behaviors include physical activity. The YRBSS includes national, state, and local school-based surveys of representative samples of ninth- through twelfth-grade students. These surveys are conducted every two years, usually during the spring semester.

Three variables from the YRBSS are relevant for this paper:

1. the percentage of students who attend physical education (PE) classes daily;
2. the percentage of students, labeled inactive, who did not participate in at least 20 min of vigorous physical activity on three or more of the past seven days and did not do at least 30 min of moderate physical activity on five or more of the past seven days; and
3. the percentage of students who exercised or participated in vigorous activity defined as physical activities that made them sweat and breathe hard for at least 20 min on three or more days of the past seven days.

CURRENT PATTERNS   In 2001, 24.2% of male students and 37.9% of female students were classified as inactive using the definition above. Inactivity among youth

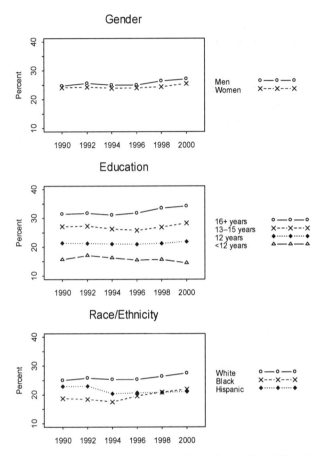

Figure 1   Trends in recommended physical activity, United States, 1990–2000.

increases by grade level from 24.3% in ninth grade to 38.9% in twelfth grade. In addition, inactivity is highest among Black youth (36.4%) and lowest among White youth (29.3%).

TIME TRENDS   On the basis of available data from YRBS, rates of physical activity among youth appear to be relatively stable over the past decade, at least by the vigorous activity metric. In 1993, 65.8% of students in grades 9–12 exercised or participated in physical activities that made them sweat and breathe hard for at least 20 min on three or more of the past seven days, compared with 64.6% in 2001. Over the 1991–2001 time frame, the percentage of students who attended PE class daily decreased from 41.6% to 32.2%, which suggests that the average amount of physical activity during school time is probably declining.

TABLE 1 Summary of key variables and rates of change

Variable	Years	Subgroup	Absolute % change	Relative % change	Annual compound %
Physical activity (%)					
Meets physical activity recommendation	1990–2000	Both sexes	1.9	7.8	0.75
Meets physical activity recommendation	1990–2000	Women	1.4	5.8	0.57
Meets physical activity recommendation	1990–2000	Men	2.4	9.7	0.93
Meets physical activity recommendation	1990–2000	<12 years education	−1.2	−7.6	−0.79
Meets physical activity recommendation	1990–2000	College education	2.8	8.9	0.86
Employment and occupation (%)					
Work in low physical activity occupation	1950–2000	Both sexes	19.3	82.8	1.19
Work in high physical activity occupation	1950–2000	Both sexes	−7.8	−25.2	−0.57
Travel behavior					
Average daily vehicle miles traveled per person (miles)	1950–2000	Both sexes	18.5	224.0	2.39
Proportion of trips to work by walking (%)	1960–2000	Both sexes	−7.4	−71.2	−2.99
Proportion of trips to work by public transit (%)	1960–2000	Both sexes	−8.9	−68.5	−2.78
Land use					
U.S. residents living in suburbs (%)	1950–2000	Both sexes	26.7	114.6	1.54
Sedentary behavior					
Daily television viewing (h/day)	1950–2000	Households	2.9	61.4	0.96

Employment and Occupation

National data on employment and occupation are available from the Bureau of Labor Statistics and the U.S. Census Bureau. The Bureau of Labor Statistics houses two relevant data sources: the Current Population Survey (CPS), which has monitored the U.S. labor force and employment/unemployment rates since 1940; and the Occupational Employment Statistics, which began in 1988 but the data from which are comparable only beginning in 1997 and are not useful for monitoring historical trends. The U.S. decennial census has collected detailed information on employment, occupation, and industry since the 1800s. Occupation is classified according to workers' specific functions, whereas industry is classified according to the work setting and economic sector. Thus, type of occupation is the preferred categorization for examining activity level at work or on the job.

OVERVIEW OF THE CPS AND ITS EMPLOYMENT INDEX   The CPS is a monthly household survey of the civilian, noninstitutionalized population 16 years and older, which measures employment status by sex, age, race, and other demographic characteristics (53). The CPS is the most complete source of national employment and unemployment statistics, as well as various economic indicators used to monitor emerging trends in labor supply, labor force participation, hours, and wages and earnings of various demographic groups.

OVERVIEW OF THE U.S. CENSUS AND ITS OCCUPATION CLASSIFICATION   Census respondents were asked what kind of work they were doing, and, beginning in 1970, what were their most important activities or duties. The information provided is then coded into the current Census Bureau occupational structure using computer programs. Unfortunately, the Census Bureau occupational classification system has changed frequently over the years, making comparisons across sequential census impractical. Since 1950, the classification system has changed three times, including significant reorganizations in 1980 and 2000. Researchers at the University of Minnesota Population Center have recoded all occupational data into the 1950 classification system to enhance comparability across years (37). Technical papers published by the U.S. Census Bureau were used from 1960 to 1990 to track occupations back to the 1950 classification. In 2000, occupations were recoded into the 1950-based classification using only job titles and good judgment. We obtained 1950-based occupational data in aggregate format from the University of Minnesota Population Center's Integrated Public Use Microdata Series Web site (37).

We then categorized occupations by activity level on the basis of the occupation description. In a study by King et al. (23), 498 occupations from the NHANES III (1988–1994) database were independently reviewed by a six-member committee and categorized as high occupational activity, low occupational activity, or uncertain activity level, according to the current occupation description provided by the U.S. Department of Labor (52). A high- or low-activity classification required agreement by all six committee members. To categorize the 1950-based Census occupations as high, low, or uncertain activity levels we matched the occupation titles to those used by King et al. (23). Each occupation was assigned the same activity level across all years. As a result, we did not account for the fact that the activity level of some occupations may have changed over time (e.g., some occupations classified as low activity today may have required more active work in the past).

One limitation of the Census data is that the universe eligible to respond to occupation questions changed over time. For example, in 1950, eligible respondents included those aged 14 or older who were currently in the labor force, whereas from 1960 to 1970, the respondents were eligible if they had worked in the previous 10 years. From 1980 to 2000 the eligible universe included persons aged 16 or older who had worked in the previous 5 years.

CURRENT PATTERNS   According to the 2002 Current Population Survey, the civilian, noninstitutionalized population aged 16 years and older consisted of 217.6 million persons, of which 144.9 million were in the labor force (66.6% participation rate). Labor force participation rates were higher in men (74.1%) as compared with women (59.6%). Overall, the ratio of men to women in the labor force was 53.5% to 46.5%. The unemployment rate in 2002 was 5.8%. Full- and part-time employment also differed by gender, with more women (25.3%) employed part time than men (10.6%).

Comparable with the CPS data, the 2000 Census reported an eligible population of 216.9 million persons aged 16 or older, of which 136.7 million were in the labor force (63.0% participation rate). Among those in the labor force, 42.6% or 58.2 million were in low-activity occupations, and 22.6% or 30.9 million were in high-activity occupations in their current or most recent job. Unfortunately, the occupation data was obtained in aggregate format and cannot be broken down by gender or other demographic subgroups.

TIME TRENDS   Over the last half century, the surge of women entering the labor force has substantially transformed the structure and characteristics of the U.S. civilian labor force. In terms of actual numbers of people, the total civilian labor force more than doubled over the past 50 years, from 62.2 million in 1950 to 142.5 million in 2000. During the same time period the number of men in the labor force increased by a factor of 1.7, whereas the number of women increased by a factor of 3.6. As a result, the ratio of men to women in the labor force has also changed substantially, from 70:30 in 1950 to nearly 50:50 in 2000. Overall, the participation rate of men has fallen slightly from 86% in 1950 to 75% in 2000, whereas participation among women nearly doubled from 34% to 60% during the same time period. Most of these changes in labor force participation occurred between 1950 and 1980, with only relatively minor changes observed in the past 20 years.

Agricultural employment, typically associated with high activity levels, has also declined substantially over the past half decade, from 12.2% in 1950 to less than 2% in 2000. These figures are based on U.S. Census data that do not include migrant workers who are not U.S. citizens.

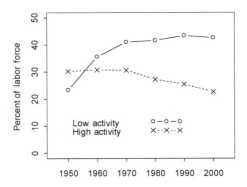

Figure 2 Trends in occupational activity, United States, 1950–2000.

The percent of the labor force in high-activity occupations remained steady at ~30% from 1950 to 1970 and then over the next 30 years began to decline slowly to the most recent estimate of 22.6% in 2000 (Figure 2). The number of persons employed in high-activity occupations grew with the increasing population from 20.8 million in 1950 to 25.2 million in 1970 to 30.9 million in 2000. The percent of labor force in low-activity occupations experienced a large increase from 23.3% in 1950 to 41.0% in 1970. Since then, this proportion has remained relatively stable. The number of persons employed in low-activity occupations was 16 million in 1950, 33.7 million in 1970, and 58.2 million in 2000.

In 1950, there were approximately 30% more persons in high-activity occupations than low-activity occupations, compared with 2000 when there were approximately twice as many persons employed in low-activity occupations than high-activity occupations. These estimates are likely conservative because they do not account for changes in activity level within occupations over time. Relative change and annual compound change over this time period are much larger for low-activity occupations than for high-activity occupations (Table 1).

Travel Behavior

Studies of travel behavior rely primarily on diaries that provide information on trips and related activities (18, 55). The most comprehensive national data source on travel behavior is the National Household Transportation Survey (NHTS) (formerly called the National Personal Transportation Survey), which is based on travel diary methods. Travel diaries provide detailed information that can be used to estimate trip frequencies, trip lengths, travel times, and mode choices. Activity diaries are structured around activities that household members engage in throughout the day while at home, shopping, and at work.

OVERVIEW OF THE NHTS AND ITS TRAVEL BEHAVIOR INDEXES   The NHTS is a nationally representative sample of households used to derive statistically reliable travel estimates at the national level (55, 56). Using computer-assisted telephone interviewing, each household in the sample was assigned a specific 24-hour travel day. Diaries were then kept to record all travel by all household members for the assigned day. In addition a 28-day travel period was assigned to collect data on longer commutes, long-distance travel, airport access, and overnight stays. In the final 2001 NHTS data set, there are approximately 66,000 households, including 26,000 in the national sample and 40,000 from add-on areas in which a state or local area funds collection of local data to give statewide or area-specific estimates of travel behavior. Daily travel surveys were conducted in 1969, 1977, 1983, 1990, 1995, and 2001. Of particular relevance to this study, the NHTS allows researchers to estimate person-trips by mode of travel (e.g., walking, private vehicle, public transit).

Vehicle Miles Traveled (VMT) data are reported as part of the Highway Statistics series and Traffic Volume Trends produced by the Federal Highway Administration (56). Annual VMT estimates are based on travel reported by the various states to the Federal Highway Administration's Highway Performance Monitoring System. The VMT is a metric used to measure vehicle travel made by a private vehicle, such as an automobile, van, pickup truck, or motorcycle. Each mile traveled is counted as one vehicle mile regardless of the number of persons in the vehicle (56). A weakness of the VMT data involves the inconsistent reporting standards for compact pickups, small utility vehicles, and minivans (41). Although the national offices have attempted to account for this potential bias, the direction and magnitude of reporting error are difficult to ascertain.

CURRENT PATTERNS   In the United States, the most recent NHTS estimates a mean of 1.9 personal vehicles per household. Households have a mean of 1.8 drivers who are 15 years and older. Thus, it appears that as of 2001, U.S. households on average have more vehicles than drivers (55). According to the 2000 Census data, 18.3% of households had three or more vehicles, 38.6% had two vehicles, 33.8% had one vehicle, and 9.4% of households did not own a vehicle. This overall increase in automobile ownership parallels an increase in the fraction of households with two or more automobiles. In turn, this increase in automobile ownership parallels increases in disposable personal income. For example, per capita income increased 48% from 1970 to 1997, after adjustment for inflation (http://www.ers.usda.gov/publications/sb965/sb965e.pdf).

Daily travel in the United States totaled about 4 trillion miles in 2001. On a daily basis, the typical person traveled an average of 40 miles, most of it (35 miles) in a personal vehicle. On the basis of the 2001 NHTS, the largest proportion of trips (45% of all trips) was taken for family and personal reasons such as shopping and running errands. Social and recreational trips were the next most common (27%), followed by commute trips to work and back (15%), and trips made for school and church (10%). Adults drove a personal vehicle for an average of 55 min and 29 miles per day. Men and women each average four trips per day, yet men drive further (38 versus 21 miles) and also spend more time driving (67 versus 44 min).

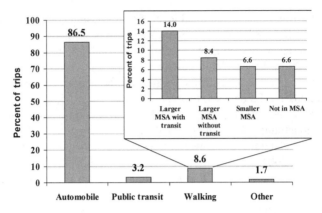

Figure 3   Utilitarian person-trips by mode and walking trips by residential location, 2001.

Nearly all person-trips are taken by automobile in the United States (Figure 3). Residents in larger urban areas (over 1 million people) with rail transit systems are much more likely to walk for utilitarian purposes than are persons who live in other areas that do not have rail transit systems. However, the higher likelihood of walking in metropolitan statistical areas (MSAs) with transit may also be due to the higher walkability of these cities. The likelihood of walking or biking is inversely related to the number of automobiles per household, regardless of income level (Figure 4). There are important differences in mode choice by race/ethnicity. For example, walking for nonwork-related travel is twice as likely in Blacks (10.6% of person-trips), Asians (10.8%), and Hispanics (9.8%), when compared with Whites (5.1%) (54). Also, commute times are higher for minority groups when compared with Whites.

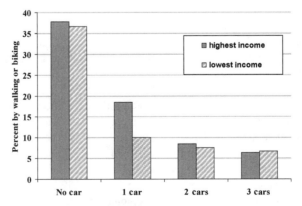

Figure 4   Relationship between automobile ownership and walking or biking trips by income level, 2001.

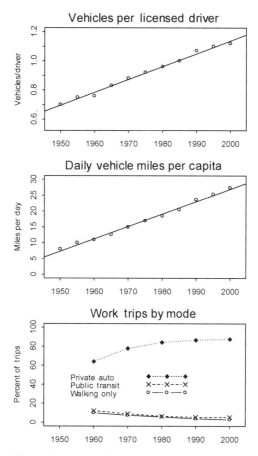

Figure 5 Trends in transportation activity and automobile dependence, 1950–2000.

TIME TRENDS   There has been a steady, linear, upward trend in vehicles per licensed driver and in daily VMT per person over the past half century (Figure 5). The relative change in VMT from baseline is more than 200%, with an annual change among the highest of the key variables considered in this paper (Table 1). On the basis of linear regression ($R^2 = 0.99$), daily VMT per person increased by 0.4 miles per year over the past 50 years. For daily travel to work, the proportion of trips by automobile increased from 67% in 1960 to 88% in 2000, while work-trips by walking or public transit declined.

Land Use

Recent attention has focused on the potential impacts of urban sprawl on rates of physical inactivity and obesity (13). The definition of sprawl often includes scattered or leapfrog development, commercial strip development, uniform low-density development, and/or single-use development (13). As one crude measure of urban sprawl, the proportion of the U.S. population living in suburbs was ascertained. In the U.S. Census, a suburb is described as the area inside a metropolitan area but outside the central city (i.e., the largest city in a metropolitan area).

OVERVIEW OF THE AMERICAN HOUSING SURVEY   The American Housing Survey collects data through in-person interviews on housing (including apartments, single-family homes, mobile homes, and vacant housing units), household characteristics, income, housing and neighborhood quality, housing costs, equipment and fuels, size of housing unit, and recent moves (50). National data are collected in odd num-bered years, and data for each of 47 selected metropolitan areas are currently col-lected about every 6 years. The national sample covers an average of 55,000 hous-ing units. Each metropolitan area sample covers 4100 or more housing units. Final data are weighted according to a number of factors including probability of selec-tion, noninterview due to refusal or no one being home, and demographic factors.

CURRENT PATTERNS   Several important patterns emerge from the 2001 Ameri-can Housing Survey for the United States. In particular, we examined variables related to the built environment that may encourage or discourage walking and bicycling. For example, 62.5% of survey respondents reported having satisfactory neighborhood shopping within one mile of their home (56). Among U.S. residents with children 13 years or younger, 56.8% had a public elementary school within one mile of their housing unit. Over half (55.2%) of respondents reported having access to public transportation. Unfortunately, these detailed data on the neighbor-hood environment are available only for 1997, 1999, and 2001, making trend data extremely limited.

TIME TRENDS   From 1950 to 1980, there was a relatively steep, linear trend ($R^2 = 0.96$) showing a higher proportion of Americans living in the suburbs (Figure 6). This trend has moderated since 1980. Overall, from 1950 to 2000, the proportion of U.S. residents living in the suburbs has more than doubled. On the basis of the linear trend, the proportion living in the suburbs has increased 5.3% every 10 years.

Sedentary Activities and Time Use

Several other data sets were used to assemble data on sedentary activities (e.g., television viewing) and other common time-use activities.

The most comprehensive and long-term data on television viewing is avail-able from Nielsen Media Research (30). In the sampling, meters are placed in a sample of 5100 households in the United States, randomly selected and recruited by Nielsen Media Research. Nielsen Media Research uses the U.S. Census Bu-reau's decennial (updated annually) census counts of all housing units in the na-tion. Sample housing units are randomly selected within each sample area. Each

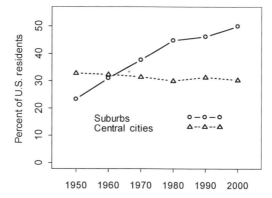

Figure 6   Trends in the proportion of U.S. residents living in suburbs and central cities, 1950–2000.

occupied housing unit is a household. This sampling method is designed to give each occupied household a chance to be selected for the Nielsen sample.

Another data source recently presented by Sturm (45) is the breakdown of "sedentary" industry output compiled by the Bureau of Economic Analysis. Industry output is measured in gross domestic product and represents each private industry's contribution to the nation's output (24). Comparable annual data are available from 1977 to 2000, although some of the classifications change over time. For the industries of interest, comparable numbers (adjusted to 1996 dollars) are available from 1987 to 2000.

Time diaries have been used to estimate how Americans spend their time (36). Researchers used a microbehavioral approach in which each part of a question is broken into easier and answerable components. Methodologic studies have confirmed the reliability of the diary method (36). These data are available for 1965, 1975, 1985, and 1995. Information was collected on the basis of national probability samples, with sample sizes ranging from 1200 to 5300. Data shown are confined to the 18- to 64-year-old sector of the population because that is the only age range for which data are available at all four time points.

TIME TRENDS   In 1950, only about 10% of U.S. households had a television (34). Now 98% of all households in America have at least one television. Television viewing has increased in a linear fashion since 1950, with an approximate doubling of average viewing hours per day (Figure 7). Following a linear trend ($R^2 = 0.96$), the average U.S. household increased its TV watching by 36 min every 10 years. The annual compound change is nearly a 1% increase every year (Table 1).

Economic data by industry show a growth in sales for sporting goods and bicycle shops from 1987 to 2000. However, the growth is much sharper for sedentary

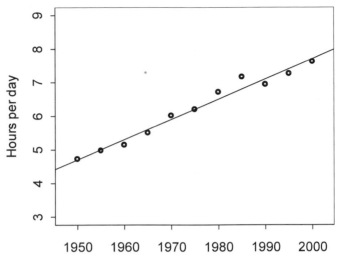

Figure 7   Average daily television viewing of U.S. residents, 1950–2000.

industries such as sales in radio and television stores. Similarly, both active sports clubs and more sedentary sports have grown over the same time period, with steeper growth for sports that people watch compared with those in which they participate.

Several common daily activities can be described by gender (36). From 1965 to 1995 slight increases were noted among women for paid work and time spent in recreation (Figure 8). A slight decline was noted in time spent eating, and a larger decline was observed for hours per week spent doing household work. Declines from 1965 to 1995 were observed among men for paid work and time spent eating. Increases were noted for time spent watching television, doing household work,

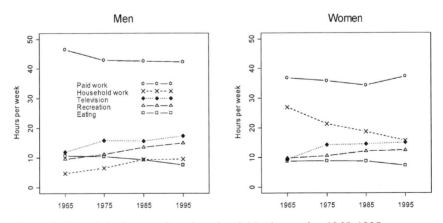

Figure 8   Trends in time use for selected activities by gender, 1965–1995.

and in recreation. Related data from the Harris Poll suggests that the percentage of adults whose favorite pastime involves exercise (e.g., gardening, walking, housework, yard work) has declined from 38% in 1995 to 29% in 2003 (47).

SUMMARY

We have provided data on several important patterns and long-term trends. Changes in total physical activity levels have been broadly affected by major structural changes in society and in the economy over the last half century—the twentieth century can be characterized as the century of technological changes in the workplace (decline of physically active occupations), in the home (advent of labor-saving devices), and in transport systems (widespread use of the automobile).

When examining these data, a number of limitations should be kept in mind. For many variables (e.g., physical activity behavior), reliable data were not available over multiple decades. Further, for data that were available, they usually could not be disaggregated by gender, race, or socioeconomic status. Because data were from a variety of sources and reported at varying intervals, formal time-series analyses could not be conducted.

Despite the limitations, several provocative patterns and trends emerge that may serve as a basis for recommendations to increase population rates of physical activity. These patterns are briefly summarized below.

Population-Wide Declines in Physical Activity

Although leisure-time physical activity has increased slightly over the past decade, the rates of household activity in women and occupational activity in both genders have declined substantially. In addition, transport activity is declining at a more modest rate. Taken together, these data suggest the total burden of inactivity is increasing. Trends according to major type of physical activity follow these patterns on the basis of the available data:

- leisure-time physical activity: level or slightly increasing;
- work-related activity: declining;
- transportation activity: declining;
- activity in the home: declining; and
- sedentary activity: increasing; therefore,
- total physical activity: declining.

Diverging Rates of Leisure-Time Activity by Subgroup

Despite slight increases in leisure-time physical activity over time, not all segments of the population are benefiting equally. As rates improve for the highly educated, rates are level or declining for less-educated segments of the U.S. population.

Need to Better Understand Gender-Specific Patterns in Activity

Important gender differences observed across time deserve further investigation. For example, there is a significant decline in housework activity over time among women. Because this type of activity accounts for a significant percentage of total activity in women (2), it is likely to be an important contributor to total activity.

Need to Better Understand Determinants of Walking for Transportation

Large differences were noted in the rates of walking for transportation across metropolitan statistical areas, with more than a twofold difference between rates in larger MSAs with transit compared with smaller MSAs or non-MSAs. A better understanding of the reasons for these differences should provide leads for persons conducting interventions.

High Rates of Automobile Dependence and Migration to the Suburbs

On average, U.S. households now have more automobiles than registered drivers, and the likelihood of walking or biking is inversely related to the number of automobiles per household. There is a strong linear increase in VMT per person over the past half century. There also is a strong and consistent trend toward Americans living in suburbs.

Declines in Walking for Transportation

In parallel with increasing automobile ownership and linear increases in VMT, rates of walking for transportation and the frequency in use of mass transit by the U.S. populace have declined.

Barriers to Youth Activity

For youth, there are significant barriers to becoming more active. Among households with children, just over half (57%) had a school within one mile of their home. Supporting data from parents notes that long distances to travel is the most often cited barrier to walking or biking to school among their children (7). The second most important barrier to youth activity was danger from traffic.

Measurement and Surveillance Challenges

To adequately monitor trends into the future, several surveillance and measurement challenges are beginning to be addressed. Newer measures of physical activity will assess both utilitarian and recreational activity domains. We also need to capture all sedentary activities (e.g., video game use) among all segments of the population.

IMPLICATIONS FOR POLICY AND PRACTICE

The patterns and trends in physical activity described in this paper are likely to be influenced by numerous policies and practices at national, state, and local levels. Policy makers, researchers, and public health practitioners should consider several issues when addressing the topics in our review (see below).

- Focused attention and action is needed on how to make the suburbs more activity-friendly through improved mixed-use development, siting of smaller and more common parks and schools, inclusion of greenspace in developments, and connectivity of neighborhoods. Our automobile-oriented daily lives and urban sprawl development have helped to create a less activity-oriented society. Movements such as Smart Growth (43) and the Congress for the New Urbanism (11) are attempting to promote activity-friendly land use development. In part, this involves promotion of principles and policies that support more walkable, mixed-use neighborhoods.

- Policies and practices are needed to put more physical activity back in the daily lives of children. Only one third of youth attended daily PE class in 2001, yet we know that when implemented properly, physical education in schools has a positive effect on activity rates (21). In addition, a return to smaller, neighborhood schools may encourage children to walk or bike to school. Programs such as Safe Routes to School (49) increasingly are being implemented to bring routine activity back into the school day.

- Considering the high rate of sedentary activity (television, video games, computer use), national media campaigns are needed to encourage activity. One promising such endeavor is CDC's VERB campaign (9), which is helping young people to realize that physical activity can be fun, cool, and a part of everyday life.

- Given the high proportion of persons employed in low activity occupations, it is important for employers to find ways of encouraging activity in the work environment. This may include incentives for walking or biking to work and creating more activity-friendly work environments (e.g., providing exercise facilities and/or allowing time for physical activity during the work day). In addition, placement of point-of-decision prompts to encourage stair use instead of elevator or escalator use is an effective method for promoting workplace activity (21).

- There have been promising developments for measuring physical activity. More recent questionnaire data such as the newly modified BRFSS and the International Physical Activity Questionnaire will allow researchers and practitioners to estimate rates of physical activity by domain (e.g., separating recreational activity from transportation activity) (12). There is also a strong need for a population-based surveillance system that tracks policies that enable or impede physical activity, similar to systems that have been developed for tobacco policies (1, 10).

CONCLUSION

Although difficult to precisely quantify owing to the lack of long-term data, a combination of characteristics of the built environment and increases in the proportion of the population engaging in sedentary activities put the majority of the American population at high risk of physical inactivity. A complex interaction of cultural, social, economic, and familial issues have likely set the stage for these changing physical activity trends. Creative, multicomponent approaches will be needed to address the high burden of inactivity.

ACKNOWLEDGMENTS

An earlier version of this paper was prepared for the Transportation Research Board and the Institute of Medicine Committee on Physical Activity, Health, Transportation, and Land Use. The authors appreciate the helpful review comments from the Committee members. They are also grateful for the advice and analytic assistance from Sandra Ham and Drs. Susan Handy, George King, and Joseph Schofer.

The *Annual Review of Public Health* is online at
http://publhealth.annualreviews.org

LITERATURE CITED

1. Alciati MH, Frosh M, Green SB, Brownson RC, Fisher PH, et al. 1998. State laws on youth access to tobacco in the United States: measuring their extensiveness with a new rating system. *Tob. Control* 7:345–52

2. Brownson RC, Eyler AA, King AC, Brown DR, Shyu Y-L, Sallis JF. 2000. Patterns and correlates of physical activity among women aged 40 years and older, United States. *Am. J. Public Health* 90:264–70

3. Brownson RC, Jones DA, Pratt M, Blanton C, Heath GW. 2000. Measuring physical activity with the Behavioral Risk Factor Surveillance System. *Med. Sci. Sports Exerc.* 32:1913–18

4. Caspersen CJ, Merritt RK. 1995. Physical activity trends among 26 states, 1986–1990. *Med. Sci. Sports Exerc.* 27:713–20

5. Caspersen CJ, Powell KE, Christenson GM. 1985. Physical activity, exercise, and physical fitness: definitions and distinctions for health-related research. *Public Health Rep.* 100:126–31

6. Cent. Dis. Control Prev. 2001. Physical activity trends–United States, 1990–1998. *MMWR* 50:166–69

7. Cent. Dis. Control Prev. 2003. Physical activity levels among children aged 9–13 years–United States, 2002. *MMWR Morb. Mortal. Wkly. Rep.* 52:785–88

8. Cent. Dis. Control Prev. 2003. Prevalence of physical activity, including lifestyle activities among adults–United States, 2000–2001. *MMWR Morb. Mortal. Wkly. Rep.* 52:764–69

9. Cent. Dis. Control Prev. 2004. *National Campaign to Get Kids Physically Active is Working.* Atlanta, GA: Cent. Dis. Control Prev.

10. Chriqui JF, Frosh M, Brownson RC, Shelton DM, Sciandra RC, et al. 2002. Application of a rating system to state clean indoor air laws (USA). *Tob. Control* 11:26–34

11. Congr. New Urbanism. 2001. *The Coming Demand.* San Francisco: Congr. New Urbanism

12. Craig CL, Marshall AL, Sjostrom M, Bauman AE, Booth ML, et al. 2003. International physical activity questionnaire: 12-country reliability and validity. *Med. Sci. Sports Exerc.* 35:1381–95

13. Ewing R, Schmid T, Killingsworth R, Zlot A, Raudenbush S. 2003. Relationship between urban sprawl and physical activity, obesity, and morbidity. *Am. J. Health Promot.* 18:47–57

14. Frank L, Engelke P, Schmid T. 2003. *Health and Community Design. The Impact of the Built Environment on Physical Activity.* Washington, DC: Island

15. Gentry EM, Kalsbeek WD, Hogelin GC, Jones JT, Gaines KL, et al. 1985. The behavioral risk factor surveys: II. Design, methods, and estimates from combined state data. *Am. J. Prev. Med.* 1:9–14

16. Giles-Corti B, Donovan RJ. 2002. The relative influence of individual, social and physical environment determinants of physical activity. *Soc. Sci. Med.* 54:1793–812

17. Hahn RA, Teutsch SM, Rothenberg RB, Marks JS. 1990. Excess deaths from nine chronic diseases in the United States, 1986. *JAMA* 264:2654–59

18. Handy SL, Boarnet MG, Ewing R, Killingsworth RE. 2002. How the built environment affects physical activity: views from urban planning. *Am. J. Prev. Med.* 23:64–73

19. Hoehner CM, Brennan LK, Brownson RC, Handy SL, Killingsworth R. 2003. Opportunities for integrating public health and urban planning approaches to promote active community environments. *Am. J. Health Promot.* 18:14–20

20. Jackson RJ. 2003. The impact of the built environment on health: an emerging field. *Am. J. Public Health* 93:1382–84

21. Kahn EB, Ramsey LT, Brownson RC, Heath GW, Howze EH, et al. 2002. The effectiveness of interventions to increase physical activity. A systematic review (1,2). *Am. J. Prev. Med.* 22:73–107

22. Killingsworth R, Earp J, Moore R. 2003. Supporting health through design: challenges and opportunities. *Am. J. Health Promot.* 18:1–2

23. King GA, Fitzhugh EC, Bassett DR Jr, McLaughlin JE, Strath SJ, et al. 2001. Relationship of leisure-time physical activity and occupational activity to the prevalence of obesity. *Int. J. Obes. Relat. Metab. Disord.* 25:606–12

24. Lum S, Moyer B, Yuskavage R. 2000. Improved estimates of gross product by industry for 1947–98. *Surv. Curr. Bus.* June:24–54

25. Macera CA, Pratt M. 2000. Public health surveillance of physical activity. *Res. Q. Exerc. Sport* 71:S97–103

26. McGinnis JM. 1992. The public health burden of a sedentary lifestyle. *Med. Sci. Sports Exerc.* 6:S196–S200

27. McGinnis JM, Foege WH. 1993. Actual causes of death in the United States. *J. Am. Med. Assoc.* 270:2207–12

28. Mokdad AH, Marks JS, Stroup DF, Gerberding JL. 2004. Actual causes of death in the United States, 2000. *JAMA* 291:1238–45

29. Muller PO. 1995. Transportation and urban form: stages in the spatial evolution of the American metropolis. In *The Geography of Urban Transportation*, ed. S Hanson, pp. 26–52. New York: Guilford

30. Nielsen Media Res. 2003. Nielsen Media Research. Accessed 23 November http://www.nielsenmedia.com/

31. Pate R, Pratt M, Blair S, Haskell W, Macera C, et al. 1995. Physical activity and public health: a recommendation from the Centers for Disease Control and Prevention and the American College of Sports Medicine. *JAMA* 273:402–7

32. Powell KE, Blair SN. 1994. The public health burden of sedentary living habits: theoretical but realistic estimates. *Med. Sci. Sports Exerc.* 26:851–56

33. Pratt M, Macera CA, Wang G. 2000. Higher direct medical costs associated with physical inactivity. *Physician Sportsmedicine* 28:63–70

34. Putnam RD. 1995. Tuning in, tuning out: the strange disappearance of social capital in America. *Polit. Sci. Polit.* 28:664–83

35. Remington PL, Smith MY, Williamson DF, Anda RF, Gentry EM, Hogelin GC. 1988. Design, characteristics, and usefulness of state-based behavioral risk factor surveillance: 1981–1987. *Public Health Rep.* 103:366–75

36. Robinson JP, Godbey G. 1999. *Time for Life. The Surprising Ways Americans Use Their Time.* University Park: Penn. Univ. Press

37. Ruggles S, Sobek M, Alexander T. 2003. *Integrated Public Use Microdata Series: Version 3.0, Historical Census Projects.* Minneapolis: Univ. Minn. Press. http://www.ipums.org

38. Saelens BE, Sallis JF, Frank LD. 2002. Environmental correlates of walking and cycling: findings from the transportation, urban design and planning literatures. *Ann. Behav. Med.* 25:80–91

39. Schilling J, Linton L. 2004. *The public health roots of zoning and modern land development codes: in search of active living's legal genealogy.* Presented at Active Living Res. Annu. Conf., San Diego, CA

40. Schrank D, Lomax T. 2003. *The 2003 Annual Urban Mobility Report*, Texas Transportation Institute. College Station: Tex. A&M Univ. Syst.

41. Shelton TST. 1995. *Research Note. Revised Vehicle Miles of Travel for Passenger Cars and Light Trucks, 1975 to 1993*, US Dep. Transp. Natl. Cent. Stat. Analysis., Washington, DC

42. Siegel PZ, Brackbill RM, Frazier EL, Mariolis P, Sanderson LM, et al. 1991. Behavioral risk factor surveillance, 1986–1990. *MMWR* 40:1–23

43. Smart Growth Netw. 2002. *Getting to Smart Growth: 100 Policies for Implementation.* Washington, DC: Smart Growth Netw.

44. Stephens T. 1987. Secular trends in adult physical activity: exercise boom or bust? *Res. Q. Exerc. Sport* 58:94–105

45. Sturm R. 2004. The economics of physical activity: societal trends and rationales for interventions. *Am. J. Prev. Med.* 27(Suppl. 3):126–35

46. Talbot LA, Fleg JL, Metter EJ. 2003. Secular trends in leisure-time physical activity in men and women across four decades. *Prev. Med.* 37:52–60

47. Taylor H. 2003. *Large declines Since 1995 in Favorite Activities Which Require Physical Exercise.* Rochester, NY: Harris Interact.

48. Taylor HL. 1983. Physical activity: Is it still a risk factor? *Prev. Med.* 12:20–24

49. Transp. Altern. 2004. Safe Routes to School. Accessed 23 April http://www.saferoutestoschool.org/

50. US Census Bur. 2003. *The American Housing Survey.* Washington, DC: US Census Bur.

51. US Dep. Health Hum. Serv. 1996. *Physical Activity and Health. A Report of the Surgeon General.* Atlanta, GA: US Dep. Health Hum. Serv.; Cent. Dis. Control Prev.

52. US Dep. Labor. 1998. *Standard Occupational Classification*, Bureau of Labor Statistics, Washington, DC

53. US Dep. Labor. 2004. *Current Population Survey.* Washington, DC: Bur. Labor Stat.

54. US Dep. Transp. 2000. *Travel Patterns of*

People of Color. Washington, DC: Fed. Highway Adm., US Dep. Transp. (Prepared by Battelle)

55. US Dep. Transp. Bur. Transp. Stat. 2003. *NHTS 2001 Highlights Report*. Washington, DC: US Dep. Transp. Bur. Transp. Stat.

56. US Dep. Transp. Bur. Transp. Stat. 2003. *TransStats*. Washington, DC: Bur. Transp. Stat.

57. Waksberg J. 1978. Sampling methods for random digit dialing. *J. Am. Stat. Assoc.* 73:40–46

Annu. Rev. Public Health 2005. 26:445–67
doi: 10.1146/annurev.publhealth.26.021304.144532
Copyright © 2005 by Annual Reviews. All rights reserved
First published online as a Review in Advance on October 26, 2004

Primary Prevention of Diabetes: What Can Be Done and How Much Can Be Prevented?

Matthias B. Schulze[1] and Frank B. Hu[1,2,3]

Departments of Nutrition[1] and Epidemiology,[2] Harvard School of Public Health, Boston, Massachusetts 02115; email: mschulze@mail.dife.de, frank.hu@channing.harvard.edu
[3]Channing Laboratory, Department of Medicine, Brigham and Women's Hospital and Harvard Medical School, Boston, Massachusetts 02115

■ **Abstract**   Although it is widely believed that type 2 diabetes mellitus is the result of a complex interplay between genetic and environmental factors, compelling evidence from epidemiologic studies indicates that the current worldwide diabetes epidemic is largely due to changes in diet and lifestyle. Prospective cohort studies and randomized clinical trials have demonstrated that type 2 diabetes can be prevented largely through moderate diet and lifestyle modifications. Excess adiposity is the most important risk factor for diabetes, and thus, maintaining a healthy body weight and avoiding weight gain during adulthood is the cornerstone of diabetes prevention. Increasing physical activity and reducing sedentary behaviors such as prolonged TV watching are important both for maintaining body weight and improving insulin sensitivity. There is increasing evidence that the quality of fat and carbohydrate plays a more important role than does the quantity, and thus, public health strategies should emphasize replacing saturated and trans fats with unsaturated fats and replacing refined grain products with whole grains. Recent studies have also suggested a potential role for coffee, dairy, nuts, magnesium, and calcium in preventing diabetes. Overall, a healthy diet, together with regular physical activity, maintenance of a healthy weight, moderate alcohol consumption, and avoidance of sedentary behaviors and smoking, could nearly eliminate type 2 diabetes. However, there is still a wide gap between what we know and what we practice in the field of public health; how to narrow that gap remains a major public health challenge.

INTRODUCTION

Diabetes mellitus is a group of metabolic diseases whose common feature is an elevated blood glucose level resulting from defects in insulin secretion, insulin action, or both. Type 2 diabetes mellitus accounts for 90%–95% of all diabetes cases, and it develops when the production of insulin is insufficient to overcome the underlying abnormality of increased resistance to its action. In contrast, type 1 diabetes mellitus is characterized by an absolute deficiency of insulin secretion resulting from autoimmune destruction of pancreatic beta cells. Though both forms

0163-7525/05/0421-0445$20.00

of diabetes are believed to be the products of complex interplay between genetic susceptibility and environmental factors, for type 1 diabetes there are few known modifiable environmental risk factors. Type 2 diabetes, in contrast, has increased rapidly during the past few decades worldwide, from ~35 million people affected in 1985 to ~171 million in 2000 (4). Investigators believe that changes in environmental factors are responsible for the growing epidemic of type 2 diabetes because the genetic background is unlikely to have changed during this short time period. The diabetes epidemic closely parallels the worldwide epidemic of obesity (2); while genotypes resulting in a thrifty metabolism may have been an advantage in times of nutrient scarcity, these same genes—when combined with an increasingly inactive and hypercaloric lifestyle in most parts of the world—may now contribute to obesity and diabetes (90).

Diabetes is associated with serious health consequences. It is a major risk factor for coronary heart disease (CHD) and stroke. In fact, the vast majority of diabetic patients die of cardiovascular complications. Diabetes is also the leading cause of blindness, kidney failure, and nontraumatic amputations, resulting from microvascular complications. The economic toll of diabetes is enormous. For example, in 2002, direct medical and treatment costs and indirect costs due to diabetes-related disability and mortality in the United States exceeded $132 billion (3). The economic burden will continue to rise as researchers predict an increase from 171 million diabetic individuals worldwide in 2000 to 370 million by the year 2030 (146). Because there is no cure for diabetes, primary prevention through diet and lifestyle modification is of paramount importance.

In this chapter, we review epidemic and clinical trial evidence concerning the preventability of diabetes through diet and lifestyle as well as through pharmacological means. We also review the epidemiologic evidence concerning individual risk factors for the development of diabetes and discuss public health implications for primary prevention of diabetes at both individual and population levels.

PREVENTABILITY OF TYPE 2 DIABETES MELLITUS

Epidemiologic Evidence

Strong epidemiologic evidence indicates that diabetes is associated with lifestyle. People who migrate to Westernized countries, with their more sedentary lifestyles and "Westernized" diets, have greater risk of developing type 2 diabetes than do their counterparts, who remain in the native countries (80). Populations undergoing Westernization in the absence of migration, such as North American Indians (35) and Western Samoans (17, 42), also have experienced dramatic rises in obesity and type 2 diabetes. Meanwhile, numerous prospective cohort studies have suggested that the combination of a Western diet and lifestyle is primarily responsible for the increased risk of diabetes (133).

Although a large body of evidence from epidemiologic studies has implicated individual dietary and lifestyle factors in the development of type 2 diabetes in diverse populations, few studies have examined multiple risk factors simultaneously. Using data from the Nurses' Health Study, Hu and colleagues (47) defined a low-risk group according to five variables: body-mass index (BMI; the weight in kilograms divided by the square of the height in meters) of less than 25, a diet high in cereal fiber and polyunsaturated fat and low in trans fat and glycemic load (which reflects the effect of diet on the blood glucose level), engagement in moderate-to-vigorous physical activity for at least half an hour per day, no current smoking, and the consumption of an average of at least a half-serving of an alcoholic beverage per day. As compared with the rest of the cohort, women in the low-risk group (3.4% of the women) had a relative risk (RR) of diabetes of 0.09 [95% confidence interval (CI): 0.05–0.17]. A total of 91% of the cases of diabetes in this cohort (95% CI: 83%–95%) could be attributed to the five factors listed above (Figure 1). These data provide strong epidemiologic evidence that the majority of type 2 diabetes cases could be prevented by the adoption of a healthier lifestyle.

Lifestyle Trials

The preventability of diabetes has been demonstrated by several randomized trials (Table 1). In a Chinese trial, 577 subjects who had impaired glucose tolerance (IGT) were randomly assigned to either the control group or to three different

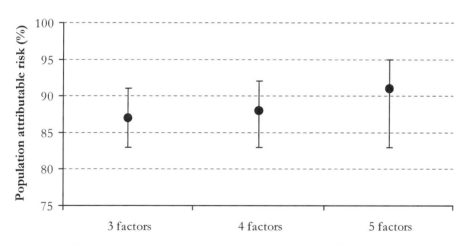

Low-risk groups defined by combinations of modifiable risk factors

Figure 1   Population attributable risk of type 2 diabetes mellitus in the Nurses' Health Study for Groups defined by combinations of modifiable risk factors. Adapted from Hu et al. (47). 3 factors: healthy dietary score (high polyunsaturated:saturated fat ratio, high in cereal fiber, low in trans fat, low in glycemic load), BMI < 25.0, moderate-to-vigorous exercise ≥30 min/day. 4 factors: 3 factors above plus nonsmoking. 5 factors: 4 factors above plus alcohol use ≥5 g/day.

intervention groups (diet, exercise, or diet plus exercise) (96). Participants in the diet-intervention group were prescribed a diet with a specific fat content and with individual goals for cereal, vegetables, meat, milk, and oil intake. Compared with the control group, the diet alone, exercise alone, and diet-plus-exercise interventions were associated with 31%, 46%, and 42% reductions, respectively, in risk of developing diabetes. In the Finnish Diabetes Prevention Study (132), 522 persons with IGT were randomly assigned to either a control group or an intervention group, in which each individual received counseling aimed at reducing weight, total fat intake, and saturated fat intake and increasing both intake of fiber and physical activity. The intervention resulted in an overall risk reduction of 58%. In the U.S.-based Diabetes Prevention Program (64), 3234 nondiabetic persons with IGT were randomly assigned to placebo, metformin (a biguanide that lowers blood glucose levels primarily by decreasing hepatic glucose production) (850 mg twice daily), or a lifestyle-modification program with the goals of at least a 7% weight loss and at least 150 min of physical activity per week. In this study, 50% of the participants in the lifestyle-intervention group had achieved the goal of weight loss of 7% or more by the end of the curriculum (at 24 weeks), and 38% had a weight loss of at least 7% at the time of the most recent visit; the percentage of participants who met the goal of at least 150 min of physical activity per week was 74% at 24 weeks and 58% at the most recent visit. During 2.8 years of follow-up, the lifestyle intervention reduced diabetes incidence by 58% (95% CI, 48%–66%) as compared with the control group. Lifestyle intervention was equally effective in both men and women and in different ethnic groups.

Drug Trials

Several trials have evaluated the efficacy of drugs in the prevention or delay of type 2 diabetes. In the Diabetes Prevention Program (64), 3234 subjects with IGT were randomly assigned to a lifestyle-intervention group, a metformin intervention group (850 mg twice daily), or a placebo group. The metformin group experienced a 31% diabetes risk reduction over a 3-year intervention period compared with the controls, although this effect was considerably smaller than that observed for the lifestyle-intervention group (58%).

In the Study to Prevent Non-Insulin-Dependent Diabetes Mellitus (STOP-NIDDM) (13), a multicenter trial in Austria, Canada, Germany, Denmark, Finland, Israel, Norway, Spain, and Sweden, 1429 subjects with IGT were randomly assigned to either an acarbose intervention or a placebo group. Acarbose is an alpha-glucosidase inhibitor that decreases the absorption of carbohydrates from the intestine, resulting in a slower and lower rise in blood glucose, particularly after meals. Over 3 years of intervention, the acarbose intervention group experienced a 25% diabetes risk reduction compared with the placebo group.

Troglitazone, a thiazolidinedione, was used as drug intervention in the Troglitazone in Prevention of Diabetes study (TRIPOD) (8). The primary mechanism

TABLE 1 Randomized trials on diet and lifestyle and prevention of type 2 diabetes

	Da-Qing study (96)	Finnish Diabetes prevention study (132)	Diabetes prevention program (64)
Study population			
N, sex	577 men and women with IGT	522 men and women with IGT	3234 men and women with IGT
Age	>25 years (mean = 45.0)	40–65 years (mean = 55)	>25 years (mean = 50.6)
Country	China	Finland	U.S.A.
Interventions			
Weight reduction goal	BMI = 23 for overweight subjects in diet group	≥ 5%	7%
Intervention arms	diet alone exercise alone diet + exercise control	lifestyle intervention control	lifestyle intervention metformin control
Dietary intervention	25%–30% energy from fat; 55%–65% energy from carbohydrate; specific advice on cereal, vegetable, meat, milk, and oil intake in subjects with BMI ≥ 25	<30% energy from fat; <10% saturated fat; fiber ≥ 15g/1000 kcal; frequent intake of whole-grain products, vegetables, fruits, low-fat milk and meat products, soft margarines and vegetable oils	25% fat, low-calorie diet; healthy eating based on U.S.D.A. Food Guide Pyramid
Lifestyle intervention	1 unit physical activity daily (5–30 min depending on intensity); 2 units per day if possible for those <50 years of age with no evidence of cardiovascular disease	moderate exercise ≥30 min daily	150 min/week physical activity
Follow-up (years)	6	3.2	2.8
Outcomes			
Weight change	Weight loss in all groups in subjects developing diabetes; weight gain in nondiabetics in control, diet, and activity groups; weight loss in nondiabetics in diet + exercise group	Intervention group: −4.2 kg (−4.7%) Control group: −0.8 kg (−0.9%)	Lifestyle intervention group: −5.6 kg Metformin group: −2.1 kg Control group: −0.1 kg
Diabetes risk reduction with intervention compared with controls	Diet only: 31% Exercise only: 46% Diet + exercise: 42%	58%	Lifestyle intervention group: 58% Metformin group: 31%

of action of thiazolidinediones involves binding to the peroxisome proliferator-activated receptor gamma, a transcription factor that regulates the expression and release of mediators of insulin resistance originating particularly in adipose tissue (e.g., free fatty acids, tumor necrosis factor alpha, resistin, adiponectin), resulting in net improvement in insulin sensitivity (124). Two hundred sixty-six women with a history of gestational diabetes and at high risk of developing type 2 diabetes (as determined by 5 oral glucose tolerance tests) were randomly assigned to troglitazone treatment (400 mg/d) or placebo, and during 3.5 years, treatment with troglitazone resulted in a 55% lower diabetes risk compared with treatment with placebo.

Post-hoc analyses of drug intervention trials with cardiovascular diseases as primary outcomes suggest that antihypertensive and cholesterol-lowering medications can prevent type 2 diabetes. Among 5720 patients in the Heart Outcomes Prevention Evaluation (HOPE) trial without known diabetes but with vascular disease at baseline, patients randomized to receive treatment with ramipril (an angiotensin-converting enzyme inhibitor) had a RR of 0.66 (95% CI: 0.51–0.85) to develop type 2 diabetes over a 4.5-year period compared with those who received placebo (151). A 30% diabetes risk reduction was observed with pravastatin therapy among 5974 participants in the West of Scotland Coronary Prevention Study (WESCOPS) (31). In the Losartan Intervention For Endpoint reduction in hypertension study (LIFE), fewer hypertensive patients with left ventricular hypertrophy developed diabetes mellitus if they were treated with losartan (an angiotensin II antagonist) than if they were treated with atenolol (a beta-blocker) (RR: 0.75, 95% CI: 0.63 to 0.88) (70).

These trials provide evidence that type 2 diabetes can be prevented through pharmacological means in high-risk populations. However, drug treatments were less efficacious than lifestyle modifications and can cause side effects. In contrast, a healthy diet and lifestyle is effective in not only preventing diabetes but also reducing risk of other chronic diseases such as CHD (122) and colon cancer (118).

MAJOR LIFESTYLE RISK FACTORS FOR DIABETES

Although multifactorial intervention trials have demonstrated the preventability of diabetes, they cannot tease apart the role of individual risk factors. Over the past several decades, numerous epidemiologic studies have contributed to our understanding of these risk factors.

Obesity

Excessive body weight, even at average levels for the U.S. population, increases the risk of diabetes. In the Nurses' Health Study (47), the single most important risk factor for type 2 diabetes was overweight and obesity; the RRs were 38.8 for

35 kg/m^2 or greater and 20.1 for 30.0 to 34.9 kg/m^2, as compared with less than 23 kg/m^2. Even a BMI within a normal range (23–24.9 kg/m^2) substantially elevated the risk (RR = 2.67). In this cohort of women, 61% (95% CI: 58%–64%) of type 2 diabetes cases could be attributed to overweight and obesity (using 25 kg/m^2 as a cut point). Similarly, in the Womens' Health Study (145), the RRs for developing type 2 diabetes were 3.22 (95% CI: 2.69–3.87) for overweight and 9.06 (95% CI: 7.60–10.8) for obese women compared with normalweight women. The magnitude of the association with BMI was much stronger than with physical activity in this study, a finding confirmed among Finnish men and women (50).

Abdominal obesity, as assessed by waist circumference or waist-to-hip ratio (WHR), predicts risk of diabetes independent of BMI (10, 61, 78, 92, 143). In the Nurses' Health Study (10), controlling for BMI and other potentially confounding factors, the RR for the 90th percentile of WHR ($\geq$0.86) versus the tenth percentile ($\leq$0.70) was 3.1 (95% CI: 2.3–4.1), and the RR for the 90th percentile of waist circumference ($\geq$36.2 inches or 92 cm) versus the tenth percentile ($\leq$26.2 inches or 67 cm) was 5.1 (95% CI: 2.9–8.9).

Weight gain during adulthood, even at modest levels (e.g., less than 5 kg), is associated with increased risk of diabetes independent of initial body weight. In the Nurses' Health Study (16), compared with women with stable weight (those who gained or lost less than 5 kg between age 18 years and 1976) and after adjusting for age and BMI at age 18 years, the RR for diabetes among women who had a weight gain of 5.0 to 7.9 kg was 1.9 (95% CI: 1.5–2.3). The corresponding RRs were 2.7 (95% CI: 2.1–3.3) for women who gained 8.0 to 10.9 kg and 12.3 (95% CI: 10.9–13.8) for those who gained 20.0 kg or more. In contrast, women who lost more than 5.0 kg reduced their risk for diabetes mellitus by 50% or more. Similarly, for every kilogram of weight gained, risk increased by 7.3% among men in the Health Professionals Follow-Up Study (65). Also noteworthy, although weight cycling is strongly associated with BMI, it does not appear to be independently predictive of developing diabetes (27).

Physical Activity

Convincing epidemiologic data support the role of physical activity in preventing diabetes. Physical activity is clearly a cornerstone of weight maintenance. Aerobic exercise by overweight and obese adults results in modest weight loss independent of the effect of caloric reduction through dieting (1). However, only part of the beneficial effect of physical activity on diabetes is mediated through body weight. Physical activity is clearly associated with increased insulin sensitivity (22, 82, 139). A reduced risk of developing diabetes with increased activity has been demonstrated in several prospective studies (37, 39, 45, 47, 48, 50, 51, 66, 79, 93, 139, 145). In most studies, a significant inverse association between physical activity and diabetes remained even after adjustment for BMI. Besides the benefits of vigorous activity, daily walking for >30 min is associated with a 20%–45% risk reduction (45, 46, 48, 51, 139, 145), and a faster walking pace predicted lower risk independent of the time spent walking (45, 48, 139).

Sedentary behaviors such as prolonged television watching are strongly associated with obesity, weight gain, and risk of diabetes, with the increased risk not entirely explained by the decreased physical activity and unhealthy eating patterns associated with television watching (46). In the Health Professionals' Follow-Up Study (45), men who watched TV more than 40 h per week had a nearly threefold increase in the risk of type 2 diabetes compared with those who spent less than 1 h per week watching TV. In the Nurses' Health Study (46), each 2-h/day increment in TV watching was associated with a 23% (95% CI: 17%–30%) increase in obesity and a 14% (95% CI: 5%–23%) increase in risk of diabetes. In contrast, each 1 h/day of brisk walking was associated with a 24% (95% CI, 19%–29%) reduction in obesity and a 34% (95% CI, 27%–41%) reduction in diabetes risk. It was estimated that 30% (95% CI, 24%–36%) of new cases of obesity and 43% (95% CI, 32%–52%) of new cases of diabetes could be prevented by adopting a relatively active lifestyle (<10 h/wk of TV watching and ≥30 min/day of brisk walking). Thus, public health campaigns to reduce the risk of obesity and type 2 diabetes should promote not only increasing exercise levels but also decreasing sedentary behaviors, especially prolonged TV watching.

Smoking

Several prospective studies have demonstrated that smoking is associated with a modestly increased risk of developing diabetes (23, 25, 60, 104, 105, 107 140, 147). Although earlier studies did not detect a significant positive effect (6, 9, 83, 84, 91, 94, 150), most have not focused on smoking and diabetes in their major hypotheses, and the majority have lacked the power to detect the relatively small but important effect (102). Although smoking cessation is associated with a modest increase in weight, it increases insulin sensitivity and improves the lipoprotein profile (24). Prospective studies clearly demonstrated that the beneficial effects of smoking cessation on diabetes risk outweigh the adverse effects on weight gain (140, 147).

Alcohol

Moderate alcohol consumption (1–3 drinks/day) has been consistently associated with lower incidence of diabetes compared with abstinence or occasional alcohol consumption (5, 11, 18, 21, 25, 36, 41, 43, 44, 47, 59, 76, 87, 89, 104, 121, 125, 130, 138, 141, 142, 144). Most studies have observed a U-shaped association, with heavy alcohol consumption being associated with increased risk compared with moderate consumption (21, 36, 59, 89, 130, 138, 141, 144). Five experimental studies investigated the effect of alcohol consumption on insulin sensitivity. One study with 51 postmenopausal women showed a significant increase in insulin sensitivity after 8 weeks of moderate alcohol consumption (20). In another study among 23 healthy middle-aged men, insulin sensitivity seemed to increase over a 17-day period in an insulin-resistant subgroup but not among men with normal insulin sensitivity (117). However, the other three intervention trials found no effect of alcohol consumption on insulin sensitivity (19, 28, 152).

MAJOR DIETARY FACTORS FOR DIABETES

Amount and Types of Fat

Higher total fat intake has been hypothesized to contribute to diabetes through two major pathways. First, a high percentage of fat in the diet may promote weight gain and the development of obesity. Second, a high percentage of fat in the diet may cause insulin resistance, independent of obesity. The first hypothesis has been hotly debated within recent years (53, 148). Although in short-term studies, a modest reduction in body weight has been seen typically in individuals assigned to diets with a lower percentage of calories from fat, recently published weight-loss trials on low-carbohydrate-high-fat/protein diets suggest greater weight loss with high-fat diets than with low-fat diets (30, 112). Compensatory mechanisms appear to operate such that in the long term, fat consumption within the range of 18%–40% of energy appears to have little if any effect on body fat (148). Although some investigators argue that high-fat diets tend to be more energy-dense, which in turn leads to passive overconsumption (53), the replacement of fat generally by simple sugars in many processed foods in industrialized countries has not led to a decrease in energy density of diets. Furthermore, high-fat diets are not necessarily energy-dense. The Mediterranean diet, for example, is based predominantly on energy-diluted foods, e.g., vegetables, fruits, and legumes but contains moderate to high amounts of fat, predominantly in the form of vegetable oils.

Results from metabolic studies on the relationship between total fat intake and insulin sensitivity in humans—with no change in the fatty acid profile—are inconsistent and generally do not support the hypothesis that high-fat diets have detrimental effects on insulin sensitivity (69). Similarly, whereas some earlier prospective observational studies found a positive association between total fat intake and diabetes risk (26, 81), most large cohort studies with validated food-frequency questionnaires suggest no association (15, 38, 85, 109–111, 136).

More important than the total fat intake may be the specific types of fat consumed (49). Substituting unsaturated fat for saturated fat increases insulin sensitivity in intervention studies in diabetic (126), overweight (75), and healthy subjects (137). High intake of vegetable fat or polyunsaturated fat is inversely associated with diabetes risk in the Nurses' Health Study and the Iowa Women's Study, two large cohort studies among women (85, 110). A high polyunsaturated:saturated fat ratio was significantly associated with diabetes risk in the EPIC-Norfolk Study, although the association was attenuated after adjustment for BMI (38). In the Health Professionals Follow-Up Study (136), a significant inverse association between polyunsaturated fat and diabetes was observed only among lean men. Trans-fatty acids, formed by hardening of unsaturated fatty acids, substantially increased diabetes risk among women in the Nurses' Health Study (110), but this association was not observed in other cohorts (85, 136). Although one intervention study observed increased postprandial insulinemia with a high-trans-fat diet (20% of energy from trans-fat) (14), other intervention studies did not observe any appreciable effects of trans-fatty acids on insulin sensitivity or glucose metabolism (68, 74, 75).

Quality and Quantity of Carbohydrates

Low-fat, high-carbohydrate diets generally produce high postprandial glucose and insulin responses. However, similar to total fat, the total percentage of energy derived from carbohydrates in the diet generally has not been found to predict diabetes risk (86, 109, 111, 114). Metabolic consequences of carbohydrate intake depend not only on their quantity but also on their quality. The glycemic response of a given carbohydrate load depends on the food sources, which has led to the development of the glycemic index, ranking foods by their ability to raise postprandial blood glucose levels (52). The glycemic index quantifies the glycemic response by a standard amount of carbohydrates from a food relative to the response by the same amount of carbohydrates from white bread or glucose. The overall glycemic index of a diet has been associated with an increased diabetes risk in some prospective observational studies (109, 111, 114), although findings are inconsistent so far (86, 123). However, the relevance of the concept of glycemic index is indirectly supported by the reduction in diabetes incidence observed with acarbose treatment, an alpha-glucosidase inhibitor that slows down the digestion of carbohydrates (13).

Effects of carbohydrate-rich foods on insulin resistance and diabetes risk may also depend on fiber content and type. Several epidemiologic studies found that diets rich in whole grains (33, 72, 86, 88) or cereal fiber (47, 86, 88, 109, 111, 114, 123) may protect against type 2 diabetes (Figure 2). Controlled feeding studies have found benefits of whole grains on insulin sensitivity and glucose metabolism compared with refined grains (12, 32, 62, 99), although this finding has not been observed in all studies (57). This effect may be partially mediated by positive effects on body weight—studies generally support an inverse association between intake of whole grains and body weight (101). In addition, fiber tends to slow down gastrointestinal absorption, resulting in a lower glycemic index of whole-grain products compared with their refined-grain counterparts; however, other mechanisms by which whole grains influence glucose metabolism are likely to play a role as well, e.g., short-chain fatty acid production (127) and micronutrient content (71).

Micronutrients

Magnesium is an important component of whole grains and other unprocessed foods, such as nuts and green leafy vegetables. Its intake has substantially decreased in industrialized countries owing to overprocessing of foods and adoption of Western diets. Hypomagnesemia is a frequent condition in patients with type 2 diabetes (129). Hypomagnesemia has been associated with a reduction of tyrosine-kinase activity at the insulin receptor level, which may result in the impairment of insulin action and development of insulin resistance (97). Higher magnesium intakes have been associated with a decreased risk of developing type

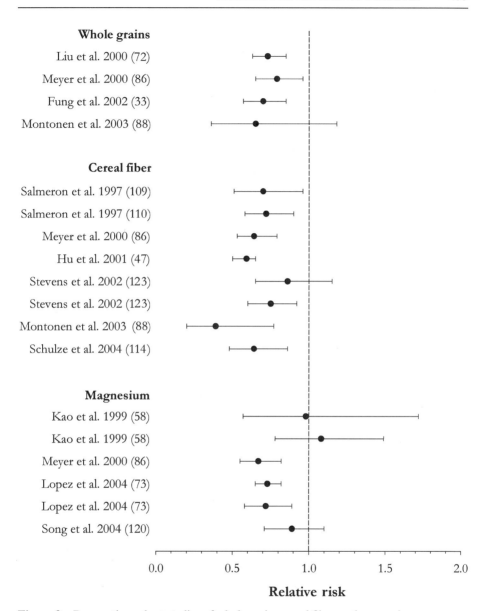

Figure 2   Prospective cohort studies of whole grain, cereal fiber, and magnesium consumption and risk of type 2 diabetes mellitus.

2 diabetes in most (73, 86, 109, 111, 120) but not all (58) prospective studies (Figure 2).

Iron is a transitional metal that can catalyze the conversion of poorly reactive free radicals into highly active free radicals, which may play a role in the development of diabetes. Iron excess seems to contribute initially to insulin resistance by decreasing glucose uptake by muscles and subsequently to decreased insulin synthesis and secretion in the pancreas (149). Increased total body iron stores have been associated with an increased risk of type 2 diabetes (55). However, only heme-iron intake from red meat, but not nonheme iron, was positively associated with risk of type 2 diabetes in two prospective studies (54, 67). This association may have been confounded by other components of red meat or dietary exposures associated with it. Therefore, evidence is limited in support of the hypothesis that a lower dietary iron intake may be important in the prevention of diabetes. Still, measurement of body iron stores may be helpful in identifying those at high risk who would possibly benefit from lifestyle or therapeutic interventions that can lower iron stores in the body.

Longitudinal observational studies and small controlled trials in humans suggest that increasing dietary calcium or dairy intake may prevent future weight gain (98), but the results are inconsistent and more studies are clearly needed. In addition to its potential effects on weight gain, dietary calcium has been inversely associated with insulin resistance (100). However, the strong correlation between calcium and dairy intake in observational studies makes it impossible to clearly separate the potential effect of calcium from that of other components of dairy products.

Individual Foods

The relationship between consumption of specific foods and diabetes risk has been examined in recent years. An inverse association between coffee consumption and risk of type 2 diabetes has been observed in several prospective cohort studies (106, 108, 131, 134), but not in all (113). The beneficial effect of long-term coffee consumption on the development of diabetes has been attributed to caffeine, but other constituents of coffee, e.g., potassium, niacin, magnesium, and antioxidant substances, may have beneficial effects on glucose metabolism and insulin resistance as well.

Frequent consumption of meat, in particular processed meat, has been consistently shown to increase the risk of diabetes in prospective studies (34, 116, 119, 136). Although processed meats are a major component of the so-called Western diet pattern in these study populations, these associations have been found to be independent of the Western pattern (34, 116). Furthermore, although the associations between red meat consumption and diabetes risk were largely attenuated by controlling for fat intake, processed meats remained significantly associated with risk (116), indicating that constituents of processed meats other than fatty acids, e.g., nitrite or advanced glycation end products, may be relevant in the development of diabetes.

Recent findings from prospective studies also indicate that consumption of nuts (56) and dairy products (100) may have beneficial effects in the development of diabetes. Fruit and vegetable consumption was inversely associated with risk of diabetes in the National Health and Nutrition Examination Survey (29) but not among older women in the Iowa Women's Health Study (86).

Several epidemiologic studies found that diets rich in whole grains may protect against type 2 diabetes (33, 72, 86, 88). Controlled feeding studies have found benefits of whole grains to insulin sensitivity and glucose (99) compared with refined grains.

Sugar-sweetened beverages receive growing attention as potential contributors to the obesity and diabetes epidemic (7). Energy contained in beverages seems less well-detected by the body, and subsequent food intake is poorly adjusted to account for the energy intake from beverages. Sugar-sweetened beverages have been associated with weight gain in clinical studies (103, 128) and observational studies among children (77) and adults (115). The high sugar loads from sugar-sweetened beverages may also have detrimental effects on glucose metabolism leading to diabetes, beyond their potential contribution to obesity (115). In the Nurses' Health Study II, frequent consumption of sugar-sweetened soft drinks (one serving or more per day) was associated with a 40% increase in diabetes risk after controlling for body mass index and other diabetes risk factors (115).

Overall Dietary Patterns

Recently, two prospective studies have reported the role of overall dietary patterns in predicting risk of diabetes (34, 135). A prudent pattern (characterized by high consumption of vegetables, fruits, fish, poultry, and whole grains) was associated with a modest risk reduction in both studies, whereas a Western pattern (characterized by high consumption of red meat, processed meat, French fries, high-fat dairy products, refined grains, and sweets and desserts) was associated with an increased risk for type 2 diabetes. In contrast, in the Nurses' Health Study, Hu et al. (47) found that an a priori–defined pattern score based on the intake of cereal fiber, polyunsaturated fatty acids, trans-fatty acids, and glycemic load had a tremendous effect on diabetes incidence. Women within the highest quintile of the pattern score had a RR of 0.49 (95% CI: 0.42–0.56) compared with women in the lowest quintile.

PUBLIC HEALTH IMPLICATIONS

Translating Knowledge into Practice

The past decade has witnessed many advances in our understanding of diabetes risk factors. However, there is still a wide gap between what we know and what we practice in the field of public health. Thus, an important public health priority is to narrow this gap. Obesity control is clearly the key to diabetes prevention; measures aimed at reducing or preventing overweight and obesity are particularly relevant in reducing diabetes risk. Lifestyle modifications with regard to changing diet and activity, balancing energy intake and expenditure, and making healthy food and lifestyle choices are therefore cornerstones of diabetes prevention at the individual level, and such information needs to be communicated to the public and translated into practice. The changes required to reduce the risk of diabetes at the population level are, however, unlikely to be achieved without major environmental changes to facilitate appropriate choices by individuals (2). Competing interests in school

(school lunch programs, funding sources, school boards) and work environments may be major barriers to modification of diet and activity patterns in children and adults. Urban environments may not facilitate activity behaviors owing to the lack of sidewalks, bike paths, athletic fields, etc. Heavy marketing of energy-dense, micronutrient-poor foods and beverages, particularly to children, clearly conflicts with attempts to promote healthy food choices. Whether healthy food choices are available and affordable, particularly to individuals of lower socioeconomic status, may greatly affect the adoption of healthy eating behaviors. A broad-based public health perspective working at various levels—the individual, the work, school, and home environments, in communities, nationally, and internationally—is therefore needed to stem the tide of the diabetes epidemic.

Cost-Effectiveness of Lifestyle Changes

It is necessary to evaluate the cost-effectiveness of preventive interventions to help health systems and policy makers implement prevention strategies into efficient clinical and public health practice. The Diabetes Prevention Program Research Group evaluated in detail the costs associated with the two different interventions, lifestyle modifications and metformin (40). The direct medical costs per capita during the 3-year intervention period (including the intervention itself and care outside the study protocol) were $2191 in the metformin group and $2269 in the lifestyle-intervention group compared with the placebo group, which was about $750 per capita and per year for both interventions. These costs could be substantially reduced by the use of less-expensive generic metformin and a more cost-effective delivery of the lifestyle intervention (40). A recent study by Palmer et al. (95) projected the long-term health and economic implications of these interventions in five industrialized countries (Australia, France, Germany, Switzerland, and the United Kingdom). Both metformin and lifestyle interventions were projected to lead to improvements in life expectancy and an increase in diabetes-free years of life. Implementation of the interventions could lead to cost savings in all countries, with the exception of the United Kingdom, where a minor increase in costs was observed. Even in the United Kingdom, the projected cost-effectiveness (€5400 and €6381 per life-year gained from metformin and lifestyle intervention) lay within a range clearly considered cost-effective (63). Thus, widespread implementation of dietary and lifestyle interventions, as well as drug interventions, in high-risk groups for the prevention of diabetes carries no obvious drawbacks. Although lifestyle and drug interventions are both cost-effective for high-risk populations, lifestyle modifications will likely have much broader benefits on health because the same target diet and lifestyle also reduce risk of other chronic diseases including cardiovascular disease and certain forms of cancer. Unlike drug treatments, lifestyle interventions have few side effects. For low-risk populations, community-based lifestyle interventions are the only viable option because drug interventions would be impractical and unethical in these populations.

SUMMARY AND CONCLUSIONS

Compelling evidence from metabolic studies, large prospective observational studies, and clinical trials indicate that unhealthy diets, obesity, and sedentary lifestyles are major contributors to the diabetes epidemic. Obesity is the strongest risk factor for diabetes, and maintenance of a healthy weight by avoiding energy overconsumption and engaging in regular physical activity is clearly the key to diabetes prevention. However, the relationship between diet and obesity remains controversial. With regard to dietary fat, long-term trials have not produced clear evidence to support the hypothesis that low-fat diets are more effective for weight maintenance than are moderate-fat diets (148). Because total fat generally has also not been associated with diabetes risk in observational studies, nor with insulin resistance in metabolic studies, there is no good evidence supporting the effectiveness of low-fat diets in diabetes prevention. The type and quality of fat and carbohydrates may be more important than the total amount. Substitution of unsaturated fat for saturated and trans fats and of whole grain foods for refined grain foods are effective and important strategies to prevent diabetes. A diet rich in fruits, vegetables, legumes, whole grains, and healthy sources of protein (poultry and fish), and containing unsaturated vegetable fats as the main source of fat, but that is low in red and processed meats, refined grains, and sugar-sweetened beverages can offer significant protection against type 2 diabetes. Such diets, with favorable fatty acid composition and high amounts of fiber and micronutrients, may be beneficial also in weight maintenance (2).

Physical activity reduces diabetes risk by helping to maintain a healthy body weight and by improving insulin sensitivity. Even moderate activities, e.g., regular walking, offer substantial benefits. Sedentary behaviors like TV watching, in contrast, promote weight gain and diabetes risk. Avoidance of smoking and consumption of a moderate amount of alcohol have benefits also with regard to risk reduction. A healthy diet, together with regular physical activity, maintenance of a healthy body weight, consumption of moderate amounts of alcohol, and avoidance of sedentary behaviors and smoking, is likely to prevent most type 2 diabetes cases.

The *Annual Review of Public Health* is online at
http://publhealth.annualreviews.org

LITERATURE CITED

1. 1998. Natl. Inst. Health. Clinical guidelines on the identification, evaluation, and treatment of overweight and obesity in adults—the evidence report. *Obes. Res.* 6(Suppl. 2):S51–209
2. 2002. Diet, nutrition and the prevention of chronic diseases: report of a joint WHO/FAO expert consultation. *WHO Tech. Rep. Ser. No. 916*, Geneva, Switz.
3. 2003. Economic costs of diabetes in the U.S. in 2002. *Diabetes Care* 26:917–32
4. 2003. *The World Health Report 2002*. Geneva, Switz.: WHO
5. Ajani UA, Hennekens CH, Spelsberg A,

Manson JE. 2000. Alcohol consumption and risk of type 2 diabetes mellitus among US male physicians. *Arch. Intern. Med.* 160:1025–30

6. Balkau B, King H, Zimmet P, Raper LR. 1985. Factors associated with the development of diabetes in the Micronesian population of Nauru. *Am. J. Epidemiol.* 122:594–605

7. Bray GA, Nielsen SJ, Popkin BM. 2004. Consumption of high-fructose corn syrup in beverages may play a role in the epidemic of obesity. *Am. J. Clin. Nutr.* 79:537–43

8. Buchanan TA, Xiang AH, Peters RK, Kjos SL, Marroquin A, et al. 2002. Preservation of pancreatic beta-cell function and prevention of type 2 diabetes by pharmacological treatment of insulin resistance in high-risk hispanic women. *Diabetes* 51:2796–803

9. Butler WJ, Ostrander LD Jr, Carman WJ, Lamphiear DE. 1982. Diabetes mellitus in Tecumseh, Michigan. Prevalence, incidence, and associated conditions. *Am. J. Epidemiol.* 116:971–80

10. Carey VJ, Walters EE, Colditz GA, Solomon CG, Willett WC, et al. 1997. Body fat distribution and risk of non-insulin-dependent diabetes mellitus in women. The Nurses' Health Study. *Am. J. Epidemiol.* 145:614–19

11. Carlsson S, Hammar N, Grill V, Kaprio J. 2003. Alcohol consumption and the incidence of type 2 diabetes: a 20-year follow-up of the Finnish twin cohort study. *Diabetes Care* 26:2785–90

12. Chandalia M, Garg A, Lutjohann D, von Bergmann K, Grundy SM, Brinkley LJ. 2000. Beneficial effects of high dietary fiber intake in patients with type 2 diabetes mellitus. *N. Engl. J. Med.* 342:1392–98

13. Chiasson JL, Josse RG, Gomis R, Hanefeld M, Karasik A, Laakso M. 2002. Acarbose for prevention of type 2 diabetes mellitus: the STOP-NIDDM randomised trial. *Lancet* 359:2072–77

14. Christiansen E, Schnider S, Palmvig B,

Tauber-Lassen E, Pedersen O. 1997. Intake of a diet high in trans monounsaturated fatty acids or saturated fatty acids. Effects on postprandial insulinemia and glycemia in obese patients with NIDDM. *Diabetes Care* 20:881–87

15. Colditz GA, Manson JE, Stampfer MJ, Rosner B, Willett WC, Speizer FE. 1992. Diet and risk of clinical diabetes in women. *Am. J. Clin. Nutr.* 55:1018–23

16. Colditz GA, Willett WC, Rotnitzky A, Manson JE. 1995. Weight gain as a risk factor for clinical diabetes mellitus in women. *Ann. Intern. Med.* 122:481–86

17. Collins VR, Dowse GK, Toelupe PM, Imo TT, Aloaina FL, et al. 1994. Increasing prevalence of NIDDM in the Pacific island population of Western Samoa over a 13-year period. *Diabetes Care* 17:288–96

18. Conigrave KM, Hu BF, Camargo CA Jr, Stampfer MJ, Willett WC, Rimm EB. 2001. A prospective study of drinking patterns in relation to risk of type 2 diabetes among men. *Diabetes* 50:2390–95

19. Cordain L, Melby CL, Hamamoto AE, O'Neill DS, Cornier MA, et al. 2000. Influence of moderate chronic wine consumption on insulin sensitivity and other correlates of syndrome X in moderately obese women. *Metabolism* 49:1473–78

20. Davies MJ, Baer DJ, Judd JT, Brown ED, Campbell WS, Taylor PR. 2002. Effects of moderate alcohol intake on fasting insulin and glucose concentrations and insulin sensitivity in postmenopausal women: a randomized controlled trial. *JAMA* 287:2559–62

21. de Vegt F, Dekker JM, Groeneveld WJ, Nijpels G, Stehouwer CD, et al. 2002. Moderate alcohol consumption is associated with lower risk for incident diabetes and mortality: the Hoorn Study. *Diabetes Res. Clin. Pract.* 57:53–60

22. Duncan GE, Perri MG, Theriaque DW, Hutson AD, Eckel RH, Stacpoole PW. 2003. Exercise training, without weight loss, increases insulin sensitivity and postheparin plasma lipase activity in

previously sedentary adults. *Diabetes Care* 26:557–62

23. Eliasson B, Asplund K, Nasic S, Rodu B. 2004. Influence of smoking and snus on the prevalence and incidence of type 2 diabetes amongst men: the northern Sweden MONICA study. *J. Intern. Med.* 256:101–10

24. Eliasson B, Attvall S, Taskinen MR, Smith U. 1997. Smoking cessation improves insulin sensitivity in healthy middle-aged men. *Eur. J. Clin. Invest.* 27:450–56

25. Feskens EJ, Kromhout D. 1989. Cardiovascular risk factors and the 25-year incidence of diabetes mellitus in middle-aged men. The Zutphen Study. *Am. J. Epidemiol.* 130:1101–8

26. Feskens EJ, Virtanen SM, Rasanen L, Tuomilehto J, Stengard J, et al. 1995. Dietary factors determining diabetes and impaired glucose tolerance. A 20-year follow-up of the Finnish and Dutch cohorts of the Seven Countries Study. *Diabetes Care* 18:1104–12

27. Field AE, Manson JE, Laird N, Williamson DF, Willett WC, Colditz GA. 2004. Weight cycling and the risk of developing type 2 diabetes among adult women in the United States. *Obes. Res.* 12:267–74

28. Flanagan DE, Pratt E, Murphy J, Vaile JC, Petley GW, et al. 2002. Alcohol consumption alters insulin secretion and cardiac autonomic activity. *Eur. J. Clin. Invest.* 32:187–92

29. Ford ES, Mokdad AH. 2001. Fruit and vegetable consumption and diabetes mellitus incidence among U.S. adults. *Prev. Med.* 32:33–39

30. Foster GD, Wyatt HR, Hill JO, McGuckin BG, Brill C, et al. 2003. A randomized trial of a low-carbohydrate diet for obesity. *N. Engl. J. Med.* 348:2082–90

31. Freeman DJ, Norrie J, Sattar N, Neely RD, Cobbe SM, et al. 2001. Pravastatin and the development of diabetes mellitus: evidence for a protective treatment effect in the West of Scotland Coronary Prevention Study. *Circulation* 103:357–62

32. Fukagawa NK, Anderson JW, Hageman G, Young VR, Minaker KL. 1990. High-carbohydrate, high-fiber diets increase peripheral insulin sensitivity in healthy young and old adults. *Am. J. Clin. Nutr.* 52:524–28

33. Fung TT, Hu FB, Pereira MA, Liu S, Stampfer MJ, et al. 2002. Whole-grain intake and the risk of type 2 diabetes: a prospective study in men. *Am. J. Clin. Nutr.* 76:535–40

34. Fung TT, Schulze MB, Manson JE, Willett WC, Hu FB. 2004. Dietary patterns, meat intake and the risk of type 2 diabetes in women. *Arch. Intern. Med.* In press

35. Gohdes D, Kaufman S, Valway S. 1993. Diabetes in American Indians. An overview. *Diabetes Care* 16:239–43

36. Gurwitz JH, Field TS, Glynn RJ, Manson JE, Avorn J, et al. 1994. Risk factors for non-insulin-dependent diabetes mellitus requiring treatment in the elderly. *J. Am. Geriatr. Soc.* 42:1235–40

37. Haapanen N, Miilunpalo S, Vuori I, Oja P, Pasanen M. 1997. Association of leisure time physical activity with the risk of coronary heart disease, hypertension and diabetes in middle-aged men and women. *Int. J. Epidemiol.* 26:739–47

38. Harding AH, Day NE, Khaw KT, Bingham S, Luben R, et al. 2004. Dietary fat and the risk of clinical type 2 diabetes: the European prospective investigation of Cancer-Norfolk study. *Am. J. Epidemiol.* 159:73–82

39. Helmrich SP, Ragland DR, Leung RW, Paffenbarger RS Jr. 1991. Physical activity and reduced occurrence of non-insulin-dependent diabetes mellitus. *N. Engl. J. Med.* 325:147–52

40. Hernan WH, Brandle M, Zhang P, Williamson DF, Matulik MJ, et al. 2003. Costs associated with the primary prevention of type 2 diabetes mellitus in the diabetes prevention program. *Diabetes Care* 26:36–47

41. Hodge AM, Dowse GK, Collins VR, Zimmet PZ. 1993. Abnormal glucose tolerance and alcohol consumption in three populations at high risk of non-insulin-dependent diabetes mellitus. *Am. J. Epidemiol.* 137:178–89

42. Hodge AM, Dowse GK, Toelupe P, Collins VR, Imo T, Zimmet PZ. 1994. Dramatic increase in the prevalence of obesity in western Samoa over the 13 year period 1978–1991. *Int. J. Obes. Relat. Metab. Disord.* 18:419–28

43. Holbrook TL, Barrett-Connor E, Wingard DL. 1990. A prospective population-based study of alcohol use and non-insulin-dependent diabetes mellitus. *Am. J. Epidemiol.* 132:902–9

44. Howard AA, Arnsten JH, Gourevitch MN. 2004. Effect of alcohol consumption on diabetes mellitus: a systematic review. *Ann. Intern. Med.* 140:211–19

45. Hu FB, Leitzmann MF, Stampfer MJ, Colditz GA, Willett WC, Rimm EB. 2001. Physical activity and television watching in relation to risk for type 2 diabetes mellitus in men. *Arch. Intern. Med.* 161:1542–48

46. Hu FB, Li TY, Colditz GA, Willett WC, Manson JE. 2003. Television watching and other sedentary behaviors in relation to risk of obesity and type 2 diabetes mellitus in women. *JAMA* 289:1785–91

47. Hu FB, Manson JE, Stampfer MJ, Colditz G, Liu S, et al. 2001. Diet, lifestyle, and the risk of type 2 diabetes mellitus in women. *N. Engl. J. Med.* 345:790–97

48. Hu FB, Sigal RJ, Rich-Edwards JW, Colditz GA, Solomon CG, et al. 1999. Walking compared with vigorous physical activity and risk of type 2 diabetes in women: a prospective study. *JAMA* 282:1433–39

49. Hu FB, van Dam RM, Liu S. 2001. Diet and risk of Type II diabetes: the role of types of fat and carbohydrate. *Diabetologia* 44:805–17

50. Hu G, Lindstrom J, Valle TT, Eriksson JG, Jousilahti P, et al. 2004. Physical activity, body mass index, and risk of type 2 diabetes in patients with normal or impaired glucose regulation. *Arch. Intern. Med.* 164:892–96

51. Hu G, Qiao Q, Silventoinen K, Eriksson JG, Jousilahti P, et al. 2003. Occupational, commuting, and leisure-time physical activity in relation to risk for Type 2 diabetes in middle-aged Finnish men and women. *Diabetologia* 46:322–29

52. Jenkins DJ, Wolever TM, Taylor RH, Barker H, Fielden H, et al. 1981. Glycemic index of foods: a physiological basis for carbohydrate exchange. *Am. J. Clin. Nutr.* 34:362–66

53. Jequier E, Bray GA. 2002. Low-fat diets are preferred. *Am. J. Med.* 113(Suppl. 9B):41–46

54. Jiang R, Ma J, Ascherio A, Stampfer MJ, Willett WC, Hu FB. 2004. Dietary iron intake and blood donations in relation to risk of type 2 diabetes in men: a prospective cohort study. *Am. J. Clin. Nutr.* 79:70–75

55. Jiang R, Manson JE, Meigs JB, Ma J, Rifai N, Hu FB. 2004. Body iron stores in relation to risk of type 2 diabetes in apparently healthy women. *JAMA* 291:711–17

56. Jiang R, Manson JE, Stampfer MJ, Liu S, Willett WC, Hu FB. 2002. Nut and peanut butter consumption and risk of type 2 diabetes in women. *JAMA* 288:2554–60

57. Juntunen KS, Laaksonen DE, Poutanen KS, Niskanen LK, Mykkanen HM. 2003. High-fiber rye bread and insulin secretion and sensitivity in healthy postmenopausal women. *Am. J. Clin. Nutr.* 77:385–91

58. Kao WH, Folsom AR, Nieto FJ, Mo JP, Watson RL, Brancati FL. 1999. Serum and dietary magnesium and the risk for type 2 diabetes mellitus: the Atherosclerosis Risk in Communities Study. *Arch. Intern. Med.* 159:2151–59

59. Kao WH, Puddey IB, Boland LL, Watson RL, Brancati FL. 2001. Alcohol consumption and the risk of type 2 diabetes mellitus: atherosclerosis risk in communities study. *Am. J. Epidemiol.* 154:748–57

60. Kawakami N, Takatsuka N, Shimizu H,

Ishibashi H. 1997. Effects of smoking on the incidence of non-insulin-dependent diabetes mellitus. Replication and extension in a Japanese cohort of male employees. *Am. J. Epidemiol.* 145:103–9

61. Kaye SA, Folsom AR, Sprafka JM, Prineas RJ, Wallace RB. 1991. Increased incidence of diabetes mellitus in relation to abdominal adiposity in older women. *J. Clin. Epidemiol.* 44:329–34

62. Keenan JM, Pins JJ, Frazel C, Moran A, Turnquist L. 2002. Oat ingestion reduces systolic and diastolic blood pressure in patients with mild or borderline hypertension: a pilot trial. *J. Fam. Pract.* 51: 369

63. Klonoff DC, Schwartz DM. 2000. An economic analysis of interventions for diabetes. *Diabetes Care* 23:390–404

64. Knowler WC, Barrett-Connor E, Fowler SE, Hamman RF, Lachin JM, et al. 2002. Reduction in the incidence of type 2 diabetes with lifestyle intervention or metformin. *N. Engl. J. Med.* 346:393–403

65. Koh-Banerjee P, Wang Y, Hu FB, Spiegelman D, Willett WC, Rimm EB. 2004. Changes in body weight and body fat distribution as risk factors for clinical diabetes in US men. *Am. J. Epidemiol.* 159:1150–59

66. Kriska AM, Saremi A, Hanson RL, Bennett PH, Kobes S, et al. 2003. Physical activity, obesity, and the incidence of type 2 diabetes in a high-risk population. *Am. J. Epidemiol.* 158:669–75

67. Lee DH, Folsom AR, Jacobs DR Jr. 2004. Dietary iron intake and Type 2 diabetes incidence in postmenopausal women: the Iowa Women's Health Study. *Diabetologia* 47:185–94

68. Lichtenstein AH, Erkkila AT, Lamarche B, Schwab US, Jalbert SM, Ausman LM. 2003. Influence of hydrogenated fat and butter on CVD risk factors: remnant-like particles, glucose and insulin, blood pressure and C-reactive protein. *Atherosclerosis* 171:97–107

69. Lichtenstein AH, Schwab US. 2000. Relationship of dietary fat to glucose metabolism. *Atherosclerosis* 150:227–43

70. Lindholm LH, Ibsen H, Borch-Johnsen K, Olsen MH, Wachtell K, et al. 2002. Risk of new-onset diabetes in the Losartan Intervention For Endpoint reduction in hypertension study. *J. Hypertens.* 20:1879–86

71. Liu S. 2002. Intake of refined carbohydrates and whole grain foods in relation to risk of type 2 diabetes mellitus and coronary heart disease. *J. Am. Coll. Nutr.* 21:298–306

72. Liu S, Manson JE, Stampfer MJ, Hu FB, Giovannucci E, et al. 2000. A prospective study of whole-grain intake and risk of type 2 diabetes mellitus in US women. *Am. J. Public Health* 90:1409–15

73. Lopez-Ridaura R, Willett WC, Rimm EB, Liu S, Stampfer MJ, et al. 2004. Magnesium intake and risk of type 2 diabetes in men and women. *Diabetes Care* 27:134–40

74. Louheranta AM, Turpeinen AK, Vidgren HM, Schwab US, Uusitupa MI. 1999. A high-trans fatty acid diet and insulin sensitivity in young healthy women. *Metabolism* 48:870–75

75. Lovejoy JC, Smith SR, Champagne CM, Most MM, Lefevre M, et al. 2002. Effects of diets enriched in saturated (palmitic), monounsaturated (oleic), or trans (elaidic) fatty acids on insulin sensitivity and substrate oxidation in healthy adults. *Diabetes Care* 25:1283–88

76. Lu W, Jablonski KA, Resnick HE, Jain AK, Jones KL, et al. 2003. Alcohol intake and glycemia in American Indians: the strong heart study. *Metabolism* 52:129–35

77. Ludwig DS, Peterson KE, Gortmaker SL. 2001. Relation between consumption of sugar-sweetened drinks and childhood obesity: a prospective, observational analysis. *Lancet* 357:505–8

78. Lundgren H, Bengtsson C, Blohme G, Lapidus L, Sjostrom L. 1989. Adiposity and adipose tissue distribution in relation

to incidence of diabetes in women: results from a prospective population study in Gothenburg, Sweden. *Int. J. Obes.* 13:413–23

79. Manson JE, Rimm EB, Stampfer MJ, Colditz GA, Willett WC, et al. 1991. Physical activity and incidence of non-insulin-dependent diabetes mellitus in women. *Lancet* 338:774–78

80. Manson JE, Spelsberg A. 1994. Primary prevention of non-insulin-dependent diabetes mellitus. *Am. J. Prev. Med.* 10:172–84

81. Marshall JA, Hoag S, Shetterly S, Hamman RF. 1994. Dietary fat predicts conversion from impaired glucose tolerance to NIDDM. The San Luis Valley Diabetes Study. *Diabetes Care* 17:50–56

82. Mayer-Davis EJ, D'Agostino R Jr, Karter AJ, Haffner SM, Rewers MJ, et al. 1998. Intensity and amount of physical activity in relation to insulin sensitivity: the Insulin Resistance Atherosclerosis Study. *JAMA* 279:669–74

83. McPhillips JB, Barrett-Connor E, Wingard DL. 1990. Cardiovascular disease risk factors prior to the diagnosis of impaired glucose tolerance and non-insulin-dependent diabetes mellitus in a community of older adults. *Am. J. Epidemiol.* 131:443–53

84. Medalie JH, Papier CM, Goldbourt U, Herman JB. 1975. Major factors in the development of diabetes mellitus in 10,000 men. *Arch. Intern. Med.* 135:811–17

85. Meyer KA, Kushi LH, Jacobs DR Jr, Folsom AR. 2001. Dietary fat and incidence of type 2 diabetes in older Iowa women. *Diabetes Care* 24:1528–35

86. Meyer KA, Kushi LH, Jacobs DR Jr, Slavin J, Sellers TA, Folsom AR. 2000. Carbohydrates, dietary fiber, and incident type 2 diabetes in older women. *Am. J. Clin. Nutr.* 71:921–30

87. Monterrosa AE, Haffner SM, Stern MP, Hazuda HP. 1995. Sex difference in lifestyle factors predictive of diabetes in Mexican-Americans. *Diabetes Care* 18:448–56

88. Montonen J, Knekt P, Jarvinen R, Aromaa A, Reunanen A. 2003. Whole-grain and fiber intake and the incidence of type 2 diabetes. *Am. J. Clin. Nutr.* 77:622–69

89. Nakanishi N, Suzuki K, Tatara K. 2003. Alcohol consumption and risk for development of impaired fasting glucose or type 2 diabetes in middle-aged Japanese men. *Diabetes Care* 26:48–54

90. Neel JV. 1962. Diabetes mellitus: a "thrifty" genotype rendered detrimental by "progress"? *Am. J. Hum. Genet.* 14:353–62

91. Ohlson LO, Larsson B, Bjorntorp P, Eriksson H, Svardsudd K, et al. 1988. Risk factors for type 2 (non-insulin-dependent) diabetes mellitus. Thirteen and one-half years of follow-up of the participants in a study of Swedish men born in 1913. *Diabetologia* 31:798–805

92. Ohlson LO, Larsson B, Svardsudd K, Welin L, Eriksson H, et al. 1985. The influence of body fat distribution on the incidence of diabetes mellitus. 13.5 years of follow-up of the participants in the study of men born in 1913. *Diabetes* 34:1055–58

93. Okada K, Hayashi T, Tsumura K, Suematsu C, Endo G, Fujii S. 2000. Leisure-time physical activity at weekends and the risk of Type 2 diabetes mellitus in Japanese men: the Osaka Health Survey. *Diabet. Med.* 17:53–58

94. Paffenbarger RS Jr, Wing AL. 1973. Chronic disease in former college students. XII. Early precursors of adult-onset diabetes mellitus. *Am. J. Epidemiol.* 97:314–23

95. Palmer AJ, Roze S, Valentine WJ, Spinas GA, Shaw JE, Zimmet PZ. 2004. Intensive lifestyle changes or metformin in patients with impaired glucose tolerance: modeling the long-term health economic implications of the diabetes prevention program in Australia, France, Germany,

Switzerland, and the United Kingdom. *Clin. Ther.* 26:304–21

96. Pan XR, Li GW, Hu YH, Wang JX, Yang WY, et al. 1997. Effects of diet and exercise in preventing NIDDM in people with impaired glucose tolerance. The Da Qing IGT and Diabetes Study. *Diabetes Care* 20:537–44

97. Paolisso G, Barbagallo M. 1997. Hypertension, diabetes mellitus, and insulin resistance: the role of intracellular magnesium. *Am. J. Hypertens.* 10:346–55

98. Parikh SJ, Yanovski JA. 2003. Calcium intake and adiposity. *Am. J. Clin. Nutr.* 77:281–87

99. Pereira MA, Jacobs DR Jr, Pins JJ, Raatz SK, Gross MD, et al. 2002. Effect of whole grains on insulin sensitivity in overweight hyperinsulinemic adults. *Am. J. Clin. Nutr.* 75:848–55

100. Pereira MA, Jacobs DR Jr, Van Horn L, Slattery ML, Kartashov AI, Ludwig DS. 2002. Dairy consumption, obesity, and the insulin resistance syndrome in young adults: the CARDIA Study. *JAMA* 287:2081–89

101. Pereira MA, Ludwig DS. 2001. Dietary fiber and body-weight regulation. Observations and mechanisms. *Pediatr. Clin. N. Am.* 48:969–80

102. Perry IJ. 2001. Commentary: smoking and diabetes—accumulating evidence of a causal link. *Int. J. Epidemiol.* 30:554–55

103. Raben A, Vasilaras TH, Moller AC, Astrup A. 2002. Sucrose compared with artificial sweeteners: different effects on ad libitum food intake and body weight after 10 wk of supplementation in overweight subjects. *Am. J. Clin. Nutr.* 76:721–29

104. Rimm EB, Chan J, Stampfer MJ, Colditz GA, Willett WC. 1995. Prospective study of cigarette smoking, alcohol use, and the risk of diabetes in men. *Br. Med. J.* 310:555–59

105. Rimm EB, Manson JE, Stampfer MJ, Colditz GA, Willett WC, et al. 1993. Cigarette smoking and the risk of diabetes

in women. *Am. J. Public Health* 83:211–14

106. Rosengren A, Dotevall A, Wilhelmsen L, Thelle D, Johansson S. 2004. Coffee and incidence of diabetes in Swedish women: a prospective 18-year follow-up study. *J. Intern. Med.* 255:89–95

107. Sairenchi T, Iso H, Nishimura A, Hosoda T, Irie F, et al. 2004. Cigarette smoking and risk of type 2 diabetes mellitus among middle-aged and elderly Japanese men and women. *Am. J. Epidemiol.* 160:158–62

108. Salazar-Martinez E, Willett WC, Ascherio A, Manson JE, Leitzmann MF, et al. 2004. Coffee consumption and risk for type 2 diabetes mellitus. *Ann. Intern. Med.* 140:1–8

109. Salmeron J, Ascherio A, Rimm EB, Colditz GA, Spiegelman D, et al. 1997. Dietary fiber, glycemic load, and risk of NIDDM in men. *Diabetes Care* 20:545–50

110. Salmeron J, Hu FB, Manson JE, Stampfer MJ, Colditz GA, et al. 2001. Dietary fat intake and risk of type 2 diabetes in women. *Am. J. Clin. Nutr.* 73:1019–26

111. Salmeron J, Manson JE, Stampfer MJ, Colditz GA, Wing AL, Willett WC. 1997. Dietary fiber, glycemic load, and risk of non-insulin-dependent diabetes mellitus in women. *JAMA* 277:472–77

112. Samaha FF, Iqbal N, Seshadri P, Chicano KL, Daily DA, et al. 2003. A low-carbohydrate as compared with a low-fat diet in severe obesity. *N. Engl. J. Med.* 348:2074–81

113. Saremi A, Tulloch-Reid M, Knowler WC. 2003. Coffee consumption and the incidence of type 2 diabetes. *Diabetes Care* 26:2211–12

114. Schulze MB, Liu S, Rimm EB, Manson JE, Willett WC, Hu FB. 2004. Glycemic index, glycemic load, and dietary fiber intake and incidence of type 2 diabetes in younger and middle-aged women. *Am. J. Clin. Nutr.* 80:348–56

115. Schulze MB, Manson JE, Ludwig DS,

Colditz GA, Stampfer MJ, et al. 2004. Sugar-sweetened beverages, weight gain, and incidence of type 2 diabetes in young and middle-aged women. *JAMA* 292:927–34

116. Schulze MB, Manson JE, Willett WC, Hu FB. 2003. Processed meat intake and incidence of Type 2 diabetes in younger and middle-aged women. *Diabetologia* 46:1465–73

117. Sierksma A, Patel H, Ouchi N, Kihara S, Funahashi T, et al. 2004. Effect of moderate alcohol consumption on adiponectin, tumor necrosis factor-alpha, and insulin sensitivity. *Diabetes Care* 27:184–89

118. Slattery ML. 2000. Diet, lifestyle, and colon cancer. *Semin. Gastrointest. Dis.* 11:142–46

119. Song Y, Manson JE, Buring JE, Liu S. 2004. A prospective study of red meat consumption and type 2 diabetes in middle-aged and elderly women: the Women's Health Study. *Diabetes Care* 27:2108–15

120. Song Y, Manson JE, Buring JE, Liu S. 2004. Dietary magnesium intake in relation to plasma insulin levels and risk of type 2 diabetes in women. *Diabetes Care* 27:59–65

121. Stampfer MJ, Colditz GA, Willett WC, Manson JE, Arky RA, et al. 1988. A prospective study of moderate alcohol drinking and risk of diabetes in women. *Am. J. Epidemiol.* 128:549–58

122. Stampfer MJ, Hu FB, Manson JE, Rimm EB, Willett WC. 2000. Primary prevention of coronary heart disease in women through diet and lifestyle. *N. Engl. J. Med.* 343:16–22

123. Stevens J, Ahn K, Juhaeri Houston D, Steffan L, Couper D. 2002. Dietary fiber intake and glycemic index and incidence of diabetes in African-American and white adults: the ARIC study. *Diabetes Care* 25:1715–21

124. Stumvoll M, Haring HU. 2002. Glitazones: clinical effects and molecular mechanisms. *Ann. Med.* 34:217–24

125. Sugimori H, Miyakawa M, Yoshida K, Izuno T, Takahashi E, et al. 1998. Health risk assessment for diabetes mellitus based on longitudinal analysis of MHTS database. *J. Med. Syst.* 22:27–32

126. Summers LK, Fielding BA, Bradshaw HA, Ilic V, Beysen C, et al. 2002. Substituting dietary saturated fat with polyunsaturated fat changes abdominal fat distribution and improves insulin sensitivity. *Diabetologia* 45:369–77

127. Thorburn A, Muir J, Proietto J. 1993. Carbohydrate fermentation decreases hepatic glucose output in healthy subjects. *Metabolism* 42:780–85

128. Tordoff MG, Alleva AM. 1990. Effect of drinking soda sweetened with aspartame or high-fructose corn syrup on food intake and body weight. *Am. J. Clin. Nutr.* 51:963–69

129. Tosiello L. 1996. Hypomagnesemia and diabetes mellitus. A review of clinical implications. *Arch. Intern. Med.* 156:1143–48

130. Tsumura K, Hayashi T, Suematsu C, Endo G, Fujii S, Okada K. 1999. Daily alcohol consumption and the risk of type 2 diabetes in Japanese men: the Osaka Health Survey. *Diabetes Care* 22:1432–37

131. Tuomilehto J, Hu G, Bidel S, Lindstrom J, Jousilahti P. 2004. Coffee consumption and risk of type 2 diabetes mellitus among middle-aged Finnish men and women. *JAMA* 291:1213–19

132. Tuomilehto J, Lindstrom J, Eriksson JG, Valle TT, Hamalainen H, et al. 2001. Prevention of type 2 diabetes mellitus by changes in lifestyle among subjects with impaired glucose tolerance. *N. Engl. J. Med.* 344:1343–50

133. van Dam RM. 2003. The epidemiology of lifestyle and risk for type 2 diabetes. *Eur. J. Epidemiol.* 18:1115–25

134. van Dam RM, Feskens EJ. 2002. Coffee consumption and risk of type 2 diabetes mellitus. *Lancet* 360:1477–78

135. van Dam RM, Rimm EB, Willett WC, Stampfer MJ, Hu FB. 2002. Dietary

patterns and risk for type 2 diabetes mellitus in U.S. men. *Ann. Intern. Med.* 136:201–9

136. van Dam RM, Willett WC, Rimm EB, Stampfer MJ, Hu FB. 2002. Dietary fat and meat intake in relation to risk of type 2 diabetes in men. *Diabetes Care* 25:417–24

137. Vessby B, Unsitupa M, Hermansen K, Riccardi G, Rivellese AA, et al. 2001. Substituting dietary saturated for monounsaturated fat impairs insulin sensitivity in healthy men and women: The KANWU Study. *Diabetologia* 44:312–19

138. Wannamethee SG, Camargo CA Jr, Manson JE, Willett WC, Rimm EB. 2003. Alcohol drinking patterns and risk of type 2 diabetes mellitus among younger women. *Arch. Intern. Med.* 163:1329–36

139. Wannamethee SG, Shaper AG, Alberti KG. 2000. Physical activity, metabolic factors, and the incidence of coronary heart disease and type 2 diabetes. *Arch. Intern. Med.* 160:2108–16

140. Wannamethee SG, Shaper AG, Perry IJ. 2001. Smoking as a modifiable risk factor for type 2 diabetes in middle-aged men. *Diabetes Care* 24:1590–95

141. Wannamethee SG, Shaper AG, Perry IJ, Alberti KG. 2002. Alcohol consumption and the incidence of type II diabetes. *J. Epidemiol. Community Health* 56:542–48

142. Watanabe M, Barzi F, Neal B, Ueshima H, Miyoshi Y, et al. 2002. Alcohol consumption and the risk of diabetes by body mass index levels in a cohort of 5,636 Japanese. *Diabetes Res. Clin. Pract.* 57:191–97

143. Wei M, Gaskill SP, Haffner SM, Stern MP. 1997. Waist circumference as the best predictor of noninsulin dependent diabetes mellitus (NIDDM) compared to body mass index, waist/hip ratio and other anthropometric measurements in Mexican Americans—a 7-year prospective study. *Obes. Res.* 5:16–23

144. Wei M, Gibbons LW, Mitchell TL, Kampert JB, Blair SN. 2000. Alcohol intake and incidence of type 2 diabetes in men. *Diabetes Care* 23:18–22

145. Weinstein AR, Sesso HD, Lee IM, Cook NR, Manson JE, et al. 2004. Relationship of physical activity vs body mass index with type 2 diabetes in women. *JAMA* 292:1188–94

146. Wild S, Roglic G, Green A, Sicree R, King H. 2004. Global prevalence of diabetes: estimates for the year 2000 and projections for 2030. *Diabetes Care* 27:1047–53

147. Will JC, Galuska DA, Ford ES, Mokdad A, Calle EE. 2001. Cigarette smoking and diabetes mellitus: evidence of a positive association from a large prospective cohort study. *Int. J. Epidemiol.* 30:540–46

148. Willett WC, Leibel RL. 2002. Dietary fat is not a major determinant of body fat. *Am. J. Med.* 113(Suppl. 9B):47–59

149. Wilson JG, Lindquist JH, Grambow SC, Crook ED, Maher JF. 2003. Potential role of increased iron stores in diabetes. *Am. J. Med. Sci.* 325:332–39

150. Wilson PW, Anderson KM, Kannel WB. 1986. Epidemiology of diabetes mellitus in the elderly. The Framingham Study. *Am. J. Med.* 80:3–9

151. Yusuf S, Gerstein H, Hoogwerf B, Pogue J, Bosch J, et al. 2001. Ramipril and the development of diabetes. *JAMA* 286:1882–85

152. Zilkens RR, Burke V, Watts G, Beilin LJ, Puddey IB. 2003. The effect of alcohol intake on insulin sensitivity in men: a randomized controlled trial. *Diabetes Care* 26:608–12

Annu. Rev. Public Health 2005. 26:469–500
doi: 10.1146/annurev.publhealth.26.021304.144542
Copyright © 2005 by Annual Reviews. All rights reserved
First published online as a Review in Advance on January 11, 2005

PSYCHOSOCIAL FACTORS AND CARDIOVASCULAR DISEASES

Susan A. Everson-Rose[1,2,3] and Tené T. Lewis[1]

Departments of Preventive Medicine[1] and Psychology[2] and Rush Institute for Healthy Aging,[3] Rush University Medical Center, Chicago, Illinois 60612; email: Susan_A_Everson@rush.edu, Tene_T_Lewis@rush.edu

Key Words depression, anger, hostility, stress, pathophysiological mechanisms

■ **Abstract** Rapidly accruing evidence from a diversity of disciplines supports the hypothesis that psychosocial factors are related to morbidity and mortality due to cardiovascular diseases. We review relevant literature on (*a*) negative emotional states, including depression, anger and hostility, and anxiety; (*b*) chronic and acute psychosocial stressors; and (*c*) social ties, social support, and social conflict. All three of these psychosocial domains have been significantly associated with increased risk of cardiovascular morbidity and mortality. We also discuss critical pathophysiological mechanisms and pathways that likely operate in a synergistic and integrative way to promote atherogenesis and related clinical manifestations. We conclude by discussing some of the important challenges and opportunities for future investigations.

OVERVIEW

Traditional cardiovascular risk factors, including smoking, high blood pressure, high cholesterol, and diabetes, do not fully account for or explain the excess burden of cardiovascular diseases (CVD) in the population. Most individuals who develop CVD have at least one of these risk factors (67); nevertheless, other factors contribute to the development and progression of CVD. Several psychosocial characteristics are importantly related to coronary heart disease (CHD), hypertension, stroke, and other cardiovascular disorders. Indeed, the literature on this topic is quite expansive. The purpose of this review is to provide a selected summary of key findings in this literature. We note some of the classic studies and historical developments important to the field and focus on prospective, epidemiological studies, with clinical endpoints [e.g., myocardial infarction (MI), CVD mortality, stroke] and/or subclinical cardiovascular disease (e.g., carotid atherosclerosis, coronary calcification) as the outcome. We begin with current statistics on the impact and cost of CVD, outline and review the literature on three important psychosocial domains that have received much of the research attention, discuss key pathophysiological mechanisms and pathways by which psychosocial factors may

0163-7525/05/0421-0469$20.00

influence CVD, and discuss some future directions likely to be critical to advancing the field.

CARDIOVASCULAR DISEASE BURDEN

Cardiovascular diseases are the leading cause of death and disability in the United States and in most countries around the world (4, 16). In 1999, an estimated 17 million persons worldwide succumbed to CVD (16). In 2001, the most recent year for which U.S. mortality data are available, more than 38% of all deaths that occurred in the United States were attributed to CVD; nearly three quarters of these deaths were due specifically to CHD and stroke. In total numbers, more women than men die from CVD each year in the United States. Indeed, while mortality due to CVD has declined steadily among men in the past 25 years, CVD mortality among women has remained relatively constant (4). This event is, at least in part, due to the fact that women typically survive to older ages, when CVD is most prevalent.

Cardiovascular diseases are the leading cause of death among nearly all race or ethnic groups in the United States. However, African American men and women experience disproportionately higher rates of hypertension, CHD, MI, and stroke than do Caucasians and a greater prevalence of these disorders occurs at younger ages (4, 144). Among females, Mexican Americans also have a greater prevalence of CVD than do Caucasians (4). The incidence of many chronic diseases, including CHD, stroke, hypertension, and heart failure, likely will increase in the coming decades as our population ages (16, 28). Moreover, the rapidly increasing prevalence of obesity and type 2 diabetes occurring in all segments of the U.S. population (149) likely will contribute to a growing epidemic of CVD in the United States in future years. The projected direct and indirect costs of CVD for 2004 are more than $386 billion (4). Clearly, the personal, economic, and population impact of cardiovascular diseases is enormous, making CVD one of the largest public health problems of the twenty-first century.

NEGATIVE EMOTIONS, PSYCHOSOCIAL STRESS, AND SOCIAL FACTORS RELATED TO CARDIOVASCULAR DISEASES

A broad range of psychological and social characteristics have been investigated in relation to CVD and related risk factors. Indeed, clinical anecdotes and historical observations have ascribed etiological importance to emotional and personality factors in the manifestation of CVD for many centuries (see 35 for a review). We have chosen to focus on three psychosocial domains in this review: (*a*) negative emotional states—here defined as depression or depressive symptoms, anger and hostility, and anxiety; (*b*) chronic psychosocial stressors, particularly occupation or work-related stress, and acute life stress; and (c) social factors—specifically social ties, social support, and social conflict. Research on these domains has dominated much of the literature. Table 1 lists sample items from some of the most commonly used questionnaire measures assessing these three psychosocial domains. We do not cover research on socioeconomic position or social class and health. The impact of socioeconomic position on nearly all aspects of health is one of the most widely observed and enduring observations in all of public health (92); however, this vast literature is beyond the scope of this review.

Negative Emotional States and Cardiovascular Disease Risk

In the past 15–20 years, understanding of the contribution of negative emotional states to CVD and CVD-related health outcomes has grown exponentially. Research has typically focused on (a) depression or depressive symptoms, (b) anger and hostility, or (c) anxiety. Each of these areas is reviewed separately, below.

DEPRESSION AND DEPRESSIVE SYMPTOMS   Major depressive disorder, current depressive symptoms, and a history of depression all have been associated with increased risk of CVD morbidity and mortality. The earliest reports of an association between depression and mortality appeared in the 1930s when it was noted that depressed psychiatric inpatients had a higher incidence of CHD-related death than did nonpsychiatric controls (64, 129). More recent studies of psychiatric patients similarly found high rates of CVD mortality in patients with unipolar or bipolar depression (213, 218). Among cardiac patients, it has long been recognized clinically that rates of depression are high among patients after suffering an MI, that depression adversely impacts the prognosis of CVD, and that there are high rates of sudden cardiovascular death in depressed patients (176). These observations have been confirmed in empirical studies with cardiac patients (9, 21, 61).

Epidemiological evidence on the cardiovascular consequences of depression or depressive symptoms comes from selected and unselected population samples that have included both male and female participants ranging in age from young adulthood to older ages. In 1993, Anda and colleagues (5) reported that depressed affect, measured by 4 items from the General Health Questionnaire, was significantly associated with a 50%–60% excess risk of fatal and nonfatal ischemic heart disease (IHD) after adjusting for traditional coronary risk factors over 12 years of follow-up of more than 2800 initially healthy men and women from the National Health Examination Follow-up Survey (NHEFS). Subsequently, a number of population- or community-based studies have reported similar findings. Results from several well-controlled studies are noted below.

Pratt and colleagues (169) reported that a diagnosis of major depression was significantly related to a 4.5-fold increased risk of self-reported MI, and a history of dysphoria predicted a 2.7-fold increased risk of self-reported MI in a sample of 1551 adults drawn from the general population and who were initially free of heart disease. Depressive symptoms, measured by the Center for Epidemiological

TABLE 1   Sample items included in commonly used scales assessing psychosocial factors

Psychosocial factor

Depressive symptoms (CES-D, Radloff 1977) (170)
"I felt that I could not shake off the blues, even with help from my family and friends."
"I had trouble keeping my mind on what I was doing."
"I felt that everything I did was an effort."
"I had crying spells."
"I felt sad."

Hopelessness (Everson et al. 1996) (45)
"It is impossible for me to reach the goals that I would like to strive for."
"The future seems to me to be hopeless and I can't believe things are changing for the better."

Anxiety (trait) (Spielberger 1980) (202)
"I am a steady person."
"I feel nervous and restless."
"I get in a state of turmoil or tension as I think over my recent concerns and interests."
"I worry too much over something that does not matter."

Hostility/cynical distrust (Cook & Medley 1954) (27)
"I think most people would lie to get ahead."
"It is safer to trust nobody."
"No one cares much what happens to you."
"Most people make friends because friends are likely to be useful to them."
"Most people are honest chiefly through fear of being caught."

Anger-in (Spielberger et al. 1985) (203)
"I am irritated more than people are aware."
"I pout or sulk."
"I harbor grudges."
"I am seething inside but don't show it."

Anger-out (Spielberger et al. 1985) (203)
"I do things like slam doors."
"I say nasty things."
"I strike out at whatever infuriates me."
"If someone annoys me, I'm apt to tell him or her how I feel."

Social connections (Kaplan et al. 1988) (93)
"What is your current marital status?"
"How often do you visit friends and relatives?"
"How many people usually come to see your or call you per day?"
"How often do you go to meetings of clubs, associations, or societies?"

Emotional support (Seeman & Berkman 1988) (188)
"Can you count on someone to provide you with *emotional* support (talking over problems or helping you make a difficult decision)?"
"Could you have used more emotional support than you needed?"

Availability of emotional support/attachment (Orth-Gomér et al. 1993) (160)
"Someone special, whom [you] can lean on"
"Someone to share feelings with"
"Someone to confide in"
"Someone to hold and comfort [you]"

(Continued)

TABLE 1 (*Continued*)

Psychosocial factor

Job strain (Karasek et al. 1998) (96)
  "Do you have time enough to do your work?"
  "Do you have to work fast?"
  "Are there conflicting demands in your job?"
  "Do you learn new things in your job?"
  "Is your job monotonous?"
  "Can you influence how your work is to be performed?"

Effort-reward imbalance (Siegrist et al. 2004) (198)
  "I have constant pressure due to a heavy work load."
  "I have a lot of responsibility in my job."
  "People close to me say I sacrifice too much for my job."
  "I experience adequate support in difficult situations."
  "My job promotion prospects are poor."
  "Considering all my efforts and achievements, I receive the respect and prestige I deserve
    at work."
  "Considering all my efforts and achievements, my salary/income is adequate."

Studies Depression (CES-D) Scale, predicted greater than 70% excess risk of incident CHD in women and men and 2.34-fold greater CHD mortality in men in adjusted analyses after nearly 10 years of follow-up in the first National Health and Nutrition Examination Survey (54). Most recently, data from the Women's Health Initiative Observational Study, which followed a multi-ethnic sample of nearly 94,000 women aged 50–79 years for approximately 4 years, found that current depressive symptoms, measured by a short form of the CES-D, were associated with a significant 1.5-fold higher risk of death, after controlling for education, income, and traditional coronary risk factors (216). Depressive symptoms also have been linked to incident stroke (89, 157), stroke mortality (52), and incident hypertension (31).

Hopelessness is one symptom of depression that appears to have particularly adverse effects on health. In their report from the NHEFS, Anda et al. (5) reported that the single item on hopelessness from their measure of depressed affect predicted a more than twofold risk of fatal and nonfatal IHD and was a stronger predictor than the complete measure. In the San Antonio Heart Study, high levels of hopelessness predicted all-cause and CVD mortality in Mexican Americans and Caucasians (204). Everson and colleagues (45) found that hopelessness predicted a twofold increase in CVD mortality, MI, and all-cause mortality over six years of follow-up in a population sample of middle-aged Finnish men from the Kuopio Ischemic Heart Disease (KIHD) study, after controlling for demographic characteristics, cardiovascular risk factors, and overall depressive symptoms. Hopelessness also was related to accelerated progression of intimal-medial thickening (IMT) in the carotid arteries and threefold greater risk of incident hypertension over four years in the KIHD study (48, 49).

Some studies have failed to support the hypothesis that depressive symptoms are associated with greater CVD morbidity or mortality (113, 146, 175). Moreover, studies have varied in the extent to which they adequately controlled for potential confounding variables such as concurrent health status and behavioral risk factors. As reviewed above, however, a number of methodologically sound studies have consistently identified a positive association between depression or depressive symptoms using a variety of assessment tools in a number of different populations.

Nonetheless, because the majority of published studies have not included racial or ethnic minorities, less is known about the impact of depressive symptoms on CVD in these populations. Available evidence suggests that depressive symptoms may confer greater CVD risk in African Americans, particularly with respect to hypertension and stroke outcomes. Data from the Coronary Artery Risk Development in Young Adults (CARDIA) study showed that high scores on the CES-D were associated with 2.8-fold increased risk of hypertension after 5 years of follow-up among African Americans but not among Caucasians (31), although more recent data from CARDIA with 15 years of follow-up did not show racial differences in psychosocial risk factors for hypertension (226). Two reports from the NHEFS found that negative affect (symptoms of anxiety and depression) predicted twice the risk of incident hypertension and a 1.73-fold greater risk of stroke over 7–22 years of follow-up, with the strongest associations observed among African Americans (88, 89). Interestingly, studies suggest that African Americans, compared with Caucasians, report higher levels of depressive symptoms (86, 215) but no difference in the prevalence of major depressive disorder (86, 104), although earlier reports suggest the prevalence of depressive disorder was lower among African Americans (105). With the documented higher rates of CVD among African Americans and other minorities, further work is needed to assess the impact of depressive symptoms and other psychosocial characteristics among racial and ethnic minority populations.

ANGER AND HOSTILITY   Investigations into the effects of anger and hostility on risk for CVD have a long history. Early psychoanalytic and psychodynamic literature described episodes of anger, hostility, or other strong emotions or personality characteristics, such as aggressiveness and a need to be hard-driving and tough-minded, in patients with heart disease or hypertension (1, 7, 39). These observations, together with the need to provide a clearer definition and assessment of what was deemed "coronary-prone behavior," motivated work in the 1950s and 1960s on what came to be called the Type A behavior pattern. On the basis of observations of their own cardiac patients, Rosenman & Friedman described the Type A individual as one who was exceedingly hard-driving and ambitious, competitive, time-urgent, and unusually quick-tempered and tightly wound (62). Their initial work suggested that Type A men and women had higher cholesterol levels and greater evidence of CHD, compared with those who were "Type B" (62). This distinction led to the Western Collaborative Group Study, a prospective study of more than 3100 middle-aged men, which established Type A as a risk factor for CHD (179). In that study, Type A men were twice as likely as Type B men to develop CHD in the subsequent 8.5 years—a level of risk equivalent to that conferred by any traditional coronary risk factors. This now classic work on the Type A behavior pattern was critical in advancing our understanding of psychosocial factors in relation to CVD risk. Indeed, Type A was the first psychosocial factor to be accepted by the medical community as a recognized coronary risk factor (28).

Shortly following the medical community's acceptance of the Type A behavior pattern, studies with negative findings began to appear in the literature (171, 193, 194). Because many of the historical observations had focused on anger, hostility, and aggressive qualities as predisposing factors in CHD and hypertension, attention then turned to identifying whether these aspects or features of Type A were the important or "toxic" components (35).

Hostility is typically characterized by a suspicious, mistrustful attitude or disposition toward interpersonal relationships and the wider environment; it is considered to be enduring, i.e., a personality trait. Anger is an emotion that is considered one component of a broader, multidimensional construct that includes hostility and aggressive behavior (201, 203). Anger usually is triggered in response to perceptions of unjust events or actions and has both trait and situational aspects.

In the past two decades, numerous studies have investigated hostility and anger, measured with various instruments, in relation to risk of hypertension, stroke, and CVD morbidity and mortality, with both positive and null findings. The literature reported and quality of studies are quite mixed, and many studies used selected samples (3, 10, 72, 73, 119). However, a meta-analytic review of 45 studies published in 1996 concluded that hostility is an independent risk factor for CHD and all-cause mortality (147). A number of studies investigating hostility and/or anger and incident CVD have been published since then; the majority reported positive associations. Selected findings from these more recent studies are noted below.

A recent case-control study from the Multiple Risk Factor Intervention Trial showed that men at high risk for CVD who scored high on a behavioral rating of hostility were more likely to die from CVD in the intervening 16 years than were men who were low in hostility, after adjustment for coronary risk factors (139). In the Normative Aging Study, each 1-point increase in hostility scores predicted a 6% increased risk of incident CHD over 3 years (155), and after 7 years of follow-up, men with high levels of anger (upper 20% of the distribution) at baseline had experienced 2.5 times more incident coronary events (nonfatal MI, fatal CHD, angina pectoris) than had men with low levels of anger (lowest 20%) (100). In the KIHD study, hostility predicted a more than twofold increased risk of MI and CV mortality over nine years (50), which was largely explained by behavioral risk factors in subsequent adjusted analyses. In contrast, anger expression style (i.e., "anger-out") was associated with twice the risk of incident stroke over eight years of follow-up (47), and both "anger-out" and "anger-in" were associated with a significantly increased four-year risk of incident hypertension in the KIHD study

(46) in adjusted analyses. Recent data from CARDIA found that individuals scoring in the upper quartile on hostility and the time urgency–impatience component of Type A behavior experienced 80% excess risk of cumulative 15-year incidence of hypertension in the total sample (226). The Atherosclerosis Risk in Communities (ARIC) study found that anger predicted incident CHD (223) and incident stroke (222), after adjusting for age, sex, and race/ethnicity.

Some studies have found that hostility and anger are associated with subclinical cardiovascular disease. High hostility scores and high trait anger and anger-in were associated with the extent and severity of carotid atherosclerosis 10 years later in a sample of 200 healthy postmenopausal women (140). Among middle-aged men in the KIHD study, high hostility scores together with high levels of anger control were associated with a twofold greater progression of carotid atherosclerosis over two years (90). Finally, Iribarren and colleagues (82) reported that higher hostility was associated with greater coronary artery calcification ten years later in a subset of participants from the CARDIA study.

Taken together, the available evidence, especially from methodologically strong population-based studies, indicates that anger and hostility do increase the risk of CVD in healthy populations. A review by Hemingway & Marmot (74), however, concluded that prospective data in patients with documented CHD indicate that anger and hostility are not strong predictors of recurrent events or mortality in coronary patients. Moreover, as noted above, the vast majority of research in this area has been limited to men, especially Caucasian men. Although the few studies that have included women have generally reported positive findings, it remains to be seen whether anger and hostility will be clearly and consistently associated with CVD risk in women as well as in ethnic minorities.

ANXIETY   Studies with psychiatric and coronary patients and community-based samples suggest that anxiety disorders may be associated with greater mortality, particularly sudden cardiac death, and greater cardiovascular morbidity. Early evidence suggested that psychiatric patients with panic disorder had increased mortality rates (29). Among coronary patients, higher levels of anxiety have been associated with poorer prognosis and greater recurrence of cardiac events post-MI (60, 205); however, findings are inconsistent. Frasure-Smith & Lesperance (59) found that higher trait anxiety predicted greater cardiac-related mortality in a sample of nearly 900 MI patients, but this effect was nonsignificant following adjustment for disease severity. Two earlier studies found that high anxiety levels were protective in coronary patients (15, 76).

Several epidemiologic studies support the hypothesis that high levels of anxiety increase risk for CHD, although most of these studies are limited to men. Men with high levels of anxiety had nearly four times greater risk of fatal CHD over 10 years than did men with low levels of anxiety after adjusting for traditional CVD risk factors (69). Similarly, phobic anxiety predicted 2.45-fold greater risk of fatal CHD in a sample of nearly 34,000 male health professionals initially free of disease (98). In the Normative Aging Study, men with at least two self-reported anxiety symptoms had increased risk of cardiac death, compared with men with no symptoms of anxiety, although only a small number of events occurred (102). In separate analyses from that study (109), men who reported high levels of worrying had a more than twofold increased risk of nonfatal MI after 20 years of follow-up.

Among women, epidemiologic evidence regarding the association between anxiety and CVD risk is weaker and more limited. Symptoms of anxiety were associated with significantly greater risk of incident MI and cardiac death after 20 years among homemakers but not among employed women in more than 700 initially healthy women from the Framingham Heart Study (41). Baseline levels of trait anxiety were not related to mean levels of carotid IMT 10 years later in a sample of 200 healthy postmenopausal women (140). More recently, a study of more than 700 French men and women without a history of MI or angina found that individuals with sustained high levels of anxiety over 2 years showed greater 4-year increases in carotid artery IMT relative to those who were not anxious, although this association was only marginally significant among women ($p = 0.07$) after multivariate adjustment, and relatively few men ($n = 29$) or women ($n = 47$) reported sustained high anxiety levels (164).

In sum, studies examining the influence of anxiety on CVD risk among men are generally positive, but the association among women is weaker, and some clinical evidence suggests anxiety may be protective. Moreover, because this work has been limited largely to Caucasian samples, it is unclear whether anxiety is related to CVD risk in minority populations.

Psychosocial Stressors and Cardiovascular Disease Risk

Research on the role of psychosocial stressors in CVD also has a long history. Early epidemiologic and sociologic observations noted the impact of stressors such as poverty, poor housing, and work conditions on the health of populations (177). In addition, Cannon and Selye, two prominent physiologists working in the early half of the twentieth century, made critical theoretical and empirical observations that have motivated much of the research on the effects of stress on health. Cannon (20) identified the fight-or-flight response, a set of physiological responses to threat or challenge, and Selye (191) was the first to recognize that severe, prolonged stress could lead to tissue damage and disease. Their observations have stimulated research in many disciplines that has helped elucidate the physiologic pathways by which psychosocial factors may increase risk of CVD.

OCCUPATIONAL/WORK-RELATED STRESSORS   Epidemiological studies of stress and CVD often have focused on occupational or work-related stressors. The job strain model posits that high job demands coupled with low job control have a particularly deleterious effect on cardiovascular health (95, 110). The more recent effort-reward imbalance model suggests that high efforts (high demands and/or high involvement) in the presence of low rewards (low pay, low esteem, few career opportunities, and/or job insecurity) may have a hazardous influence on cardiovascular health (196, 198). Although not unequivocal (78, 114), a number of large-scale, prospective studies have found positive associations between overall job strain and CVD morbidity and mortality (95, 110, 210); the low control aspect of the job strain model had the most consistent negative effects (17, 186).

Other studies have found significant associations between effort-reward imbalance and indices of CVD, including progression of atherosclerosis (51, 125) and new coronary events (196, 197). In a sample of 6895 men and 3413 women from the Whitehall II cohort, Bosma and colleagues (17) found that effort-reward imbalance and aspects of job strain (low job control) independently predicted cardiovascular outcomes, conferring a 1.56- to 2.38-fold greater risk of new coronary disease over 5 years of follow-up. Consequently, researchers have begun to combine information from the two models to improve estimation of cardiovascular outcomes (165). Recent studies have found significant associations between a more generalized measure of work stress and CVD mortality (138) as well as job insecurity (also a component of the effort-reward imbalance model) and incident CHD (117). On average, job strain, effort-reward imbalance, and other occupational stressors have consistently predicted cardiovascular outcomes for men, but less consistently for women (114, 161).

ACUTE PSYCHOSOCIAL STRESSORS   Other types of psychosocial stressors also predict CVD endpoints. Historically, anecdotal observations and case studies have often noted that the development of cardiac disease follows an experience of acute stress (44, 66). For example, bereavement was associated with increased mortality from IHD and all causes in a sample of more than 95,000 men and women (94). Fairly severe acute life stressors, such as earthquakes and terrorist attacks, also are associated with increased sudden cardiac death (97, 120, 211). In 1991, following the Iraqi missile attack on Israel, Kark et al. (97) noted a 58% increase in total population mortality, largely attributable to out-of-hospital deaths due to CVD. Loer and colleagues (120) conducted a comprehensive review of county coroner records the week before, the day of, and the week following the Northridge, California, earthquake in 1994. They observed a sharp increase in the number of sudden cardiac deaths—from an average of 4.6 deaths during the week preceding the earthquake to 24 deaths on the day of the earthquake.

CHRONIC PSYCHOSOCIAL STRESSORS   Relatively few studies have examined the relationship between chronic, nonoccupational daily life stressors and the onset or exacerbation of CVD. In a sample of more than 73,000 Japanese men and women initially free of CVD, women who reported high levels of (nonspecific) daily life stress had a 1.6- to 2-fold higher age-adjusted risk of death from CVD after 8 years of follow-up compared with women with low stress levels (83). Results for men were less pronounced: Men with moderate daily life stress had higher rates of MI compared with their low-stress counterparts, but no associations were observed between daily life stress and other CVD endpoints.

Two reports from the Nurses Health Study show a strong association between another chronic stressor, caregiving, and incident CHD, including mortality, in women. Women caring for an ill spouse for 9 or more hours a week had nearly twice the risk of incident CHD over 4 years (116). Women who reported high levels of caregiving for non-ill children (more than 21 hours a week) or grandchildren (more than 9 hours a week) also experienced increased CHD risk (115), compared with women without caregiving responsibilities.

In summary, a number of psychosocial stressors are prospectively associated with incidence and progression of CVD. Most studies have examined chronic stressors in the form of work stress or caregiving and produced fairly consistent results. These effects may be patterned by gender; occupational stressors appear to influence outcomes more for men, whereas other types of stressors (daily life stress, caregiving) may influence CVD risk in women. In addition, with few exceptions (83), studies examining clinical outcomes have largely focused on samples of Caucasian men and, more recently, Caucasian women. Further work is needed to determine whether associations between psychosocial stressors and CVD outcomes vary by ethnicity.

Social Ties, Social Support, Social Conflict, and Cardiovascular Disease Risk

In the 1960s and 1970s, investigations into the influence of environmental conditions, social stress, and status on chronic diseases, such as hypertension and CHD, proliferated (79, 87, 208, 209). In addition, theoretical and empirical work on the importance of social relationships to the health and well-being of individuals and communities (14, 24, 80) was rapidly expanding. We review here the literature on three related social stressors: social ties, social support, and social conflict.

SOCIAL TIES Epidemiological studies have consistently found associations between social ties and CVD (19, 93, 159). Social isolation has been defined as living alone or being unmarried (23, 225), and/or having little social contact with relatives, friends, and other social groups (19, 93). Socially isolated individuals typically have higher rates of CVD morbidity (159) and mortality (19, 43, 93). In a study of 32,624 initially healthy men, socially isolated men experienced a nearly twofold greater risk of CVD mortality over 4 years, compared with socially integrated men (99). Further analyses of the same cohort revealed similar associations after 10 years of follow-up; socially isolated men have a twofold greater risk of fatal CHD, compared with nonisolated men (43).

Kaplan and colleagues (93) found that Finnish men in the lowest two quintiles on a scale measuring social connectedness were at an increased risk of CVD mortality compared with men in the highest quintile. Similarly, coronary patients with small social networks (three or fewer individuals) were found to have a 2.4-fold higher rate of mortality over 5 years, compared with those with larger networks, after adjusting for age and disease severity (19).

Most epidemiological studies in this area have assessed objective indices of social isolation in the form of marital status and number of social contacts; subjective measures of social isolation also may be associated with CVD endpoints. A prospective study of 1290 patients undergoing coronary bypass surgery found that patients who agreed with the statement "I feel lonely" prior to surgery had a significant 2.61-fold increased mortality after 30 days and a 1.78-fold increased risk 5 years later, compared with patients who did not feel lonely (75).

SOCIAL SUPPORT   Social ties measure quantitative aspects of an individual's social behavior, whereas social support captures the qualitative aspects of social interactions. Several major subtypes of social support have been described (emotional, instrumental, and informational); however, emotional support has been the most commonly assessed subtype in the CVD literature. Emotionally supportive relationships, characterized by high degrees of caring, sympathy, understanding, and esteem support (160, 188), have shown to be cardio-protective (108, 178, 214). Conversely, low levels of emotional support have been associated with a number of negative cardiovascular health outcomes (214, 225). In one study, low levels of emotional support from close friends were associated with a significant 3.1-fold increased risk of incident MI and CHD mortality over 6 years of follow-up in a sample of 736 initially healthy men, after controlling for other potential risk factors (160).

Low levels of emotional support appear to be particularly harmful in individuals who are already ill. In a sample of 194 male and female patients hospitalized for acute MI, Berkman and colleagues (13) observed a 2.9-fold increase in mortality over the course of 6 months in individuals reporting low levels of emotional support. Absence of a close confidante conferred a three-fold greater risk of mortality in a group of male and female patients with pre-existing CAD (225). More recently, Krumholz et al. (108) observed a 3-fold greater risk of fatal and non-fatal CVD in a sample of 292 male and female heart failure patients without emotional support.

SOCIAL CONFLICT   Research on social relationships has focused primarily on the positive, health-enhancing effects of social networks and social support. However, there is a growing recognition that social relationships have both positive and negative aspects (56, 57). Although some investigators speculate that social conflict may be associated with poorer health outcomes, few studies have prospectively examined these issues with respect to CVD. A specific form of social conflict—marital distress—may be associated with CVD morbidity and mortality. In a study of 292 female coronary patients aged 30–62 years, women who reported severe marital stress had a 3-fold greater likelihood of recurrent coronary events (defined as cardiac death, hospitalization for recurrent AMI, and revascularization) over a 4-year follow-up, compared with women who reported low or no marital stress, after controlling for demographic, behavioral, and disease status variables (161). Matthews & Gump (138) reported that marital dissolution was associated with a significant 1.37-fold greater risk of CVD mortality over 9 years of follow-up in a sample of nearly 11,000 men.

Taken together, these findings suggest that social factors (networks, supports, and conflicts) have a relatively consistent impact on CVD; the strongest effects have been observed in populations already affected by or at risk for CVD. The majority of studies exploring the impact of social factors on CVD have included primarily samples of Caucasian men (93, 99, 138, 160) and, to a lesser extent, Caucasian women (13, 14, 161). Less is known about the role of social factors in CVD risk in minority populations.

PATHOPHYSIOLOGICAL MECHANISMS

The rapid growth of research on psychosocial factors and CVD morbidity and mortality over the past few decades has brought about a greater focus on the pathophysiological mechanisms or pathways by which psychosocial factors influence disease development and progression. A number of important and potentially interrelated physiological mechanisms may underlie the observed associations. These represent direct pathophysiological effects of negative emotions, stress, and social factors that can contribute to disease. Activation of the hypothalamic-pituitary-adrenal (HPA) axis and autonomic nervous system (ANS), serotonergic dysfunction, secretion of proinflammatory cytokines, and platelet activation, reviewed below, are four critical mechanisms by which psychosocial factors may contribute to atherogenesis. Figure 1 presents a proposed integrative model that illustrates some of the interrelationships among these mechanisms and the pathways through which psychosocial factors may lead to atherosclerosis and related clinical outcomes. The relationship between psychosocial factors and CVD is highly complex and multifactorial. Environmental, social, and behavioral pathways also have important influences on this relationship; however, such pathways are not depicted because the focus in this review is on putative and recognized biologic pathways.

HPA and ANS Activation

Psychosocial factors may influence cardiovascular function and promote atherogenesis through the HPA axis and/or the ANS, which are activated in response to fear, anxiety, depression, anger, and stress (142, 151, 173). Chronic dysregulation of the HPA axis, which occurs in depression (166, 173), can result in hormonal and neuroendocrine alterations, including hypercortisolemia or excess glucocorticoid secretion (190). Even small increases in glucocorticoids sustained over time can contribute to hypertension, insulin resistance, visceral obesity, coagulation changes, and increased lipid levels, all of which are precursors to CVD (25, 151). Other research has found that hostile individuals have higher circulating levels of catecholamines (206), greater cardiovascular reactivity (i.e., exaggerated blood pressure and heart rate responses) to psychological challenge (207), and higher cortisol levels (167) than do their nonhostile counterparts. Similarly, chronic stress such as job strain has been associated with higher levels of blood pressure

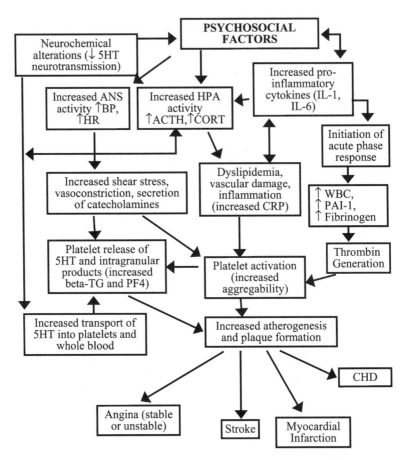

Figure 1 Proposed physiological mechanisms and pathways linking psychosocial factors and atherogenesis and related outcomes. (Adapted from Reference 133). Abbreviations: 5H, serotonin; ANS, autonomic nervous system; BP, blood pressure; HR, heart rate; ACTH, adrenocorticotropin hormone; CORT, cortisol; IL-1, interleukin-1; IL-6, interleukin-6; CRP, C-reactive protein; WBC, white blood cell count; PAI-1, plasminogen activator inhibitor; ß-TG, beta-thromboglobulin; PF4, platelet-factor 4; CHD, coronary heart disease.

(137, 185) and increased blood pressure over time (121). Social factors also may influence the HPA axis and ANS activation. The presence of social support during stressful situations attenuates blood pressure and heart rate responses to stress in women (65, 91) and reduces cortisol reactivity in men (107). Poor-quality relationships and low social support have been associated with higher levels of epinephrine (58, 189). In animal models, social isolation and chronic social stress have been associated with excess cortisol secretion, HPA dysfunction, altered autonomic activity, and endothelial damage (182, 217, 224).

Serotonergic Dysfunction

Abnormalities in serotonergic function may be another mechanism by which negative emotional states and stress influence atherogenesis. Serotonin is critical in the regulation of mood, emotions, and behavior. Preclinical investigations and clinical studies indicate that depression is associated with serotonergic dysfunction in the central nervous system (8, 30, 145) and in peripheral circulating platelets (162). Moreover, both central and peripheral serotonergic mechanisms influence thrombovascular processes. Serotonin has known vasoactive properties and is involved in thrombogenesis, platelet activation, and hypertension (33, 55, 184). Most of the circulating serotonin in the blood is contained within platelets (68). Serotonin secreted by platelets activated at the site of vascular injury contributes to smooth muscle cell proliferation, vasospasms, and thrombus formation (32). Depressed patients, especially those with high levels of anxiety, showed serotonin-stimulated increases in platelet intracellular calcium, which is involved in platelet activation and maintenance of blood pressure (34). Chronic stress also can produce alterations in serotonin levels and function (143, 144). Serotonergic dysregulation plays a critical role in aggressive behavior and impulsivity and may be associated with high levels of anger and hostility (124, 131). Current hostility and lifetime history of aggressive behavior in adults with major depression have been associated with high levels of platelet serotonin (130), and increasing levels of hopelessness have been associated with high whole blood serotonin levels in a population-based sample of older adults (53). Central and peripheral indices of serotonergic function appear to be inversely associated with one another; however, the human and animal data supporting this association are limited (141, 195), and the mechanisms by which these two systems may be related are unknown at the present time.

Secretion of Pro-Inflammatory Cytokines

Inflammatory processes play a critical, early role in atherogenesis. Indeed, the likely primary event in atherogenesis is injury to the arterial endothelium (180). Endothelial injury and damage can result from fluid mechanical forces or large shear stress gradients in the vasculature (36); traditional coronary risk factors, including cigarette smoking, high cholesterol, diabetes, and hypertension (180); as well as infectious agents (156). Endothelial injury results in the induction of cytokines, vasoactive molecules, and growth factors that stimulate the endothelium to have procoagulant rather than anticoagulant properties, which initiates an acute phase response and resultant cascade of atherogenic changes (181). Psychosocial factors, including stress and negative emotional states, can adversely affect these inflammatory processes, particularly via the action of proinflammatory cytokines. This pathway is clearly bidirectional (see Figure 1). Cytokines can induce behavioral and psychological expressions of stress, including negative emotional states. The pro-inflammatory cytokines IL-1 and IL-6 stimulate the HPA axis, initiating a classic stress response that results in elevated circulating glucocorticoids (11, 183). Cytokines also induce "sickness behavior," fatigue, anorexia, anhedonia, and decreased psychomotor activity (103), which are recognized symptoms of depression. Increased plasma concentrations of IL-1, IL-6, and other cytokines have been observed in patients with major depression, with a concomitant increase in acute phase proteins significantly associated with IL-6 (128, 200). Human and animal models indicate that IL-6 levels are increased under conditions of psychological and social stress (106, 163, 228).

Platelet Activation

Markovitz & Matthews (133) initially proposed that enhanced platelet response to psychological stress is a key mechanism whereby psychosocial stress may trigger acute ischemic events and contribute to the development and progression of CVD. Figure 1 is an adaptation and extension of their proposed model, which incorporates additional mechanisms discussed in this review. Platelets play a central role in hemostasis, thrombosis, and the development of atherosclerosis and acute coronary syndromes (118). Depressive symptoms have been associated with increased platelet activation and exaggerated platelet reactivity in patients with major depression (152, 153). Patients with IHD and comorbid depression showed increased plasma concentrations of platelet-specific proteins, β-thromboglobulin (β-TG), and platelet factor-4 (PF4), compared with nondepressed patients with IHD or healthy control subjects (111). Hostility similarly has been associated with increased β-TG (134) and platelet activation among CHD patients but not among healthy controls (132). Anger expression has been positively correlated with platelet aggregability (219). The relation between psychosocial factors and platelet activation and/or reactivity may be mediated, at least in part, by alterations in serotonergic function (133).

Other Mechanisms

Other pathophysiological mechanisms may play a role in explaining how various psychological or social factors influence CVD risk. Altered autonomic control of the heart appears to be important, particularly concerning negative emotional states. Several studies have reported that patients who are depressed or have anxiety disorder have reduced heart rate variability and impaired or poor vagal control (22, 101). Similarly, research suggests that hostile men have diminished vagal control of cardiac function, compared with nonhostile men (199). This evidence indicates that negative emotions may promote arrhythmogenesis. Recent findings support this hypothesis. Anger triggered ventricular arrhythmias in patients with implantable defibrillators (112), and anger and hostility predicted incident atrial fibrillation in men but not women in the Framingham Offspring Study (42). Earlier studies suggested that acute psychological distress precedes arrhythmias (18, 172). Animal studies have reported that cardiac arrhythmias are more frequent in social compared with nonsocial stress (192).

Psychosocial factors also may indirectly influence CVD development and progression through nonphysiological pathways. It is well-documented that individuals who are anxious, depressed, angry, or hostile, or who have more stressful lives or are more socially isolated, frequently have poor behavioral risk profiles or less healthy lifestyles, including higher rates of smoking, more sedentary lifestyles, excess consumption of alcohol, and poor compliance with medical regimens (6, 98, 123). However, the majority of studies published to date have found that the excess CVD risk associated with psychosocial characteristics is not adequately explained by these factors and largely persists following statistical adjustment for known cardiovascular risk factors. Thus, our focus here has been on biologically plausible physiological mechanisms by which psychosocial factors can influence CVD.

RECOMMENDATIONS FOR FUTURE STUDIES

A number of important and emerging issues provide impetus to and a framework for future investigations into the role of psychosocial factors and risk for CVD. We have identified seven areas of research that we believe are particularly promising and briefly describe each of these areas below.

Investigating the Impact of Differential Exposure to Psychological Stress on CVD Risk Among Minorities

A majority of studies to date have included only male participants and largely Caucasian populations. This is particularly true in studies of clinical cardiovascular endpoints, although a growing number of studies have included women and ethnic minority samples. African Americans may be more susceptible to the adverse cardiovascular consequences of negative emotions, especially hypertension and stroke (31, 88, 89). Minority populations also experience a disproportionate burden of CVD (4). Several researchers have argued that ethnic disparities in CVD are a result primarily of ethnic differences in exposure to psychosocial stress (e.g., poverty, chronic stress, discrimination, negative emotions) (85, 221). African Americans frequently report greater exposure to discrimination (187, 212, 221), negative life events (84, 187), higher rates of hostility (2, 81), and more depressive symptomatology (86) than do Caucasians. Hispanics also have a higher prevalence of major depressive disorder (148, 154) than do Caucasians. Differential exposure rates to psychosocial stress may confer an increased vulnerability to clinical manifestations of CVD; however, few studies have investigated these relationships.

Understanding Psychosocial Factors that May Uniquely Influence Minority and Immigrant Populations

Certain psychological or social factors may be especially relevant to the experience of minority or immigrant populations. There is growing interest in the cardiovascular consequences of chronic social status stressors in the form of discrimination and unfair treatment, although no prospective epidemiological investigations of these associations have been reported. Available cross-sectional data suggest that reports of discrimination may be associated with higher levels of IMT (212) and, in some instances, hypertension (220), although evidence to date has been inconsistent (70). Degree of acculturation also may be particularly significant in the development of CVD among immigrant populations. Greater acculturation has been associated with greater prevalence of CHD in Japanese Americans (136) and first-generation Indian immigrants (150) and greater prevalence of stroke among Mexican Americans (158). These effects have not been examined prospectively.

Examining Multiple Psychological and Social Influences That Impact People's Lives

Numerous psychological and social influences affect individuals' lives and ultimately their health. Empirical research to date rarely reflects this; most investigations have focused on only one or perhaps two psychological characteristics or social factors and have ignored interrelationships among these factors and how they jointly affect cardiovascular health. However, available evidence is suggestive. In the KIHD study, men who reported feeling hopeless, hostile, and socially isolated experienced greater progression of carotid artery IMT over four years (127) and were nearly three times as likely to suffer an MI or CVD death over eight years of follow-up (126), compared with men with none of these characteristics. Moreover, the health outcomes of the men with all three psychosocial risk factors was significantly worse than among men with one or two characteristics. Other work found that the effects of perceived stress on cardiovascular function were pronounced among those with low social support but buffered in those with high social support (26). Among post-MI patients, a pattern of high stress, social isolation, and limited education predicted mortality in men (181), and suppressed emotions and economic disadvantage predicted mortality in women (168). Such intriguing findings emphasize the need to study reciprocal or intercorrelated relationships among individuals' psychological characteristics and their social environments.

Understanding Neighborhood Effects on CVD Risk and Health Outcomes

A burgeoning literature has documented important neighborhood effects on health. Residents in a low social environment experienced significantly higher 11-year mortality risk than did residents of a high social environment, after adjusting for individual education, income, race, health status, and behavioral risk factors (227). Living in a disadvantaged neighborhood increased the risk of incident CHD over nine years of follow-up in the ARIC study, after considering age and personal socioeconomic indicators (38). Neighborhood environments likely impact health via psychosocial and behavioral characteristics (174). These and related findings point to the potential significance of multilevel analyses of psychosocial determinants of cardiovascular health (37, 135).

Exploring Continuing Scientific Advances in the Measurement of CVD

In the past 15 years there has been a dramatic growth in studies using noninvasive assessment techniques (e.g., B-mode ultrasonography, electron beam tomography), as such technology has become available, to detect early indications of atherosclerotic changes. These technological advances have enabled investigators to examine whether and to what extent psychosocial factors are important early in the disease process. This trend will continue as advances in the measurement of CVD are made. Knowledge gleaned from such work can help inform future intervention and prevention efforts.

Investigating Pathophysiological Mechanisms that Underlie the Associations between Psychosocial Characteristics and CVD Risk

Continued refinement of pathophysiological mechanisms and pathways is needed as we achieve greater understanding of the complexity of mechanisms that link psychosocial factors and CVD. One integrative hypothesis has been put forth recently. Harris & Matthews (71) proposed that interactions between endothelial function and ANS regulation, including sympathetic and parasympathetic activity, may be one mechanism by which psychosocial factors are related to CVD. Further understanding of pathophysiological mechanisms will help identify effective interventions that may lead to a reduction in CVD mortality and morbidity.

Examining the Efficacy of Psychosocial Interventions to Reduce Disease Risk and Prevent the Development of CVD

The literature on psychosocial interventions dates back more than 25 years and is decidedly mixed. Two meta-analytic reviews recently concluded that psychosocial interventions in post-MI patients reduce cardiac morbidity and mortality (40, 122); yet relatively few large, well-controlled clinical trials have been conducted. The most promising early results were from the Recurrent Coronary Prevention Project, which found that type A behavior modification and group counseling successfully reduced type A behavior and hostility and reduced the risk of recurrent coronary events in a sample of 1013 MI patients, of whom 592 received the intervention (63). Most recently, findings from the Enhancing Recovery in Coronary Heart Disease trial, a comparison of cognitive behavioral therapy for depression and/or social isolation versus usual care in 2481 post-MI patients from 8 clinical settings, showed that although the intervention improved the psychosocial risk of participants, it had no impact on coronary outcomes (12). Further research is needed to explore the efficacy of psychosocial interventions in reducing the risk of recurrent events among patients with CVD and in preventing coronary events in at-risk individuals. Much also remains to be learned about the psychophysiological mechanisms by which psychosocial interventions may reduce cardiac events.

SUMMARY

In this review, we have summarized some of the rapidly accruing findings relating psychosocial factors to CVD morbidity and mortality. Population-based and community studies, studies of psychiatric and cardiac patients, and experimental investigations from varied scientific disciplines, including epidemiology, cardiology, psychiatry, sociology, psychology, and physiology, have contributed to this literature. Taken together, this breadth and diversity of scientific work on the role of psychological and social characteristics in the development and progression of CVD make the relative consistency of the findings all the more remarkable. Indeed, these observations highlight the temporality and strength of the relationships between psychosocial factors and CVD, coherence and consistency of the findings, and the biologic plausibility of the associations. Each of these features strengthens the hypothesis that psychosocial factors are causally related to CVD (77).

We focused on three psychosocial domains: negative emotional states (depression, anger and hostility, and anxiety); chronic and acute psychosocial stressors, especially job stress; and three related social factors (social ties, social support, social conflict). Although not unequivocal, available evidence indicates that these psychosocial domains all are associated with increased risk of CVD morbidity and mortality. Moreover, accumulating data show that these psychosocial characteristics have direct pathophysiological effects. These pathophysiological mechanisms are multifactorial and undoubtedly act in an integrative and synergistic fashion to promote atherogenesis and its clinical manifestions (Figure 1). The work reviewed here has contributed greatly to our knowledge and understanding about psychosocial factors and risk for CVD. Nonetheless, many opportunities for future research remain. Some of the most important challenges facing future work in this area include identifying the impact of psychosocial factors in ethnic minority populations, who suffer a disproportionate burden of CVD; expanding conceptual and empirical models to determine how interrelated psychological and social factors relate to CVD risk; utilizing multilevel models to explore the complexity of psychosocial determinants of cardiovascular health; keeping pace with scientific advances in CVD measurement techniques; further refining our understanding of pathophysiological mechanisms and pathways linking psychosocial factors to CVD; and exploring the efficacy and utility of interventions to reduce psychosocial risk and thereby decrease risk of CVD morbidity and mortality.

The *Annual Review of Public Health* is online at
http://publhealth.annualreviews.org

LITERATURE CITED

1. Alexander F. 1939. Emotional factors in essential hypertension. *Psychosom. Med.* 1:173–79

2. Allen J, Markovitz J, Jacobs DR Jr, Knox SS. 2001. Social support and health behavior in hostile black and white men

and women in CARDIA. Coronary Artery Risk Development in Young Adults. *Psychosom. Med.* 63:609–18

3. Almada SJ, Zonderman AB, Shekelle RB, Dyer AR, Daviglus ML, et al. 1991. Neuroticism and cynicism and risk of death in middle-aged men: the Western Electric Study. *Psychosom. Med.* 53:165–75

4. Am. Heart Assoc. 2003. *Heart Disease and Stroke Statistics—2004 Update.* Dallas, TX: Am. Heart Assoc.

5. Anda R, Williamson D, Jones D, Macera C, Eaker E, et al. 1993. Depressed affect, hopelessness, and the risk of ischemic heart disease in a cohort of U.S. adults. *Epidemiology* 4:285–94

6. Anda RF, Williamson DF, Escobedo LG, Mast EE, Giovino GA, Remington PL. 1990. Depression and the dynamics of smoking: a national perspective. *JAMA* 264:1541–45

7. Arlow JA. 1945. Identification of mechanisms in coronary occlusion. *Psychosom. Med.* 7:195–209

8. Asberg M, Traskman L, Thoren P. 1976. 5-HIAA in the cerebrospinal fluid: a biochemical suicide predictor? *Arch. Gen. Psychiatry* 33:1193–97

9. Barefoot JC, Helms MJ, Mark DB, Blumenthal JA, Califf RM, et al. 1996. Depression and long-term mortality risk in patients with coronary artery disease. *Am. J. Cardiol.* 78:613–17

10. Barefoot JC, Larsen S, von der Leith L, Schroll M. 1995. Hostility, incidence of acute myocardial infarction, and mortality in a sample of older Danish men and women. *Am. J. Epidemiol.* 142:477–84

11. Berkenbosch R, Oers J, Rey A, Tilders F, Besedovsky H. 1987. Corticotropin-releasing factor-producing neurons in the rat activated by interleukin-1. *Science* 238:524–26

12. Berkman LF, Blumenthal J, Burg M, Carney RM, Catellier D, et al. 2003. Effects of treating depression and low perceived social support on clinical events after myocardial infarction: the Enhancing Recovery in Coronary Heart Disease Patients (ENRICHD) Randomized Trial. *JAMA* 289:3106–16

13. Berkman LF, Leo-Summers L, Horwitz RI. 1992. Emotional support and survival after myocardial infarction. A prospective, population-based study of the elderly. *Ann. Intern. Med.* 117:1003–9

14. Berkman LF, Syme SL. 1979. Social networks, host resistance, and mortality: a nine-year follow-up study of Alameda County residents. *Am. J. Epidemiol.* 109:186–204

15. Blumenthal JA, Thompson LW, Williams RB Jr, Kong Y. 1979. Anxiety-proneness and coronary heart disease. *J. Psychosom. Res.* 23:17–21

16. Bonow RO, Smaha LA, Smith SC Jr, Mensah GA, Lenfant C. 2002. World Heart Day 2002: the international burden of cardiovascular disease: responding to the emerging global epidemic. *Circulation* 106:1602–5

17. Bosma H, Peter R, Siegrist J, Marmot M. 1998. Two alternative job stress models and the risk of coronary heart disease. *Am. J. Public Health* 88:68–74

18. Brodsky MA, Sato DA, Iseri LT, Wolff LJ, Allen BJ. 1987. Ventricular tachyarrhythmia associated with psychological stress. The role of the sympathetic nervous system. *JAMA* 257:2064–67

19. Brummett BH, Barefoot JC, Siegler IC, Clapp-Channing NE, Lytle BL, et al. 2001. Characteristics of socially isolated patients with coronary artery disease who are at elevated risk for mortality. *Psychosom. Med.* 63:267–72

20. Cannon WB. 1935. Stresses and strains of homeostasis (Mary Scott Newbold Lecture). *Am. J. Med. Sci.* 189:1–14

21. Carney RM, Rich MW, Freedland KE, Saini J, teVelde A, et al. 1988. Major depressive disorder predicts cardiac events in patients with coronary artery disease. *Psychosom. Med.* 50:627–33

22. Carney RM, Saunders RD, Freedland KE, Stein P, Rich MW, Jaffe AS. 1995.

Association of depression with reduced heart rate variability in coronary artery disease. *Am. J. Cardiol.* 76:562–64

23. Case RB, Moss AJ, Case N, McDermott M, Eberly S. 1992. Living alone after myocardial infarction. Impact on prognosis. *JAMA* 267:515–19

24. Cassel J. 1976. The contribution of the social environment to host resistance: the Fourth Wade Hampton Frost Lecture. *Am. J. Epidemiol.* 104:107–23

25. Chrousos GP, Gold PW. 1998. A healthy body in a healthy mind—and vice versa—the damaging power of 'uncontrollable' stress. *J. Clin. Endocrinol. Metab.* 83:1842–45

26. Cohen S, Wills TA. 1985. Stress, social support, and the buffering hypothesis. *Psychol. Bull.* 98:310–57

27. Cook WW, Medley D. 1954. Proposed hostility and pharisaic virtue scales for the MMPI. *J. Appl. Psychol.* 38:414–18

28. Cooper T, Detre T, Weiss SM. 1981. Coronary-prone behavior and coronary heart disease: a critical review. The review panel on coronary-prone behavior and coronary heart disease. *Circulation* 63:1199–215

29. Coryell W, Noyes R, Clancy J. 1982. Excess mortality in panic disorder. A comparison with primary unipolar depression. *Arch. Gen. Psychiatry* 39:701–3

30. Csernansky JG, Sheline YI. 1993. Abnormalities of serotonin metabolism and nonpsychotic psychiatric disorders. *Ann. Clin. Psychiatry* 5:275–82

31. Davidson K, Jonas BS, Dixon KE, Markovitz JH. 2000. Do depression symptoms predict early hypertension incidence in young adults in the CARDIA study? Coronary artery risk development in young adults. *Arch. Intern. Med.* 160:1495–500

32. De Clerck F. 1991. Effects of serotonin on platelets and blood vessels. *J. Cardiovasc. Pharmacol.* 17:S1–5

33. De Clerck F. 1990. The role of serotonin in thrombogenesis. *Clin. Physiol. Biochem.* 8:40–49

34. Delisi SM, Konopka LM, O'Connor FL, Crayton JW. 1998. Platelet cystolic calcium response to serotonin in depressed patients and controls: relationship to symptomology and medication. *Biol. Psychiatry* 43:327–34

35. Dembroski TM, Czajkowski SM. 1989. Historical and current developments in coronary-prone behavior. In *In Search of Coronary-Prone Behavior: Beyond Type A*, ed. AW Siegman, TM Dembroski, pp. 21–39. Hillsdale, NJ: Erlbaum

36. DePaola N, Gimbrone MA Jr, Davies PF, Dewey CF Jr. 1992. Vascular endothelium responds to fluid shear stress gradients. *Arterioscler. Thromb.* 12:1254–57

37. Diez Roux AV. 2001. Investigating neighborhood and area effects on health. *Am. J. Public Health* 91:1783–89

38. Diez Roux AV. 2004. Estimating neighborhood health effects: the challenges of causal inference in a complex world. *Soc. Sci. Med.* 58:1953–60

39. Dunbar F. 1943. *Psychosomatic Diagnosis.* New York: Hoeber

40. Dusseldorp E, van Elderen T, Maes S, Meulman J, Kraaij V. 1999. A meta-analysis of psychoeducational programs for coronary heart disease patients. *Health Psychol.* 18:506–19

41. Eaker ED, Pinsky J, Castelli WP. 1992. Myocardial infarction and coronary death among women: psychosocial predictors from a 20-year follow-up of women in the Framingham Study. *Am. J. Epidemiol.* 135:854–64

42. Eaker ED, Sullivan LM, Kelly-Hayes M, D'Agostino RB Sr, Benjamin EJ. 2004. Anger and hostility predict the development of atrial fibrillation in men in the Framingham Offspring Study. *Circulation* 109:1267–71

43. Eng PM, Rimm EB, Fitzmaurice G, Kawachi I. 2002. Social ties and change in social ties in relation to subsequent

total and cause-specific mortality and coronary heart disease incidence in men. *Am. J. Epidemiol.* 155:700–9

44. Engel GL. 1971. Sudden and rapid death during psychological stress. Folklore or folk wisdom? *Ann. Intern. Med.* 74:771–82

45. Everson SA, Goldberg DE, Kaplan GA, Cohen RD, Pukkala E, et al. 1996. Hopelessness and risk of mortality and incidence of myocardial infarction and cancer. *Psychosom. Med.* 58:113–21

46. Everson SA, Goldberg DE, Kaplan GA, Julkunen J, Salonen JT. 1998. Anger expression and incident hypertension. *Psychosom. Med.* 60:730–35

47. Everson SA, Kaplan GA, Goldberg DE, Lakka TA, Sivenius J, Salonen JT. 1999. Anger expression and incident stroke: prospective evidence from the Kuopio ischemic heart disease study. *Stroke* 30:523–28

48. Everson SA, Kaplan GA, Goldberg DE, Salonen JT. 2000. Hypertension incidence is predicted by high levels of hopelessness in Finnish men. *Hypertension* 35:561–67

49. Everson SA, Kaplan GA, Goldberg DE, Salonen R, Salonen JT. 1997. Hopelessness and 4-year progression of carotid atherosclerosis. The Kuopio Ischemic Heart Disease Risk Factor Study. *Arterioscler. Thromb. Vasc. Biol.* 17:1490–95

50. Everson SA, Kauhanen J, Kaplan GA, Goldberg DE, Julkunen J, et al. 1997. Hostility and increased risk of mortality and acute myocardial infarction: the mediating role of behavioral risk factors. *Am. J. Epidemiol.* 146:142–52

51. Everson SA, Lynch JW, Chesney MA, Kaplan GA, Goldberg DE, et al. 1997. Interaction of workplace demands and cardiovascular reactivity in progression of carotid atherosclerosis: population based study. *Br. Med. J.* 314:553–58

52. Everson SA, Roberts RE, Goldberg DE, Kaplan GA. 1998. Depressive symptoms and increased risk of stroke mortality over a 29-year period. *Arch. Intern. Med.* 158:1133–38

53. Everson-Rose SA, Karavolos K, Musselman DL, Owens MJ, Ritchie J, et al. 2004. Hopelessness is related to whole blood serotonin levels in middle-aged and older adults. *Psychosom. Med.* 66:A26 (Abstr.)

54. Ferketich AK, Schwartzbaum JA, Frid DJ, Moeschberger ML. 2000. Depression as an antecedent to heart disease among women and men in the NHANES I study. *Arch. Intern. Med.* 160:1261–68

55. Fetkovska N, Amstein R, Ferracin F, Regenass M, Buhler FR, Pletscher A. 1988. 5HT-kinetics and sensitivity of human blood platelets: variations with age, gender and platelet number. *Thromb. Haemost.* 60:486–90

56. Finch JF, Okun MA, Barrera M Jr, Zautra AJ, Reich JW. 1989. Positive and negative social ties among older adults: measurement models and the prediction of psychological distress and well-being. *Am. J. Community Psychol.* 17:585–605

57. Fiore J, Becker J, Coppel DB. 1983. Social network interactions: a buffer or a stress. *Am. J. Community Psychol.* 11:423–39

58. Fleming R, Baum A, Gisriel MM, Gatchel RJ. 1982. Mediating influences of social support on stress at Three Mile Island. *J. Hum. Stress* 8:14–22

59. Frasure-Smith N, Lesperance F. 2003. Depression and other psychological risks following myocardial infarction. *Arch. Gen. Psychiatry* 60:627–36

60. Frasure-Smith N, Lesperance F, Talajic M. 1995. The impact of negative emotions on prognosis following myocardial infarction: Is it more than depression? *Health Psychol.* 14:388–98

61. Frasure-Smith N, Lesperance F, Talajio M. 1995. Depression and 18-month prognosis after myocardial infarction. *Circulation* 91:999–1005

62. Friedman M, Rosenman RH. 1971. Type A behavior pattern: its association with coronary heart disease. *Ann. Clin. Res.* 3:300–12

63. Friedman M, Thoresen CE, Gill JJ, Ulmer D, Powell LH, et al. 1986. Alteration of type A behavior and its effect on cardiac recurrences in post myocardial infarction patients: summary results of the recurrent coronary prevention project. *Am. Heart J.* 112:653–65

64. Fuller RG. 1935. What happens to mental patients after discharge from the hospital? *Psychiatr. Q.* 9:95–104

65. Gerin W, Milner D, Chawla S, Pickering TG. 1995. Social support as a moderator of cardiovascular reactivity in women: a test of the direct effects and buffering hypotheses. *Psychosom. Med.* 57:16–22

66. Greene WA, Goldstein S, Moss AJ. 1972. Psychosocial aspects of sudden death. A preliminary report. *Arch. Intern. Med.* 129:725–31

67. Greenland P, Knoll MD, Stamler J, Neaton JD, Dyer AR, et al. 2003. Major risk factors as antecedents of fatal and nonfatal coronary heart disease events. *JAMA* 290:891–97

68. Guicheney P, Baudouin-Legros M, Valtier D, Meyer P. 1987. Reduced serotonin content and uptake in platelets from patients with essential hypertension: Is a ouabain-like factor involved? *Thromb. Res.* 45:289–97

69. Haines AP, Imeson JD, Meade TW. 1987. Phobic anxiety and ischaemic heart disease. *Br. Med. J.* 295:297–99

70. Harrell JP, Hall S, Taliaferro J. 2003. Physiological responses to racism and discrimination: an assessment of the evidence. *Am. J. Public Health* 93:243–48

71. Harris KF, Matthews KA. 2004. Interactions between autonomic nervous system activity and endothelial function: a model for the development of cardiovascular disease. *Psychosom. Med.* 66:153–64

72. Hearn MD, Murray DM, Luepker RV. 1989. Hostility, coronary heart disease, and total mortality: a 33-year follow-up study of university students. *J. Behav. Med.* 12:105–21

73. Helmers KF, Krantz DS, Howell RH, Klein J, Bairey CN, Rozanski A. 1993. Hostility and myocardial ischemia in cornary artery disease patients: evaluation by gender and ischemic index. *Psychosom. Med.* 55:29–36

74. Hemingway H, Marmot M. 1999. Evidence based cardiology: psychosocial factors in the aetiology and prognosis of coronary heart disease. Systematic review of prospective cohort studies. *Br. Med. J.* 318:1460–67

75. Herlitz J, Wiklund I, Caidahl K, Hartford M, Haglid M, et al. 1998. The feeling of loneliness prior to coronary artery bypass grafting might be a predictor of short-and long-term postoperative mortality. *Eur. J. Vasc. Endovasc. Surg.* 16:120–25

76. Hermann C, Brand-Driehorst S, Buss U, Ruger U. 2000. Effects of anxiety and depression on 5-year mortality in 5,057 patients referred for exercise testing. *J. Psychosom. Res.* 48:455–62

77. Hill AB. 1965. The environment and disease: association or causation? *Proc. R. Soc. Med.* 58:295–300

78. Hlatky MA, Lam LC, Lee KL, Clapp-Channing NE, Williams RB, et al. 1995. Job strain and the prevalence and outcome of coronary artery disease. *Circulation* 92:327–33

79. House JS. 1974. Occupational stress and coronary heart disease: a review and theoretical integration. *J. Health Soc. Behav.* 15:12–27

80. House JS, Robbins C, Metzner HL. 1982. The association of social relationships and activities with mortality: prospective evidence from the Tecumseh Community Health Study. *Am. J. Epidemiol.* 116:123–40

81. Hughes JW, Sherwood A, Blumenthal JA, Suarez EC, Hinderliter AL. 2003. Hostility, social support, and adrenergic receptor responsiveness among African-American and white men and women. *Psychosom. Med.* 65:582–87

82. Iribarren C, Sidney S, Bild DE, Liu K, Markovitz JH, et al. 2000. Association of

hostility with coronary artery calcification in young adults—The CARDIA study. *JAMA* 283:2546–51

83. Iso H, Date C, Yamamoto A, Toyoshima H, Tanabe N, et al. 2002. Perceived mental stress and mortality from cardiovascular disease among Japanese men and women: the Japan Collaborative Cohort Study for Evaluation of Cancer Risk Sponsored by Monbusho (JACC Study). *Circulation* 106:1229–36

84. Ituarte PH, Kamarck TW, Thompson HS, Bacanu S. 1999. Psychosocial mediators of racial differences in nighttime blood pressure dipping among normotensive adults. *Health Psychol.* 18:393–402

85. Jackson JS, Brown TN, Williams DR, Torres M, Sellers SL, Brown K. 1996. Racism and the physical and mental health status of African Americans: a thirteen year national panel study. *Ethn. Dis.* 6:132–47

86. Jackson-Triche ME, Greer SJ, Wells KB, Rogers W, Camp P, Mazel R. 2000. Depression and health-related quality of life in ethnic minorities seeking care in general medical settings. *J. Affect. Disord.* 58: 89–97

87. James SA, Kleinbaum DG. 1976. Socioecologic stress and hypertension related mortality rates in North Carolina. *Am. J. Public Health* 66:354–58

88. Jonas BS, Lando JF. 2000. Negative affect as a prospective risk factor for hypertension. *Psychosom. Med.* 62:188–96

89. Jonas BS, Mussolino ME. 2000. Symptoms of depression as a prospective risk factor for stroke. *Psychosom. Med.* 62: 463–71

90. Julkunen J, Salonen R, Kaplan GA, Chesney MA, Salonen JT. 1994. Hostility and the progression of carotid atherosclerosis. *Psychosom. Med.* 56:519–25

91. Kamarck TW, Manuck SB, Jennings JR. 1990. Social support reduces cardiovascular reactivity to psychological challenge: a laboratory model. *Psychosom. Med.* 52: 42–58

92. Kaplan GA, Keil JE. 1993. Socioeco-

nomic factors and cardiovascular disease: a review of the literature. *Circulation* 88:1973–98

93. Kaplan GA, Salonen JT, Cohen RD, Brand RJ, Syme SL, Puska P. 1988. Social connections and mortality from all causes and from cardiovascular disease: prospective evidence from eastern Finland. *Am. J. Epidemiol.* 128:370–80

94. Kaprio J, Koskenvuo M, Rita H. 1987. Mortality after bereavement: a prospective study of 95,647 widowed persons. *Am. J. Public Health* 77:283–87

95. Karasek R, Baker D, Marxer F, Ahlbom A, Theorell T. 1981. Job decision latitude, job demands, and cardiovascular disease: a prospective study of Swedish men. *Am. J. Public Health* 71:694–705

96. Karasek R, Brisson C, Kawakami N, Houtman I, Bongers P, Amick B. 1998. The Job Content Questionnaire (JCQ): an instrument for internationally comparative assessments of psychosocial job characteristics. *J. Occup. Health Psychol.* 3:322–55

97. Kark JD, Goldman S, Epstein L. 1995. Iraqi missile attacks on Israel. The association of mortality with a life-threatening stressor. *JAMA* 273:1208–10

98. Kawachi I, Colditz GA, Ascherio A, Rimm EB, Giovannucci E, et al. 1994. Prospective study of phobic anxiety and risk of coronary heart disease in men. *Circulation* 89:1992–97

99. Kawachi I, Colditz GA, Ascherio A, Rimm EB, Giovanucci E, et al. 1996. A prospective study of social networks in relation to total mortality and cardiovascular disease in men in the USA. *J. Epidemiol. Community Health* 50:245–51

100. Kawachi I, Sparrow D, Spiro AI, Vokonas P, Weiss ST. 1995. A prospective study of anger and coronary heart disease: The Normative Aging Study. *Circulation* 84:2090–95

101. Kawachi I, Sparrow D, Vokonas PS, Weiss ST. 1995. Decreased heart rate variability in men with phobic anxiety (data from the

Normative Aging Study). *Am. J. Cardiol.* 75:882–85

102. Kawachi I, Sparrow D, Vokonas PS, Weiss ST. 1994. Symptoms of anxiety and risk of coronary heart disease. The Normative Aging Study. *Circulation* 90:2225–29

103. Kent S, Bluthe RM, Dantzer R, Hardwick AJ, Kelley KW, et al. 1992. Different receptor mechanisms mediate the pyrogenic and behavioral effects of interleukin 1. *Proc. Natl. Acad. Sci. USA* 89:9117–20

104. Kessler RC, Berglund P, Demler O, Jin R, Koretz D, et al. 2003. The epidemiology of major depressive disorder: results from the National Comorbidity Survey Replication (NCS-R). *JAMA* 289:3095–105

105. Kessler RC, McGonagle KA, Zhao S, Nelson CB, Hughes M, et al. 1994. Lifetime and 12-month prevalence of DSM-III-R psychiatric disorders in the United States. Results from the National Comorbidity Survey. *Arch. Gen. Psychiatry* 51:8–19

106. Kiecolt-Glaser JK, Preacher KJ, MacCallum RC, Atkinson C, Malarkey WB, Glaser R. 2003. Chronic stress and age-related increases in the proinflammatory cytokine IL-6. *Proc. Natl. Acad. Sci. USA* 100:9090–95

107. Kirschbaum C, Klauer T, Filip S, Hellhammer DH. 1995. Sex-specific effects of social support on cortisol and subjective responses to acute psychological stress. *Psychosom. Med.* 57:23–31

108. Krumholz HM, Butler J, Miller J, Vaccarino V, Williams CS, et al. 1998. Prognostic importance of emotional support for elderly patients hospitalized with heart failure. *Circulation* 97:958–64

109. Kubzansky LD, Kawachi I, Spiro A III, Weiss ST, Vokonas PS, Sparrow D. 1997. Is worrying bad for your heart? A prospective study of worry and coronary heart disease in the Normative Aging Study. *Circulation* 95:818–24

110. Kuper H, Marmot M. 2003. Job strain, job demands, decision latitude, and risk of coronary heart disease within the White-

hall II study. *J. Epidemiol. Community Health* 57:147–53

111. Laghrissi-Thode F, Wagner W, Pollock B, Johnson P, Finkel M. 1997. Elevated platelet factor 4 and b-thromboglobulin plasma levels in depressed patients with ischemic heart disease. *Biol. Psychiatry* 42:290–95

112. Lampert R, Joska T, Burg MM, Batsford WP, McPherson CA, Jain D. 2002. Emotional and physical precipitants of ventricular arrhythmia. *Circulation* 106:1800–5

113. Lane D, Carroll D, Ring C, Beevers DG, Lip GY. 2001. Mortality and quality of life 12 months after myocardial infarction: effects of depression and anxiety. *Psychosom. Med.* 63:221–30

114. Lee S, Colditz G, Berkman L, Kawachi I. 2002. A prospective study of job strain and coronary heart disease in US women. *Int. J. Epidemiol.* 31:1147–53

115. Lee S, Colditz G, Berkman L, Kawachi I. 2003. Caregiving to children and grandchildren and risk of coronary heart disease in women. *Am. J. Public Health* 93:1939–44

116. Lee S, Colditz GA, Berkman LF, Kawachi I. 2003. Caregiving and risk of coronary heart disease in U.S. women: a prospective study. *Am. J. Prev. Med.* 24:113–19

117. Lee S, Colditz GA, Berkman LF, Kawachi I. 2004. Prospective study of job insecurity and coronary heart disease in US women. *Ann. Epidemiol.* 14:24–30

118. Lefkovits J, Plow EF, Topol EJ. 1995. Mechanisms of disease—platelet glycoprotein IIb/IIIa receptors in cardiovascular medicine. *N. Engl. J. Med.* 332:1553–59

119. Leon GR, Finn SE, Murray D, Bailey JM. 1988. Inability to predict cardiovascular disease from hostility scores or MMPI items related to type A behavior. *J. Consult. Clin. Psychol.* 56:597–600

120. Leor J, Kloner RA. 1996. The Northridge earthquake as a trigger for acute myocardial infarction. *Am. J. Cardiol.* 77:1230–32

121. Light KC, Turner JR, Hinderliter AL. 1992. Job strain and ambulatory work blood pressure in healthy young men and women. *Hypertension* 20:214–18

122. Linden W, Stossel C, Maurice J. 1996. Psychosocial interventions for patients with coronary artery disease: a meta-analysis. *Arch. Intern. Med.* 156:745–52

123. Lobstein DD, Mosbacher BJ, Ismail AH. 1983. Depression as a powerful discriminator between physically active and sedentary middle-aged men. *J. Psychosom. Res.* 27:69–76

124. Lucki I. 1998. The spectrum of behaviors influenced by serotonin. *Biol. Psychiatry* 44:151–62

125. Lynch J, Krause N, Kaplan GA, Salonen R, Salonen JT. 1997. Workplace demands, economic reward, and progression of carotid atherosclerosis. *Circulation* 96:302–7

126. Lynch JW, Kaplan GA, Everson SA, Salonen JT. 1997. Psychosocial risk factor clustering and the risk of all-cause and cardiovascular mortality and acute myocardial infarction. *Ann. Behav. Med.* 18:S073 (Abstr.)

127. Lynch JW, Kaplan GA, Everson SA, Salonen JT. 1997. Socioeconomic and psychosocial factors in the progression of carotid atherosclerosis. *Can. J. Cardiol.* 13(Suppl. B):B156 (Abstr.)

128. Maes M, Scharpe S, Meltzer H, Bosmans E, Suy E, et al. 1993. Relationships between interleukin-6 activity, acute phase proteins and HPA-axis function in severe depression. *Psychiatry Res.* 49:11–27

129. Malzberg B. 1937. Mortality among patients with involuntional melancholia. *Am. J. Psychiatry* 93:1231–38

130. Mann JJ, McBride PA, Anderson GM, Mieczkowski TA. 1992. Platelet and whole blood serotonin content in depressed inpatients: correlations with acute and life-time psychopathology. *Biol. Psychiatry* 32:243–57

131. Manuck SB, Flory JD, McCaffery JM, Matthews KA, Mann JJ, Muldoon MF. 1998. Aggression, impulsivity, and central nervous system serotonergic responsivity in a nonpatient sample. *Neuropsychopharmacology* 19:287–99

132. Markovitz JH. 1998. Hostility is associated with increased platelet activation in cornary heart disease. *Psychosom. Med.* 60:586–91

133. Markovitz JH, Matthews KA. 1991. Platelets and coronary heart disease—potential psychophysiological mechanisms. *Psychosom. Med.* 53:643–68

134. Markovitz JH, Matthews KA, Kiss J, Smitherman TC. 1996. Effects of hostility on platelet reactivity to psychological stress in coronary heart disease patients and in healthy controls. *Psychosom. Med.* 58:143–49

135. Marmot M. 2000. Multilevel approaches to understanding social determinants. In *Social Epidemiology*, ed. LF Berkman, I Kawachi, pp. 349–67. New York: Oxford Univ. Press

136. Marmot MG, Syme SL. 1976. Acculturation and coronary heart disease in Japanese-Americans. *Am. J. Epidemiol.* 104:225–47

137. Matthews KA, Cottington EM, Talbott E, Kuller LH, Siegel JM. 1987. Stressful work conditions and diastolic blood pressure among blue collar factory workers. *Am. J. Epidemiol.* 126:280–91

138. Matthews KA, Gump BB. 2002. Chronic work stress and marital dissolution increase risk of posttrial mortality in men from the Multiple Risk Factor Intervention Trial. *Arch. Intern. Med.* 162:309–15

139. Matthews KA, Gump BB, Harris KF, Haney TL, Barefoot JC. 2004. Hostile behaviors predict cardiovascular mortality among men enrolled in the multiple risk factor intervention trial. *Circulation* 109:66–70

140. Matthews KA, Owens JF, Kuller LH, Sutton-Tyrrell K, Jansen-McWilliams L. 1998. Are hostility and anxiety associated with carotid atherosclerosis in

healthy postmenopausal women? *Psychosom. Med.* 60:633–38

141. McBride PA, Anderson GM, Hertzig ME, Sweeney JA, Kream J, et al. 1989. Serotonergic responsivity in male young adults with autistic disorder. Results of a pilot study. *Arch. Gen. Psychiatry* 46:213–21

142. McEwen BS. 1997. Hormones as regulators of brain development: life-long effects related to health and disease. *Acta Paediatr. Suppl.* 422:41–44

143. McEwen BS, Mendelson S. 1993. Effects of stress on the neurochemistry and morphology of the brain: counter-regulation versus damage. In *Handbook of Stress: Theoretical and Clinical Aspects,* ed. L Goldberger, S Breznitz, pp. 101–26. New York: Free Press

144. McGee D, Cooper R, Liao Y, Durazo-Arvizu R. 1996. Patterns of comorbidity and mortality risk in blacks and whites. *Ann. Epidemiol.* 6:381–85

145. Meltzer H. 1989. Serotonergic dysfunction in depression. *Br. J. Psychiatry* 155: 25–31

146. Mendes de Leon CF, Krumholz HM, Seeman TS, Vaccarino V, Williams CS, et al. 1998. Depression and risk of coronary heart disease in elderly men and women: New Haven EPESE, 1982–1991. Established Populations for the Epidemiologic Studies of the Elderly. *Arch. Intern. Med.* 158:2341–48

147. Miller TQ, Smith TW, Turner CW, Guijarro ML, Hallet AJ. 1996. A meta-analytic review of research on hostility and physical health. *Psychol. Bull.* 119:322–48

148. Minsky S, Vega W, Miskimen T, Gara M, Escobar J. 2003. Diagnostic patterns in Latino, African American, and European American psychiatric patients. *Arch. Gen. Psychiatry* 60:637–44

149. Mokdad AH, Bowman BA, Ford ES, Vinicor F, Marks JS, Koplan JP. 2001. The continuing epidemics of obesity and diabetes in the United States. *JAMA* 286:1195–200

150. Mooteri SN, Petersen F, Dagubati R, Pai RG. 2004. Duration of residence in the United States as a new risk factor for coronary artery disease (The Konkani Heart Study). *Am. J. Cardiol.* 93:359–61

151. Musselman DL, Evans DL, Nemeroff CB. 1998. The relationship of depression to cardiovascular disease: epidemiology, biology, and treatment. *Arch. Gen. Psychiatry* 55:580–92

152. Musselman DL, Marzec UM, Manatunga A, Penna S, Reemsnyder A, et al. 2000. Platelet reactivity in depressed patients treated with paroxetine— preliminary findings. *Arch. Gen. Psychiatry* 57:875–82

153. Musselman DL, Tomer A, Manatunga AK, Knight BT, Porter MR, et al. 1996. Exaggerated platelet reactivity in major depression. *Am. J. Psychiatry* 153:1313–17

154. Myers HF, Lesser I, Rodriguez N, Mira CB, Hwang WC, et al. 2002. Ethnic differences in clinical presentation of depression in adult women. *Cultur. Divers. Ethn. Minor. Psychol.* 8:138–56

155. Niaura R, Todaro JF, Stroud L, Spiro A III, Ward KD, Weiss S. 2002. Hostility, the metabolic syndrome, and incident coronary heart disease. *Health Psychol.* 21:588–93

156. Nieto FJ. 1998. Infections and atherosclerosis: new clues from an old hypothesis? *Am. J. Epidemiol.* 148:937–48

157. Ohira T, Iso H, Satoh S, Sankai T, Tanigawa T, et al. 2001. Prospective study of depressive symptoms and risk of stroke among Japanese. *Stroke* 32:903–8

158. Ontiveros J, Miller TQ, Markides KS, Espino DV. 1999. Physical and psychosocial consequences of stroke in elderly Mexican Americans. *Ethn. Dis.* 9:212–17

159. Orth-Gomér K, Horsten M, Wamala SP, Mittleman MA, Kirkeeide R, et al. 1998. Social relations and extent and severity of coronary artery disease. The Stockholm Female Coronary Risk Study. *Eur. Heart J.* 19:1648–56

160. Orth-Gomér K, Rosengren A, Wilhelmsen L. 1993. Lack of social support and incidence of coronary heart disease in middle-aged Swedish men. *Psychosom. Med.* 55:37–43

161. Orth-Gomér K, Wamala SP, Horsten M, Schenck-Gustafsson K, Schneiderman N, Mittleman MA. 2000. Marital stress worsens prognosis in women with coronary heart disease: The Stockholm Female Coronary Risk Study. *JAMA* 284:3008–14

162. Owens MJ, Nemeroff CB. 1994. Role of serotonin in the pathophysiology of depression: focus on the serotonin transporter. *Clin. Chem.* 40:288–95

163. Papanicolaou DA, Wilder RL, Manolagas SC, Chrousos GP. 1998. The pathophysiologic roles of interleukin-6 in human disease. *Ann. Intern. Med.* 128:127–37

164. Paterniti S, Zureik M, Ducimetiere P, Touboul PJ, Feve JM, Alperovitch A. 2001. Sustained anxiety and 4-year progression of carotid atherosclerosis. *Arterioscler. Thromb. Vasc. Biol.* 21:136–41

165. Peter R, Siegrist J, Hallqvist J, Reuterwall C, Theorell T. 2002. Psychosocial work environment and myocardial infarction: improving risk estimation by combining two complementary job stress models in the SHEEP Study. *J. Epidemiol. Community Health* 56:294–300

166. Plotsky PM, Owens MJ, Nemeroff CB. 1998. Psychoneuroendocrinology of depression: hypothalamic-pituitary-adrenal axis. *Psychoneuroendocrinology* 21:293–307

167. Pope MK, Smith TW. 1991. Cortisol excretion in high and low cynically hostile men. *Psychosom. Med.* 53:386–92

168. Powell LH, Shaker LA, Jones BA, Vaccarino LV, Thorsen CE, Patillo JR. 1993. Psychosocial predictors of mortality in 83 women with premature acute myocardial infarction. *Psychosom. Med.* 55:426–33

169. Pratt LA, Ford DE, Crum RM, Armenian HK, Gallo JJ, Eaton WW. 1996. Depression, psychotropic medication, and risk of myocardial infarction. Prospective data form the Baltimore ECA follow-up. *Circulation* 94:3123–29

170. Radloff L. 1977. The CES-D Scale: a self-report depression scale for research in the general population. *Appl. Psychol. Meas.* 1:385–401

171. Ragland DR, Brand RJ. 1988. Type A behavior and mortality from coronary heart disease. *N. Engl. J. Med.* 318:65–69

172. Reich P, DeSilva RA, Lown B, Murawski BJ. 1981. Acute psychological disturbances preceding life-threatening ventricular arrhythmias. *JAMA* 246:233–35

173. Ritchie JC, Nemeroff CB. 1991. Stress, the hypothalamic-pituitary-adrenal axis, and depression. In *Stress, Neuropeptides, and Systemic Disease*, ed. JA McCubbin, PG Kaufmann, CB Nemeroff, pp. 181–97. San Diego, CA: Academic

174. Robert SA. 1999. Neighborhood socioeconomic context and adult health. The mediating role of individual health behaviors and psychosocial factors. *Ann. NY Acad. Sci.* 896:465–68

175. Roberts RE, Kaplan GA, Camacho TC. 1990. Psychological distress and mortality: evidence from the Alameda County Study. *Soc. Sci. Med.* 31:527–36

176. Roose SP, Dalack GW. 1992. Treating the depressed patient with cardiovascular problems. *J. Clin. Psychiat.* 53(Suppl.):25–31

177. Rosen G. 1963. The evolution of social medicine. In *Handbook of Medical Sociology*, ed. HE Freeman, S Levine, LG Reeder, pp. 1–61. Englewood Cliffs, NJ: Prentice Hall

178. Rosengren A, Wilhelmsen L, Orth-Gomér K. 2004. Coronary disease in relation to social support and social class in Swedish men. A 15 year follow-up in the study of men born in 1933. *Eur. Heart J.* 25:56–63

179. Rosenman RH, Brand RJ, Jenkins D, Friedman M, Straus R, Wurm M. 1975. Coronary heart disease in the Western

Collaborative Group Study: final follow-up experience of 8 1/2 years. *JAMA* 233: 872–77

180. Ross R. 1993. The pathogenesis of atherosclerosis: a perspective for the 1990s. *Nature* 362:801–9

181. Ruberman W, Weinblatt E, Goldberg JD, Chaudhary BS. 1984. Psychosocial influences on mortality after myocardial infarction. *N. Engl. J. Med.* 311:552–59

182. Sanchez MM, Aguado F, Sanchez-Toscano F, Saphier D. 1995. Effects of prolonged social isolation on responses of neurons in the bed nucleus of the stria terminalis, preoptic area, and hypothalamic paraventricular nucleus to stimulation of the medial amygdala. *Psychoneuroendocrinology* 20:525–41

183. Sapolsky R, Rivier C, Yamamoto G, Plotsky P, Vale W. 1987. Interleukin-1 stimulates the secretion of hypothalamic corticotropin-releasing factor. *Science* 238:522–24

184. Saxena PR, Villalon CM. 1990. Cardiovascular effects of serotonin agonists and antagonists. *J. Cardiovasc. Pharmacol.* 15:S17–34

185. Schlussel YR, Schnall PL, Zimbler M, Warren K, Pickering TG. 1990. The effect of work environments on blood pressure: evidence from seven New York organizations. *J. Hypertens.* 8:679–85

186. Schnall PL, Landsbergis PA, Baker D. 1994. Job strain and cardiovascular disease. *Annu. Rev. Public Health* 15:381–411

187. Schulz A, Israel B, Williams D, Parker E, Becker A, James S. 2000. Social inequalities, stressors and self reported health status among African American and white women in the Detroit metropolitan area. *Soc. Sci. Med.* 51:1639–53

188. Seeman TE, Berkman LF. 1988. Structural characteristics of social networks and their relationship with social support in the elderly: who provides support. *Soc. Sci. Med.* 26:737–49

189. Seeman TE, Berkman LF, Blazer D, Rowe JW. 1994. Social ties and support and neuroendocrine function: The MacArthur Studies of Successful Aging. *Ann. Behav. Med.* 16:95–106

190. Seeman TE, Singer BH, Rowe JW, Horwitz RI, McEwen BS. 1997. Price of adaptation-allostatic load and its health consequences. MacArthur Studies of Successful Aging. *Arch. Intern. Med.* 157:2259–68

191. Selye H. 1956. *The Stress of Life.* New York: McGraw-Hill

192. Sgoifo A, Koolhaas JM, Musso E, De Boer SF. 1999. Different sympathovagal modulation of heart rate during social and nonsocial stress episodes in wild-type rats. *Physiol. Behav.* 67:733–38

193. Shekelle RB, Gale M, Norusis M. 1985. Type A score (Jenkins Activity Survey) and risk of recurrent coronary heart disease in the Aspirin Myocardial Infarction Study. *Am. J. Cardiol.* 56:221–25

194. Shekelle RB, Hulley SB, Neaton JD, Billings JH, Borhani NO, et al. 1985. The MRFIT behavior pattern study. II. Type A behavior and incidence of coronary heart disease. *Am. J. Epidemiol.* 122:559–70

195. Shively CA, Brammer GL, Kaplan JR, Raleigh MJ, Manuck SB. 1991. The complex relationship between behavioral attributes, social status, and whole blood serotonin in male *Macaca fascicularis*. *Am. J. Primatol.* 23: 99–112

196. Siegrist J. 1996. Adverse health effects of high-effort/low-reward conditions. *J. Occup. Health Psychol.* 1:27–41

197. Siegrist J, Peter R, Junge A, Cremer P, Seidel D. 1990. Low status control, high effort at work and ischemic heart disease: prospective evidence from blue-collar men. *Soc. Sci. Med.* 31:1127–34

198. Siegrist J, Starke D, Chandola T, Godin I, Marmot M, et al. 2004. The measurement of effort-reward imbalance at work: European comparisons. *Soc. Sci. Med.* 58:1483–99

199. Sloan RP, Shapiro PA, Bigger JT Jr,

Bagiella E, Steinman RC, Gorman JM. 1994. Cardiac autonomic control and hostility in healthy subjects. *Am. J. Cardiol.* 74:298–300

200. Sluzewska A, Rybakowski J, Bosmans E, Sobieska M, Berghmans R, et al. 1996. Indicators of immune activation in major depression. *Psychiatry Res.* 64:161–67

201. Smith TW. 1992. Hostility and health: current status of a psychosomatic hypothesis. *Health Psychol.* 11:139–50

202. Spielberger CD. 1980. *Preliminary Manual for the State-Trait Personality Inventory.* Palo Alto, CA: Consult. Psychol. Press

203. Spielberger CD, Johnson EH, Russell SF, Crane R, Jacobs GA, Worden TJ. 1985. The experience and expression of anger: construction and validation of an anger expression scale. In *Anger and Hostility in Cardiovascular and Behavioral Disorders*, ed. MA Chesney, RH Rosenman, pp. 5–30. New York: Hemisphere

204. Stern SL, Dhanda R, Hazuda HP. 2001. Hopelessness predicts mortality in older Mexican and European Americans. *Psychosom. Med.* 63:344–51

205. Strik JJ, Denollet J, Lousberg R, Honig A. 2003. Comparing symptoms of depression and anxiety as predictors of cardiac events and increased health care consumption after myocardial infarction. *J. Am. Coll. Cardiol.* 42:1801–7

206. Suarez EC, Kuhn CM, Schanberg SM, Williams RB, Zimmermann EA. 1998. Neuroendocrine, cardiovascular, and emotional responses of hostile men: the role of interpersonal challenge. *Psychosom. Med.* 60:78–88

207. Suls J, Wan CK. 1993. The relationship between trait hostility and cardiovascular reactivity: a quantitative review and analysis. *Psychophysiology* 30:615–26

208. Syme SL, Berkman LF. 1976. Social class, susceptibility and sickness. *Am. J. Epidemiol.* 104:1–8

209. Syme SL, Hyman MM, Enterline PE. 1965. Cultural mobility and the occurrence of coronary heart disease. *J. Health Hum. Behav.* 6:178–89

210. Theorell T, Tsutsumi A, Hallquist J, Reuterwall C, Hogstedt C, et al. 1998. Decision latitude, job strain, and myocardial infarction: a study of working men in Stockholm. The SHEEP Study Group. Stockholm Heart Epidemiology Program. *Am. J. Public Health* 88:382–88

211. Trichopoulos D, Katsouyanni K, Zavitsanos X, Tzonou A, Dalla-Vorgia P. 1983. Psychological stress and fatal heart attack: the Athens 1981 earthquake natural experiment. *Lancet* 1:441–44

212. Troxel WM, Matthews KA, Bromberger JT, Sutton-Tyrrell K. 2003. Chronic stress burden, discrimination, and subclinical carotid artery disease in African American and Caucasian women. *Health Psychol.* 22:300–9

213. Tsuang MT, Woolson RF, Fleming JA. 1980. Causes of death in schizophrenia and manic-depression. *Br. J. Psychiatry* 136:239–42

214. Uchino BN, Cacioppo JT, Kiecolt-Glaser JK. 1996. The relationship between social support and physiological processes: a review with emphasis on underlying mechanisms and implications for health. *Psychol. Bull.* 119:488–531

215. Ulbrich PM, Warheit GJ, Zimmerman RS. 1989. Race, socioeconomic status, and psychological distress: an examination of differential vulnerability. *J. Health Soc. Behav.* 30:131–46

216. Wassertheil-Smoller S, Shumaker S, Ockene J, Talavera GA, Greenland P, et al. 2004. Depression and cardiovascular sequelae in postmenopausal women. The Women's Health Initiative (WHI). *Arch. Intern. Med.* 164:289–98

217. Watson SL, Shively CA, Kaplan JR, Line SW. 1998. Effects of chronic social separation on cardiovascular disease risk factors in female cynomolgus monkeys. *Atherosclerosis* 137:259–66

218. Weeke A, Juel K, Vaeth M. 1987. Cardio-vascular death and manic-depressive psy-chosis. *J. Affect. Disord.* 13:287–92

219. Wenneberg SR, Schneider RH, Walton KG, MacLean CRK, Levitsky DK, et al. 1997. Anger expression correlates with platelet aggregation. *Behav. Med.* 22:174–77

220. Williams DR, Neighbors H. 2001. Racism, discrimination and hypertension: evidence and needed research. *Ethn. Dis.* 11:800–16

221. Williams DR, Yu Y, Jackson J, Anderson NB. 1997. Racial differences in physical and mental health. Socio-economic status, stress and discrimination. *J. Health Psychol.* 2:335–51

222. Williams JE, Nieto FJ, Sanford CP, Couper DJ, Tyroler HA. 2002. The association between trait anger and incident stroke risk: the Atherosclerosis Risk in Communities (ARIC) Study. *Stroke* 33:13–19

223. Williams JE, Nieto FJ, Sanford CP, Tyroler HA. 2001. Effects of an angry temperament on coronary heart disease risk: The Atherosclerosis Risk in Communities Study. *Am. J. Epidemiol.* 154:230–35

224. Williams JK, Kaplan JR, Manuck SB. 1993. Effects of psychosocial stress on endothelium-mediated dilation of atherosclerotic arteries in cynomolgus monkeys. *J. Clin. Invest.* 92:1819–23

225. Williams RB, Barefoot JC, Califf RM, Haney TL, Saunders WB, et al. 1992. Prognostic importance of social and economic resources among medically treated patients with angiographically documented coronary artery disease. *JAMA* 267:520–24

226. Yan LL, Liu K, Matthews KA, Daviglus ML, Ferguson TF, Kiefe CI. 2003. Psychosocial factors and risk of hypertension: the Coronary Artery Risk Development in Young Adults (CARDIA) study. *JAMA* 290:2138–48

227. Yen IH, Kaplan GA. 1999. Neighborhood social environment and risk of death: multilevel evidence from the Alameda County Study. *Am. J. Epidemiol.* 149:898–907

228. Zhou D, Kusnecov AW, Shurin MR, De-Paoli M, Rabin BS. 1993. Exposure to physical and psychological stressors elevates plasma interleukin 6: relationship to the activation of hypothalamic-pituitary-adrenal axis. *Endocrinology* 133:2523–30

Annu. Rev. Public Health 2005. 26:501–12
doi: 10.1146/annurev.publhealth.26.021304.144351
First published online as a Review in Advance on October 14, 2004

ABORTION IN THE UNITED STATES

Cynthia C. Harper, Jillian T. Henderson,
and Philip D. Darney
*Center for Reproductive Health Research and Policy, Department of Obstetrics,
Gynecology, and Reproductive Sciences, University of California, San Francisco,
California 94143; email: harperc@obgyn.ucsf.edu, hendersonj@obgyn.ucsf.edu,
darneyp@obgyn.ucsf.edu*

Key Words legal restrictions, access to services, medical abortion, socioeconomic
disparities

■ **Abstract**   Abortion is an extremely safe and common medical procedure. In the
United States, over one million women had an abortion in the year 2000. Advances in
early abortion techniques have helped to increase the proportion of early procedures,
the safest type. Abortion rates have been declining since the early nineties among adults
and adolescents, but rates among poor, minority women remain high. State restrictions
to abortion have a larger impact on poor women and young women. Restrictions and
regulations have also resulted in the concentration of abortion services in specialized
clinics. These clinics are subject to harassment. The expansion of abortion services
to more types of providers could increase access, as well as integrate abortion into
women's health care.

LEGAL CHANGES AND STATE RESTRICTIONS

Since the passage of *Roe v. Wade* in 1973, many legal challenges to abortion rights
have been mounted. The 1992 decision *Planned Parenthood v. Casey* upheld the
right to abortion but, at the same time, gave states the right to enact restrictions that
do not create an "undue burden" for women seeking abortion. This decision encouraged numerous legal and regulatory restrictions on abortion. These restrictions
tend to have a greater effect on women who are at the highest risk of unintended
pregnancy, namely poor women and young women. The restrictions also often
define the clinical settings where services can be delivered. State regulatory restrictions, including zoning rules, state licensing, and inspection requirements,
explain the concentration of abortions in specialized abortion clinics (24).

In addition to targeted regulations, abortion restrictions that impede access
to services include state-mandated waiting periods and counseling topics, such
as showing women sonographic or other images of fetal development, parental
involvement for minors, and insurance restrictions. Although many states require
some kind of counseling, five states (Louisiana, Mississippi, Utah, Wisconsin, and
Indiana) require counseling in person at least 18 h before the procedure, which

means women must make at least two trips to the office or clinic (3). This type of requirement is particularly burdensome for women who have to travel some distance to reach a clinic, including women who live in the 87% of counties, mostly rural, that do not have abortion services (24).

Most states require parental consent or notification for minors,[1] but provide the option of seeking a court order exempting minors from the requirement. The regulations are complex, ranging from consent, notification, judicial bypass, involvement of other adult relatives, to exceptions for medical emergencies or abuse, assault, incest or neglect (4). Such extensive variation in different laws means that few minors are likely to be aware of all requirements.

Coverage of abortion costs is limited. The federal Medicaid program pays for abortion only for life endangerment, incest, or rape, as required by the Hyde Amendment [1977]. Only 18 states cover abortion under Medicaid for reasons beyond rape, incest, and life endangerment, as of December 2002. South Dakota, however, will cover Medicaid recipients only for life endangerment and not for incest or rape (5). State prohibitions on coverage for abortion exist for both public employee plans and private insurance plans. In Colorado and Kentucky, abortion coverage is never given for public employees, not even when life is at risk. In four states (Idaho, Kentucky, Missouri, and North Dakota), private insurance can cover abortion only in cases of life endangerment (6).

Federal Restrictions

During the 1990s several states passed a ban on a procedure referred to as "partial-birth" abortion, though the accepted medical term is dilation and extraction (D&X), a procedure used rarely in second-trimester terminations. The procedure accounted for approximately 0.17% or 2000 abortions in the year 2000 (19). In *Stenberg v. Carhart*, in 2000, the Supreme Court declared unconstitutional Nebraska's law criminalizing "partial-birth" abortion because the law lacked an exception to protect health and was written so broadly as to confuse D&X with other second-trimester procedures including dilation and evacuation (D&E). Whereas state courts blocked 18 state bans, in other states the bans were unchallenged (5).

The legal movement to ban D&X culminated in the passage of the federal Partial Birth Abortion Act. The Act went into effect in November 2003. However, hospitals and physicians immediately began to challenge the constitutionality of the ban because it potentially includes many different types of procedures that may be medically necessary (7). The Justice Department responded by issuing subpoenas for medical records of patients who have had abortions. However, the clinics and hospitals have stated that the subpoena violates the patient-privacy

---

[1]Thirty-three states require parental consent or notification: Alabama, Arkansas, Arizona, Delaware, Georgia, Iowa, Idaho, Indiana, Kansas, Kentucky, Louisiana, Massachusetts, Maryland, Michigan, Minnesota, Missouri, Mississippi, North Carolina, North Dakota, Nebraska, Ohio, Pennsylvania, Rhode Island, South Carolina, South Dakota, Tennessee, Texas, Utah, Virginia, Wisconsin, West Virginia, and Wyoming.

provisions of the Health Insurance Portability and Accountability Act (HIPAA), and the Justice Department has amended its request for patient records and lists of physicians who provide abortion at the plaintiff institutions (34). The Federal District Court in San Francisco recently rejected the constitutionality of the ban, but decisions are pending in other cases and appeals are likely to bring the legislation before the Supreme Court.

Clinics Under Siege

Harassment and violence have aroused fear in women seeking abortions and are significant factors in the decline in the numbers of abortion providers over the past few decades. In response to clinic harassment and violence, in 1994 the federal government enacted the Freedom of Access to Clinic Entrances Act, prohibiting property damage, use of force or threat of force, or obstruction of someone entering a clinic. Several states have passed specific legislation to ensure the federal act is upheld (8). However, harassment is still common, particularly at larger clinics. Eighty percent of providers of 440 or more abortions per year reported harassment in 2000, 28% reported picketing with physical contact with patients, 18% reported vandalism, 14% reported picketing homes of staff, and 15% reported receiving bomb threats. Aside from picketing, other types of harassment have declined since implementation of the act to protect clinics (24).

In addition to harassment, there have also been attempts to arouse fear in women seeking services by linking abortion to the risk of breast cancer. Although scientific evidence does not support this link (14, 15), it took a full panel of experts to remove misleading information from the Web site of the National Cancer Institute. However, the misinformation did not stop at the Web site; several states enacted legislation that required the inclusion of misleading breast cancer information as part of "informed consent" for abortion. In some states it is also required to include photographs of developing fetuses and descriptions of mental and physical risks not proven to be associated with abortion.

SERVICES

Advances in medicine and other areas have helped to improve abortion services in spite of the myriad factors that work to block access. Abortion in the early first trimester (before eight weeks) is far more accessible than in the past, and the choice of methods has expanded to include several regimens of medical abortion and manual uterine aspiration. Advancements in abortion clinic protocols, such as the requirement of fewer clinic visits and provision of all types of contraception, including emergency contraception, have increased convenience for women and efficiency for clinics and decreased costs (32, 37). Clinical research on abortion continues to improve the safety of the various procedures and opens up new possibilities for the future as well (21, 36). Scientific progress in abortion research and improvements in services are important for women's health because induced abortion is among the most common medical procedures in the United States. In the year 2000 there were 1.31 million abortions. Nearly half of American women will have one or more in their lifetimes (19).

Although abortion is a common procedure, the abortion rate has been declining over time since the early nineties. In 1973, when abortion was first made legal throughout the United States, there were 16.3 abortions per 1000 women aged 15–44; the rate increased to 29.3 in 1982 and fell to 21.3 in 2000 (19). The adolescent abortion rate has been declining since 1987, and from the mid-nineties to 2000, it declined at a faster rate than that of adult women (28). Almost 90% of abortions occur in the first trimester (by 12 weeks gestation), and more than 98% are done by 20 weeks gestation (19).

The majority of abortions in the United States are provided in freestanding clinics. Clinics provided 93% of abortions in 2000; specialized abortion clinics provided 71%. Hospitals provided 5%, down from 22% in 1980. Physicians' offices accounted for only 2% of abortions (19). Although this service delivery model has been satisfactory for many years, it has also served to isolate abortion from the broader spectrum of women's health care and has made providers and clients more susceptible to antiabortion harassment and violence. If abortion services were integrated into mainstream medical care, harassment and violence would be less common.

Demographic Characteristics

Data from a nationally representative survey of women undergoing abortions in 2000–2001 showed the overall adolescent abortion rate (aged 15–19 years) to be 25 per 1000 women aged 15–19; the younger adolescents, ages 15–17 years, had a rate of 15 per 1000; and ages 18–19 years had a rate of 39 per 1000. Women aged 20–24 years had the highest rate of 47 per 1000. Higher rates among young women ages 18–24 years are due to lower usage of effective contraception in that age range than in older women, as well as to higher fecundity (28).

Women who are unmarried (single or cohabiting) are more likely to have abortions than are married women. Low-income women also have more abortions because they have far more unintended pregnancies than do high-income women. Abortion rates in the year 2000 among low-income women were 44 per 1000 compared with 10 per 1000 among high income. Abortion rates fell for high- and middle-income women from the mid-nineties to the year 2000, but they increased among low-income and Medicaid recipients, including low-income teenagers. Black women are more likely to have unintended pregnancies than are women in other racial/ethnic groups, and thus they are more likely to have abortions. The abortion rate is 49 per 1000 for blacks, 33 per 1000 for Hispanics, 31 per 1000 for Asians, and 13 per 1000 for whites (28).

Safety

After legalization, deaths and morbidity caused by abortion experienced a steep and rapid decline (12, 18, 42). Data from the Abortion Mortality Surveillance

System of the Centers for Disease Control and Prevention show that the risk of death associated with abortion is low, at 0.6 per 100,000 abortions. The risk of death from childbirth is 11 times greater than the risk of death from abortion. The causes of death from abortion are equally distributed among hemorrhage, infection, embolism, and anesthesia complications. The risk of major complications is less than 1%, and there is no evidence of subsequent childbearing problems among women who have had abortions (18).

Early procedures are extremely safe. Most deaths result from abortion during more advanced gestational periods. Bartlett et al. (9) estimated the relative risk of abortion-related mortality at higher gestations compared with abortions at 8 weeks or less. The relative risk was 14.7 at 13–15 weeks gestation, 29.5 at 16–20 weeks, and 76.6 at 20+ weeks (95% CI 32.5, 180.8). The authors concluded that up to 87% of deaths in women having abortions may have been avoided if the pregnancy had been terminated before 8 weeks gestation. Increased access to abortion services, and particularly early abortion services, may help to decrease abortion-related deaths.

Early Abortion

Before 1990 provision of early abortion was rare. However, a growing proportion of providers now offer very early abortion: Whereas only 7% of providers offered early abortion in 1993, 37% did in 2000. Abortion clinics are more likely to offer very early abortion than are other providers. The proportion of abortions performed in early pregnancy (up to 6 weeks gestational age) increased from 14% in 1992 to 22% in 1999 (19).

Research has shown high rates of success at early gestational ages with both medical and surgical abortion owing to advances such as vaginal ultrasonography and highly sensitive urine pregnancy tests (17). Manual uterine aspiration, a non-electric aspiration technique used in low-resource settings for postabortion care, has recently been shown to be an acceptable and effective method in the United States as well (20). Manual uterine aspiration can be used for early abortion and as a backup for failed medical abortions.

Medical Abortion

In September 2000, the U.S. Food and Drug Administration (FDA) approved mifepristone for abortion in the United States. While methotrexate had been available earlier for medical abortion, its use was off-label and infrequent. Distribution of mifepristone began in November 2000, and in the first half of 2001, there were approximately 37,000 medical abortions, or 6% of all abortions. One third of abortion providers offered medical abortion in that time period: 72% of these used mifepristone, and the rest used methotrexate. Medical abortion was more likely to be available from large clinics that already used surgical methods than from doctors' offices or hospitals. The average cost of a medical abortion in nonhospital facilities in 2000 was $490 (24). By comparsion, the inflation-adjusted cost of surgical abortion remained steady until the late nineties, and then began to rise;

the average client paid $319 for surgical abortion at 10 weeks in 1997 and $373 in 2001 (24).

Research has shown that medical abortion can be provided in any physician's office or medical facility and that it could be done successfully by all types of providers (10). Because the method requires no surgical training, primary care physicians, family practice physicians, internists, and adolescent health specialists could offer medical abortion (26). The involvement of nurse practitioners and physicians' assistants, along with more streamlined protocols such as home use of misoprostol, can reduce the cost of medical abortions. The expansion of abortion services outside of specialized clinics also means that abortions could take place in privacy, outside of the scrutiny of picketers and protesters (11, 22).

However, integrating medical methods of abortion into mainstream medical practice will take some experimentation and flexibility. The FDA-approved labeling is restrictive (use within 7 weeks gestational age, mifepristone dose 600 mg; misoprostol oral dose in person in physician's office; follow-up visit for exam). In addition, other requirements such as sonographic evaluation, backup for surgical abortion, and direct ordering of the drug rather than availability through pharmacies have hindered the expansion to providers who do not perform surgical abortions (27).

Both research and clinical practice have shown more convenient and efficient approaches to be safe and effective, including a 200-mg, rather than a 600-mg, dose of mifepristone, vaginal rather than oral misoprostal, and fewer clinic visits (35, 37, 38). Most providers in the United States have adopted the newer, convenient protocols, giving a dose of 200 mg mifepristone (83%) and allowing the client to take misoprostol at home (84%) (24). The experience in Europe with medical abortion has shown that although it has taken a long time to integrate services into the health care system, once this integration happens over half of women seeking early abortion choose medical abortion. The availability of medical abortion services in Europe has not increased overall abortion rates, although women have begun to seek abortions earlier in the pregnancy.

ACCESS TO ABORTION

Geography

Many women in need of an abortion face obstacles to services. For example, women encounter bureaucratic barriers such as state laws requiring waiting periods and parental consent prior to obtaining an abortion. Another barrier to access is the absence of physicians who do abortions. The number of abortion providers has declined substantially since rising to a peak level in 1982 (24). The percentage of counties without an abortion provider has remained high since 1973. Yet more counties than ever lack an abortion provider: 87% of counties had no abortion provider as of the year 2000, and these counties contain over one third of the population of women aged 15–44 (19). Consequently, nearly one quarter (24%) of women seeking an abortion travel 50 miles or more to find a capable physician (24). Long travel distances, along with mandatory wait periods, can delay services (28).

Counties without an abortion provider usually are in a rural region. Just 3% of nonmetropolitan counties have an abortion provider. Abortion providers are more likely to be found in urban areas; nonetheless, over one third of metropolitan areas have no abortion provider. Women in the northeast and the western regions of the United States are served by a greater number of abortion providers than are women in other regions; these regions also have less-restrictive laws, and abortion rates are higher. Some variation in state abortion rates can be attributed to women's travel from states that have fewer providers or more-restrictive policies and gestational limits to states where they can receive care (25). An example is the decline in the Wisconsin abortion rate after the passage of a two-day mandatory delay law and a concomitant rise in Illinois.

Providers and Training

Currently the majority of abortion providers are physicians specializing in obstetrics and gynecology (OB-GYN). A smaller proportion of providers who offer abortions are family practice physicians and general internists. Interest in offering medication abortion was relatively high among obstetrician gynecologists, family practice physicians, and even nonphysician providers (APNs, CNMs, PAs) prior to the approval of mifepristone (23). Consequently, in states permitting nonphysician clinicians to offer first-trimester abortions (e.g., Colorado, Maine, and California), small numbers of nurse practitioners (NP), physician assistants (PA), and certified nurse midwives (CNM) have sought training and are beginning to provide first-trimester abortions.

Abortion training opportunities, which had remained at low levels for more than two decades, have begun to increase, though primarily as an optional rather than a mandatory component of medical education. More OB-GYN residency programs are including abortion training as a routine part of medical education (2). For example, all public hospitals offering OB-GYN residencies in New York City must now provide abortion training; California passed similar legislation in 2002 applying to state-supported residencies. In 1991–1992, 70% of residency programs in obstetrics and gynecology offered first-trimester abortion training; however, only 12% of OB-GYN residency programs included the training as a standard component of medical education (33). Residency programs in family medicine are also beginning to incorporate abortion training, but levels of training among family practice residents remain low: Only 12% of residencies provided the option in 1994 (41). A survey found that 29% offered optional or routine training in first-trimester abortion, but only 15% of chief residents had any clinical experience providing abortion (39). Changes to graduate medical education requirements and the development of new fellowship programs in family planning may increase the availability of abortion training. The likelihood that a physician will offer abortion services is highly associated with the training they receive during residency (1, 40).

FUTURE PROSPECTS

Early Abortion

New abortion techniques and medical protocols that have recently been developed are expanding the options women have for obtaining abortions in the early weeks of an unwanted pregnancy. The benefits for women are substantial, as are the potential benefits for abortion access. Expanded abortion options in the first eight weeks of pregnancy are available using either medication or manual uterine aspiration. The availability of medication abortion is increasing, but only approximately one third of abortion facilities offer it (24). A survey of National Abortion Federation (NAF) members in 2000 found that 59% of sites were offering early surgical or medication abortion (11), and in early 2002, two thirds of NAF members were offering medication abortion (30). The expansion of medication abortion services in France, Great Britain, and Sweden provide some insight into the potential for the United States because these countries approved mifepristone years ago and have observed the diffusion of the new option (30), though in a much-less-contested political environment. In each of these countries, medical abortion became more accessible over time. Given the size of the United States and the absence of providers in most counties, medication abortion has the potential to increase access.

Unique barriers to offering medical abortion and strategies to overcome them have been identified for the United States (13). The opportunities to make abortion available in new settings and to expand the number of providers increase with these new options, but they will not be realized without organizational and financial assistance to training programs wanting to establish new services.

Contraceptive Use

A recent nationally representative study of contraceptive use among women obtaining abortions found that more than half of women were using some kind of contraceptive (either consistently or inconsistently) in the month they became pregnant (29). Low-income women were more likely to report difficulty accessing contraceptive services as one reason for their nonuse or inconsistency. Reductions in Medicaid health insurance coverage and stagnating Title X funding for reproductive health services and supplies are undoubtedly decreasing access to contraceptives in many states. Women and couples need a range of contraceptive options and comprehensive information to help them select and use a method that suits their needs.

Sixteen percent of all women obtaining abortions became pregnant because they were not expecting to have sex (29). Research suggests that increased emphasis on abstinence as a method of contraception may result in increased demand for abortion; although theoretical effectiveness is high, use effectiveness is low. Emergency contraception use may be responsible for some of the decline in the abortion rate during the nineties (29).

Sociodemographics, Social Disparities, and Abortion

Public health researchers and policy makers are increasingly attentive to social disparities in health and health care access in the United States (43). But little attention is paid to trends in abortion and how they are affecting women differently by race and class. In recent years, the rate of abortion has risen among low-income women (those living below 200% of the federal poverty line) so that these women account for over half of all abortions obtained in the United States, although they comprise only 15% of the population. Abortion rates among black and Hispanic women have risen in recent years, whereas rates fell for white women. Access to information, education, quality health care, and contraceptive methods and services may contribute to the disparity in rates. Policies and programs that help women avoid unintended pregnancy are important public health measures, but maintaining access to abortion services is also critical to the lives of women with limited resources.

Changes in welfare policy in the United States may affect abortion access and incidence. The 1996 Personal Responsibility and Work Opportunity Reconciliation Act (P.L. 104–193) introduced new U.S. welfare policy that included work requirements and permitted states to place caps on the amount of money a woman could receive irrespective of her family size. The reform to welfare policy was driven, in part, by public perceptions that poor women were having additional children to get more money from the government. Twenty-three states implemented the family cap policies, which were intended to discourage women reliant on Temporary Assistance for Needy Families (TANF) from having more children. The act may reduce women's capacity to support children and might increase rates of abortion. Research on the impact of welfare reform and family cap policies on abortion rates is limited but has not found such an association thus far (16, 31). The increase in abortion rates for poor women that has occurred in recent years, as overall rates have fallen, could be partially a result of the economic pressures poor families increasingly face; but no evidence supports the assumption that poor families have changed their childbearing patterns because of changes in welfare policy. Broadening the abortion rights platform to include the right to bear children and to support wanted children with profamily policies could result in reductions in the abortion rate for low-income women if some of these women are having abortions for economic reasons. Conversely, if they want fewer children for other reasons, such as work opportunity, rates may not change.

Women over the age of 25 comprise a greater proportion of the population of women having abortions than they did in 1973. Increases in the mean age for women at first marriage, as well as changes in the U.S. age structure, may have contributed to this shift. In addition, women under the age of 18 have faced increasing challenges to their autonomy and access to confidential abortion services with more states mandating parental involvement. The impact of parental involvement laws on abortion rates is difficult to estimate. Teen pregnancy rates have fallen overall in recent years, so declines in abortion rates for this age group do not necessarily reflect reduced access to services. Comparisons of abortion rates in states with parental consent laws and states without parental consent laws are also difficult to interpret since some women cross state lines to obtain abortions.

FUTURE

Interpreting the 30 years of trend data on legal abortion incidence is challenging but important because the sources of change in abortion rates have very different public health implications. Increased use of more effective contraceptives, for example, would support a positive interpretation of a downward trend. A decline due to decreased access to abortion, however, could have detrimental effects on the health of women and children. Similarly, if legal restrictions were responsible, women might be unable to gain access to safe abortion and rely on unsafe, clandestine sources. As more effective long-acting contraceptives are utilized, there is potential for the abortion rate to decline. Access to health services and contraception, however, is not evenly distributed in the United States, and it is likely that reductions in the need for abortion will occur among the most privileged segments of the population. Such a demographic shift may further undermine support for access to safe and legal abortion.

The reasons women unintentionally become pregnant are many, and pregnancy is not always avoidable. Therefore, abortion will continue to be an important component of women's health care even with the advent of better methods of contraception. New developments in abortion technology and practice are encouraging because they have the potential to increase access to earlier (and hence safer) abortion. Integrating abortion care into settings where it has not been available and increasing the number of providers may be more possible with medical abortion than it has been in the past with surgical abortion.

The public health implications of legal and safe access to abortion are clear. Women's lives are saved when they are able to terminate unwanted pregnancies as early as possible and in safe medical conditions. Legalizing abortion in the United States has allowed women to get abortions earlier and has dramatically decreased the rate of complications and deaths related to induced abortion. Furthermore, the legality of abortion has allowed researchers to develop and improve the technologies and procedures that make abortion safer than it has ever been (12). Unfortunately, abortion remains highly contested in U.S. society and politics and is also stigmatized within medicine.

The *Annual Review of Public Health* is online at
http://publhealth.annualreviews.org

REFERENCES

1. Aiyer AN, Ruiz G, Steinman A, Ho GYF. 1991. Influence of physician attitudes on willingness to perform abortion. *Obstet. Gynecol.* 93:576–80

2. Almeling R, Tews L, Dudley S. 2000. Abortion training in U.S. obstetrics and gynecology residency programs, 1998. *Fam. Plann. Perspect.* 32:268–71

3. Alan Guttmacher Inst. 2004a. *State Policies in Brief: Mandatory Counseling and Waiting Periods for Abortion.* New York: AGI

4. Alan Guttmacher Inst. 2004b. *State Policies in Brief: Parental Involvement in Minors' Abortions.* New York: AGI

5. Alan Guttmacher Inst. 2004c. *State Policies in Brief: Restricting Insurance Coverage of Abortion.* New York: AGI

6. Alan Guttmacher Inst. 2004d. *State Policies in Brief: State Funding of Abortion Under Medicaid.* New York: AGI

7. Alan Guttmacher Inst. 2004e. *State Policies in Brief: Bans on "Partial-Birth Abortion."* New York: AGI

8. Alan Guttmacher Inst. 2004f. *State Policies in Brief: Protecting Access to Clinics.* New York: AGI

9. Bartlett LA, Berg CJ, Shulman HB, Zane SB, Green CA, et al. 2004. Risk factors for legal induced abortion-related mortality in the United States. *Obstet. Gynecol.* 103:729–37

10. Beckman LJ, Harvey SM, Satre SJ. 2002. The delivery of medical abortion services: the views of experienced providers. *Women's Health Issues* 12:103–12

11. Benson J, Clark KA, Gerhardt A, Randall L, Dudley S. 2003. Early abortion services in the United States: a provider survey. *Contraception* 67:287–94

12. Cates WJ, Grimes DA, Schulz KF. 2003. The public health impact of legal abortion: 30 years later. *Perspect. Sex. Reprod. Health* 35:25–28

13. Coeytaux F, Moore K, Gelberg L. 2003. Convincing new providers to offer medical abortion: What will it take? *Perspect. Sex. Reprod. Health* 35:44–47

14. Collab. Group Horm. Factors Breast Cancer. 2004. Breast cancer and abortion: collaborative reanalysis of data from 53 epidemiological studies, including 83,000 women with breast cancer from 16 countries. *Lancet* 363:1007–16

15. Comm. Gynecol. Pract. Am. Coll. Obstet. Gynecol. 2003. ACOG committee opinion.

Induced abortion and breast cancer: Number 285, August 2003. *Int. J. Gynaecol. Obstet.* 83:233–35

16. Donovan P. 1998. Does the family cap influence birthrates?: Two new studies say "no". *Guttmach. Rep. Pub. Pol.* 1:10–11

17. Edwards J, Carson SA. 1997. New technologies permit safe abortion at less than six weeks' gestation and provide timely detection of ectopic gestation. *Am. J. Obstet. Gynecol.* 176:1101–6

18. Elam-Evans L, Strauss LT, Herndon J, Parker WY, Bowens SV, et al. 2003. Abortion Surveillance, United States, 2000. *MMWR* 52:1–32

19. Finer LB, Henshaw SK. 2003. Abortion incidence and services in the United States in 2000. *Perspect. Sex. Reprod. Health* 35:6–15

20. Goldberg AB, Dean G, Kang MS, Darney PD. 2004. Manual versus electric vacuum aspiration for early first-trimester abortion: a controlled study of complication rates. *Obstet. Gynecol.* 103:101–7

21. Grossman D, Ellertson C, Grimes DA, Walker D. 2004. Routine follow-up visits after first tri-mester induced abortion. *Obstet. Gynecol.* 103:738–45

22. Harper C, Ellertson C, Winikoff B. 2001. Could American women use mifepristone safely with less medical supervision? *Contraception* 65:133–42

23. Henry J. Kaiser Family Found. 1998. *Two National Surveys: Views of Americans and Health Care Providers on Medical Abortion: What They Know, What They Think, and What They Want.* Menlo Park, CA: The Foundation

24. Henshaw SK, Finer LB. 2003. The accessibility of abortion services in the United States, 2001. *Perspect. Sex. Reprod. Health* 35:16–24

25. Herndon J, Strauss LT, Whitehead S, Parker WY, Bartlett L, Zane S. 2002. Abortion Surveillance—United States 1998. *Cent. Dis. Control, MMWR* 51:1–32

26. Joffe C. 2003. Roe v. Wade at 30: What are

the prospects for abortion provision? *Perspect. Sex. Reprod. Health* 35:29–33

27. Joffe C, Weitz TA. 2003. Normalizing the exceptional: incorporating the "abortion pill" into mainstream medicine. *Soc. Sci. Med.* 56:2353–66

28. Jones RK, Darroch JE, Henshaw S. 2002. Patterns in the socioeconomic characteristics of women obtaining abortions in 2000–2001. *Perspect. Sex. Reprod. Health* 34:226–35

29. Jones RK, Darroch JE, Henshaw SK. 2002. Contraceptive use among U.S. women having abortions in 2000–2001. *Perspect. Sex. Reprod. Health* 34:294–303

30. Jones RK, Henshaw S. 2002. Mifepristone for early medical abortion: experiences in France, Great Britain and Sweden. *Perspect. Sex. Reprod. Health* 34:154–61

31. Joyce T, Kaestner R, Korenman S, Henshaw S. 2004. *Family cap provisions and changes in births and abortions.* Work. Pap. 10214, Natl. Bur. Econ. Res.

32. Kirin U, Amin P, Penketh RJ. 2004. Self-administration of misoprostol for termination of pregnancy: safety and efficacy. *J. Obstet. Gynaecol.* 24:155–56

33. MacKay HT, McKay AP. 1995. Abortion training in obstetrics and gynecology residency programs in the United States, 1991–1992. *Fam. Plann. Perspect.* 27:112–15

34. McLellan F. 2004. US judges seek medical records in abortion cases. *Lancet* 363:626

35. Newhall EP, Winikoff B. 2000. Abortion with mifepristone and misoprostol: regimens, efficacy, acceptability and fu-

ture directions. *Am. J. Obstret. Gynecol.* 183:S44–53

36. Schaff EA, Fielding SL, Westhoff C, Ellertson C, Eisinger SH, et al. 2000. Vaginal misoprostol administered 1, 2 or 3 days after mifepristone for early medical abortion. *JAMA* 284:1948–53

37. Schaff E, Eisinger S, Stadalius L, Franks P, Gore B, Poppema S. 1999. Low dose mifepristone 200 mg and vaginal misoprostol for abortion. *Contraception* 59:1–6

38. Schaff EA, Fielding SL, Eisinger SH, Stadalius LS, Fuller L. 2000. Low-dose mifepristone followed by vaginal misoprostol at 48 hours for abortion up to 63 days. *Contraception* 61:41–46

39. Steinauer JE, DePineres T, Robert AM, Westfall J, Darney P. 1997. Training family practice residents in abortion and other reproductive health care: a nationwide survey. *Fam. Plann. Perspect.* 29:222–27

40. Steinauer JE, Landy U, Jackson RA, Darney PD. 2003. The effect of training on the provision of elective abortion: a survey of five residency programs. *Am. J. Obstet. Gynecol.* 188:1161–63

41. Talley PP, Bergus GR. 1996. Abortion training in family medicine residency training programs. *Fam. Pract.* 28:245–48

42. Tietze C. 1975. The effect of legalization of abortion on population growth and public health. *Fam. Plann. Perspect.* 7:123–27

43. U.S. Dep. Health Hum. Serv. 2000. *Healthy People 2010: Understanding and Improving Health.* Washington, DC: US Gov. Print. Off. 2nd ed.

Annu. Rev. Public Health 2005. 26:513–59
doi: 10.1146/annurev.publhealth.25.050503.153958

PATIENT PERCEPTIONS OF THE QUALITY OF HEALTH SERVICES

Shoshanna Sofaer and Kirsten Firminger

School of Public Affairs, Baruch College, New York, NY 10010;
email: shoshanna_sofaer@baruch.cuny.edu

Key Words patient satisfaction, performance reporting, patient experiences, patient expectations, consumer satisfaction

■ **Abstract** As calls are made for a more patient-centered health care system, it becomes critical to define and measure patient perceptions of health care quality and to understand more fully what drives those perceptions. This chapter identifies conceptual and methodological issues that make this task difficult, including the confusion between patient perceptions and patient satisfaction and the difficulty of determining whether systematic variations in patient perceptions should be attributed to differences in expectations or actual experiences. We propose a conceptual model to help unravel these knotty issues; review qualitative studies that report directly from patients on how they define quality; provide an overview of how health plans, hospitals, physicians, and health care in general are currently viewed by patients; assess whether and how patient health status and demographic characteristics relate to perceptions of health care quality; and identify where further, or more appropriately designed, research is needed.

> Our aim is to find out what patients want, need and experience in health care, not what professionals (however well-motivated) believe they need or get.
>
> *Through the Patient's Eyes* (23)

INTRODUCTION

Purpose and Content of this Chapter

In its groundbreaking work *Crossing the Quality Chasm*, the Institute of Medicine identified providing patient-centered care as one of six aims of the health care system (35). Further, among its simple rules to achieve quality are two rules stating that "[c]ustomization based on patients' needs and values" is needed and that "[t]he patient is the source of control" of interactions with the health care delivery system[1] (35). These are just two of the many signs that, within health care, the

---

[1] Note that the report calls for such control at the microlevel of interactions between patients and providers/facilities. It apparently did not consider the potential of patient control at the governance level of health care practice and policy.

513

role of patients has gained greater significance for many, though not all, providers, policy makers, and researchers. Nevertheless, our understanding of patient perceptions of quality is still in its childhood, if not its infancy, in part because patients themselves still have fairly inchoate and pliable understandings of what quality means and, as noted in Hibbard & Peters' earlier *Annual Review* chapter (31), tend to have constructed rather than stable preferences about health related choices.

The purpose of this review is to summarize what we do and do not know about several, though not all, aspects of patient perceptions of health care quality. We begin by putting the issues into an intellectual and policy context. We then address conceptual issues that plague us in trying to understand the sources and consequences of patient perceptions, including the confusion between patient perceptions and patient satisfaction. We propose a conceptual model as a framework to guide both our review and our recommendations for further study. We then review a series of qualitative studies that (unlike most closed-ended surveys) permit researchers to hear more directly from patients, in their own languages, how they define quality and what is important to them about quality in health care. We briefly confirm that indeed patient perspectives on quality are somewhat, though not entirely, distinct from those of clinicians and that little if any systematic attention has been paid to the stability of patient perceptions and thus to the criteria patients use in making assessments of quality.

The next section reviews existing data, primarily from a variety of patient experience and/or satisfaction surveys, to provide an overview of how health plans, hospitals, physicians, and health care in general are viewed currently by patients. Next, we examine research that has analyzed whether, how, and in what direction key demographic characteristics of survey respondents, and their health statuses, are related to their reports and ratings of health care. In the course of these discussions, we point out the attribution difficulties and other interpretative problems inherent in such studies. We end with an overall assessment of the field and point out areas where further, or more appropriately designed, research is needed on this important topic.

Intellectual and Policy Context

At least two major intellectual forces are driving attention to patient perceptions of quality. They are (*a*) the dominance of market-oriented approaches to reforms in health care delivery and cost; and (*b*) the emergence of a normative perspective on clinical practice that emphasizes the need to deliver patient-centered care (e.g., 13, 23, 47, 49, 54, 55).

Those espousing a market-oriented approach to health policy take the position that the health care system will operate more effectively and efficiently, producing greater value (high quality for the price) if the market failures historically found in health care are identified and reduced. This orientation emerged as the nation rejected voluntary efforts such as community health planning, which died in the early 1980s (73). Historically, health care was seen as a monopoly with power concentrated in the hands of providers, especially physicians, who had and still have considerable ability to determine what type and volume of services will be provided, to whom, in which settings and facilities (80). The first significant break in this pattern emerged when those who purchase health care coverage and services for actual patients (i.e., employers, labor unions, and public agencies), in reaction to substantial and continuing cost increases, began to recognize that they could play a far more aggressive role in driving down costs. Early business and health coalitions did not appear to have much of an impact on their original target, reducing cost inflation (6), except when they focused on protecting themselves against cost-shifts from public-coverage programs to private payers (4). More recently, however, purchaser coalitions both huge (e.g., the Pacific Business Group on Health) and more moderate in size (e.g., the Central Florida Health Care Coalition, the Buyer's Health Care Action Group in Minnesota) as well as individual behemoths of industry such as General Motors, General Electric, and Xerox have been far more effective in negotiating premium prices, benefit structures, and quality targets with health plans and, more recently, directly with provider systems.

Did this shift in market power lead to a focus on patients (i.e., employees, covered lives) or to a focus on prices paid by purchasers of coverage and care, including health plans themselves? It appears that, at least on the level of rhetoric, this realignment of market forces made users of care more relevant. Purchasers naturally desire both to protect their bottom line and to serve the interests of those for whom they are making sizable premium contributions. In addition, they too want to improve the effectiveness of the marketplace, which has traditionally been viewed as having failed because the patient, at the point of service, has little awareness of the cost consequences of their behaviors (30, 65). Further, employers want the health care they purchase to improve the health and productivity of their work force. Public purchasers of care, for populations such as people with Medicaid or with Medicare, also see themselves both as protecting the health of these constituencies and, especially in the Medicare program, paying increasing attention to how the behavior of individual beneficiaries in a market context can drive plans and providers to offer greater value. Thus, to at least some extent, focus on a market orientation to health policy increases the focus on the person choosing and using health care coverage and services, the person who is, or may become, a patient.

The other major driver of attention to patients has been, in fact, the movement toward patient-centered care. For many years, the Federal government supported community health planning and eventually mandated that consumers be in the majority in the governance of planning agencies. Since the demise of that effort, those concerned that our health system reflects democratic values, that the public should be the major beneficiary, may have shifted focus to the experience of patients. Indeed, the world of medical care was becoming increasingly difficult for patients to navigate. Specialization led to fragmentation of care, an increasingly noticeable absence of care coordination, and little recognition that the patient was a whole, multi-faceted human being (23). In spite of growing evidence of the significant effect of psychosocial and behavioral factors in the onset and presentation and prognosis of many illnesses (26), a biomedical model remained dominant in medical practice. In a country with growing population diversity, care was nevertheless increasingly standardized (and not necessarily in compliance with practice guidelines) rather than customized to individual patient and family needs or preferences. As chronic disease became more prevalent, the need for ongoing, productive relationships between patients and physicians and other providers became more critical (90); yet evidence has grown that what is termed patient adherence to medical advice was sketchy at best, often because of failures in the physician-patient relationship (3, 7, 24). In sum, late twentieth-century medical civilization had an increasing number of discontents.

Following are two final and related points about this growing focus on the centrality of the patient. First, a patient focus has always been a hallmark of advocates who historically have been concerned about achieving equal access to health care. Such advocates are often uncomfortable about market-oriented strategies for health care reform. For them, a strong patient orientation means emphasizing patient protection through strong regulatory action. They typically distrust market-oriented strategies, which are seen as putting the most vulnerable patient populations at great risk. Contrast this with the emphasis of many purchasers on patient empowerment, which when operationalized often means simultaneously providing patients with more choices while putting them at greater financial risk, all to encourage them to act prudently in their own self interest (77). Thus, though the notions of patient-centered care and a consumer-driven health system (30) have gained currency, this does not mean stakeholders and analysts agree about what these terms mean or why it is important to pay attention to patient perceptions of quality.

Second, a greater focus on the patient is linked to the drive for greater accountability, or transparency, in health care. The issue of accountability has several significant implications for examinations of patient perceptions of quality. For example, it raises the question of exactly whom patients hold responsible for the quality of the care they receive, and thus whose quality should be measured. It is difficult to gather information on quality from patients if they do not believe that the questioner is asking questions about the right individual or entity. In addition, the public reporting of quality measures associated with a more accountable health care system requires care in the development of instruments to provide a patient perspective on the quality of plans and providers. The authors hope that this review helps move the field toward ever more patient-driven measures, which reflect patient definitions of quality rather than only clinical or managerial views of what questions about quality patients should be asked.

Why are patient perceptions of quality important? There are two perspectives one can take in answering this question. First, one can be normative and say that patient perceptions of quality are inherently meaningful and should be a primary focus of attention within the health care system. Second, one can take the position that we have to pay attention to patient perceptions because they are powerful drivers of outcomes important to various other stakeholders, outcomes such as patient choice of plan or provider, patient adherence to medical advice (3, 7, 24), patient complaints (86), grievances (28), the level and seriousness of malpractice claims (32, 33), or, perhaps most important, actual health and functional status outcomes (7, 10a, 13a, 22a, 26a, 40a, 81, 52, 52a). We presume to take both positions in this paper, to posit that patient perceptions have both inherent and instrumental value.

However, we recognize that there is far from unanimity on the importance of patient perceptions of quality. Skeptics still voice concern that patients simply do not know enough (or perhaps even care enough) about medicine to have perceptions of health care quality that should be taken seriously by the delivery system. Some will grudgingly admit that patient perceptions may be important when it comes to service quality in health care, things like how easy it is to get an appointment or how politely patients are treated by the office staff. But these skeptics believe that it is important that patients get the right diagnostic and treatment services, delivered the right way, at the right time, in the right kind of facility, by properly trained clinicians, so that they maximize their chances for having positive health outcomes. And many patients would agree with this statement. Jane Austen makes a critical distinction, in her novel *Sense and Sensibility*, between ignorance (not knowing something) and stupidity (being incapable of learning anything). Although patients are often ignorant about some elements of what it takes to maximize health care quality and health outcomes, they are not stupid. Knowledge about what it takes to maximize quality is not inherently incomprehensible to patients (when we as professionals know it ourselves). This review, in fact, moves toward the conclusion that a truly complete understanding of patient perceptions of quality will not emerge until we have more effectively educated patients about the pathways through which positive health outcomes are achieved.

THE NATURE OF PATIENT PERCEPTIONS OF QUALITY

Conceptual Issues

For many years, patient satisfaction has been widely studied. Considerable effort has gone into developing survey instruments to measure patient satisfaction. Until the recent drive toward accountability, there were two major uses of such instruments: first, in research studies in which patient satisfaction was considered an outcome, either to assess the value of a new intervention or to identify patient characteristics that appear to influence quality assessment; second, by health plans, hospitals, and other providers to assess the satisfaction of their members or patients with their services. The results of such surveys were rarely reported publicly, except in advertising campaigns.

PATIENT PERCEPTIONS VERSUS PATIENT SATISFACTION   The terms perceptions and satisfaction have often been used interchangeably (95). This can lead to considerable conceptual confusion. Satisfaction is an example of a perception, but it is by no means the only example. Satisfaction can be defined as fulfilling expectations, needs, or desires (72). In their comprehensive review of the literature on patient satisfaction, Crow and colleagues (16) stated that two conclusions follow from this definition: (*a*) Satisfaction does not imply superior service, only adequate or acceptable service; and (*b*) satisfaction is a relative concept—therefore, what satisfies one person may dissatisfy another. Even though satisfaction is not the only form of patient assessment of care, patient satisfaction and its correlates are predominant in quality care assessment studies. Most reviews of the literature have been critical of its use since there is rarely any theoretical or conceptual development of patient satisfaction, little standardization, low reliability, and uncertain validity of measures (16, 57).

Crow identifies three bases for the conceptual development of patient satisfaction and its measurement: expectation theories; evaluations of health services attributes; and economics, in particular, utility. These authors also point to a fourth possibility, a holistic approach that incorporates a wide range of determinants of satisfaction and emphasizes feedback loops between expectations and experiences (16, 59, 83, 84).

EXPECTATION THEORIES   Satisfaction is based on the difference between what one expects and what occurs (42, 68, 88). Within the disconfirmation paradigm (25, 50, 56), satisfaction is determined by the difference between a patient's standard of expectancies, ideals, or norms and the same patient's perceptions of their experiences of care, with satisfaction arising from either confirming positive expectation or disconfirming negative expectations. A fourth type of expectation is labeled an uninformed expectation, in which patients are not capable or are reluctant to communicate their expectations, either because they may not have any expectations or because they do not wish to substantiate their feelings or cannot express them (22, 57). Given the potential for uninformed expectations, Crow notes that patients should be educated about appropriate expectations for care (particularly technical features) and motivated to judge the quality of care they are receiving (16).

HEALTH SERVICE ATTRIBUTES   Many studies of satisfaction subdivide their measures (or items) according to Donabedian's classic differentiation of structure, process, and outcome (18). Structure is the patient/consumer's rating of the physical environment and physical facilities in which the service occurs. Process measures address, for example, the patient's rating of interpersonal interactions with service personnel and of personnel with each other. Specific attributes include, for example, responsiveness, friendliness, empathy, courtesy, competence, and availability. Outcome-related measures or items ask about the patient's perception of the results of process, including symptom reduction or resolution, improvement in functioning, or resolution of underlying problems. Note that Donabedian was attempting to subdivide criteria for assessing the quality of health care. His categorization has been very useful to various kinds of health professionals, but there is no reason to think it would be particularly useful to help us understand the dimensionality of patient's experiences of health care or serve as the most useful framework for organizing the wide array of criteria they may use in judging health care quality.

ECONOMICS   In economic terms, satisfaction is defined by the utility of a product or service that a person purchases for its utility-generating attributes (65). As in expectation theories, satisfaction depends on the difference between the experience of the actual utility and the utility the consumer expected. Different consumers have different preferences and therefore will purchase different products defined by a variety of characteristics. Most consumers work within limited budgets and make trade-offs based on their priorities (16), although they may not do so consciously.

Studies of patient satisfaction have contributed to our understanding of how patient perceptions affect the patient's own behavior. For example, studies have shown that patients who report being more satisfied with their care are more positive, more compliant and cooperative, and are more likely to participate in their treatment procedures (3, 7, 21, 24). However, there have also been critiques of the use of satisfaction as a measure of quality. If satisfaction is a result of both expectations and experiences, we can never be sure if variations in ratings from one patient to another are a result of differences in their expectations or in their experiences. Thus, someone with relatively low expectations may be "satisfied" with an experience of care that a person with high expectations would find totally unacceptable. This is a serious problem in today's environment, when, as often as not, we are trying to assess patients' perceptions either to identify better performers (so we can choose or reward them) or to identify where improvements in quality are needed.

Furthermore, if satisfaction is, as Crow states, an indicator simply of "acceptable" care, then how much do we learn about the quality of an enterprise when we find out that its customers are merely "satisfied" with it? As many have noted, patient satisfaction surveys are frequently prone to ceiling effects, which have the unfortunate consequence of making it difficult to distinguish those providing simply adequate services from those providing superior care (67). In this context, it may be more important to know about the level of dissatisfaction (14). For example, patients may report being satisfied even if they feel that there were problems with the care that they had received (20). For instance, Irurita found that patients qualified their statements about the quality of their nursing care, such as "...you just had to wait. It wasn't through them being lazy, it was being pushed, busy...They need more staff, so they're not rushing off and leaving you...They can only spread themselves so far" (36).

In addition, many satisfaction surveys include global ratings of their patients' overall satisfaction with an experience of care, a health plan, or a provider. It appears to be cognitively (and perhaps even emotionally) difficult for some patients to give global ratings of satisfaction because their experiences of care vary over time and across different providers. This has led many survey developers to shift their attention from ratings of satisfaction to reports of experiences. As Epstein and his colleagues note (20) it may be more useful to ask patients about specific time periods and experiences with their care, documenting both reports of their care and the rating, or value, that patients placed on that experience. In studies of potential users of the patient survey results, lay people have reported that they prefer to know specific aspects of other patients' experiences, instead of their overall ratings of satisfaction, when they are choosing health care providers. For instance, they want to know how long patients waited to see their doctors, rather than "how satisfied" they were with the waiting times, since their need or expectation of care may differ from another patient's need (19). Asking very specific questions may also minimize the subjectivity and the confounding of patient expectations and their ratings (67).

To support greater conceptual clarity, we present the following framework for examining patient perceptions of quality.

In this model, patient perceptions of quality are in response to their experiences, whether a single episode of care or a number of episodes over time. These perceptions result from the interaction of the patient's expectations and their experiences. Then, as patients apply their own definitions and/or criteria regarding quality, their perceptions of the quality of the care they received crystallize. It is important, however, to recognize that these definitions or criteria are rarely if ever consciously articulated or named by the individual. They are typically implicit rather than explicit.

The model identifies several factors that influence patients' expectations. These include the reputation of the entity in question; the nature, number, and seriousness of the patient's health needs; the extent of choice available; the patient's previous experiences; social and cultural norms that are both general (e.g., whether it is appropriate or acceptable to be critical of those with greater education or authority) and health specific (e.g., whether it is appropriate or acceptable for lay persons to be critical of medical professionals); patient attitudes (e.g., their sense of entitlement, the extent to which they are fatalistic); patient demographics (e.g., age, gender); and last, but certainly not least, the extent to which the patient has knowledge of what s/he should expect [e.g., knowing that a baseline history and physical should include questions about smoking history and careful (preferably multiple) readings of blood pressure].

Note that patient experiences are present at two points in the model. On the right-hand side of the model, the patient's specific experience of seeking and using services is the experience against which expectations are compared. On the left-hand side, the patient's previous experience(s) help shape those expectations. Also note that the term satisfaction is missing from the model. This is by design. We believe that being satisfied is only one way of characterizing patient perceptions of quality and that it is not a particularly useful way. Instead, we believe research is needed to help identify other more useful characterizations that relate to the concerns of, and preferably use the language of, patients themselves.

FINDINGS FROM STUDIES OF PATIENT DEFINITIONS OF QUALITY

What Do We Know About How Patients Themselves Define Quality?

A sizable literature addresses how patients rate the quality of their care. It is important to distinguish, however, between studies that use concepts and measures derived from the perspective of clinicians, researchers, or administrators (such as many patient satisfaction studies) and those that actually attempt to learn more directly from patients what health care quality means to them. Terms such as quality are inherently value-laden; one could argue that definitions of quality are socially constructed. Given the socialization and values of health professionals, one would expect to find at least some variation between their perspectives, definitions, and criteria and those of patients. We identified a limited number of studies (eleven to be exact) that were likely designed to determine patients' own definitions of quality care. They are typically small-scale, qualitative studies using patient interviews and focus groups (1, 2, 12, 23, 34, 36, 38, 46, 62, 64, 82). This methodological choice is understandable; using an inherently open-ended approach is entirely appropriate when we are in what Kaplan has called the "context of discovery" (41, 74, 75).

These studies have elicited a wide range of specific definitions offered by patients themselves. In some cases the researchers, and in other cases we ourselves, have categorized these specific definitions into several categories or dimensions and named them using terms familiar to health professionals. The categories are patient-centered care; access; communication and information; courtesy and emotional support; technical quality; efficiency of care/organization; and structure and facilities. Table 1 presents each of the studies in detail, giving information about the studies' purposes, designs, and methods and about the dimensions elicited, as well as measures within those dimensions, as communicated in the language of patients. We review these studies dimension by dimension.

PATIENT-CENTERED CARE   Across the qualitative studies, patients defined quality through what has been termed patient-centered care. For patients in these studies, quality included having their physical and emotional needs met; receiving individualized care; being involved with their care and decision-making about their care; having doctors, nurses, and staff who have personalized knowledge of the patient, who respect and know about the patient's health beliefs, including beliefs regarding non-Western health practices, who build rapport with the patient, show respect for the patient, listen to the patient, and anticipate the patient's needs; protecting patient privacy and confidentiality; having nurses who act as advocates for the patient; giving equal care for all patients; and involving family and friends in the care of the patient.

TABLE 1 Definitions of quality elicited from patients

Citation	Year	Purpose	Study design and methods	Study findings: measures
Anderson et al. (1)	2001	Examine women's concepts and definitions of health care quality	Study site: United States Sample: $N = 137$ women $N = 47$ African American $N = 52$ Caucasian $N = 20$ Asian $N = 18$ Latina Methods: 18 focus groups stratified by age (18–34, 35–54, and >55) and race/ethnicity	**Patient-centered care** Understanding women's health care and health needs, such as reproductive heath and childbirth Respect for and knowledge of nontraditional medical practices Privacy, such as security of records, disclosure of information **Access** Support in understanding and using health care system Accessing appointments **Communication and information** Communication abilities of providers Patient-physician interactions **Courtesy and emotional support** Sensitivity and caring Courtesy Social support, including friends and family **Efficiency of care/organization** Care coordination and comprehensiveness, including referrals **Technical quality** Provider clinical skills, including knowledge, training, and experience Treatment and prevention for specific diseases and health issues (e.g., diabetes and breast cancer) **Structure and facilities** Environment, such as room temperature, seating, décor, and privacy

		Purpose	Study details / Methods	Findings
Attree (2)	2001	Explore patients' and relatives' perceptions of care and their criteria for evaluating care	Study site: United Kingdom Sample: $N = 34$ acute medical patients Purposive sample 18 males, 16 females Age range 19–89 19–39 = 5 40–49 = 12 60–89 = 17 Methods: Semi-structured qualitative interviews	**Patient-centered care** Patient focused Involves patients Acknowledges patients' individuality and provides individualized care Care related to patient's need Needs anticipated and help offered willingly Patients known as people Providers take and spend time with patient **Access** Available and accessible to patients **Communication and information** Open communication and information flow **Courtesy and emotional support** Encourages a close, sociable relationship Demonstrates kindness, concern, compassion, and sensitivity Patient feeling cared for and about Develops bond/rapport **Technical quality** Holistic care
Concato & Feinstein (12)	1997	Ask patients to describe important attributes of their primary health care	Study site: United States Sample: $N = 202$ patients Randomly selected Age Median = 69 Male $N = 200$ Female $N = 2$ Methods: Short open-ended interview	**Patient-centered care** Physician's attentiveness to patient's individual concerns **Access** Affordability/costs of care **Courtesy and emotional support** Amiability of physician Attitude of the clerical staff

(Continued)

TABLE 1 (*Continued*)

Citation	Year	Purpose	Study design and methods	Study findings: measures
				Efficiency of care/organization Waiting time in clinics Waiting time or efficiency at the pharmacy **Technical quality** Physician's diligence **Structure and facilities** Parking Location and proximity of clinics
Gerteis et al. (23)	1993	Ask patients what it is about their interaction with providers, systems, and institutions that matters to them and affects them, either positively or negatively.	Study site: United States Sample: 3 focus groups; 50 patient interviews Methods: 3 focus groups; open-ended telephone interviews based on focus group findings	**Patient-centered care** Respect for patients' values, preferences, and expressed needs, including patients' quality of life, involvement in decision making, dignity, needs, and autonomy **Communication and information** Provides information on clinical status, progress, and prognosis and processes of care Provides information and education to facilitate autonomy, self-care, and health promotion **Courtesy and emotional support** Emotional support and alleviation of fear and anxiety, including anxiety over clinical status, treatment, and prognosis, over the impact of the illness on self and family, and over the financial impact of the illness Involvement of family and friends, such as accommodating family and friends, involving family in decision making, supporting the family as caregiver, recognizing the needs of the family

| Infante et al. (34) | 2004 | Explore the perceptions of patients with chronic conditions about the nature and quality of their care in general practice | Study site: New South Wales and South Australia
Sample: $N = 76$ consumers
Age $M = 63.4$
45 females, 31 males
Methods:
12 focus groups | **Efficiency of care/organization**
Care coordination and comprehensiveness, including referrals
Coordination and integration of care, including coordination and integration of clinical care; ancillary and support services; and front-line patient care
Transition and continuity, such as information, coordination and planning, and support
Technical quality
Physical comfort, including pain management and help with activities of daily living
Structure and facilities
Surroundings and hospital environment
Patient-centered care
Trusts and believes patients
Respects patients and treats each as an individual
Is accessible by telephone and has time for patients
Access
Convenient consultation times
Home visits
Access to services and time management
Access to other specialists and providers
Communication and information
Has good interpersonal skills, including good listener and communicates well
Provides patient education
Guides patients through the different stages of their chronic conditions |

(Continued)

TABLE 1 (*Continued*)

Citation	Year	Purpose	Study design and methods	Study findings: measures
				Courtesy and emotional support:
				Caring and compassionate
				Friendly receptionists
				Technical quality
				Clinical skills
				Good diagnostician
				Knowledgeable and up-to-date
				Holistic approach
				Efficiency of care/organization
				Good triage system
				Short waiting times
				Recall/reminder system in place
				Referrals for patients when necessary
				Continuity of care
				Structure and facilities
				Variety of clinical services
				Practice nurse and manager
				Quiet room for sicker patients
				Comfortable reception area
				Computerized
				Bulk-billing
Irurita (36)	1999	Exploring the adult patient's perspective of quality nursing care	Study site: Western Australia Sample: $N = 23$ patients	**Patient-centered care** Doing more than the job was perceived to require Ensuring physical and emotional comfort

		Methods: Post-discharge interviews supplemented by information from field notes, quality assurance surveys, biographical data sheets, and relevant literature	Being available and dependable, enhancing a sense of security Using appropriate touch Developing an effective nurse-patient relationship Has sufficient time to meet patients' needs **Communication and information** Communication and coordination Knowing what to expect and understanding hospital routine **Courtesy and emotional support** Demonstrating empathy and compassion Being friendly to patients **Technical quality** Technically competent **Efficiency of care/organization** Consistency of caregiver **Structure and facilities** Staffing levels Organizational factors including type of hospital Level of funding for the hospital
Jun et al. (38)	1998	Examine what patients (and physicians and administrators) perceive to be the key attributes of quality Study site: United States Sample: $N = 6$ patients 2 males, 4 females Age range 30–75 years Methods: Focus group interviews collecting detailed patient feedback on their feelings, attitudes, and perceptions about service quality	**Patient-centered care** Understanding of the patient Responsiveness Time spent with patient Privacy Consistency/equal treatment **Access** Convenience Visibility in the community **Communication and information**

(Continued)

TABLE 1 (*Continued*)

Citation	Year	Purpose	Study design and methods	Study findings: measures
				Technical complexity explained
				Interaction
				Courtesy and emotional support
				Caring and positive attitude
				Efficiency of care/organization
				Teamwork
				Collaboration internal and external to the hospital
				Accurate billing
				Technical quality
				Professionalism
				Education
				Continual improvement
				Patient outcomes
Larrabee & Bolden (46)	2001	Identify good nursing care from the patients' perspective	Study site: United States Sample: $N = 199$ patients Convenience sample: 107 men, 92 women Age $M = 39$ 85.4% African American 28% Medicaid 42% No insurance Methods: Short open-ended interview: Patients were asked to respond to the question "What is good nursing care?"	**Patient-centered care** Providing for patient needs Checking on patient Responding to patients' requests Respecting patients Treating patients with patience **Communication and information** Giving accurate information **Courtesy and emotional support** Treating patients nicely Having a positive attitude Being there for the patient Showing care or concern

| Ngo-Metzger et al. (62) | 2003 | Examine factors contributing to quality of care from the perspective of Chinese and Vietnamese American patients with limited English language skills | Study site: United States
Sample: $N = 122$ Chinese American ($N = 66$) and Vietnamese American ($N = 56$) patients
Chinese Age $M = 57$
Vietnamese Age $M = 51$
Methods: 12 focus groups (6 conducted in Vietnamese, 4 in Cantonese, 2 in Mandarin), 6 all-male and 6 all-female groups. | **Efficiency of care/organization**
Providing prompt care
Technical quality
Providing pain relief/comfort
Being competent
Using knowledgeable skills
Striving for excellence
Structure and facilities
Providing pleasant environment

Patient-centered care
Providers know about and respect non-Western health beliefs and practices
Providers discuss patient's health beliefs and practices in nonjudgmental manner
Patients treated with respect by interpreters
Providers and staff show respect and dignity
Providers spend enough time with patient
Adequate time spent with interpreter
Access
Access to care
Access to professional, culturally appropriate interpreters
Gender-concordant interpreters for sensitive issues
Interpreter access for nonscheduled visits and for after-hour phone calls
Staff help patient understand and navigate the medical system |

(Continued)

TABLE 1 (*Continued*)

Citation	Year	Purpose	Study design and methods	Study findings: measures
				Urgent care without needing scheduled appointments
				Medical care within walking distance or accessible by public transportation
				Communication and information
				Providers listen to what patient has to say
				Complete and accurate translations
				Written medication labels in patient's native language
				Effective communication of health-related information
				Education regarding lifestyle behaviors and preventative care
				Prompt communication about test results
				Courtesy and emotional support
				Respect for patients preferences and shows emotional support
				Providers and staff display empathy and support in nonverbal ways
				Providers ask about how your family or living situation may affect your health
				Efficiency of care/organization
				Continuity and transition (e.g., arrangement for follow-up appointments)
				Staff arrange follow-up appointments, tests, and referrals for patients

			Providers coordinate care for evaluation and treatment
			Providers communicate with others who may be involved in the patient's care
			Staff provide assistance in other areas (housing, welfare, immigration, etc. . .)
			Providers help patient obtain health-related assistance and support services
			Interpreter services available at the time of referrals
			Appointments as soon as patients' wanted
			Short waiting time during office visit
Radwin (64)	2000	Analyze theoretically oncology patients' perceptions of the attributes and outcomes of quality nursing care	Study site: United States Sample: $N = 22$ patients Purposive sample 7 males, 15 women Age ranged from 27–82 years Methods: Semi-structured schedule guided qualitative interviews	**Patient-centered care** Attentiveness and addressed patients needs promptly Partnership (with patients, e.g., in decision making) Individualization of care Rapport (e.g., knew some things about the nurse) **Courtesy and emotional support** Caring approach with patient Show concern and be nurturing **Efficiency of care/organization** Continuity (e.g., repeated encounters with the same nurse) Coordination (among providers) **Technical quality** Professional knowledge, including experiential knowledge and technical competence

(Continued)

TABLE 1 (*Continued*)

Citation	Year	Purpose	Study design and methods	Study findings: measures
Stichler & Weiss (82)	2000	Define quality from the perspectives of patients (among others) associated with a hospital-based women's service line and determine how they evaluate a hospital's quality	Study site: United States Sample: $N = 39$ patients receiving services in a variety of settings within a hospital-based women's service line Methods: Qualitative semistructured interview	Outcomes that included increased fortitude and sense of well-being **Patient-centered care** Take a personal interest in patient Treat the patient "right" Is attentive, anticipatory, and responsive to the patient Responds to patient requests in a timely manner **Courtesy and emotional support** Generally friendly and helpful **Efficiency of care/organization** Efficiency within the patient care environment An obvious flow and organization to the work A desire to "be ready" and keep things moving on schedule **Technical quality** Strong professional demeanor Technical skill Assurance of accuracy in diagnoses Diagnostics tests Provision of effective treatment Achievement of expected results **Structure and facilities** Clean and comfortable environment Quality of the food Availability of security in the hospital and grounds Availability of parking

ACCESS   Many but not all studies also report patient concerns about access, such as having doctors, nurses, and staff who make themselves available and accessible to the patient; having access to specialists; having care that is affordable; having convenient places and times for visits; having providers who make home visits; having access to gender-concordant, professionally trained, and culturally appropriate interpreter services; having access to urgent care; and having help from staff in navigating the health system.

COMMUNICATION AND INFORMATION   Almost all the studies reported patient interest in the quality of communication and information. This category includes open communication and information flow; providers with good interpersonal communication skills such as listening carefully and attentively and explaining complex technical information clearly; provision of information on clinical status, progress, prognosis, and processes of care; provision of information on what to expect (for example, hospital routines); prompt communication of test results; complete and accurate translations, including written prescription labels in the patient's native language; and education to facilitate patient autonomy, self-care, and health promotion.

COURTESY AND EMOTIONAL SUPPORT   Patients defined quality in terms of and based on the social and emotional characteristics of interactions with providers and office staff. They wanted everyone not only to be courteous, but also to show sensitivity and kindness, to be caring, and to express compassion and sympathy for the patient. It was important for them to have emotional security and feel trust in their caregivers to help reduce feelings of vulnerability and anxiety. Overall, they wanted the doctors, nurses, and staff to be friendly. It is somewhat difficult to distinguish this dimension from patient-centered care.

EFFICIENCY OF CARE/EFFECTIVE ORGANIZATION   Patients expected care to be efficient, with coordination between the many individuals and organizations involved in their care, such as multiple providers within a hospital, between generalists and specialists, across facilities, and between their providers and their health plans. They also felt the need for care from the same providers over time, a need that is linked to their desire for aspects of patient-centered care such as personalized knowledge of the patient and the building of trust and rapport. Accurate billing, efficient referral processes, short waiting times for appointments and at ancillary settings like the pharmacy were also mentioned as a sign of an efficient organization. A study with Asian patients emphasized the need for help in obtaining a wide range of nonmedical services such as housing, welfare, immigration, etc.

TECHNICAL QUALITY   Patients mentioned features that can easily be related to what clinicians often refer to as the technical quality of care. Across these studies, patients expressed a desire for technically knowledgeable, competent, and experienced providers who are well educated; provide effective treatments, accurate diagnoses, and diligent and efficient services and treatment; and present themselves in a professional manner. In one study patients said they wanted providers to "strive for excellence." Patients also defined quality as having good health outcomes and improved quality of life.

Some clinicians and researchers have expressed concern about patients' ability to assess a health care provider's technical quality (5, 20). Although patients do not have the expertise of a trained professional, they do have the capacity to report whether their doctors delivered tests and treatments appropriate to their diagnosis, age, gender, or family health status. For example, when a diabetic patient visits her doctor's office, was she checked for blood sugar level, possible kidney problems, high blood pressure, or high cholesterol? Did she receive a foot exam? Patients' ability to rate technical quality may be improved if they are more educated in the basic expectations they should have of their health status and possible health risks. Additionally, being informed may help patients to take part in the decision making about their care (20). If patients do not know about tangible indicators of the technical quality of care they are receiving, they may use proxy indicators, such as building cleanliness, instead. For example, when patients were asked "Did your GP work according to the newest medical developments?," Jung and colleagues found that patients evaluated their care through the general practitioner's (GP) actions but not their affective performance. General medical-technical competence was evaluated by the patient through the following behaviors: "examined well; observed well; worked according to certain order: first listening, judgments only after examination; examinations and actions done in proper way, gave good solutions; knew answers, causes, what to do, what patient could expect, and shows no doubts in diagnosing" (39).

STRUCTURE AND FACILITIES   Patients evaluate quality of the health care organizations' structures and facilities, including easy access, parking availability, safety and security in and around the facility, cleanliness and comfort, quality of food provided, a quiet and pleasant environment, a variety of clinical services available, use of up-to-date technology such as computers, and the visibility of the care provider in the community. Some patients mentioned such classic features of structure as the ownership of the facility, the funding levels, and the staffing levels.

Developing Instruments Using Patient Definitions and Perceptions

Another sign of the focus on patient-centered care is that, increasingly, surveys of patient perceptions are being developed using data collected through the kinds of qualitative studies described above. Indeed, the work described by Gerteis and colleagues (23) resulted in the development of an entire family of patient satisfaction surveys for various kinds of facilities, known as the Picker surveys[2]. Similarly,

---

[2]The Picker Institute was formed to develop such surveys and eventually became a major survey vendor. The organization was sold in 2001 to the National Research Corporation, which now offers these and other surveys to a wide range of facilities.

several other patient satisfaction surveys that are widely used today indicate in their marketing materials that they used, among other sources, feedback from patients in focus groups to develop their instruments (63).

Since 1994, the Agency for Healthcare Research and Quality (AHRQ, then known as the Agency for Health Care Research and Policy) has carried out an initiative to develop and rigorously test another family of instruments to get a consumer perspective on health care quality. The CAHPS® initiative, as it is now called, began in 1994 and 1995 with the explicit goal of developing reliable and valid survey instruments that would gather information from consumers, which would then be publicly reported. A standard survey used across health plans of all kinds was intended to make it possible for consumers to compare health plans with each other and introduce a greater emphasis on quality into decisions in the marketplace. In addition to commissioning an in-depth examination of existing satisfaction surveys, the agency conducted a set of focus groups with consumers around the country. In these groups, consumers identified not just what information about health plan quality they would most like to have, but also what information about health plan quality about which other consumers were in a particularly good position to report (15). The dimensions identified in these groups have guided the development of multiple surveys of health plans, for people with Medicare, for people with Medicaid, for children as well as adults, for people seeking help with mental health problems, for people with chronic conditions, for people who prefer to use Spanish, and more recently to assess not only health plans but also medical groups, nursing homes, hospitals, and dialysis centers. These surveys include dimensions that emerged frequently in the qualitative studies discussed above, such as how clinicians interact and communicate with patients. In addition, consumers mentioned several aspects of access to care, including issues that become especially salient in a managed care environment, such as being able to find a regular doctor a patient is happy with, as well as more traditional issues such as wait times to get appointments and in the office.

The development of CAHPS® illustrates a significant trend in the development of instruments to collect information from consumers/patients: the trend to ask people to report on their experiences rather than to provide a rating of their satisfaction. Although CAHPS instruments typically ask for overall ratings, a major contribution of these surveys is their emphasis on patient reports. In addition, the range of items includes questions about whether specific services (e.g., a flu shot) have or have not been received, which can be seen as taking a step in the direction of asking patients about the technical quality of care.

How Do Patient Definitions and Ratings of Quality Differ from those of Providers?

We have argued that patient perceptions of quality can be very different from those of providers. What is the evidence? Three studies have been conducted that identify significant differences between how patients and clinicians view quality. Lynn & McMillen (51) conducted a study to examine whether nurses know what patients think is important about nursing care. Using a measure developed from qualitative interviews with patients, they surveyed 448 patients and 350 nurses, asking them to rank ~90 different items in order of importance as a determinant of patient assessments of nursing quality. Nurses were found to overestimate the importance of trust, empathy, nurse competence, nurse's examination of patients, and explanations of status to the patient. Patients gave significantly higher ratings to 46 of the 90 items than did the nurses and gave high ranks to several very concrete items: nurse is skillful, especially with needles (ranked second most important by patients compared with a ranking of eighth by nurses); equipment needed for patient care is available (ranked third versus fifty-second); nurse gives patient's medication on time (fourth versus forty-second); and nurse is there when patient needs her/him (ninth versus fourteenth).

In their study comparing patients' and physicians' ratings of the importance of various determinants of the quality of care, Laine and colleagues (44) found that both groups concurred that clinical skill is the most important determinant. However, patients and physicians disagreed significantly about the relative importance of the provision of information, with patients ranking it second and physicians ranking it sixth most important. Similarly, a Dutch study conducted by Jung and colleagues (40) compared patient and GP evaluations of care and found differences in ratings of care but substantial similarity in ranking performance with respect to different features of care. Thus, GPs were more critical of the care provided than were their patients; GPs also underestimated how positively the patients rated their care. In ranking the features they felt were most positive, the correlation between patient and GP was 0.76 (p < 0.001). However, GPs rated their performance more positively on waiting time and being able to talk to the GP on the telephone, whereas patients rated GP performance more positively on the communication of information and support. Thus, evidence states that patients' perceptions are in fact distinctive and that these perceptions may lead to different assessments of the quality of care.

How Stable are Patient Definitions and Ratings of Quality?

If patient definitions of quality are not stable over time, it willl be difficult both to develop a health care system that patients perceive as high quality and to provide comparative quality information that is meaningful. However, we could find only one study that examined issues related to this. Jackson and colleagues (37) studied 500 retired military patients who were walk-in patients seeing new physicians because of a symptom. Patient ratings of the quality of the visit went up over time: 52% rated their overall care as excellent immediately postvisit, 59% gave an excellent rating two weeks later, and 63% gave this rating three months later. Of greater interest, there was some change in the determinants of satisfaction, and of dissatisfaction, over these three points in time. The researchers began by identifying the expectations and concerns of the patients prior to the visit; 98% articulated at least one specific previsit expectation, including a desire for an explanation of the cause of their symptom(s) (80%), a prescription (66%), information about the anticipated time for recovery (62%), a diagnostic test (56%), or a subspecialty referral (47%). Sixty-four percent were concerned that their symptom might represent a serious illness.

Multi-variate analysis revealed that 26% of the variance in immediate postvisit satisfaction was determined by age (older patients were more likely to give a high satisfaction rating), better functional status, having no unmet expectations, and getting an explanation of symptom cause and likely duration. Two weeks later, predictors of satisfaction shifted. Those with a shorter symptom duration, whose symptoms had improved, who were less worried about having a serious illness, who felt the symptom had not lasted longer than expected and had not required another physician visit, and who reported having no unmet expectations, were more satisfied. These predictors were stable from two weeks to three months. Thus, initial satisfaction is linked to patient-physician interaction, whereas over time and distance from the interaction itself satisfaction shifts to the course and impact of the patient's symptoms.

Sofaer et al. (76, 78) conducted a quasi-experimental evaluation of an innovative approach to provide people with Medicare information about the financial consequences of their health care coverage decisions. All participants were enrolled in a three-hour workshop covering the same topics but using different materials. In examining the entire sample, she found that participants' rankings of the importance of different features of health were changed after exposure to the workshop. Prior to the intervention, the feature "choice of provider" was fourth most important, whereas after the intervention it became second most important. The educational intervention included a discussion of the features of newly available Medicare options, such as Health Maintenance Organizations (HMOs), including the fact that HMO members would be limited to a network of providers rather than having free choice of provider. This appears to have given greater salience, and thus importance, to "choice of provider" as a feature. One can argue that choice was important to this group all along but that they did not realize it was at risk, rather than something that could be taken for granted, until they were presented with information.

WHAT'S THE SCORE? FINDINGS ON HOW PATIENTS RATE HEALTH CARE QUALITY

Health Plans

The single best source of information in the United States on how patients rate the quality of their health plans is the National CAHPS® Benchmarking Database (NCBD). The most recent compilation of ratings and composite reports based on CAHPS® surveys conducted around the United States and reported to the NCBD was published in 2004 (94) and presents results of surveys in 2003 of 220 commercial health plans, 181 Medicaid plans, 49 SCHIP plans, and 295 Medicare plans. This includes 69 Medicaid plans that conducted surveys of children's care (by definition SCHIP surveys address children's care). CAHPS® surveys are analyzed and reported to the public using composites of multiple items that relate to dimensions of care identified through consumer testing (53). On the composite "getting needed care" the average scores ranged from a low of 67% of adults in Medicaid reporting that this was "not a problem" to 83% of parents responding for their children enrolled in SCHIP. In contrast, scores on the composite "getting care quickly" were much lower. These ranged from 55% of people with Medicare and of children in Medicaid reporting they always got care quickly to 44% of adults in Medicaid and 45% of adults in commercial plans saying they always got care quickly enough.

Another CAHPS® composite addresses "doctors who communicate well." On this feature, positive responses range from 58% of respondents in SCHIP and adult commercial plans to 68% of people with Medicare and 71% of children in Medicaid. As noted earlier, CAHPS® surveys include several overall ratings, where people are asked to give a number from 0 for the "worst possible" to 10 for the "best possible." On these measures, the distribution is skewed to the higher ratings; many observers think this reflects an underlying problem of ceiling effects. Ratings of 9–10 for the personal doctor range from 52% in adult commercial plans to 66% for children in Medicaid and 65% for people with Medicare. Ratings of 9–10 for specialists similarly range from 67% for people with Medicare to 56% for adults in commercial plans and 57% for adults with Medicaid. Overall ratings of health care follow a very similar pattern. However, overall ratings of the health plans themselves look somewhat different and have a much wider range of positive responses. Less than half, 41%, of adults in commercial plans rate their health plans a 9 or a 10, whereas 20% give their plan a rating from 0 to 6. In contrast, 70% of those in SCHIP gave the highest ratings, whereas only 8% gave ratings from 0 to 6.

Obviously, the purpose of CAHPS® surveys is to make far more finely grained comparisons of individual health plans. However, the national results show both that there are important differences across health plans serving different subgroups of the population and that although there may be ceiling effects, especially in the ratings of providers, there is much room for improvement.

However, how do we interpret these results if variations in scores on such surveys can be explained by other factors? For example, Carlson and colleagues (8), using the Consumer Assessment of Behavioral Health Survey (CAHBS), compared the responses of members of commercial and five public-managed behavioral health plans. Although unadjusted global ratings of commercial and public plans were statistically significant, significant differences disappeared when the analysis controlled for patient characteristics such as educational level, self-reported health and mental health status, use patterns, and whether coverage paid for all or only some of the costs of care. Does this mean there really are no differences in patient perceptions of plan quality? Or does it mean that people with different personal characteristics or patterns of using care do not get the same kind of care? At present, it is impossible to know. It may well make sense to control for the level of benefits in a plan, but what about controlling for the education level of its members?

Similarly, Landon et al. (45) examined the relationship between structural features of health plans and patients' assessments of quality reported on CAHPS® Medicare Managed Care surveys by 82,583 people with Medicare from 182 plans. The strongest predictors of performance were ownership and national affiliation; for-profit and national health plans scored lower on almost all of the outcome variables. Clearly, these kinds of comparisons cannot be explained away as easily but rather need to be examined further.

Solomon et al. (79) used a major field test of a survey from the CAHPS® family, "G-CAHPS" or "Group-CAHPS," which was under development, to analyze the variation in patient-reported quality among health care across health plans, regional service organizations (RSOs), medical groups, and practice sites.[3] They found that patient-reported quality is strongly influenced by the site of care. Practice sites accounted for at least 60% of explained variation for eight of nine composites for which there were between-site differences, for three of four global rating items, and for the willingness of a patient to recommend the medical group to others. Medical groups have influence on getting access to needed care, timeliness of care, and global ratings of care. Health plans accounted for much less of the variation in patient-reported quality, except for measures of office staff and advice composites and global ratings of specialists and office staff. This finding demonstrates another complexity involved in measuring patient perceptions: making appropriate attributions regarding the level(s) of the system that can or should be held accountable for patients' experiences of care.

Reporting on a national sample telephone survey, conducted in both English and Spanish, of adults under age 65 on Consumer Experiences with Health Plans, Schlesinger et al. (70) found that 51% of their 2500 respondents reported having at least one problem that they attributed in part to their health plan. Of the 1278 people reporting a problem, nearly 10% said it had caused a serious decline in their health, 8.5% said it significantly delayed treatment; and 8.5% said it caused them to incur large out-of-pocket expenses.

Another national sample telephone survey, this time of 3080 people with Medicare who had been or were in managed care plans, was conducted by Nelson and colleagues (61). This survey emphasized access concerns related to the structure of managed care plans that can have quality consequences. In this study, the "old old," those 85 years of age or older, the nonelderly disabled, African Americans, and those reporting they were in worse health than one year ago were significantly more likely to report at least one kind of quality-related access problem, less likely to rate their overall care as excellent, and less likely to recommend the plan to

---

[3]Note that this study did not report actual scores, but only analyzed sources of variation in scores across different levels of a single, large, health care plan, Partners Community Healthcare, Inc.

family members or friends with a serious or chronic health problem. The authors interpret these variations as indicating that Medicare managed care plans are not doing as good a job in serving the needs of more vulnerable groups compared with those with fewer or more complex health care needs.

Hospitals

Cleary et al. (9) conducted a nationwide survey of 6455 adults using one of the earliest version of a Picker survey. Eighty percent of respondents reported their overall satisfaction with their care as excellent or very good. Only 6.5% would not recommend the hospital to family and/or friends and only 15.3% were angry about their care while they were in the hospital. The authors found that the total number of patient-reported problems with care was the strongest predictor of overall patient evaluation of care (9).

Recently, more public reports of hospital quality from the patient perspective are being issued. One such report is the result of a voluntary initiative sponsored by the California Health Care Foundation. Called the PEP-C project (for Patients' Evaluation of Performance), the 2003 Technical Report has results from surveys of nearly 35,000 patients discharged from 181 acute care hospitals in California, compared with results from 176,443 respondents in 446 hospitals from 49 states and the District of Columbia. Scores are calibrated from 1 to 100, low to high. We report only the national scores, which have been adjusted for self-reported health status, gender, and education. When all dimensions of care are combined, the national overall score is 72. Nationwide, hospitals are doing best on physical comfort (82), involving family and friends (76), and coordination of care [see also (76)]. They are doing worst on emotional support (65), transition to home (69), and providing information and education [see also (69)]. The score on respecting patient preferences is 74. Clearly, there is considerable room for improvement on all these patient-centered dimensions of quality.

Physicians

Patient perceptions of the quality of physicians is, to some extent, expressed in items included in surveys of their experiences in health plans and medical groups, as discussed above. In addition, studies of patient experiences in primary care often examine physicians in particular. More research is now being conducted to acquire patient reports on physicians, both generalists and specialists, which has not yet resulted in published findings.

Safran and her colleagues (69) have developed, field tested, and refined a measure of primary care, the Primary Care Assessment Survey (PCAS), and report results from two longitudinal studies. They note that an important element of primary care, as defined by the Institute of Medicine, is "whole-person care." On this element—which includes whether the primary care physician (PCP) knows the patient's entire medical history, their responsibilities at work and at home, what worries them most about their health, and the patient as a person, including their values and beliefs—primary care is not doing very well, according to the authors. Thus, less than half of patients in the general adult population and among those 65 or older rate their PCP as excellent or very good across these items.

Perhaps more troubling, these authors report a general decline in patients' reports of primary care experiences from 1996 to 1999 for a study of Massachusetts adults who retained the same PCP (58) and for a study of people with Medicare from 1998 to 2000. In the Massachusetts study, all items assessing physician-patient interaction declined except physician's knowledge of the patient. In the Medicare study, there were declines in patient reports on communication, interpersonal treatment, and thoroughness of the physical examination, as well as in financial access, visit-based continuity, and integration of care. Even here with an instrument that focuses on reports rather than ratings, given the lack of research on the stability (or instability) of expectations and preferences over time, it is difficult to know whether these declines reflect changes in objective circumstances, changes in expectations, or perhaps patient unhappiness over the lack of improvement over time in aspects of care on which they have provided feedback.

International Comparisons

The Commonwealth Fund has supported a multinational study comparing the United States with Australia, Canada, New Zealand, and the United Kingdom using patient reported measures of quality (11). One set of items assessed care received from a regular doctor or physician. The United States ranked best on doctors making clear the specific goals for treatment (80% of Americans reported U.S. doctors did this) and tied for first rank with New Zealand on doctors asking for ideas and opinions about treatment and care (53% did this). The United States ranked poorly (fourth or fifth) on doctors spending enough time with patient (21% of patients said they did not feel the doctor spent enough time, compared with 10% in the best-performing nation), being accessible by phone or in person (23% of patients said they were not accessible, compared with 9% in the best-performing nation), and on listening carefully to patient's health concerns (17% of patients said they did not listen carefully, compared with only 8% in the highest ranking nation).

Another set of items addressed patient-reported perceptions of medication and medical errors. There was little variation across the five countries in this area. However, the United States ranked the lowest, reporting twice as many medication or medical errors that caused a serious health consequence than did the highest rated country, the United Kingdom (18% versus 9%). Adults in the United States were much more likely to report taking multiple medications. Those taking more medications were more likely to report errors.

Several items looked at the timeliness of care. On the one hand, U.S. patients do not face long waits for surgery or hospital admissions—the United States ranked first on those items. On the other hand, we rank fourth on having to wait more than five days for an appointment or experiencing delays or problems while discharge arrangements were made. In terms of what Davis and her colleagues (17) term efficiency, the United States does very poorly indeed. The United States ranked last on all aspects of what many might call problems in the organization and coordination of care, which considers experiences over a two-year period: being sent for a duplicate test (22% reported this experience), having to tell the same story to multiple health professionals (57%), and having medical records or test results not reach the physician's office in time for an appointment (25%). Finally, on three of four items categorized as "effectiveness" the United States ranks last. These items include not getting a recommended test, treatment, or follow-up visit because of cost (26% of Americans reported this experience), not filling a prescription because of cost (35%), and skipping doses to make medicine last longer (16%). Although the United States performs best in terms of having a doctor who reviews all the patient's medications, 30% of Americans reported their physician did not do this for them.

The World Health Organization (WHO) has conducted an ambitious and some-what controversial project to compare the health care systems of countries at all stages of development across the globe. One element of this comparative assessment is termed health system responsiveness (59). As part of this effort, the WHO created a World Health Survey, which questioned citizens about their experiences in the following domains of responsiveness: autonomy; choice; communication; confidentiality; dignity; quality of basic amenities; prompt attention; and access to family and community support (89). In 1999, the United States ranked first among all nations rated on this element of the assessment. This result starkly contrasts its poor performance on other dimensions considered by WHO, including fairness in resource allocation, decision making, and health status. The score for the United States on their index was 8.10 (uncertainty interval 7.32–8.96). This score compares with scores of 6.98 for Canada, 6.81 for Australia, 6.51 for the United Kingdom, 5.37 for the Russian Federation, 5.20 for China, and 3.73 for Niger (96).

Findings on Factors Influencing Patient Responses to Care

Several studies (including some summarized above) have examined whether and how patient characteristics such as age, race/ethnicity, gender, socioeconomic status, physical and mental health status, attitudes, and expectations of care may also influence patient perceptions of quality of care.[4] The enduring difficulty of these studies is that it is rarely possible to determine if such systematic differences should be attributed to differences in patient expectations, perceptions, or the actual care received. Further, the results of the research have often been inconsistent and

---

[4]Hall & Dornan (27) conducted a meta-analysis of patients' sociodemographic characteristics as they relate to satisfaction with medical care. This meta-analysis largely confirms the results reported here.

contradictory. These studies are summarized in Table 2 and are discussed briefly here.

The most consistent findings relate to age, with older patients reporting more positively (8, 9, 29, 66) across health plans, both commercial and public (Medicaid, Medicare). Overall, research indicates also that patients in better health (which can be defined to include not only physical health status but also disability, low quality of life, and psychological distress) give higher ratings to their care (10, 16, 29, 43, 66, 87), although this may not hold for dimensions directly related to care, including daily care, medical care, and information (87). However, Wensing and colleagues (93) note in their review that the meaning of the relationship between health status and patient perceptions is unclear. Do patients who have better compliance to their doctor's advice have better health outcomes and report higher satisfaction? Do doctors respond more negatively to patients in poorer health?

When examining race and ethnicity, one first-order concern is methodological. The reliability and validity of surveys conducted with diverse cultural and linguistic participants can be compromised by problems in the quality of translations, culturally based differences in the interpretation of questions, differences among cultural groups in styles or patterns of responses, and the minimum levels of literacy needed to fully understand questions. Morales (57) reports that although there are methods to test and adjust surveys to take into account these potential problems, these methods are not used often. In their review of the literature on racial and ethnic differences in assessment of care, he and his colleagues found that, although some research reports that race and ethnicity does not influence satisfaction with care, the more recent research has found differences. Morales' own studies (57), showed lower ratings of communication with providers among Latinos who communicate primarily in Spanish, as well as lower ratings (compared with whites) across the board among Asian/Pacific Islanders and among Latinos concerning access to care, promptness of care, and health plan customer service. In contrast, African Americans reported better provider communication and office staff helpfulness than did Whites. Note that these differences were not found among overall ratings of personal doctors, specialists, and overall health care, although they were found on more specific questions. Are we to put more stock in the more specific report questions or in the more general ratings? Taira and colleagues (85) found that Asian respondents' assessments of care were significantly lower than were Whites on 9 of 11 dimensions in the PCAS discussed earlier (77). Asian patients also scored significantly lower than did African Americans on eight dimensions and significantly lower than did Latinos on four dimensions. Given the number of control variables, as well as extensive testing of the validity and reliability of the PCAS across racial and ethnic groups, we must consider these findings as suggesting that cultural norms may play a role in shaping patient expectations and the criteria they use for translating their perceptions into quality assessments, as reflected in our model (see Figure 1).

LaVeist and colleagues (48) studied satisfaction, using their own instrument, in a sample of white and African American patients with a chronic heart condition.

TABLE 2 Patient characteristics and patient perception of quality

Citation	Year	Site, sample, and method	Result
			Age
Carlson et al. (8)	2002	**Study site:** United States **Sample:** $N = 1963$ patients in public assistance and commercial health plans **Method:** Consumer Assessment of Behavioral Health Services Questionnaire	Carlson et al. found that older patients in both public assistance and commercial plans rated their care and health plans more highly than did younger patients.
Cleary et al. (9)	1992	**Study site:** United States **Sample:** $N = 6455$ discharged patients **Method:** Picker telephone survey	Controlling for total problem score, age was significantly correlated with overall evaluation; younger patients reported more problems of care, specifically physical care, pain management, and family involvement. Age did not figure in reports of problems with communication, emotional support, and education.
Haviland et al. (29)	2003	**Study site:** United States **Sample:** $N = 120,855$ 84% White, 6% African American, 3% Latino, 1% Asian **Method:** Mailed Healthcare Market Guide (HCMG) Survey	Haviland and colleagues found that ratings of satisfaction were higher among those who were older and in better health.

Roohan et al. (66)	2003	**Study site:** New York **Sample:** $N = 15,106$ commercial and Medicaid enrollees 7.07% ages 18–24, 18.94% ages 25–34, 29.36% ages 35–44, 26.09% ages 45–54, 19.55% ages 55–64 **Method:** Commercial managed care CAHPS and Medicaid managed care CAHPS surveys	Respondents 55–64 years of age rated their health plans higher than did younger respondents.

Health status

Cleary et al. (10)	1991	**Study site:** United States **Sample:** $N = 6455$ discharged patients **Method:** Picker telephone survey	Cleary and his colleagues found that poor health was the strongest predictor of a number of problems with hospital care even when controlling for age, income, and patient preferences.
Crow et al. (16)	2002	**Sample:** $N = 37$ studies addressing methodological issues, $N = 139$ articles on the determinants of satisfaction **Method:** systematic review of the literature on patient satisfaction	In their review of 31 observational studies that examined the relationship between health status and satisfaction, Crow and colleagues found that poorer physical health status, disability, low quality of life, and psychological distress are related to lower reported satisfaction.

(*Continued*)

TABLE 2 (*Continued*)

Citation	Year	Site, sample, and method	Result
Haviland (29)	2003	**Study site:** United States **Sample:** $N = 120,855$ 84% White, 6% African American, 3% Latino, 1% Asian **Method:** Mailed Healthcare Market Guide (HCMG) Survey	Ratings of health care were likely to be more positive among those in better health.
Krupat et al. (43)	2000	**Study site:** United States **Sample:** $N = 3602$ surgical patients **Method:** Picker/Commonwealth telephone interview	In their analysis of satisfaction and problems involving communication of information among surgical patients, Krupat and colleagues found that healthier patients were more satisfied with their care.
Roohan et al. (66)	2003	**Study site:** New York **Sample:** $N = 15,106$ commercial and Medicaid enrollees 19.91% in excellent health, 39.7% very good health, 30.81% good health, 8.2% fair health, 1.38% poor health **Method:** Commercial managed care CAHPS and Medicaid managed care CAHPS surveys	Health status had the largest effect on ratings: respondents rating their health status as poor gave their health plan an average rating of 6.34 on a scale of 0 to 10, whereas those who rated their health status as excellent gave their health plan an average rating of 7.72.

Thi et al. (87)	2002	**Study site:** France **Sample:** $N = 533$ patients **Method:** Patient Judgments Hospital Quality questionnaire	Thi et al. found that the two strongest and most consistent predictors of higher satisfaction among hospital patients were older age and a higher general health perception score at admission. However, a self-reported critical and serious condition at admission was associated with higher satisfaction on dimensions directly related to care, including daily care, medical care, and information.
Wensing et al. (93)	1998	**Sample:** $N = 57$ studies on patient priorities in regard to primary health care **Method:** Systematic review and data extraction	Wensing and colleagues note in their review that the meaning of the relationship between health status and patient perceptions is unclear. Overall, Wensing et al. note that a maximum of only 10% of the variation in patients' evaluation of care was explained by health status.
Race and ethnicity			
Haviland et al. (29)	2003	**Study site:** United States **Sample:** $N = 120,855$ 84% white, 6% African American, 3% Latino, 1% Asian **Method:** Mailed Healthcare Market Guide (HCMG) Survey	Asians gave lower ratings to satisfaction with medical and were more likely to intend to switch health plans, whereas African Americans gave comparable and higher ratings than did whites on overall satisfaction with health plans and would recommend their health plan to others.
LaVeist et al. (48)	2000	**Study site:** Maryland **Sample:** $N = 1784$ cardiac patients White $N = 1003$ African American $N = 852$ **Method:** Telephone Interview	After controlling for patient gender, age, health insurance status, education, and number of nights in the hospital in the past 12 months, race still significantly predicted patient satisfaction; African Americans reported less satisfaction with care. However, when perceived racism and medical mistrust were taken into account, race no longer had significant effects on satisfaction.

(Continued)

TABLE 2   *(Continued)*

Citation	Year	Site, sample, and method	Result
Morales (57)	2001	**Study site:** United States **Sample:** $N = 28,354$ commercial and Medicaid enrollees **Method:** National CAHPS Benchmarking Database	African Americans reported better care than did whites in provider communication and office staff helpfulness. In an analysis by race/ethnicity of the five reporting domains of CAHPS, including access to needed care, provider, communication, office staff helpfulness, promptness of needed care, and health plan customer service, Asian/Pacific Islanders reported worse care than did whites in all domains. Whites reported better care than other racial/ethnic groups. However, in ratings of care (which are single items that are patients' summary evaluations of care with their personal medical providers, specialists, health care, and health plan) Asian/Pacific Islanders were similar to whites across all ratings. Latinos who completed their CAHPS survey instrument in Spanish rated communication with their medical provider the lowest, followed by Latinos who completed their survey in English, and then by whites, with statistically significant differences across all groups. This finding suggests that Latinos who communicate primarily in Spanish have a greater risk of poor communication with their providers. Latinos reported worse access to care, promptness of care, and health plan customer service than did whites. Latinos rated similar to whites in evaluation of their personal doctors, specialists, and health care and rated their health plans higher than did whites. Black and Latino patients rated their plans slightly higher than did Whites.
Roohan et al. (66)	2003	**Study site:** New York **Sample:** $N = 15,106$ commercial and Medicaid enrollees 74.53% White, 12.27% African American, 8.57% Latino, 4.63% Other **Method:** Commercial managed care CAHPS and Medicaid managed care CAHPS surveys	

Seid et al. (71)	2003	**Study site:** California **Sample:** N = 3406 parents Asian N = 1158 African American N = 458 Latino N = 11,292 White N = 479 **Method:** Surveys collected by mail, telephone, and in person. Parents' Perceptions of Primary Care Measure (P3C)	In initial bivariate analyses, Asian and Latino parents reported lower levels of primary care quality than did whites and African Americans. However, when the analysis added demographic and health status variables, as well as measures of potential access to care into the regression model (accounting for 13.3% of the variance), they found that speaking a language other than English, having a regular provider, and not having commercial insurance are very strong predictors of perceptions of care, whereas race/ethnicity per se was either eliminated as an explanatory factor (Latino) or its influence was greatly reduced (Asian).
Taira et al. (85)	2001	**Study site:** Massachusetts **Sample:** N = 6092 employees of Commonwealth of Massachusetts White N = 5390 Asian N = 114 African American N = 444 Latino N = 114 **Method:** Self-administered (mail and telephone) Primary Care Assessment Survey (PCAS)	Whites assessed their care higher than did African Americans but only financial access and longitudinal continuity reached significance; African Americans rated these measures lower than did whites. Similarly with Latinos, only financial access was assessed significantly lower than whites. Within this sample, Asian patients were better educated, younger, and had fewer chronic conditions and were more likely to be employed in professional or technical occupations than were Latinos or African American patients. Asian patients also scored significantly lower than did African Americans on eight of the measures and significantly lower than did Latinos on four of the measures. They also rated the other two measures (continuity of care and integration of services) lower but not at a statistically significant level. After controlling for patient characteristics and other confounding factors, Asian respondents' assessments of care were significantly lower than were whites' on 9 of the 11 measures, including financial access, organizational access, visit-based continuity, preventive counseling, comprehensive knowledge of patient, thoroughness of physical examination, communication, interpersonal treatment, and trust.

(Continued)

TABLE 2 *(Continued)*

Citation	Year	Site, sample, and method	Result
Weech-Maldonado et al. 2003 (91)	2003	**Study site:** United States **Sample:** $N = 49,327$ adults in Medicaid managed care plans **Method:** National CAHPS Benchmarking Database (NCBD) Mail and telephone data collection	In their analysis of adults enrolled in Medicaid managed care plans from the National CAHPS Benchmarking Database, Weech-Maldonado and colleagues found that overall racial/ethnic and linguistic minorities have lower ratings of and access to care than white, English-speaking patients, particularly with assessment of timeliness of care and staff helpfulness. However, few differences were found in ratings of health plan customer service. Among whites, Latinos, and Asians, non-English speakers had more negative reports and ratings of care.
			Education level
Carlson et al. (8)	2002	**Study site:** United States **Sample:** $N = 1963$ patients in public assistance and commercial health plans **Method:** CABHS	More educated patients in commercial plans, and in publicly sponsored behavioral health care plans, rate their health plans lower. These researchers believe these differences can be attributed either to differences in expectations of care or the reporting style of the respondents.
Roohan et al. (66)	2003	**Study site:** New York **Sample:** $N = 15,106$ commercial and Medicaid enrollees	Roohan et al. confirm that patients in Medicaid with more than a college degree rated their health plans lower than did those with less education.

			Gender
		1.42% less than eighth-grade education, 30.34% some high school or high school graduate, 49.09% some college or college graduate, 19.15% greater than 4-year college education **Method:** Commercial managed care CAHPS and Medicaid managed care CAHPS surveys	
Cleary et al. (11)	2000	**Study site:** United States **Sample:** $N = 123,000$ Medicare beneficiaries **Method:** CAHPS-MMC Survey	Minimal differences were found by Cleary and colleagues in their study of gender differences in reports of quality of Medicare managed care plans; women reported slightly more positive assessments than did men.
Weisman et al. (92)	2001	**Study site:** United States **Sample:** $N = 97,873$ commercial managed care enrollees **Method:** CAHPS questionnaire administered by NCQA as part of HEDIS 1999	Weisman and colleagues found a small but significant mean difference by gender. Women reported higher satisfaction on the rating of all experience in the the health plan and on composite scores of customer services, whereas men had higher scores on three measures: getting care quickly, how well doctors communicate, and courtesy and helpfulness of office staff.

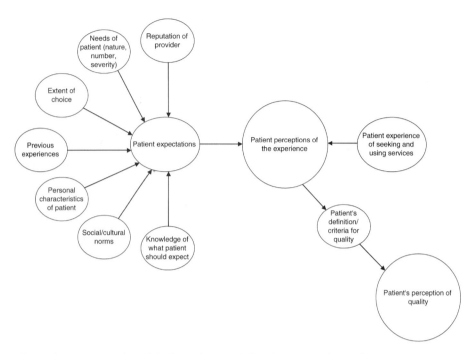

Figure 1   Conceptual model of development of patient perceptions of quality.

These authors specifically measured medical mistrust and perceived racism in the delivery of care. African Americans reported significantly higher levels of both these factors. When these variables were included in a multi-variate analysis of factors influencing satisfaction levels, race was no longer statistically significant. This study again raises the question of how variations in patient perceptions are to be interpreted. One could say that it helps explain lower satisfaction among African Americans by attributing it to perceived racism and medical mistrust, which are personal characteristics of respondents. Or one could say that, in fact, African Americans actually experience racism more frequently and have had experiences over time that lead to greater medical mistrust, thus reflecting more on the health care delivery system than on the race or ethnicity of the individual respondent. The fact that the lower satisfaction ratings by African Americans in this study stand in contrast to the higher ratings in other studies, using instruments that are more standard and administered to a sample more similar to the general adult population, further confounds our interpretive ability.

Similarly, Seid and colleagues (71) found that when they added into their regression model (accounting for 13.3% of the variance) demographic and health status variables, as well as measures of potential access to care, they found that speaking a language other than English, having a regular provider, and not having commercial insurance are very strong predictors of perceptions of care, whereas race/ethnicity per se was either eliminated as an explanatory factor (Latino) or its influence was greatly reduced (Asian). Again, this study helps us examine the black box of racial disparities by pointing to underlying structural conditions, rather than convincing us that people who happen to be Asian or Latino necessarily perceive the quality of health care in a substantially different manner than do whites. In contrast to these studies, the study by Roohan et al. (66) of respondents in Medicaid to a CAHPS® survey found that African American and Latino patients rated their plans slightly higher than did whites. Thus, the extent and nature of variations across race and ethnicity, in perceptions of health care, remain unclear, as does the issue of what drives these variations.

Two studies that examined educational level both found that more-educated patients rate their health plans lower (8, 66). Gender differences exist but are not particularly large; in general, women have slightly higher ratings than do men (11, 92). Hall & Dornan's (27) 1990 meta-analysis of patient satisfaction reported no average differences between gender in assessment of inpatient and outpatient care (27).

DISCUSSION AND RECOMMENDATIONS

Let us return to the conceptual model outlined in Figure 1 and review what we do and do not know about the development of patient perceptions of quality. We begin on the right-hand side of the model. Although there has been a good deal of research on both patient satisfaction and patient-centered care, as well as on dimensions of care such as patient-physician communication, interaction, and relationship, there has been relatively little research to explore, in a grounded manner, how patients define and perceive the quality of their health care. The situation is changing, however, because more recent measures such as the Picker and CAHPS® surveys have been developed on the basis of research using patients and consumers themselves.[5] This gives us more confidence in the validity and salience of survey results and in research that uses the results as measures of either independent or dependent variables. Methodological problems or unresolved issues still exist in current surveys, however. They include ceiling effects; uncertainty about whether instruments are reliable and valid across cultures; the continuing reliance in many surveys on ratings in which expectations are confounded with experiences; and the difficulties in collecting data from sufficiently large samples of individual physician practices or residents of smaller nursing homes, for example.

A continuing and vexing problem is that we know relatively little about whether patient definitions and perceptions of quality are stable [Jackson et al. (37) is the exception here]. Similarly, we know little about factors, including both changing

---

[5]Numerous instruments exist that address patient satisfaction with care for specific diseases and conditions. Some of these have also been based on formative work with patients. However, owing to space considerations, they are not included in this review.

experiences over time and purposeful efforts to influence expectations, that shape changes in definitions. Such studies are critically needed, especially as we begin to collect and report data on trends in patient assessments of quality.

Moving to the left-hand side of the model, we note that patient expectations have also rarely been explicitly studied [once again Jackson et al. (37) is the exception]. Instead, many studies attempt to identify how various factors directly influence patient perceptions (or more typically patient satisfaction). These factors have emphasized the demographic characteristics of patients, and aspects of their health, and as noted earlier, suffer because it is often difficult, if not impossible, to determine whether differences in ratings reflect expectations, perceptions, definitions or criteria, or experiences. One way to address this problem may be to conduct studies that explicitly compare the definitions and quality ratings of individuals with different kinds of demographic characteristics and health status, for example, or who face different kinds of choices.

Social-cultural norms have not been studied directly, even in examinations of how race and ethnicity influence reports and ratings. Some other factors that would have an influence have not received much study, including the extent of choice, provider reputation as perceived by either the patient respondent or external experts, what the patient's experience has been in the past with the plan or provider being assessed, and, as noted above, whether the patient has specific knowledge of what to expect in his/her care.

Perhaps the most important of all, the assumption persists that the technical aspects of care cannot be evaluated reliably by patients themselves. There is little doubt that patients themselves consider good health and functional status outcomes as important aspects of quality. Yet we do not believe that we should ask them, and especially publicly report, what they think about these outcomes. More work is needed to assess whether patient reports of outcomes, particularly functional status outcomes, are indeed substantially less reliable than are those of clinicians, or if in this area as in others patients focus on, and are therefore influenced by, different aspects of the experience than do clinicians. What then about patient reports of technical processes, rather than outcomes? Can we depend on patients to tell us whether specific actions were taken that are consistent with evidence-based care? What kinds of actions can they reliably report and which can they not? Additional research is needed here as well. All such research, however, will have to grapple with the uncertainty of whether to believe a medical record or the patient's report of his/her experience. We argue that unless we begin to educate patients, especially those with chronic conditions, about what they should expect from the health care system, their voices will continue to be unheard.

The growing attention to patient experience as a source of information on the quality of health care services is gratifying. However, it is clearly not enough merely to collect the data, or even to report it publicly. Ultimately, what is most critical is that we use information about patient experiences of care, whether drawn from rigorous surveys or from a one-on-one conversation between a physician and a patient, as both a goad and a guide to improve quality. The data we present here show there is considerable room for improvement. We should not continue to ignore another pathway for learning about patient experiences and perceptions: the active engagement of patients and families in quality-improvement efforts and in overall governance. Why not include patients and family members on quality-improvement teams? Why not include on hospital boards garden variety members of the public, as well as those who represent powerful stakeholders? Why not use our ingenuity both to create better-informed consumers and to provide them with opportunities to influence practice and policy more directly? If we are truly to achieve a health care system that is patient-centered, we must continue to search for creative ways to elicit, and heed, the voice of the patient.

ACKNOWLEDGMENTS

The author would like to thank Paul D. Cleary for his valuable suggestions on this paper. He is, of course, not responsible for its failings.

The *Annual Review of Public Health* is online at
http://publhealth.annualreviews.org

LITERATURE CITED

1. Anderson RT, Barbara AM, Weisman C, Scholle SH, Binko J, et al. 2001. A qualitative analysis of women's satisfaction with primary care from a panel of focus groups in the national centers of excellence in women's health. *J. Womens Health Gend. Based Med.* 10:637–47

2. Attree M. 2001. Patients' and relatives' experiences and perspectives of 'Good' and 'Not so Good' quality care. *J. Adv. Nurs.* 33:456–66

3. Bartlett JA. 2002. Addressing the challenges of adherence. *J. Acquir. Immune Defic. Syndr.* 1:S2–10

4. Bergthold L. 1984. Crabs in a bucket: the politics of health care reform in California. *J. Health Polit. Policy Law* 9:203–22

5. Blumenthal D, Epstein AM. 1996. Quality of health care. Part 6: The role of physicians in the future of quality management. *N. Engl. J. Med.* 335:1328–31

6. Brown LD, McLaughlin C. 1990. Constraining costs at the community level: a critique. *Health Aff.* 9:5–28

7. Brown R. 2001. Behavioral issues in asthma management. *Pediatr. Pulmonol. Suppl.* 21:26–30

8. Carlson MJ, Shaul JA, Eisen SV, Cleary PD. 2002. The influence of patient characteristics on ratings of managed behavioral health care. *J. Behav. Health Serv. Res.* 29:481–89

9. Cleary PD, Edgman-Levitan S, McMullen W, Delbanco TL. 1992. The relationship between reported problems and patient summary evaluations of hospital care. *Qual. Rev. Bull.* 18:53–59

10. Cleary PD, Edgman-Levitan S, Roberts M, Moloney TW, McMullen W, et al. 1991. Patients evaluate their hospital care: a national survey. *Health Aff.* 10:254–67

10a. Cleary PD, McNeil BJ. 1988. Patient satisfaction as an indicator of quality care. *Inquiry* 25:25–36

11. Cleary PD, Zaslavsky AM, Cioffi M. 2000. Sex differences in assessments of the quality of Medicare managed care. *Womens Health Issues* 10:70–79

12. Concato J, Feinstein AR. 1997. Asking patients what they like: overlooked attributes

of patient satisfaction with primary care. *Am. J. Med.* 102:399–406

13. Coulter A. 2002. After Bristol: putting patients at the centre. *BMJ* 324:648–51

13a. Covinsky KE, Rosenthal GE, Chren M, Justice AC, Fortinsky RH, et al. 1998. The relation between health status changes and patient satisfaction in older hospitalized medical patients. *J. Gen. Intern. Med.* 13:223–29

14. Coyle J, Williams B. 1999. Seeing the wood for the trees: defining the forgotten concept of patient dissatisfaction in the light of patient satisfaction research. *Int. J. Health Care Qual. Assur. Inc. Leadersh. Health Serv.* 12:i–ix

15. Crofton C, Lubalin JS, Darby C. 1999. Consumer Assessment of Health Plans Study (CAHPS). *Med. Care.* 37:MS1–9

16. Crow R, Gage H, Hampson J, Hart J, Kimber A, et al. 2002. The measurement of satisfaction with healthcare: implications for practice from a systematic review of the literature. *Health Technol. Assess.* 6:1–92

17. Davis K, Schoen C, Schoenbaum S, Audet A, Doty M, Tenney K. 2004. *Mirror, mirror on the wall: Looking at the quality of American health care through the patient's lens.* The Commonwealth Fund. http://www.cmwf.org/programs/internati onal/davis_mirrormirror_683.pdf

18. Donabedian A. 1980. Explorations in quality assessment and monitoring. *The Definition of Quality and Approaches to its Assessment*, ed. JR Griffith, 1:4–163. Washington, DC: Health Adm. Press Ann Arbor. 163 pp.

19. Edgman-Levitan S, Cleary PD. 1996. What information do consumers want and need? *Health Aff.* 15:42–56

20. Epstein KR, Laine C, Farber NJ, Nelson EC, Davidoff F. 1996. Patients' perceptions of office medical practice: judging quality through the patients' eyes. *Am. J. Med. Qual.* 11:73–80

21. Fitzpatrick R. 1991. Surveys of patient satisfaction: II—Designing a questionnaire and conducting a survey. *BMJ* 302:1129–32

22. Fitzpatrick R, Hopkins A. 1983. Problems in the conceptual framework of patient satisfaction research: an empirical exploration. *Sociol. Health Illness* 5:297–311

22a. Fremont AM, Cleary PD, Hargraves JL, Rowe RM, Jacobson NB, Ayanian JZ. 2001. Patient-centered processes of care and long-term outcomes of myocardial infarction. *J. Gen. Intern. Med.* 16:800–8

23. Gerteis M, Edgman-Levitan S, Daley J, Delbanco TL. 1993. *Through the Patient's Eyes: Understanding and Promoting Patient-Centered Care.* San Francisco: Jossey-Bass. 317 pp.

24. Golin CE, DiMatteo MR, Gelberg L. 1996. The role of patient participation in the doctor visit: implications for adherence to diabetes care. *Diabetes Care* 19:1153–64

25. Gottlieb J, Grewal D, Brown S. 1994. Consumer satisfaction and perceived quality: complementary or divergent constructs? *J. Appl. Psychol.* 79:875–85

26. Gruman JC. 1994. An expanded view of health: implications for how healthcare works. *Behav. Med.* 20:119–22

26a. Guldvog B. 1999. Can patient satisfaction improve health among patients with angina pectoris? *Int. J. Qual. Health Care.* 11:233–40

27. Hall JA, Dornan MC. 1990. Patient sociodemographic characteristics as predictors of satisfaction with medical care: a meta-analysis. *Soc. Sci. Med.* 30:811–18

28. Halperin EC. 2000. Grievances against physicians: 11 years' experience of a medical society grievance committee. *West. J. Med.* 173:235–38

29. Haviland MG, Morales LS, Reise SP, Hays RD. 2003. Do health care ratings differ by race or ethnicity? *Jt. Comm. J. Qual. Saf.* 29:134–45

30. Hertzlinger RE. 2004. *Consumer-Driven Health Care: Implications for Providers, Payers, and Policymakers.* San Francisco: Wiley. 892 pp.

31. Hibbard JH, Peters E. 2003. Supporting informed consumer health care decisions: data presentation approaches that facilitate the use of information in choice. *Annu. Rev. Public Health* 24:413–33

32. Hickson GB, Clayton EW, Githens PB, Sloan FA. 1992. Factors that prompted families to file medical malpractice claims following perinatal injuries. *JAMA* 267:1359–63

33. Hickson GB, Federspiel CF, Pichert JW, Miller CS, Gauld-Jaeger J, Bost P. 2002. Patient complaints and malpractice risk. *JAMA* 287:2951–57

34. Infante FA, Proudfoot JG, Davies GP, Bubner TK, Holton CH, et al. How people with chronic illnesses view their care in general practice: a qualitative study. *Med. J. Aust.* 181:70–73

35. Inst. Med. 2001. Crossing the quality chasm. *A New Health System for the 21st Century*, ed. R Briere, pp. 1–316. Washington, DC: National. 316 pp.

36. Irurita VF. 1999. Factors affecting the quality of nursing care: the patient's perspective. *Int. J. Nurs. Pract.* 5:86–94

37. Jackson JL, Chamberlin J, Kroenke K. 2001. Predictors of patient satisfaction. *Soc. Sci. Med.* 52:609–20

38. Jun M, Peterson R, Zsidisin G. 1998. The identification and measurement of quality in health care: focus group interview results. *Health Care Manage. Rev.* 23:81–97

39. Jung HP, Van Horne F, Wensing M, Hearnshaw H, Grol R. 1998. Which aspects of general practitioners' behaviour determine patients' evaluations of care? *Soc. Sci. Med.* 47:1077–87

40. Jung HP, Wensing M, Olesen F, Grol R. 2002. Comparison of patients' and general practitioners' evaluations of general practice care. *Qual. Saf. Health Care* 11:315–19

40a. Kane RL, Maciejewski M, Finch M. 1997. The relationship of patient satisfaction with care and clinical outcomes. *Med. Care* 35:714–30

41. Kaplan A. 1964. The conduct of inquiry. In *Methodology for Behavioral Science*, ed. L Broom, pp. 3–410. San Francisco: Chandler. 410 pp.

42. Kravitz R. 1996. Patients' expectations for medical care: an expanded formulation based on review of the literature. *Med. Care. Res. Rev.* 53:3–27

43. Krupat E, Fancey M, Cleary PD. 2000. Information and its impact on satisfaction among surgical patients. *Soc. Sci. Med.* 51:1817–25

44. Laine C, Davidoff F, Lewis CE, Nelson EC, Nelson E, et al. 1996. Important elements of outpatient care: a comparison of patients' and physicians' opinions. *Ann. Intern. Med.* 125:640–45

45. Landon BE, Zaslavsky AM, Beaulieu ND, Shaul JA, Cleary PD. 2001. Health plan characteristics and consumers' assessments of quality. *Health Aff.* 20:274–86

46. Larrabee JH, Bolden LV. 2001. Defining patient-perceived quality of nursing care. *J. Nurs. Care Qual.* 16:34–60

47. Lauver DR, Ward SE, Heidrich SM, Keller ML, Bowers BJ, et al. 2002. Patient-centered interventions. *Res. Nurs. Health* 25:246–55

48. LaVeist TA, Nickerson KJ, Bowie JV. 2000. Attitudes about racism, medical mistrust, and satisfaction with care among African American and white cardiac patients. *Med. Care Res. Rev.* 57:146–61

49. Lewin SA, Skea ZC, Entwistle V, Zwarenstein M, Dick J. 2002. Interventions for providers to promote a patient-centred approach in clinical consultations. *Cochrane Database Syst Rev.* 4:CD003267

50. Linder-Pelz S. 1982. Toward a theory of patient satisfaction. *Soc. Sci. Med.* 16:577–82

51. Lynn MR, McMillen BJ. 1999. Do nurses know what patients think is important in nursing care? *J. Nurs. Care Qual.* 13:65–74

52. Maly RC, Bourque LB, Engelhardt RF. 1999. A randomized controlled trial of

facilitating information giving to patients with chronic medical conditions: effects on outcomes of care. *J. Fam. Pract.* 48: 356–63

52a. Marshall GN, Hays RD, Mazel R. 1996. Health status and satisfaction with health care: results from the medical outcomes study. *J. Consult. Clin. Psychol.* 64:380–90

53. McGee J, Kanouse DE, Sofaer S, Hargraves JL, Hoy E, Kleimann S. 1999. Making survey results easy to report to consumers: how reporting needs guided survey design in CAHPS. Consumer Assessment of Health Plans Study. *Med. Care* 37:MS32–40

54. McLaughlin CP, Kaluzny AD. 2000. Building client centered systems of care: choosing a process direction for the next century. *Health Care Manage. Rev.* 25:73–82

55. Mead N, Bower P. 2000. Patient-centredness: a conceptual framework and review of the empirical literature. *Soc. Sci. Med.* 51:1087–110

56. Michalos A. 1985. Multiple discrepancies theory. *Soc. Indicators Res.* 16:347–413

57. Morales LS. 2001. *Assessing patient experiences with Healthcare in multi-cultural settings.* RAND http://www.rand.org/publications/RGSD/RGSD157/

58. Murphy J, Chang H, Montgomery JE, Rogers WH, Safran DG. 2001. The quality of physician-patient relationships. Patients' experiences 1996–1999. *J. Fam. Pract.* 50:123–29

59. Deleted in proof

60. Deleted in proof

61. Nelson L, Brown R, Gold M, Ciemnecki A, Docteur E. 1997. Access to care in Medicare HMOs, 1996. *Health Aff.* 16:148–56

62. Ngo-Metzger Q, Massagli MP, Clarridge BR, Manocchia M, Davis RB, et al. 2003. Linguistic and cultural barriers to care: perspectives of Chinese and Vietnamese immigrants. *J. Gen. Intern. Med.* 18:44–52

63. Press-Ganey. 2004. *Survey instruments.* http://www.pressganey.com/products_services/survey_instruments

64. Radwin L. 2000. Oncology patients' perceptions of quality nursing care. *Res. Nurs. Health* 23:179–90

65. Rice T. 1998. *The Economics of Health Reconsidered.* Chicago, IL: Health Adm. Press. 195 pp.

66. Roohan PJ, Franko SJ, Anarella JP, Dellehunt LK, Gesten FC. 2003. Do commercial managed care members rate their health plans differently than Medicaid managed care members? *Health Serv. Res.* 38:1121–34

67. Rosenthal GE, Shannon SE. 1997. The use of patient perceptions in the evaluation of health-care delivery systems. *Med. Care* 35:NS58–68

68. Ross C, Frommelt G, Hazelwood L, Chang R. 1994. The role of expectations in patient satisfaction with medical care. In *Health Care Marketing: A Foundation for Managed Quality*, ed. P Cooper, pp. 55–69. Gaithersburg, MD: Aspen

69. Safran DG. 2003. Defining the future of primary care: What can we learn from patients? *Ann. Intern Med.* 138:248–55

70. Schlesinger M, Mitchell S, Elbel B. 2002. Voices unheard: barriers to expressing dissatisfaction to health plans. *Milbank Q.* 80:709–55

71. Seid M, Stevens GD, Varni JW. 2003. Parents' perceptions of pediatric primary care quality: effects of race/ethnicity, language, and access. *Health Serv. Res.* 38: 1009–31

72. Sitzia J, Wood N. 1997. Patient satisfaction: a review of issues and concepts. *Soc. Sci. Med.* 45:1829–43

73. Sofaer S. 1988. Community health planning in the United States: a postmortem. *Fam. Community Health* 10:1–12

74. Sofaer S. 1999. Qualitative methods: What are they and why use them? *Health Serv. Res.* 34:1101–18

75. Sofaer S. 2002. Qualitative research methods. *Int. J. Qual. Health Care* 14:329–36

76. Sofaer S, Davidson BN, Goodman RD, Grier R, Kenney E, et al. 1990. Helping Medicare beneficiaries choose health insurance: the illness episode approach. *Gerontologist* 30:308–15

77. Sofaer S, Gruman J. 2003. Consumers of health information and health care: challenging assumptions and defining alternatives. *Am. J. Health Promot.* 18:151–56

78. Sofaer S, Kenney E, Davidson B. 1992. The effect of the illness episode approach on Medicare beneficiaries' health insurance decisions. *Health Serv. Res.* 27:671–93

79. Solomon LS, Zaslavsky AM, Landon BE, Cleary PD. 2002. Variation in patient-reported quality among health care organizations. *Health Care Financ. Rev.* 23:85–100

80. Starr P. 1982. The social transformation of American medicine. In *The Rise of a Sovereign Profession and the Making of a Vast Industry.* New York: Basic Books. 449 pp.

81. Stewart M, Meredith L, Brown JB, Galajda J. 2000. The influence of older patient-physician communication on health and health-related outcomes. *Clin. Geriatr. Med.* 16:25–36

82. Stichler JF, Weiss ME. 2000. Through the eye of the beholder: multiple perspectives on quality in women' s health care. *Qual. Manag. Health Care* 8:1–13

83. Strasser S, Ahorony L, Greenberger D. 1993. The patient satisfaction process: moving toward a comprehensive model. *Med. Care Rev.* 50:219–48

84. Strasser S, Davis R. 1991. *Measuring Patient Satisfaction.* Ann Arbor, MI: Health Adm. Press

85. Taira DA, Safran DG, Seto TB, Rogers WH, Inui TS, et al. 2001. Do patient assessments of primary care differ by patient ethnicity? *Health Serv. Res.* 36:1059–71

86. Taylor DM, Wolfe R, Cameron PA. 2002. Complaints from emergency department patients largely result from treatment and communication problems. *Emerg. Med.* 14:43–49

87. Thi PL, Briancon S, Empereur F, Guillemin F. 2002. Factors determining inpatient satisfaction with care. *Soc. Sci. Med.* 54:493–504

88. Thompson A, Sunol R. 1995. Expectations as determinants of patient satisfaction: concepts, theory and evidence. *Int. Qual. Health Care* 7:127–41

89. Valentine NB, DeSilva A, Kawabata K, Darby C, Murray CJL, Evans DB. 2003. Health system responsiveness: concepts, domains, and operationalization. In *Health Systems Performance Assessment: Debates, Methods, and Empiricism,* ed. CJL Murray, DB Evans, pp. 573–96. Geneva: World Health Organ. 927 pp.

90. Wagner EH, Austin BT, Von Korff M. 1996. Organizing care for patients with chronic illness. *Milbank Q.* 74:511–44

91. Weech-Maldonado R, Morales LS, Elliott M, Spritzer K, Marshall G, Hays RD. 2003. Race/ethnicity, language, and patients' assessments of care in Medicaid managed care. *Health Serv. Res.* 38:789–808

92. Weisman CS, Henderson JT, Schifrin E, Romans M, Clancy CM. 2001. Gender and patient satisfaction in managed care plans: analysis of the 1999 HEDIS/CAHPS 2.0H Adult Survey. *Womens Health Issues* 11:401–15

93. Wensing M, Jung HP, Mainz J, Olesen F, Grol R. 1998. A systematic review of the literature on patient priorities for general practice care. Part 1: Description of the research domain. *Soc. Sci. Med.* 47:1573–88

94. Westat. 2004. What consumers say about the quality of their health plan and medical care. *Natl. CAHPS Database Chartbook* 2003:34. http://ncbd.cahps.org/Home/chartbook.asp

95. Williams B. 1994. Patient satisfaction: a valid concept? *Soc. Sci. Med.* 38:509–16

96. World Health Organ. 2000. *The World Health Report 2000: Health Systems: Improving Performance.* Geneva: World Health Organ. 206 pp.

Annu. Rev. Public Health 2005. 26:561–82
doi: 10.1146/annurev.publhealth.26.021304.144703
Copyright © 2005 by Annual Reviews. All rights reserved
First published online as a Review in Advance on November 15, 2004

Toward a System of Cancer Screening in the United States: Trends and Opportunities*

Nancy Breen[1] and Helen I. Meissner[2]

[1]Health Services and Economics Branch, Applied Research Program, [2]Applied Cancer
Screening Research Branch, Behavioral Research Program, Division of Cancer Control
and Population Sciences, National Cancer Institute, Rockville, Maryland 20852-7344;
email: Breenn@mail.nih.gov, HM36D@NIH.GOV

Key Words   access, quality, cost-effectiveness

■ **Abstract**   The hard work of public health officials, physicians, and disease advocacy groups to educate Americans about the importance of early detection has resulted
in uptake of screening tests at levels equivalent to or higher than in countries with
organized cancer screening programs. However, the societal costs of high screening
rates are larger in the United States than in other countries, including higher prices for
screening, more unnecessary testing, and inefficiencies in delivery, especially in small
practices. Further, screening rates are not evenly distributed across population groups,
and the national expenditure on clinical and community research to promote cancer
screening among individuals has not been matched by research efforts that focus on
policy or clinical systems to increase screening widely throughout the population. We
identify opportunities for organizational change that improve access to use, improve
quality, and promote cost effectiveness in cancer screening delivery.

OVERVIEW

In the United States, cancer screening rates are equivalent to or higher than those
of other industrialized countries. Widespread enthusiasm in the United States for
screening is the result of the hard work of public health officials, physicians, and
disease advocacy groups to educate Americans about the importance of early detection. These efforts have likely accelerated the uptake of tests for which screening
confers a range of benefits, including the gold standard of a mortality benefit. However, these high rates of screening have been achieved at considerable societal cost.
The efforts to promote screening may also have encouraged overuse of screening
among some groups (97). Furthermore, screening rates are not evenly distributed
across the population.

---

*The U.S. Government has the right to retain a nonexclusive, royalty-free license in and to
any copyright covering this paper.

Research and dissemination efforts in the United States have focused on promoting cancer screening to individual patients, individual physicians, and, to a lesser extent, health care organizations. The national emphasis on promoting cancer screening to these specific groups has not been matched by equivalent efforts to address the broad structural and policy factors that affect the distribution and delivery of this approach to preventive care. Focusing on these broad factors is challenging, particularly when the organization and financing of health care is fragmented, as it is in the United States. However, changes to systems and policies present valuable opportunities for improving the distribution and delivery of cancer screening modalities once individual interventions have been shown effective.

In this review, we examine trends in cancer screening and the many factors that influence use of tests, including promotional interventions. The purpose of our investigation is to identify opportunities for improving the ways in which cancer screening is organized and delivered in the United States. These ways include increasing access to use, generally improving quality, and promoting cost effectiveness of services delivered. We also suggest additional directions for policy and structural interventions that could improve screening delivery. In so doing, we hope to stimulate creative thinking about cancer screening policy and improve how clinics are structured and health care is delivered. This is a critical but neglected area of research.

PERSPECTIVES ON THE BENEFITS OF CANCER SCREENING

The decision to screen for cancer should be based on well-established criteria (117). First, the disease should be an important health problem. Second, there should be a detectable preclinical phase. Third, treatment of screen-detected disease should offer advantages over and above those achieved by waiting to treat until the disease is symptomatic. Fourth, the screening test should be affordable and cost-effective. Fifth, the test must be acceptable to the target population and to health care professionals. Finally, the test must achieve an acceptable level of accuracy in the population undergoing screening. The ultimate measure of success of a cancer screening program is that it reduces disease-specific mortality in the at-risk population. For screening to be effective by this measure, it needs to be an early step in a larger care process that is conducted systematically and in a timely manner (125).

The groundbreaking 2001 Institute of Medicine (IOM) report, *Crossing the Quality Chasm*, draws on an underlying care delivery framework described by Berwick (6). This framework, which provides a useful lens through which to examine the overall health care distribution and delivery process, consists of four levels: the experience of patients; the functioning of small units (or teams) of care delivery; the functioning of the organizations that house or otherwise support care delivery; and the environment of policy, payment, regulation, accreditation, litigation, and other factors that shape the behavior, interests, and opportunities of the organizations.

The current literature already has identified important barriers to cancer screening, which individual efforts are powerless to change. These include lack of access to health care, lack of insurance coverage for preventive services, and economic pressures on physicians that result in ever-shorter office visits. The literature also shows, however, that because they establish the structural context for service delivery to patients, the three broader levels of the health care framework (care units, organizations, and environment) can do much to help reduce these barriers for patients. For example, compelling evidence suggests that systematic diffusion of guidelines, computerized reminder systems, and a system of auditing physician adherence to guidelines, along with providing routine feedback to physicians, improve the rates of recommended preventive care delivery in practices that have a clear policy supporting screening guidelines (52, 100, 116).

To fully understand trends and opportunities, as well as the specifics of distribution and delivery and the factors that may favorably affect its appropriate and equitable use, screening should be considered from a population health, or societal, perspective (70). Because it is designed to take into account everyone affected by screening programs, the societal perspective examines all significant health outcomes and costs that flow from it, regardless of who experiences the outcomes or costs (33). This perspective recognizes that resources are limited and that even health—at least to some degree—should be subject to the resource limits that constrain society. Thus, not every screening test would be reimbursed regardless of benefit. But neither would anyone be categorically excluded from getting services with a proven benefit. In short, the societal perspective is a comprehensive viewpoint that, if successful, gives appropriate weight to all significant aspects of an issue. It is from this perspective that we examine trends and opportunities for cancer screening in the United States.

TRENDS IN CANCER SCREENING

For screening to provide a maximum benefit, the population at risk needs to participate at a high level. Monitoring screening patterns and trends is critical to achieving population benefits because it enables us to identify who is getting screened and which factors may impede or facilitate the behavior. Population-based monitoring can therefore help researchers target and direct interventions so as to maximize screening rates in a population. Population-based monitoring also can be used to assess the degree to which community-based screening interventions achieve the same participation rates and beneficial outcomes as those achieved in randomized trials (106).

Trends in use of different screening modalities are influenced by a variety of factors. For example, evidence of test efficacy [as reflected by publication of U.S. Preventive Services Task Force (USPSTF) clinical guidelines] and inclusion of the procedure as a health insurance benefit (such as by Medicare) can have a significant influence on the uptake of cancer screening. Trends in use also reflect the length of time since tests were first marketed and the resources, capacity, and infrastructure available for test delivery. The availability of the equipment and staff trained to perform and evaluate the procedures are key elements that ensure adequate delivery. Trends also reflect patient and provider access to the test as influenced by financial, administrative, and geographic realities; ease of administration (for example, is specialty referral required?); and acceptability (for example, invasiveness) of the screening test.

Figure 1 shows trends in prevalence of four cancer screening tests. The Figure shows that Pap testing is the most widely used type of cancer screening. It was first introduced in the 1940s, and its widespread adoption occurred before the National Health Interview Survey (NHIS) began monitoring cancer screening, before the USPSTF guidelines, and before Medicare coverage began. After its initial diffusion, use of Pap testing increased slowly but steadily.

Figure 1 also shows that of these four tests, mammography has been the most heavily influenced by the publication of guidelines and inclusion as a covered benefit. National monitoring of mammography use began before publication of the USPSTF guidelines, and Medicare benefits followed shortly thereafter. These factors, combined with the passage of state legislation mandating private insurance

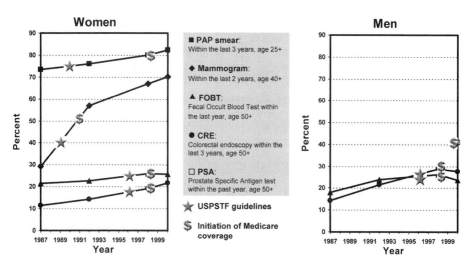

Percentages are standardized to the 2000 Projected U.S. Population by 5-year age groups.

[1] National Health Interview Survey
[2] http://healthservices.cancer.gov/seermedicare/considerations/testing.html
[3] For mammography and pap test recommendations, see U.S. Preventive Services Task Force. 1989. *Guide to Clinical Preventive Services: An Assessment of the Effectiveness of 169 Interventions.* Baltimore: Williams & Wilkins (110a). For FOBT and CRE, see U.S. Preventive Services Task Force. 1996. *Guide to Clinical Preventive Services.* Washington, DC: Off. Dis. Prev. Health Promot., US Gov. Print. Off. (110b).

Figure 1   Screening trends by gender with years of guidelines and Medicare initiation. Recent use of cancer screening tests,[1] initiation of Medicare coverage,[2] and USPSTF guidelines[3]: 1987, 1992, 1998, 2000.

coverage for mammography screening, discussed below, probably account for the documented rapid rise in reported mammography use.

Colorectal cancer screening uptake has been slower than either Pap tests or mammograms, in part because evidence of a benefit for colorectal cancer screening appeared more recently than for breast and cervical cancer screening tests (86). Another reason for the slower uptake of colorectal cancer screening may be the variety of competing tests available for this purpose. For example, one U.K. study found that uptake was slower when physicians recommended more than one screening test for a particular cancer to their patients (111). This issue may also affect the implementation of public health messages. The decline shown in Figure 1 in use of colorectal endoscopy reported by men after 1998 may be due to changes in the 2000 NHIS, when question wording was modified to reflect changes in science, technology, and physician practices. Use of prostate specific antigen (PSA) testing was already widely used in the United States when it was first measured in the 2000 NHIS, even though the efficacy of the test is fraught with uncertainty (89). Although the scientific evidence is not sufficient for USPSTF guidelines to recommend the test, it is nevertheless covered by Medicare. Randomized clinical trials to test whether PSA confers a mortality benefit are ongoing in the United States and Europe (23, 32). A recently published study questioned whether PSA could detect prostate cancer (108).

FACTORS AFFECTING THE USE OF CANCER SCREENING TESTS

For widespread screening to occur in a population, physicians and patients must know about the tests, consider them valuable, and be able to adopt them. Broad social, political, and economic systems that shape behaviors and access to resources also are critical to the widespread adoption of screening (46). As a result, factors affecting the use of cancer screening tests are frequently grouped and analyzed in terms of patients, physicians, and systems. Reviews have been conducted of the large literatures on surveillance (10, 42, 102) and behavioral intervention research on patients and providers (8, 58, 66, 74, 99, 101, 112, 113, 115, 121). Researchers also have conducted several reviews of interventions to increase recommendations for cancer screening by physicians, and they found that introducing information systems and organizational changes in staffing and procedures has consistently increased cancer screening rates (65, 99, 101).

In contrast to the large literature on factors affecting patients and providers, studies of how systemic factors affect cancer screening practices are almost nonexistent, except for a recent analysis of health plan policies and practices by Klabunde et al. (50). Little research has focused on cancer screening policy (74) except for two recent papers by Adams (1, 2) and an older paper by Holland (44), even though it is increasingly recognized that individual behavior should be considered in the context of the broader economic environment that shapes, facilitates, and limits health care delivery. In the following sections, we briefly summarize the patient and provider literature and discuss several key systemic issues that influence screening behavior.

Patient Factors

A number of factors influence the degree to which individuals receive cancer screening tests. Numerous studies have shown that patients with a usual source of care are far more likely to get screened for cancer than are other patients (10, 20, 26, 38, 64, 102, 110). Similarly, screening increases with the number of physicians seen (55), the number of appointments kept (110), the number of years of clinic attendance (63), and the receipt of regular medical check-ups (59). Cancer screening also is strongly related to use of other preventive services and behaviors (21, 59, 69, 88).

Not surprisingly, therefore, the major reason patients report not having a recent cancer screening test is lack of a physician recommendation (27, 28, 30, 35, 81, 114). Patients also report being less likely to initiate screening if they believe they cannot afford treatment if cancer is found (84). NHIS data, shown in Table 1, provides further evidence about common barriers to screening. Lack of a usual source of health care, inadequate health insurance coverage, and having recently immigrated to the United States are important patient barriers to obtaining cancer screening services (10, 47). Related barriers associated with patients not getting cancer screening services include low income, low educational attainment, rural or inner-city residence, older age, nonwhite race, and Hispanic and Asian ethnicity (102).

Cultural orientation toward preventive services shapes use among immigrants (53, 107, 109), although lack of access to health care may be a more immediate reason why immigrants in low-income populations are not screened (47, 57, 123). Clearly, solutions to these barriers, as well as to the high cost of services, are beyond an individual patient's ability to solve. Improving access to health care and providing culturally competent health services to individuals requires policy and structural interventions. For example, one recent study found that improving

TABLE 1 Cancer screening in the United States: Where are the disparities? 2000 National Health Interview Survey. From Reference 102

Barriers to screening	Pap test	Mammogram	Colorectal (women)	Colorectal (men)
Total	82%	70%	38%	41%
No health insurance	62%	38%	18%	20%
No usual source of care	58%	35%	13%	14%
Recent immigration	61%	39%	16%	20%

access to health care attenuated differences between foreign-born Latinos more than foreign-born Asians, as compared with U.S.-born whites (31).

Physician Factors

The behavioral literature on cancer screening has shown that physicians who have better general prevention knowledge and lower patient volume tend to have higher referral rates (29, 37, 55, 60, 94). Higher screening referral rates also are associated with such physician characteristics as being younger in age, being an internist (versus a family practitioner) or obstetrician gynecologist, and being female (55, 60).

Although individual physician behavior and characteristics are important, systemic modifications also can improve physician recommendations. A study by Ward et al. (116) found that system-wide internal policies and structures to promote cancer screening were more powerful predictors of the extent to which Department of Veterans Affairs (VA) physicians complied with guidelines than were an individual physician's knowledge of and proclivity toward screening. Supportive systems are needed if practices are to recommend and perform cancer screening according to guidelines. Audits of compliance with feedback (5, 62), facility policy to which care providers subscribe (116), and reminder systems have improved compliancance with guidelines. In a review published in 1998, Rimer (93) recommended that reminder systems should constitute a minimum practice for all health systems because the evidence for them was overwhelming (they doubled or tripled the odds of women getting breast or cervical cancer screening).

In addition to policies and structures to support physician recommendations for cancer screening, policies and structures also must be in place to support follow-up to cancer screening. In a review of the literature on follow-up care after cancer screening, Yabroff et al. (122) found that fewer than 75% of patients screened for cancer get timely follow-up, and a recent study (48) found that 9% of women with a newly discovered breast abnormality had received no follow-up care 12 months later. O'Malley et al. (84) found that doctors would be less likely to recommend screening if they know or suspect their patient is uninsured or unable to afford or locate free follow-up care. Delays or lack of follow-up after screening undermine the purpose of screening—to prevent or detect cancer early. Interventions to address barriers to follow-up care are needed at the patient, provider, and system levels (122).

Systemic Factors

The unusual way health services are structured and financed in the United States significantly influences the delivery and distribution of health care services, including screening.

FINANCING HEALTH CARE DELIVERY   In the United States, health care is distributed through markets. Unlike other industries, most health care is paid for by insurance companies rather than by consumers, and the services covered depend on the individual patient's insurance policy. Providers do not decide which services will be covered or their level of reimbursement. The level of services offered depends on the patient's insurance coverage and profit rates in the insurance industry. Thus, most decisions about health care screening are driven, at least to some extent, by reimbursement factors rather than by science-based policy. Key exceptions are legislation mandating private insurance coverage for mammography and programs covering breast and cervical cancer screening and treatment for poor, uninsured women.

For most Americans, health insurance is an employment benefit, although about 29% of the workforce works in small companies (defined as fewer than 25 employees). About 30% (12.6 million) work in companies where health insurance is not provided and so remain uninsured. Further analysis reveals an important dynamic that economists call "market power." Large corporations use their market power to reduce premiums paid to insurance companies and prices paid to physicians, including for cancer screening for their employees. Small businesses do not have equivalent market power to do this, and, therefore, many small businesses do not pay insurance premiums for their employees. As a result, employees of small companies lack insurance as well as face higher prices for screening services. Limited insurance coverage and higher prices for services worsen health care access. In contrast, employees of large corporations, who have better health benefits, are more likely to obtain cancer screening. Even for large corporations, however, this benefit is a Pyrrhic victory. Overall, as Reinhardt points out, the highly fragmented organization of health care financing in the United States serves to allocate relatively greater market power to the supply side of the health system, resulting in higher prices for health services. Because of fragmentation among the multiple purchasers of care, U.S. prices rise above those in industrialized countries with either a single-payer system or collective bargaining among multiple payers (91). The greater market power held by the supply side of the health system also can increase demand for services beyond what is needed.

Overall costs of cancer screening are higher in the United States than anywhere else in the industrialized world. For example, in 1997, the median charge for colonoscopy in Canada was US$606, and in the United States it was US$1736 (4). For a screening mammogram, the median charge was US$77 and US$130, respectively. Inefficiencies in the delivery of screening in the United States contribute to the high cost of screening in the United States (9). Another reason is that efforts to collect monitoring and evaluation data and to conduct promotional campaigns that encourage screening are not routinely incorporated into the delivery of clinical screening services. This means that these efforts must be funded separately, adding to the overall cost of screening. The cost of malpractice insurance, which is high relative to the revenues physicians earn from practicing medicine, is a third reason. Mammography is the procedure associated with the most malpractice suits (12, 14). Prostate cancer screening may also be vulnerable to lawsuits. Although evidence is lacking that PSA testing conveys a mortality benefit, a recent *JAMA* editorial documents a malpractice suit brought by a patient who, under presumed conditions of shared decision making, did not have a PSA and then sued when he was subsequently diagnosed with prostate cancer (75).

STRUCTURING HEALTH CARE DELIVERY   Overcoming barriers related to the structure and financing of screening services requires intervention at the policy or system level. An examination of the two most prevalent models of health care service delivery in the United States—equal access providers and small entrepreneur providers—can illuminate the types of policy- or system-level interventions that could be instituted to ensure equitable access to appropriate cancer screening services.

A growing minority of Americans obtain health care through health insurance plans that have been called "equal access" providers (98) or "organized plans." These providers include group- and staff-model HMOs, the VA, and many "safety net" providers. Organized plans determine coverage as well as provide clinical services to patients. For a fixed annual fee, they offer preventive services on the basis of whether patients are eligible according to USPSTF or other clinical practice guidelines. As a result, socioeconomic disparities all along the continuum of cancer care, from screening services through follow-up and treatment, are less likely to occur in organized practice settings. For this reason, we characterize them as equal access providers. It is important to note, however, that equal access providers offer equal access only to those able to leap the cost barrier of a monthly insurance fee. Therefore these providers may systematically exclude whole groups of people, such as the unemployed, from their care.

Most patients are served by providers who work in individual or group practices as small entrepreneurs. These patients are insured by policies independent of the health care provider, and the provider has no control over what procedures are covered. Entrepreneurial plans can be grouped into several types, including Fee-For-Service (FFS) or indemnity, Network, Individual Practice Association (IPA), and Preferred Provider Organization (PPO)/Point of Service (POS). Except for FFS, all are managed care plans. What they have in common is that they provide health care only when a patient has coverage for the service.

THE FINANCING AND STRUCTURE OF CANCER SCREENING CAN LEAD TO OVERUSE AND UNDERUSE   The way that health care is structured and financed in the United States is generally thought to encourage distortions in the appropriate use of cancer screening procedures (24, 90, 120).

Overuse   Leaving decisions about screening to individual doctors and consumers adds to the demand for services, especially when patients have insurance coverage, and creates an environment where profit, rather than public health, motivates how health care is delivered. The U.S. health care service market allows screening services to be offered regardless of their scientific merit. As a result, screening services may be used too frequently or by patients for whom cancer screening is not recommended. For example, patients who can afford widely advertised full-body scans or other unproven screening tests can readily purchase them, even though they confer no medical benefit. From a population health, or societal, perspective, these expenditures appear to be a waste of resources. If reaching an entire population, including the poor, in a timely fashion is a concern, then it seems unethical to spend resources on unproven methods or to overuse procedures when the resources could be used to provide proven screening services throughout the population.

Overuse of cancer screening also leads to higher follow-up rates for American consumers compared with consumers in other countries. Higher follow-up is due to the higher relative value placed on sensitivity compared with specificity of test results (which yields a higher rate of false positive tests) in the United States (25). Though the literature on this is scant, adverse screening results leading to unnecessary follow-up procedures may reduce quality of life (11, 36).

Underuse   Investigators generally agree that the first test for prevalence of cancer is more important than subsequent screens (18). However, although cancer screening may be frequently used by those who can afford it, some high-risk populations are never screened. One of the largest groups never screened is those without health insurance. An estimated 15.2% of the population, or 43.6 million people, were without health insurance coverage during the entire year in 2002, up from 14.6% in 2001. This represents an increase of 2.4 million people (79). Lack of insurance or other resources to cover costs of screening and follow-up can preclude realizing the benefits of early detection.

Disparities in payment to physicians may further exacerbate underuse. For example, specialists are reimbursed at higher rates, both by Medicare and by private insurance plans, than are primary care physicians. Unequal reimbursement encourages physicians to specialize, locate in relatively wealthy areas, and establish their practice or business in areas with economic demand for services. In this way, disparities in payment to physicians result in shortages of doctors in inner city and rural areas and cause differentials in quality and coverage (118).

OPPORTUNITIES TO IMPROVE CANCER SCREENING IN THE UNITED STATES

Policy has great potential to affect a large number of people inasmuch as it shapes the organization, financing, and delivery of cancer screening. However, we have little data on the effect of policy on cancer screening because it is rarely evaluated in the United States. Notable exceptions include evaluations of policies to promote cervical cancer interventions implemented in the 1980s and 1990s (44, 76) and recent evaluations of various screening programs by Adams et al. (1, 2). A recent addition to these studies compared women enrolled in organized health plans with women in the surrounding community. This evaluation concluded that enrollment in an organized health plan is associated with increased likelihood of mammography and reduced odds of late-stage breast cancer (105). The following section focuses on national policies and structural interventions at the clinical and health plan level that already facilitate cancer screening. We then propose additional interventions that could potentially reduce costs while improving the quality, coverage, and delivery of cancer screening services and then detail several key research opportunities.

Building on Current Interventions

Many programs already exist that have improved cancer screening in the United States. They operate nationally and in plans and clinics delivering health care around the country. If extended, these interventions could improve cancer screening even more.

NATIONAL INTERVENTIONS   Legislation, regulation, monitoring, and funding have increased access to some types of screening. Similar policy interventions would likely yield similar results for other types of screening in the future. For example, starting in 1987, all 50 states began passing legislation mandating mammography by private health insurance plans (71). This trend in legislation was concurrent with a rapid increase in reported use of mammography (Figure 1).

The Medicare program, which provides nearly universal health insurance coverage to Americans aged 65 and older (80) and has lower administrative costs than other do health insurance programs in the United States (119), may be the most successful policy model for health insurance coverage and surveillance in the United States. As the largest purchaser of health care services in the country, Medicare is a prime example of the power of national interventions to influence screening. Medicare's coverage for Part B participants for routine cancer screening (which follows science-based guidelines, with the notable exception of the PSA test), additional screening and follow-up after suspicious screening results, and diagnosis and treatment has had a decided impact on use of these services. In addition, as the only agency to have published reimbursement rates, Medicare tends to set the standard for private insurance reimbursement in the United States.

Although the Center for Medicare and Medicaid Services (CMS) conducts no routine systematic evaluation of the use of Medicare services or patient outcomes and does not collect claims from patients in HMOs (92), several sources of Medicare data are available to researchers; these sources could provide valuable insight into the factors that foster, as well as hinder, optimal cancer screening. These include the Medicare Current Beneficiary Survey (MCBS) (3), the Consumer Assessment of Health Plans Study (CAHPS) (40), and Medicare claims data. The MCBS collects information on cancer screening, and these data can be linked to the Medicare claims data of survey participants. Analyses using these data have led to improvements in Medicare policy. For example, Medicare eliminated its deductible on mammograms after finding that healthy, poor enrollees were less likely to obtain mammography than were other women because of the annual deductible (7). Other studies have documented disparities in delivery of Medicare services (15, 16), and these findings have led CMS to examine Medicare delivery to historically underserved populations, a critical step toward taking corrective action to eliminate disparities in care. Another service Medicare could provide is a population-based registry needed for efforts to develop an organized national system of screening.

The National Breast and Cervical Cancer Early Detection Program (BCCEDP) is another excellent example of the power of national interventions to influence screening behavior. BCCEDP provides access to breast and cervical cancer screening for uninsured, poor women. First offered to states in 1991, this federal-state partnership, administered and funded by the Centers for Disease Control and Prevention in conjunction with participating states, was rapidly adopted throughout the 50 states, territories, and Indian nations (41, 67, 68). A recent study showed that the number of years since a state adopted the program significantly predicts increased mammography and cervical cancer screening (1). Despite its popularity and success, current funding for the program covers only about 21% of eligible women aged 50–64 years, and coverage varies among states (F. Tangka, CDC, personal communication, 2004).

Considerable anecdotal evidence and studies published during the 1990s suggested that even though poor and uninsured women were getting screened through these low-cost programs, they had no means for obtaining follow-up tests when results were suspicious and no means for obtaining diagnosis and treatment in a timely manner (56). The Congress passed the Breast and Cervical Cancer Prevention and Treatment Act in 2000 to address this issue. The Act provides immediate (presumed) eligibility for Medicaid to cover follow-up care for low-income, uninsured women diagnosed with cancer. Coverage details, like other aspects of Medicaid, are left to individual states.

CLINICAL AND HEALTH PLAN INTERVENTIONS   As Zapka (124) points out, insurance plans can play an important role in improving screening because they design benefits, develop and disseminate guidelines for use and reimbursement, and provide health education. The health services literature often distinguishes between HMO/managed care and FFS/indemnity plans. This distinction is important when considering cancer screening because patients with health maintenance plans are more likely than are those with indemnity plans to obtain screening (34, 45). Two reviews of the literature on performance indicators spanning 1980–2001 documented that patient satisfaction with prevention uniformly favored managed care over nonmanaged care (77, 78). In addition, managed care coverage of preventive services was more comprehensive, though findings were mixed for other types of services. A recent comparison of Medicare beneficiaries aged 65 and older in managed care and FFS settings found that managed care was better at delivering preventive services, whereas traditional Medicare was better in other aspects of care (54). These studies included all types of managed care, not just organized plans such as group- and staff-model HMOs.

In 2000, Phillips (85) surmised from Potosky's findings (87) that the inception of widespread managed care in the United States had reduced previous differences found in screening rates between group- and staff-model HMOs and indemnity plans. Yet, almost no outcome studies distinguish between group- and staff-model HMOs and other types of managed care organizations (19). A recently published survey of health plans and policies by Klabunde et al. (51) is one of the few studies that does distinguish between staff and group model HMOs and other types of managed care. This analysis found that group- and staff-model health plans were far more likely than were other types of managed care plans to have any system at all for screening delivery or monitoring (92% versus 36%). They also were significantly more likely than were other plan types to cover more than one screening modality, to have issued screening guidelines to providers, and to have issued guidelines covering more than one screening modality.

These findings suggest that policy and structural interventions to increase cancer screenings may be more feasible or successful in organized plan and practice settings because these settings can intervene at multiple levels, and therefore the interventions can have synergistic effects (124). This is particularly true when all components of the cancer continuum are targeted (125) because, as noted at the outset, cancer screening is effective in reducing cancer mortality only when it is accompanied by timely follow-up and treatment. For example, a review of health disparities in cancer treatment found that group- and staff-model HMOs and the VA system yielded similar cancer outcomes between racial-ethnic minorities and whites diagnosed with the same stage cancer (98).

Major structural changes are often more easily implemented in an organized setting than an entrepreneurial one. For example, Taplin et al. (104) found that a "team approach" in a staff-model health plan, in which a team of providers and staff organized care for a specific group of patients, did better at providing screening than did adjacent practices, largely by implementing an information system under an agreed-on plan. A meta-analysis conducted by Stone et al. (101) found that organizational change consistently increased use of cancer screening services when compared with physician-directed and patient-directed interventions. The changes tested included establishing a separate clinic devoted to screening and prevention, incorporating prevention into planned care visits, assigning staff to identify patients in need of prevention services, and arranging appointments for those patients (101). Stone concludes that decisions to use a particular approach will depend on resources, expertise, feasibility, and cost-effectiveness.

Several factors may help explain why it is easier to execute changes in organized settings than in others: the presence of research departments that disseminate scientific findings to staff; structured opportunities for discussion and debate about practices and protocols; institutional policies to screen patients for cancer; centralized administrations that allow for economies of scale; and strategic integration of prompts and reminder systems (66), goal setting, benchmarking, audits, and feedback (62).

However, some structural changes are feasible in any setting. For example, screening test use increases when reminder systems are in place. These systems can be instituted in entrepreneurial practice settings as well as organized plans. Other structural changes can increase screening rates for tests that require a referral and additional appointment (such as mammography and colorectal endoscopy) (13, 39, 72). One innovative study at a community health center introduced academic detailing and also moved sigmoidoscopy on site. Both physician referrals for and use of sigmoidoscopy by patients increased as a result (96). This finding is important because integrating screening services by moving them to the same site is against the tide in the United States. Mammography and colorectal endoscopy services usually require an additional appointment at a separate facility.

The Health Plan Employer Data and Information Set (HEDIS), a public-private surveillance effort, is an important tool that can be used to monitor the outcomes of structural interventions at the clinic and health plan level. HEDIS is a core set of health plan performance measures covering quality, access, patient satisfaction, membership, utilization, and finance, which has begun to bridge the information gap in the privately insured population younger than age 65. Designed to provide information for employers seeking cost-effective health insurance plans for their employees, HEDIS has measured ambulatory care facility compliance with breast and cervical cancer screening guidelines since its inception (22).

HEDIS cancer screening measures are based on USPSTF recommendations, supplemented with American Cancer Society guidelines when greater precision on the timing of screening is needed than USPSTF provides (82). HEDIS data, collected from nearly 600 managed care plans covering approximately 51 million Americans, show breast and cervical cancer screening rates slightly higher for managed care facilities than for those reported by the general population (83, 102). Colorectal cancer screening will become a HEDIS measure in 2005 (http://www.ncqa.org/communications/news/hedis2004pubcomm.htm).

Promulgation of clinical practice guidelines also has been widely promoted as a strategy to improve quality of cancer screening care. However, a Cochrane Review found that passive dissemination of information is generally ineffective, and policies designed to encourage more active implementation of research-based recommendations are needed to ensure changes in practice patterns (5). Studies of the promulgation of screening guidelines to physicians need to evaluate how the characteristics of different types of plans affect screening diffusion (5, 17). A recent Swedish study (49) showed that training to bring clinical practice into conformity with guidelines is possible regardless of the practice venue, although time and financial limits may constrain physician entrepreneurs from engaging in this activity without voluntary society or government help.

LOOKING TO THE FUTURE

Many of the deficiencies in the distribution and delivery of cancer screening described in this review could be rectified if clinical services were organized into larger entities that could allow providers to take advantage of economies of scale, incorporate and update new technology rapidly, and distribute services, as needed, to at-risk populations.

Although these solutions have been identified (33) and the national interventions noted in the previous section have taken advantage of them, the high price of screening and its effect on the distribution of cancer screening services still must be addressed by global policy informed by economic analysis from the societal perspective (95). Additional research could fruitfully inform these analyses. For example, research is needed to identify the types of structures and policies that maximize access, quality, and cost-effectiveness of cancer screening. Structures themselves are rarely the target of interventions, and they need to be considered. Structural aspects of health care delivery include type of delivery system, technological systems within clinical practice, organization of clinical practice, and practice patterns. When practice patterns are analyzed, the type of delivery system is rarely described clearly. A clear explanation of the type of delivery system should be routinely included in analyses of interventions because it is impossible to generalize about findings if the study context is not known.

Studies have shown that equal-access organized health plans better promote and facilitate access to high-quality, cost-effective cancer screening than do other types of health plans. Including all types of nonindemnity plans under the umbrella term "managed care" is no longer analytically useful because managed care is the primary type of health plan in the United States, and its meaning is unclear. However, managed care includes a wide variety of types of plans and structures, including staff models, Networks, IPA, and PPO/POS. To evaluate service delivery policy and structures, studies need to report the type of system within which the intervention or surveillance is conducted.

In the meantime, however, a number of existing policies could be extended to improve cancer screening in the United States:

- Legislation mandating private insurance coverage for mammography could be extended to other scientifically supported cancer screening modalities and to regular checkups, which are associated with higher cancer screening rates.

- Single payer coverage, such as Medicare, could be extended to the entire population to adequately reimburse cancer screening and clinical follow-up (43, 73).

- Extend the BCCEDP to colorectal cancer screening and extend Medicaid presumptive eligibility to colorectal cancer treatment.

- Employ standardized guidelines for cancer screening. The VA, large-group and staff-model HMOs, and HEDIS already use established guidelines, which discourage use of screening tests that have no evidence of a mortality benefit.

- Reimburse for health maintenance visits to encourage providers to discuss cancer screening and other preventive services with new enrollees.

- Extend HEDIS measures to screening follow-up, including delivery of all test results, and follow-up when results are suspicious or treatment is needed.

- Incorporate cancer screening reminder systems for patients and providers.
- Develop a national system of screening registries linked to cancer registries to monitor periodicity of use of screening services as well as use of follow-up services. The Breast Cancer Surveillance Consortium provides a model for a cancer screening registry (http://breastscreening.cancer.gov/espp.pdf).
- Standardize forms and procedures for processing private insurance claims to bring their administrative costs in line with those of Medicare.

ACKNOWLEDGMENTS

We thank Stephen Taplin, Molla Donaldson, and Jon Kerner for helpful comments on the content of this review and Anne Rodgers for superb editing.

**The *Annual Review of Public Health* is online at
http://publhealth.annualreviews.org**

LITERATURE CITED

1. Adams EK, Florence CS, Thorpe KE, Becker ER, Joski PJ. 2003. Preventive care: female cancer screening, 1996–2000. *Am. J. Prev. Med.* 25:301–7
2. Adams EK, Thorpe KE, Becker ER, Joski PJ, Flome J. 2004. Colorectal cancer screening, 1997–1999: role of income, insurance and policy. *Prev. Med.* 38:551–57
3. Adler GS. 1994. A profile of the Medicare current beneficiary survey. *Health Care Financ. Rev.* 15(4):153–63
4. Bell CM, Crystal M, Detsky AS, Redelmeier DA. 1998. Shopping around for hospital services: a comparison of the United States and Canada. *JAMA* 279:1015–17
5. Bero LA, Grilli R, Grimshaw JM, Harvey E, Oxman AD, Thomson MA. 1998. Closing the gap between research and practice: an overview of systematic reviews of interventions to promote the implementation of research findings. The Cochrane Effective Practice and Organization of Care Review Group. *BMJ* 317:465–68
6. Berwick DM. 2002. A user's manual for the IOM's 'Quality Chasm' report. *Health Aff.* 21:80–90
7. Blustein J. 1995. Medicare coverage, supplemental insurance, and the use of mammography by older women. *N. Engl. J. Med.* 332:1138–43
8. Bonfill X, Marzo M, Pladevall M, Marti J, Emparanza JI. 2001. Strategies for increasing the participation of women in community breast cancer screening. *Cochrane Database Syst. Rev.* CD002943
9. Breen N, Brown ML. 1994. The price of mammography in the United States: data from the National Survey of Mammography Facilities. *Milbank Q.* 72:431–50
10. Breen N, Wagener DK, Brown ML, Davis WW, Ballard-Barbash R. 2001. Progress in cancer screening over a decade: results of cancer screening from the 1987, 1992, and 1998 National Health Interview Surveys. *J. Natl. Cancer Inst.* 93:1704–13
11. Brodersen J, Thorsen H, Cockburn J. 2004. The adequacy of measurement of short and long-term consequences of false-positive screening mammography. *J. Med. Screen.* 11:39–44

12. Brown D. 1994. Threat of malpractice suits leaves 'no other choice' than costly tests. *Wash. Post*, Jan. 3

13. Burack RC, Gimotty PA. 1997. Promoting screening mammography in inner-city settings. The sustained effectiveness of computerized reminders in a randomized controlled trial. *Med. Care* 35:921–31

14. Burns RB, Freund KM, Moskowitz MA, Kasten L, Feldman H, McKinlay JB. 1997. Physician characteristics: Do they influence the evaluation and treatment of breast cancer in older women? *Am. J. Med.* 103:263–69

15. Burns RB, McCarthy EP, Freund KM, Marwill SL, Shwartz M, et al. 1996. Black women receive less mammography even with similar use of primary care. *Ann. Intern. Med.* 125:173–82

16. Burns RB, McCarthy EP, Freund KM, Marwill SL, Shwartz M, et al. 1996. Variability in mammography use among older women. *J. Am. Geriatr. Soc.* 44:922–26

17. Cabana MD, Rand CS, Powe NR, Wu AW, Wilson MH, et al. 1999. Why don't physicians follow clinical practice guidelines? A framework for improvement. *JAMA* 282:1458–65

18. Carlos RC, Fendrick AM. 2004. Improving cancer screening adherence: using the "teachable moment" as a delivery setting for educational interventions. *Am. J. Manag. Care* 10:247–48

19. Chuang KH, Luft HS, Dudley RA. 2004. The clinical and economic performance of prepaid group practice. In *Toward a 21st Century Health System: The Contributions and Promise of Prepaid Group Practice*, ed. AC Enthoven, LA Tollen, pp. 45–60. San Francisco: Jossey-Bass

20. Codori A-M, Petersen GM, Miglioretti DL, Boyd P. 2001. Health beliefs and endoscopic screening for colorectal cancer: potential for cancer prevention. *Prev. Med.* 33:128–36

21. Cokkinides VE, Chao A, Smith RA, Vernon SW, Thun MJ. 2003. Correlates of underutilization of colorectal cancer screening among U.S. adults, age 50 years and older. *Prev. Med.* 36:85–91

22. Corrigan JM, Nielsen DM. 1993. Toward the development of uniform reporting standards for managed care organizations: the Health Plan Employer Data and Information Set (Version 2.0). *Jt. Comm. J. Qual. Improv.* 19:566–75

23. de Koning HJ, Auvinen A, Sanchez AB, da Silva FC, Ciatto S, et al. 2002. Large-scale randomized prostate cancer screening trials: program performances in the European randomized screening for prostate cancer trial and the prostate, lung, colorectal and ovary cancer trial. *Int. J. Cancer* 97:237–44

24. Dranove D. 1988. Demand inducement and the physician/patient relationship. *Econ. Inq.* 26:281–98

25. Esserman L, Cowley H, Eberle C, Kirkpatrick A, Chang S, et al. 2002. Improving the accuracy of mammography: volume and outcome relationships. *J. Natl. Cancer Inst.* 94:369–75

26. Fajardo LL, Saint-Germain M, Meakem TJ, Rose C, Hillman BJ. 1992. Factors influencing women to undergo screening mammography. *Radiology* 184:59–63

27. Fox SA, Klos DS, Tsou CV. 1988. Underuse of screening mammography by family physicians. *Radiology* 166:431–33

28. Fox SA, Murata PJ, Stein JA. 1991. The impact of physician compliance on screening mammography for older women. *Arch. Intern. Med.* 151:50–56

29. Frazier EL, Jiles RB, Mayberry R. 1996. Use of screening mammography and clinical breast examinations among black, Hispanic, and white women. *Prev. Med.* 25:118–25

30. Friedman LC, Woodruff A, Lane M, Weinberg AD, Cooper HP, Webb JA. 1995. Breast cancer screening behaviors and intentions among asymptomatic

women 50 years of age and older. *Am. J. Prev. Med.* 11:219–23

31. Goel MS, Wee CC, McCarthy EP, Davis RB, Ngo-Metzger Q, Phillips RS. 2003. Racial and ethnic disparities in cancer screening: the importance of foreign birth as a barrier to care. *J. Gen. Intern. Med.* 18:1028–35

32. Gohagan JK, Prorok PC, Kramer BS, Cornett JE. 1994. Prostate cancer screening in the prostate, lung, colorectal and ovarian cancer screening trial of the National Cancer Institute. *J. Urol.* 152:1905–9

33. Gold MR, Siegel JE, Russell LB, Weinstein MC, eds. 1996. *Cost-Effectiveness in Health and Medicine.* New York: Oxford Univ. Press. 425 pp.

34. Gordon NP, Rundall TG, Parker L. 1998. Type of health care coverage and the likelihood of being screened for cancer. *Med. Care* 36:636–45

35. Grady KE, Lemkau JP, McVay JM, Reisine ST. 1992. The importance of physician encouragement in breast cancer screening of older women. *Prev. Med.* 21:766–80

36. Gram IT, Lund E, Slenker SE. 1990. Quality of life following a false positive mammogram. *Br. J. Cancer* 62:1018–22

37. Haggerty J, Tamblyn R, Abrahamowicz M, Beaulieu MD, Kishchuk N. 1999. Screening mammography referral rates for women ages 50 to 69 years by recently-licensed family physicians: physician and practice environment correlates. *Prev. Med.* 29:391–404

38. Harewood GC, Wiersema MJ, Melton LJ III. 2002. A prospective, controlled assessment of factors influencing acceptance of screening colonoscopy. *Am. J. Gastroenterol.* 97:3186–94

39. Harris RP, O'Malley MS, Fletcher SW, Knight BP. 1990. Prompting physicians for preventive procedures: a five-year study of manual and computer reminders. *Am. J. Prev. Med.* 6:145–52

40. Hays RD, Shaul JA, Williams VS, Lubalin JS, Harris-Kojetin LD, et al. 1999. Psychometric properties of the CAHPS 1.0 survey measures. Consumer Assessment of Health Plans Study. *Med. Care* 37:MS22–31

41. Henson RM, Wyatt SW, Lee NC. 1996. The national breast and cervical cancer early detection program: a comprehensive public health response to two major health issues for women. *J. Public Health Manag. Pract.* 2:36–47

42. Hiatt RA, Klabunde C, Breen N, Swan J, Ballard-Barbash R. 2002. Cancer screening practices from National Health Interview Surveys: past, present, and future. *J. Natl. Cancer Inst.* 94:1837–46

43. Holahan J, Moon M, Welch WP, Zuckerman S. 1991. An American approach to health system reform. *JAMA* 265:2537–40

44. Holland BK, Foster JD, Louria DB. 1993. Cervical cancer and health care resources in Newark, New Jersey, 1970 to 1988. *Am. J. Public Health* 83:45–48

45. Hsia J, Kemper E, Kiefe C, Zapka J, Sofaer S, et al. 2000. The importance of health insurance as a determinant of cancer screening: evidence from the Women's Health Initiative. *Prev. Med.* 31:261–70

46. Inst. Med. 2001. *Health and Behavior: The Interplay of Biological, Behavioral, and Societal Influences.* Washington, DC: Natl. Acad. Press. 400 pp.

47. Kagawa-Singer M, Pourat N. 2000. Asian American and Pacific Islander breast and cervical carcinoma screening rates and Healthy People 2000 objectives. *Cancer* 89:696–705

48. Kaplan CP, Crane LA, Stewart S, Juarez-Reyes M. 2004. Factors affecting follow-up among low-income women with breast abnormalities. *J. Womens Health* 13:195–206

49. Kiessling A. 2004. Participatory learning: a Swedish perspective. *Heart* 90:113–16

50. Klabunde CN, Frame PS, Meadow A, Jones E, Nadel M, Vernon SW. 2003. A national survey of primary care physicians' colorectal cancer screening recommendations and practices. *Prev. Med.* 36:352–62

51. Klabunde CN, Riley GF, Mandelson MT, Frame PS, Brown ML. 2004. Health plan policies and programs for colorectal cancer screening: a national profile. *Am. J. Manag. Care* 10:273–79

52. Kottke TE, Solberg LI, Brekke ML, Magnan S, Amundson GM. 2000. Clinician satisfaction with a preventive services implementation trial. The IMPROVE project. *Am. J. Prev. Med.* 18: 219–24

53. Lam TK, McPhee SJ, Mock J, Wong C, Doan HT, et al. 2003. Encouraging Vietnamese-American women to obtain Pap tests through lay health worker outreach and media education. *J. Gen. Intern. Med.* 18:516–24

54. Landon BE, Zaslavsky AM, Bernard SL, Cioffi MJ, Cleary PD. 2004. Comparison of performance of traditional Medicare vs Medicare managed care. *JAMA* 291:1744–52

55. Lane DS, Zapka J, Breen N, Messina CR, Fotheringham DJ. 2000. A systems model of clinical preventive care: the case of breast cancer screening among older women. *Prev. Med.* 31:481–93

56. Lantz PM, Weisman CS, Itani Z. 2003. A disease-specific Medicaid expansion for women. The Breast and Cervical Cancer Prevention and Treatment Act of 2000. *Womens Health Issues* 13:79–92

57. Laws MB, Mayo SJ. 1998. The Latina Breast Cancer Control Study, year one: factors predicting screening mammography utilization by urban Latina women in Massachusetts. *J. Community Health* 23:251–67

58. Legler J, Meissner HI, Coyne C, Breen N, Chollette V, Rimer BK. 2002. The effectiveness of interventions to promote mammography among women with his-torically lower rates of screening. *Cancer Epidemiol. Biomarkers Prev.* 11:59–71

59. Lemon S, Zapka J, Puleo E, Luckmann R, Chasan-Taber L. 2001. Colorectal cancer screening participation: comparisons with mammography and prostate-specific antigen screening. *Am. J. Public Health* 91:1264–72

60. Lurie N, Slater J, McGovern P, Ekstrum J, Quam L, Margolis K. 1993. Preventive care for women. Does the sex of the physician matter? *N. Engl. J. Med.* 329:478–82

61. Deleted in proof

62. Mandelblatt J, Kanetsky PA. 1995. Effectiveness of interventions to enhance physician screening for breast cancer. *J. Fam. Pract.* 40:162–71

63. Mandelblatt J, Traxler M, Lakin P, Kanetsky P, Kao R, Harlem Study Team. 1993. Targeting breast and cervical cancer screening to elderly poor black women: Who will participate? *Prev. Med.* 22:20–33

64. Mandelblatt JS, Gold K, O'Malley AS, Taylor K, Cagney K, et al. 1999. Breast and cervix cancer screening among multiethnic women: role of age, health, and source of care. *Prev. Med.* 28:418–25

65. Mandelblatt JS, Yabroff KR. 1999. Effectiveness of interventions designed to increase mammography use: a meta-analysis of provider-targeted strategies. *Cancer Epidemiol. Biomarkers Prev.* 8:759–67

66. Marcus AC, Crane LA. 1998. A review of cervical cancer screening intervention research: implications for public health programs and future research. *Prev. Med.* 27:13–31

67. May DS, Lee NC, Nadel MR, Henson RM, Miller DS. 1998. The National Breast and Cervical Cancer Early Detection Program: report on the first 4 years of mammography provided to medically underserved women. *Am. J. Roentgenol.* 170:97–104

68. May DS, Lee NC, Richardson LC, Gius- tozzi AG, Bobo JK. 2000. Mammogra- phy and breast cancer detection by race and Hispanic ethnicity: results from a na- tional program (United States). *Cancer Causes Control* 11:697–705

69. Mayer-Oakes SA, Atchison KA, Matthias RE, De Jong FJ, Lubben J, Schweitzer SO. 1996. Mammography use in older women with regular physi- cians: What are the predictors? *Am. J. Prev. Med.* 12:44–50

70. McCarthy BD, Yood MU, Macwilliam CH, Lee MJ. 1996. Screening mammog- raphy use: the importance of a population perspective. *Am. J. Prev. Med.* 12:91–95

71. McKinney MM, Marconi KM. 1992. Legislative interventions to increase ac- cess to screening mammography. *J. Community Health* 17:333–49

72. McPhee SJ, Bird JA, Fordham D, Rod- nick JE, Osborn EH. 1991. Promoting cancer prevention activities by primary care physicians. *JAMA* 266:538–44

73. Medicare Paym. Advis. Comm. (Med- PAC). 2002. *Assessing Medicare bene- fits. Report to the Congress.* Washington, DC

74. Meissner HI, Breen N, Coyne C, Legler J, Green D, Edwards BK. 1998. Breast and cervical cancer screening interven- tions: an assessment of the literature. *Cancer Epidemiol. Biomarkers Prev.* 7: 951–61

75. Merenstein D. 2004. A piece of my mind. Winners and losers. *JAMA* 291:15–16

76. Miller ER, Miller A. 1984. Impact of a federally funded cervical cancer screen- ing program on reducing mortality in New Jersey. *Prog. Clin. Biol. Res.* 156: 313–28

77. Miller RH, Luft HS. 1994. Managed care plan performance since 1980. A litera- ture analysis. *JAMA* 271:1512–19

78. Miller RH, Luft HS. 2002. HMO plan performance update: an analysis of the literature, 1997–2001. *Health Aff.* 21: 63–86

79. Mills RJ, Bhandari S. 2003. *Health in- surance coverage in the United States: 2002. Rep.* P60–223

80. Moon M. 2000. Medicare matters: build- ing on a record of accomplishments. *Health Care Financ. Rev.* 22:9–22

81. Natl. Cancer Inst. Breast Cancer Screen. Consort. 1990. Screening mammogra- phy: A missed clinical opportunity? Re- sults of the NCI breast cancer screening consortium and national health interview survey studies. *JAMA* 264:54–58

82. Natl. Comm. Qual. Assur. 2004. *Tech- nical Specifications 2004.* Washington, DC

83. Natl. Comm. Qual. Assur. 2004. *The State of Managed Care Quality.* Wash- ington, DC

84. O'Malley AS, Beaton E, Yabroff KR, Abramson R, Mandelblatt J. 2004. Pa- tient and provider barriers to colorec- tal cancer screening in the primary care safety-net. *Prev. Med.* 39(1):56– 63

85. Phillips KA, Fernyak S, Potosky AL, Schauffler HH, Egorin M. 2000. Use of preventive services by managed care en- rollees: an updated perspective. *Health Aff.* 19:102–16

86. Pignone M, Rich M, Teutsch SM, Berg AO, Lohr KN. 2002. Screening for col- orectal cancer in adults at average risk: a summary of the evidence for the U.S. Preventive Services Task Force. *Ann. In- tern. Med.* 137:132–41

87. Potosky AL, Breen N, Graubard BI, Par- sons PE. 1998. The association between health care coverage and the use of can- cer screening tests. Results from the 1992 National Health Interview Survey. *Med. Care* 36:257–70

88. Rakowski W, Rimer BK, Bryant SA. 1993. Integrating behavior and inten- tion regarding mammography by respon- dents in the 1990 National Health Inter- view Survey of Health Promotion and Disease Prevention. *Public Health Rep.* 108:605–24

89. Ransohoff DF, McNaughton Collins M, Fowler FJ Jr. 2002. Why is prostate cancer screening so common when the evidence is so uncertain? A system without negative feedback. *Am. J. Med.* 113:663–67

90. Reinhardt UE. 1985. The theory of physician-induced demand: reflections after a decade. *J. Health Econ.* 4:187–93

91. Reinhardt UE, Hussey PS, Anderson GF. 2004. U.S. health care spending in an international context. *Health Aff.* 23:10–25

92. Riley G, Tudor C, Chiang Y, Ingber M. 1996. Health status of Medicare enrollees in HMOs and Fee-for-Service in 1994. *Health Care Financ. Rev.* 17:65–76

93. Rimer BK. 1998. Interventions to enhance cancer screening: a brief review of what works and what is on the horizon. *Cancer* 83(Suppl. 8):1770–74

94. Roetzheim RG, Fox SA, Leake B. 1995. Physician-reported determinants of screening mammography in older women: the impact of physician and practice characteristics. *J. Am. Geriatr. Soc.* 43:1398–402

95. Russell LB. 1994. *Educated Guesses–Making Policy about Medical Screening Tests*, Vol. 1. Berkeley: Univ. Calif. Press

96. Schroy PC, Heeren T, Bliss CM, Pincus J, Wilson S, Prout M. 1999. Implementation of on-site screening sigmoidoscopy positively influences utilization by primary care providers. *Gastroenterology* 117:304–11

97. Schwartz LM, Woloshin S, Fowler FJ Jr, Welch HG. 2004. Enthusiasm for cancer screening in the United States. *JAMA* 291:71–78

98. Shavers VL, Brown ML. 2002. Racial and ethnic disparities in the receipt of cancer treatment. *J. Natl. Cancer Inst.* 94:334–57

99. Snell JL, Buck EL. 1996. Increasing cancer screening: a meta-analysis. *Prev. Med.* 25:702–7

100. Solberg LI, Kottke TE, Brekke ML, Conn SA, Magnan S, Amundson G. 1998. The case of the missing clinical preventive services systems. *Eff. Clin. Pract.* 1:33–38

101. Stone EG, Morton SC, Hulscher ME, Maglione MA, Roth EA, et al. 2002. Interventions that increase use of adult immunization and cancer screening services: a meta-analysis. *Ann. Intern. Med.* 136:641–51

102. Swan J, Breen N, Coates RJ, Rimer BK, Lee NC. 2003. Progress in cancer screening practices in the United States: results from the 2000 National Health Interview Survey. *Cancer* 97:1528–40

103. Deleted in proof

104. Taplin S, Galvin MS, Payne T, Coole D, Wagner E. 1998. Putting population-based care into practice: real option or rhetoric? *J. Am. Board Fam. Pract.* 11:116–26

105. Taplin SH, Ichikawa L, Buist DS, Seger D, White E. 2004. Evaluating organized breast cancer screening implementation: the prevention of late-stage disease? *Cancer Epidemiol. Biomarkers Prev.* 13:225–34

106. Taplin SH, Mandelson MT, Anderman C, White E, Thompson RS, et al. 1997. Mammography diffusion and trends in late-stage breast cancer: evaluating outcomes in a population. *Cancer Epidemiol. Biomarkers. Prev.* 6:625–31

107. Taylor VM, Jackson JC, Yasui Y, Kuniyuki A, Acorda E, et al. 2002. Evaluation of an outreach intervention to promote cervical cancer screening among Cambodian American women. *Cancer Detect. Prev.* 26:320–27

108. Thompson IM, Pauler DK, Goodman PJ, Tangen CM, Lucia MS, et al. 2004. Prevalence of prostate cancer among men with a prostate-specific antigen level < or = 4.0 ng per milliliter. *N. Engl. J. Med.* 350:2239–46

109. Tu S-P, Taplin SH, Barlow WE, Boyko EJ. 1999. Breast cancer screening by

Asian-American women in a managed care environment. *Am. J. Prev. Med.* 17: 55–61

110. Urban N, Anderson GL, Peacock S. 1994. Mammography screening: How important is cost as a barrier to use? *Am. J. Public Health* 84:50–55

110a. US Prev. Serv. Task Force. 1989. *Guide to Clinical Preventive Services: An Assessment of the Effectiveness of 169 Interventions.* Baltimore: Williams & Wilkins

110b. US Prev. Serv. Task Force. 1996. *Guide to Clinical Preventive Services.* Washington, DC: Off. Dis. Prev. Health Promot., US Gov. Print. Off. 2nd ed.

111. Verne JE, Aubrey R, Love SB, Talbot IC, Northover JM. 1998. Population based randomized study of uptake and yield of screening by flexible sigmoidoscopy compared with screening by faecal occult blood testing. *BMJ* 317:182–85

112. Vernon SW. 1997. Participation in colorectal cancer screening: a review. *J. Natl. Cancer Inst.* 89:1406–22

113. Vernon SW, Laville EA, Jackson GL. 1990. Participation in breast screening programs: a review. *Soc. Sci. Med.* 30: 1107–18

114. Vernon SW, Vogel VG, Halabi S, Jackson GL, Lundy RO, Peters GN. 1992. Breast cancer screening behaviors and attitudes in three racial/ethnic groups. *Cancer* 69:165–74

115. Wagner TH. 1998. The effectiveness of mailed patient reminders on mammography screening: a meta-analysis. *Am. J. Prev. Med.* 14:64–70

116. Ward MM, Vaughn TE, Uden-Holman T, Doebbeling BN, Clarke WR, Woolson RF. 2002. Physician knowledge, attitudes and practices regarding a widely implemented guideline. *J. Eval. Clin. Pract.* 8:155–62

117. Wilson JMG, Jungner G. 1968. *Principles and Practices of Screening for Diseases: Public Health Pap. 34.* Geneva: WHO

118. Wolfe BL. 1994. Reform of health care for the nonelderly poor. In *Confronting Poverty: Prescriptions for Change*, ed. S Danziger, G Sandefur, D Weinberg, pp. 253–88. Cambridge, MA: Harvard Univ. Press

119. Woolhandler S, Campbell T, Himmelstein DU. 2003. Costs of health care administration in the United States and Canada. *N. Engl. J. Med.* 349:768–75

120. Woolhandler S, Himmelstein DU. 1988. Reverse targeting of preventive care due to lack of health insurance. *JAMA* 259:2872–74

121. Yabroff KR, Mandelblatt JS. 1999. Interventions targeted toward patients to increase mammography use. *Cancer Epidemiol. Biomarkers Prev.* 8:749–57

122. Yabroff KR, Washington KS, Leader A, Neilson E, Mandelblatt J. 2003. Is the promise of cancer-screening programs being compromised? Quality of follow-up care after abnormal screening results. *Med. Care Res. Rev.* 60:294–331

123. Zambrana RE, Breen N, Fox SA, Gutierrez-Mohamed ML. 1999. Use of cancer screening practices by Hispanic women: analyses by subgroup. *Prev. Med.* 29:466–77

124. Zapka JG, Lemon SC. 2004. Interventions for patients, providers, and health care organizations. *Cancer* 101(5 Suppl.):1165–87

125. Zapka JG, Taplin SH, Solberg LI, Manos MM. 2003. A framework for improving the quality of cancer care: the case of breast and cervical cancer screening. *Cancer Epidemiol. Biomarkers Prev.* 12: 4–13

Annu. Rev. Public Health 2005. 26:583–99
doi: 10.1146/annurev.publhealth.26.021304.144501
Copyright © 2005 by Annual Reviews. All rights reserved
First published online as a Review in Advance on November 11, 2004

Impact of Nicotine Replacement Therapy on Smoking Behavior

K. Michael Cummings and Andrew Hyland

*Department of Health Behavior, Division of Cancer Prevention and Population Sciences,
Roswell Park Cancer Institute, Buffalo, New York 14263;
email: michael.cummings@roswellpark.org, Andrew.Hyland@roswellpark.org*

Key Words tobacco, smoking cessation, pharmacotherapy, NRT

■ **Abstract** This review summarizes evidence pertaining to the role of nicotine medications in smoking cessation and focuses particularly on evaluating evidence of the impact that nicotine replacement therapies (NRT) have had on altering population trends in smoking behavior. Accumulated evidence from controlled clinical trials has demonstrated that available forms of NRT (e.g., gum, transdermal patch, nasal spray, inhaler, and lozenge) increase quit rates compared with placebos by 50%–100%. However, despite the positive results from these studies, fewer than one in five smokers making a quit attempt do so with the benefit of NRT. Because not enough smokers are using NRT, the availability of NRT has not had a measurable impact on influencing population trends in smoking behavior. Among the factors contributing to the low utilization of nicotine medications are the inadequacies of the current dosage strengths and formulations of existing medications, smokers' perceptions of the high cost of the drugs, and concerns that many smokers have about safety and efficacy of nicotine medications.

INTRODUCTION

Considerable evidence supports the view that cigarette smoking is primarily maintained by an addiction to nicotine (51, 91). Nicotine creates dependence by activating the mesolimbic dopaminergic reward system, and physiologic withdrawal symptoms occur when nicotine is no longer administered (59, 67, 71). Nicotine is an agonist of neural nicotinic acetylcholine receptors (NAChRs), which are found presynaptically in the central nervous system and postsynaptically in the autonomic nervous system (73). These receptors modulate the release of neurotransmitters. As a person's exposure to nicotine increases, NAChRs also are increased, which results in nicotine tolerance (60). Thus, factors that decrease the bioavailability of nicotine are hypothesized to increase an individual's cravings and decrease the likelihood of cessation because more of the drug is needed to achieve a given level of dopamine (13). Extrapolating from this evidence has led to the development of smoking cessation treatment methods that emphasize nicotine replacement (31).

0163-7525/05/0421-0583$20.00 **583**

The present review provides a brief summary of evidence pertaining to the role of nicotine medications, alone or in combination with other therapies in smoking cessation, and a critical analysis of the impact that these medications have had on altering population trends in smoking behavior. The discussion considers the role of nicotine replacement therapy (NRT) in a comprehensive population-based program developed to reduce the harms caused by tobacco.

NICOTINE MEDICATION FOR SMOKING CESSATION

In the mid-1980s, the vast majority (>90%) of former smokers reported that they stopped smoking without using medications or receiving formal assistance or help from anyone (33). However, this statistic has changed dramatically in the past two decades with the introduction and wide-scale availability of nicotine medications (46). Two-milligram prescription-only nicotine gum was first introduced in the United States in February 1984 (17, 31). Prescription-only nicotine patches were introduced in 1992, followed by different nicotine dose and medication formulations including 4-mg nicotine gum (1992), a nasal spray (1996), inhaler (1997), and lozenge (2003) (17, 31). Table 1 provides a brief description of different nicotine medications sold in the United States.

Numerous clinical trials have assessed the efficacy of nicotine medications for smoking cessation (31, 85). A recent systematic review of studies evaluating commercially available forms of NRT (e.g., nicotine gum, the transdermal nicotine patch, nicotine nasal spray, nicotine inhaler and nicotine sublingual tablets/lozenges) concluded that these treatments increase quit rates approximately one and a half to twofold regardless of clinical setting and/or use of adjunct treatments (31, 85). Several studies have found that complete or nearly complete abstinence from smoking in the early weeks of an attempt to quit is a strong predictor of long-term cessation (39, 56, 99). Nicotine medications appear to help smokers in quitting by providing relief from nicotine withdrawal symptoms typically experienced during the first few days and weeks of abstinence from tobacco (31, 91).

In 1996, the U.S. Food and Drug Administration (FDA) made nicotine patches and gum available over the counter (OTC) in an effort to increase access to these medications (17). Shiffman and colleagues tracked sales of pharmacological aids for smoking cessation and found that nicotine gum and patch sales increased 250% in the year following approval of OTC status (81). Several new prescription nicotine (nasal spray, oral inhaler, lozenge) and nonnicotine (Zyban®) stop-smoking medications were introduced after 1996 (17). However, of the new medications introduced after 1996, only Zyban® appears to have had any impact on medication-assisted cessation attempts (17). Of the various nicotine medications sold, the nicotine patch and nicotine gum are the most frequently used stop-smoking medications (3, 17; A. Hyland, H. Rezaishiraz, G. Giovino, J.E. Bauer, K.M. Cummings, unpublished manuscript). National survey data reveal that approximately 40% of

TABLE 1   FDA-approved nicotine replacement therapies[a]

Nicotine medication	Year approved	Dose	Advantages	Disadvantages
Gum	1984 (2mg Rx) 1992 (4mg Rx) 1996 (OTC)	2 or 4 mg per piece	Oral administration; comes in different flavors	Low compliance; under dosing is common
Patch	1992 (Rx) 1996 (OTC)	16-hour patch: 15, 10, 5 mg; 24-hour patch: 21, 14, 7 mg	Once a day administration	Fixed dose; slow delivery not conducive to treating acute cravings
Nasal spray	1996 (Rx)	10 mg/ml, 0.5 mg per spray	Fast delivery of nicotine	Unpleasant side-effects discourage repeated use
Inhaler	1997 (Rx)	10 mg per cartridge	Hand-to-mouth action simulates smoking habit; comes in menthol flavor	Low compliance; under dosing is common
Lozenge	2003 (OTC)	1, 2, or 4 mg per piece	Oral administration; faster nicotine delivery than gum	Low compliance; under dosing is common

[a]OTC, over the counter; Rx, prescription.

smokers indicate that they have used some form of nicotine medication in the past (3).

A number of studies have reported on the characteristics of smokers who have used nicotine medications (21, 23, 68, 69, 90; A. Hyland, H. Rezaishiraz, G. Giovino, J.E. Bauer, K.M. Cummings, unpublished manuscript). In the period before OTC NRT, current and former smokers who reported having used prescription nicotine patches or gum were more likely to be female, Caucasian, have higher average household incomes, have private insurance, and to smoke more than a pack per day (21, 23, 68, 69, 90; A. Hyland, H. Rezaishiraz, G. Giovino, J.E. Bauer, K.M. Cummings, unpublished manuscript). The characteristics of smokers using NRT changed after nicotine patches and gum were made available OTC. In cross-sectional surveys of Massachusetts smokers in 1993 and 1999, the use of NRT in nonwhites decreased from 21% to 3% and increased from 5% to 20% in those aged 18 to 30 years, while use remained constant in other age, race, gender, and income categories (90). Longitudinal data from the Community Intervention Trial for Smoking Cessation cohort study (COMMIT) retrospectively re-created smokers' NRT use history between 1993 and 2001 (A. Hyland, H. Rezaishiraz, G. Giovino, J.E. Bauer, K.M. Cummings, unpublished manuscript). This study revealed that annual NRT usage rates nearly doubled from the three years before (1993–1995) OTC availability compared with the three-year period after OTC availability (1997–2000). Comparing usage patterns during the pre- and post-OTC periods revealed that use of NRT decreased among Hispanics and increased among those with lower desire to quit at baseline, among lighter smokers, and among those with lower annual household incomes.

On the basis of these data, it appears that part of the increased sales of NRT since becoming available OTC may be due to increasing utilization in populations that previously had lower utilization of NRT, including younger smokers, those with lower levels of daily consumption and desire to quit, and possibly those with lower incomes. However, OTC availability of nicotine patches and gum may only partially explain why NRT usage increased in younger smokers and those with lower incomes. During this same period health insurance coverage has favored nicotine medications, including state-financed public insurance programs for the poor (e.g., Medicaid) (11, 40).

EFFECT OF NRT ON QUIT RATES

A recent meta-analysis of eight studies that examined either active OTC NRT versus placebo of OTC NRT or OTC NRT versus prescription-only concluded that OTC NRT produces similar quit rates compared with NRT obtained by prescription (50). As expected, when no adjunct behavioral support was provided, quit rates were slightly lower (31, 85). However, even in the absence of a behavioral support program, evidence showed that gum and patches increased quit rates more than that seen for placebo (31, 48, 85). Given these results, one might anticipate that OTC availability of NRT would positively impact rates of smoking cessation in the population.

Estimating the impact that NRT has had on smoking behavior in the population has been difficult because of self-selection in who uses NRT and because there are many external influences on smoking behavior that may confound measurement of population-wide trends in smoking behavior. Time series analyses of national cigarette consumption and NRT sales from 1976 to 1998 suggest that sales of NRT were associated with a modest decrease in cigarette consumption immediately following the introduction of the prescription nicotine patch in 1992 (45). However, no statistically significant effect was observed after 1996, when the patch and gum became available OTC. Thus, in spite of the apparent success of OTC NRT, during the period between 1990 and 1998, population-based data reveal that annual quit rates as well as age-specific quit ratios remained stable, especially for those between the ages of 25 and 64, the age group most likely to use NRT (16).

Repeated cross-sectional surveys from Massachusetts found that quit attempts and quit rates were no different in the period after 1996 compared with before 1996 (90). Cross-sectional surveys from California indicate a greater utilization of NRT after 1996 but show little impact on quit rates (69). Only one prospective study has investigated the impact of OTC availability of NRT on quit rates (A. Hyland, H. Rezaishiraz, G. Giovino, J.E. Bauer, K.M. Cummings, unpublished manuscript). In the COMMIT study, annual use rates of the nicotine skin patch increased from an average of 3.6% between 1993 and 1995 to 6.0% between 1997 and 2000. Among those who used the patch to stop smoking, the average quit rate was 15.3% between 1993 and 1995 and 15.5% between 1997 and 2000. The same pattern was observed for use of nicotine gum. Nicotine gum use increased from 1.8% to 2.4% before and after the OTC reclassification, whereas quit rates among gum users increased from 9.7% before OTC to 14.5% after OTC. Relapse rates among patch users were slightly higher in the OTC period compared with before, whereas no difference was seen for gum users. Thus, on balance it appears that OTC reclassification has increased access to NRT without changing quit rates among those using NRT (A. Hyland, H. Rezaishiraz, G. Giovino, J.E. Bauer, K.M. Cummings, unpublished manuscript).

WHO QUITS WITH NRT?

The current clinical practice guideline for treating nicotine dependence recommends that NRT should be used by all smokers who are trying to stop smoking (31). Researchers have investigated differential effects of NRT depending on patient characteristics and comorbid conditions (e.g., depression, other substance abuse problems). Some studies have found that those who smoke in excess of a pack of cigarettes or more per day derive greater benefit from higher dosage forms of NRT; however, amount smoked daily has not been found to be a consistent effect modifier in predicting treatment success using NRT (25, 31, 42, 85). A few studies have reported that women who use NRT have lower success rates than do men (8, 66, 95). In general, the results of studies investigating patient factors that interact with NRT to predict quit rates have been equivocal, which is why the current practice guidelines recommend NRT for all smokers who are making a quit attempt (31).

A new area of research involves identifying genetic characteristics of smokers who may derive a proportionately greater benefit from NRT. One study found that quit rates were significantly higher after 12 weeks among 755 subjects in a randomized nicotine skin patch trial among those who exhibited a certain genotype of a dopamine receptor gene (DRD2). The DRD2 gene is involved in the synthesis of noradrenalin from dopamine (54). Improved understanding of how genetic factors contribute to smoking cessation could potentially lead to improved treatment matching. However, more research is needed to clarify the utility and potential cost-effectiveness of pharmacogenetic treatment–matching approaches for smoking cessation.

WHY HASN'T NRT INFLUENCED QUIT RATES MORE?

A number of reasons could explain why increased use of NRT has not influenced quit rates more substantially in the population at large. Some authors have speculated that the availability of OTC NRT has merely encouraged quit attempts by less-motivated smokers who, to begin with, are less likely to quit (69, 90; A. Hyland, H. Rezaishiraz, G. Giovino, J.E. Bauer, K.M. Cummings, unpublished manuscript). Thus, although usage rates might increase, this benefit would be offset by higher rates of relapse among those who are less committed to making a quit attempt. There is some evidence to support this view (69; A. Hyland, H. Rezaishiraz, G. Giovino, J.E. Bauer, K.M. Cummings, unpublished manuscript). Several studies have reported that NRT use increased among less-dependent and less-motivated smokers in the post-OTC period (69, 90; A. Hyland, H. Rezaishiraz, G. Giovino, J.E. Bauer, K.M. Cummings, unpublished manuscript). Audit studies of NRT purchases reveal that, for both patch and gum, most purchase episodes last a month or less (38; J.R. Hughes, J.L. Pillitteri, P.W. Callas, R. Callahan, M. Kenny, unpublished manuscript). In the COMMIT study, the OTC switch led to a decline in the median number of days the patch was used, decreasing from 30 days to 21 days (A. Hyland, H. Rezaishiraz, G. Giovino, J.E. Bauer, K.M. Cummings, unpublished manuscript). Other studies have found that it is common for smokers to report concurrent smoking while also using NRT (3, 21, 64, 68, 82). However, long-term concurrent use of NRT and smoking is rare, and most smokers who use NRT say they do so to quit smoking, not to reduce their smoking (3, 7; S. Shiffman, J.R. Hughes, unpublished manuscript).

Data do support the view that combining some type of in-person or telephone behavioral counseling support with NRT increases quit rates, especially for those using nicotine gum (31, 58, 84, 85). Counseling support appears to enhance the impact of NRT by helping smokers understand how the medications work and how to use them appropriately (31, 85). Counseling also reinforces the smoker's motivation for quitting and remaining tobacco-free. However, despite the benefits of combining behavioral counseling with NRT, most smokers quit without receiving behavioral counseling (100; A. Hyland, H. Rezaishiraz, G. Giovino, J.E. Bauer, K.M. Cummings, unpublished manuscript). In the COMMIT cohort, fewer than 10% of NRT-assisted quit attempts were accompanied by attendance in a stop-smoking program, and this percentage decreased after nicotine patches and gum were made available OTC (A. Hyland, H. Rezaishiraz, G. Giovino, J.E. Bauer, K.M. Cummings, unpublished manuscript).

Most Quit Attempts Are Made without NRT

Another reason why NRT has not had a greater impact on quit rates in the population-at-large is that most cessation attempts are still made without the benefit of nicotine medications (3, 50, 69, 90; A. Hyland, H. Rezaishiraz, G. Giovino, J.E. Bauer, K.M. Cummings, unpublished manuscript). A 2001 national telephone

survey of 1046 adult smokers revealed that although most had heard of nicotine medications (i.e., patches, 97%; gum, 94%; inhaler, 41%; nasal spray, 9%),
only 17% of those who had made a quit attempt in the past year reported using
a stop-smoking medication in their quit attempt (3). Thus, unlike a cigarette tax
hike, worksite smoking ban, or mass media campaign that might be expected to
reach nearly all smokers, NRT is reaching only a fraction of smokers (20). Among
the factors contributing to the low utilization of NRT are smokers' perceptions
of the high cost of the medications and concerns about safety and efficacy of
NRT (3, 29).

Among smokers who have never used any stop-smoking medication, cost is
the most frequently cited reasons for never use (3). An 8–12-week course of NRT
can cost anywhere between $200–$350. Increasingly, health insurance companies
are providing coverage for NRT (40). However, most insurance companies require
smokers who get NRT to obtain a prescription and/or attend a stop-smoking class
(11, 40). Many insurance companies also limit the number of courses of NRT a
person can obtain in a given time period, which may deter smokers from making
another quit attempt. OTC NRT products are also packaged in a way that make
them noncost competitive with tobacco products (93). Most tobacco products are
packaged so the user can get a one-day supply of nicotine (e.g., pack of cigarettes,
tin of moist snuff). The smallest supply of nicotine gum or patches is a one-week
supply, which requires the user to pay a minimum of $28–$35 just to obtain the
product. Most of the OTC starter kits for NRT are packaged with a minimum of
two or even four weeks of medication, requiring the consumer to spend even more
just to get started with a quit program. Although it could be argued that the initial
high cost of purchasing OTC NRT products helps separate out those smokers who
are truly motivated to quit, growing evidence suggests that the initial high cost
of obtaining the medication is a deterrent to smokers to use NRT to help them
quit (3).

Evidence from several studies shows that when cost barriers are reduced, utilization of NRT increases (1, 24, 38, 77; N. Miller, T.R. Frieden, S.Y. Liu, S.Y.
Matte, F. Mostashari, D. Deitcher, K.M. Cummings, C. Chang, U. Bauer, M.T.
Massett, unpublished manuscript). Research supports the idea that many more
smokers would be induced to try NRT if the cost were reduced or the medication
was made available for free (1, 38, 86; N. Miller, T.R. Frieden, S.Y. Liu, S.Y. Matte,
F. Mostashari, D. Deitcher, K.M. Cummings, C. Chang, U. Bauer, M.T. Massett,
unpublished manuscript). For example, in 2003, in a random sample telephone
survey of 815 adult smokers in upstate New York, 53% said they would think
seriously about quitting if offered free nicotine patches/gum (38).

In a recent cessation program sponsored by the New York City Department
of Health and Mental Hygiene, smokers of 10+ cigarettes per day who were
willing to make a commitment to quit smoking were offered a free 6-week
supply of nicotine patches (N. Miller, T.R. Frieden, S.Y. Liu, S.Y. Matte,
F. Mostashari, D. Deitcher, K.M. Cummings, C. Chang, U. Bauer, M.T. Massett,
unpublished manuscript). This unique program, marketed through a single press

release, resulted in over 400,000 calls to obtain the free nicotine patches. The offer of discounted nicotine patches in New Zealand resulted in over 80,000 calls to their government-sponsored quit line (1). A recent follow-up study of a random sample of the 35,000 participants in the New York City patch give-away program revealed that more than 87% of participants made an attempt to stop smoking and 33% were not smoking 6 months later, yielding an average cost per quit of about $300 (N. Miller, T.R. Frieden, S.Y. Liu, S.Y. Matte, F. Mostashari, D. Deitcher, K.M. Cummings, C. Chang, U. Bauer, M.T. Massett, unpublished manuscript). Population-based efforts such as those conducted in New Zealand and New York City appear to be effective in increasing the reach and utilization of NRT and thus have the potential to increase the overall quit rate in the population at large (1, 34, 86; N. Miller, T.R. Frieden, S.Y. Liu, S.Y. Matte, F. Mostashari, D. Deitcher, K.M. Cummings, C. Chang, U. Bauer, M.T. Massett, unpublished manuscript).

Although the perceived high cost of NRT is clearly a factor that can influence NRT use, cost alone is not the only explanation for the low utilization of nicotine medications by smokers. Recent studies of smokers and former smokers reveal that many smokers worry about using nicotine medications because of safety concerns (3, 29). Even though nicotine in the dosage strengths available in stop-smoking medications is fairly safe (7, 31), many smokers worry that concurrent smoking while using NRT will trigger a heart attack or may even cause cancer (3, 29). Many smokers also express skepticism about the efficacy of NRT to help them quit (3, 29). In a recent survey of 500 adult smokers, Etter & Perneger (29) found that only 16% agreed that nicotine medications help people quit smoking. Studies reveal that knowledge deficits are especially pronounced among smokers who have never used nicotine medications in the past, particularly those who are older, those who are less educated, and users of light and ultralight cigarettes (3).

In an effort to market NRT products, the pharmaceutical industry has invested heavily in consumer advertising. Much of this advertising appears to be targeted to smokers who are already primed to stop smoking on their own, which may help explain why NRT has had little impact on quit rates even though the percentage of medication-assisted quit attempts has gone up in the past decade (3; A. Hyland, H. Rezaishiraz, G. Giovino, J.E. Bauer, K.M. Cummings, unpublished manuscript). Recently, Bolton and colleagues (L.E. Bolton, J.B. Cohen & P.N. Bloom, unpublished manuscript) have speculated that advertising of stop-smoking medications may have a boomerang effect, unintentionally undermining smokers' risk perceptions about smoking and thus delaying smokers' efforts to quit. Because advertising of stop-smoking medications conveys a message that there is a remedy for addiction to tobacco, it is thought that a smoker's worry about the risks of smoking might be dampened by their belief that the medications can help them quit easily. Whether or not this boomerang effect is a real phenomena that can undermine motivation for cessation of smoking remains to be demonstrated, although a recent national survey of smokers found that 39% believed that it is easier for smokers to stop smoking today because of the availability of stop-smoking medications (22).

USE OF NRT FOR SMOKING REDUCTION

Some smokers express an interest in using NRT to cut back on their smoking but not to quit altogether (26). This is a controversial subject because the health benefits of reduced smoking appear to be minimal (87). Reducing cigarette consumption may decrease dependence and increase the likelihood of future cessation. However, smokers who reduce their consumption may feel they have lowered their disease risk due to smoking and do not need to make any more effort toward cessation. Data from clinical trials where medication is used to assist in reduction reveal that smokers who are not interested in quitting can reduce their consumption by as much as 50% and maintain this consumption level for at least 6 months or more (9, 15, 28, 94). Higher quit rates were observed among reducers in each of these studies.

Outside the clinical setting, relatively few smokers in the general population can maintain large consumption reductions over extended periods of time (30, 47, 52), and those who reduce their consumption by at least 50% may have a greater likelihood of future cessation, although these studies examine smokers who self-select for smoking reduction. Investigators do not know what impact a smoking reduction message, as opposed to a cessation-only message, would have on the general population; this topic warrants additional research.

CAN NICOTINE MEDICATIONS BE IMPROVED?

Yet another explanation for why NRT has not had a more pronounced effect on influencing population trends in smoking behavior concerns the inadequacies of the current dosage strengths and formulations of nicotine medications (6, 80). The reinforcing effect of nicotine depends on the amount of nicotine and the way in which nicotine enters the blood stream (5, 6, 27, 41, 80, 91). Nicotine in cigarette smoke is absorbed in the lungs (91). It takes ~7–10 sec for nicotine to reach the brain and for the smoker to feel the effects (91). By contrast, nicotine in gum is absorbed through the mucus membrane in the mouth and takes longer to reach the brain (6, 80). Nicotine in the patch is absorbed even more slowly through the skin and takes more than an hour to reach peak levels (5, 80). Nicotine medications designed to deliver nicotine more rapidly into the blood stream would very likely be more effective in helping smokers alleviate withdrawal symptoms when they quit, thus increasing quit rates (5, 80). The prescription nicotine nasal spray was designed precisely to deliver nicotine more rapidly than other nicotine medications (31). Placebo-controlled studies evaluating the nasal spray do show slightly higher quit rates compared with other nicotine medications, especially among more dependent smokers (31, 85). However, the downside of the nasal spray is that most smokers experience nasal and throat irritation that discourages repeated use of the product (31, 85, 92). Thus, compliance with the nasal spray is typically lower than with other types of nicotine medications (78).

A quick review of the patent literature reveals that many companies are working on developing faster nicotine-delivery medications (36, 65). A fast nicotine-delivery tablet has been developed and tested in Scotland, and a faster nicotine-delivery gum has been patented and tested in the United States (63, 70). Some public health officials have even advocated supporting wider marketing of medicinal nicotine and even oral smokeless tobacco products as a safer alternative for cigarette smoking (35, 57, 88). A number of other nicotine delivery products including nicotine aerosol inhalers, water, straws, wafers, and even lollipops have been patented and may soon find their way into the marketplace (36, 65). Tobacco manufacturers including Philip Morris, R.J. Reynolds, and Japan Tobacco hold patents for devices that could be used to deliver aerosolized nicotine into the lungs providing a potentially safer alternative to conventional cigarettes (36, 44, 78).

Another approach to improving nicotine medications is to offer them in different dosage strengths. Studies show that there is a dose-dependent relationship between NRT formulations and quit rates, although side effects become more common as the nicotine dose is increased (25, 42). There is wide individual variation in how smokers metabolize and respond to nicotine, which may help explain variation in treatment effects (54, 79). In particular, heavy smokers may not get enough nicotine from the current high-dose forms of nicotine medication now available. Some evidence supports the idea that more closely matching NRT dosage with an individual's daily biological dose of nicotine received while smoking can increase quit rates (25).

Rather than feeding one's dependence on nicotine in an effort to wean smokers from cigarettes, new therapies are now being developed and tested that treat nicotine dependence by blocking or replacing the effect of nicotine in the brain (37). Bupropion, marketed as Zyban®, is a non-nicotine medication that promotes smoking cessation by inhibiting dopamine reuptake in the brain, thereby dampening the reinforcing benefits of nicotine (31). Clinical trials support the use of bupropion for smoking cessation (31, 72). Prescription Zyban® was introduced in the United States in 1997 and has become, after nicotine patches and gum, the third most popular stop-smoking medication used by smokers (17). To date there is only one published study comparing the efficacy of bupropion with NRT. In the study by Jorenby et al. (55) quit rates were higher for bupropion alone and bupropion and patch combined at 6 and 12 months, compared with placebo and nicotine patch alone.

A number of other non-nicotine pharmacotherapies targeting nicotine receptors and the dopamine system are undergoing evaluation in human placebo-controlled trials (18, 43). One of the more interesting research efforts under way concerns the development of a vaccine for the treatment of nicotine addiction (89). The vaccine treatment is intended to block nicotine delivery to the brain, thereby removing the main reinforcement for smoking. The vaccine works by stimulating the immune system to produce antibodies that find and attach to nicotine molecules. The resulting compounds are too large to pass through the blood-brain barrier so that most of the nicotine is unable to reach the brain. Animal studies have clearly demonstrated that the vaccine can work; however, it remains unclear if human smokers will respond to the vaccine by increasing cigarette consumption to compensate for the lack of nicotine (43). Should this treatment modality work it would have profound implications for addressing the problem of nicotine dependence.

NICOTINE MAY NOT BE THE ONLY SOLUTION

Other investigators have speculated that efforts focusing solely on nicotine replacement or blockage are doomed to fail because nicotine may only partially explain smoking behavior (74). The airway sensations associated with smoking as well as the rituals of lighting, holding, and puffing on a cigarette are important reinforcing features of the act of smoking. Previous studies indicate that smokers report missing the behavioral aspects (i.e., actions that are ritualistic/repetitive) as well as the sensory cues of smoking such as taste, aroma, respiratory tract sensations/airway stimulation, and irritant reactions in the mouth, throat, and tracheo-bronchial tree (2, 12, 27, 76, 96, 97). Baldiner et al. (2) has suggested that the tar level of the product, not nicotine, seems to regulate puffing behavior. Brauer et al. (4) reviewed nine clinical trials that looked at the sensory impact of denicotinized cigarettes and concluded that denicotinized cigarettes help reduce cravings and withdrawal for cigarettes, especially among highly dependent smokers. This could be explained by classical conditioning theory, where inhalation impact turns to a conditioned stimulus as a result of being associated with nicotine exposure, which can function as an unconditioned stimulus.

Regardless of the mechanism, NRT is not entirely efficacious over the long term likely because the sensory and psychomotor aspects of smoking are inadequately addressed in cessation treatments (74). Many current cessation methods focus first on stopping smoking (which abruptly disrupts sensory and motor/behavior associated with smoking), followed by a course of nicotine replacement therapy to compensate for withdrawal symptoms, and concluding with discontinuation of the therapy to wean the smoker of the pharmacological effects resulting from the nicotine in the medication. This process, in effect, does not consider the sensorimotor cues thought to be very important in the addiction process. Several previous studies have shown that the sensory airway effects of smoking are important in relieving craving for cigarettes, as well as facilitating smoking abstinence (4, 12, 14). A sound theoretical basis predicts that smoking cessation treatments that address both sensorimotor and pharmacological aspects of a smoker's addiction will be more efficacious than either approach alone (74). Findings of one small study that combined a denicotinized cigarette (i.e., Next) and nicotine patch therapy revealed that 50% of subjects using Next in combination with a nicotine skin patch were off cigarettes after four weeks, confirmed by a breath carbon monoxide test (75).

SUMMARY

Tobacco control research literature reveals that the most potent demand reducing influences on tobacco use include interventions, such as higher cigarette taxes, smoke-free policies, comprehensive advertising bans, and paid counter-advertising campaigns, that reach the most consumers and directly impact their behavior (20, 92). This review shows that NRT has had little impact on influencing population trends in smoking behavior over the past decade. The main reason for the limited impact of NRT on smoking behavior has to do with low utilization of NRT by smokers (3).

Making NRT more accessible to smokers by providing it free and/or packaging the medication in single daily doses has the potential to vastly increase utilization (1, 34, 80, 88; N. Miller, T.R. Frieden, S.Y. Liu, S.Y. Matte, F. Mostashari, D. Deitcher, K.M. Cummings, C. Chang, U. Bauer, M.T. Massett, unpublished manuscript). Research is needed to understand better who would utilize such products, the products' effectiveness for cessation, optimal dosing and packaging, and the cost effectiveness of using different strategies to provide NRT for smokers. Counseling and behavioral therapies for smoking cessation can increase the effectiveness of NRT, yet are underutilized in clinical practice (9, 32; A. Hyland, H. Rezaishiraz, G. Giovino, J.E. Bauer, K.M. Cummings, unpublished manuscript). Research is needed to determine how to cost-effectively provide to smokers using NRT such behavioral support services perhaps via telephone quit lines and the Internet (1, 58, 84, 86; N. Miller, T.R. Frieden, S.Y. Liu, S.Y. Matte, F. Mostashari, D. Deitcher, K.M. Cummings, C. Chang, U. Bauer, M.T. Massett, unpublished manuscript). Finally, more research is needed to test the benefits and potential harms associated with producing new faster-delivery forms of nicotine medication (61, 80).

In the United States, nicotine medications are licensed only as aids for smoking cessation (16, 31). However, some other countries have permitted NRT to be used as a way to reduce smoking or temporarily treat nicotine withdrawal. Liberalizing government regulations so that cleaner forms of nicotine become more acceptable and accessible to smokers when compared with tobacco products has the potential to revolutionize the way the tobacco problem is perceived and addressed in the future (19, 88, 93).

ACKNOWLEDGMENTS

Grateful acknowledgment is extended to Maansi Bansal at Roswell Park Cancer Institute and Joe Gitchell from Pinney Associates for assisting us in compiling the literature reviewed in and for this review. We also acknowledge the support of Roswell Park Cancer Institute's NCI-funded Cancer Center Support Grant CA16056-26, which provides research support for both authors.

The *Annual Review of Public Health* is online at
http://publhealth.annualreviews.org

LITERATURE CITED

1. Backlog for Quitline. 2001. *Stop Mag.* 3:6
2. Baldiner B, Hasenfratz M, Battig K. 1995. Switching to ultra-low nicotine cigarettes: effects of different tar yields and blocking of olfactory cues. *Pharmacol. Biochem. Behav.* 50:233–39
3. Bansal M, Cummings KM, Hyland A, Giovino G. 2004. Stop smoking medications: Who uses them? Who misuses them? Who is misinformed? *Nicotine Tob. Res.* In press
4. Behm FM, Schur C, Levin ED, Tashkin DP, Rose JE. 1993. Clinical evaluation of a citric acid inhaler for smoking cessation. *Drug Alcohol Depend.* 31:131–38
5. Benowitz NL. 1988. Pharmacologic aspects of cigarette smoking and nicotine addiction. *N. Engl. J. Med.* 319:1318–30
6. Benowitz NL. 1993. Nicotine replacement therapy. What has been accomplished—can we do better? *Drugs* 45:157–70
7. Benowitz NL. 1998. *Nicotine Safety and Toxicity.* New York: Oxford Univ. Press
8. Bohadana A, Nilsson F, Rasmussen T, Martinet Y. 2003. Gender differences in quit rates following smoking cessation with combination nicotine therapy: influence of baseline smoking behavior. *Nicotine Tob. Res.* 5:111–16
9. Bolliger CT, Zellweger JP, Danielsson T, van Biljon X, Robidou A, Westin A, et al. 2000. Smoking reduction with oral nicotine inhalers: double-blind, randomized clinical trial of efficacy and safety. *BMJ* 321:329–33
10. Deleted in proof
11. Boyle RG, Solberg LI, Magnan S, Davison G, Alesci NL. 2002. Does insurance coverage for drug therapy affect smoking cessation? *Health Track.* Nov./Dec.:162–68
12. Brauer LH, Behm FM, Lane JD, Westman EC, Perkins C, Rose JE. 2001. Individual differences in smoking reward from denicotinized cigarettes. *Nicotine Tob. Res.* 3:101–9
13. Breese CR, Marks MJ, Logel J, Adams CE, Sullivan B, et al. 1997. Effect of smoking history on [3H] nicotine binding in human postmortem brain. *J. Pharmacol. Exp. Ther.* 282:7–13
14. Butschky MF, Bailey D, Henningfield JE, Pickworth WB. 1995. Smoking without nicotine delivery decreases withdrawal in 12-hour abstinence smokers. *Pharmacol. Biochem. Behav.* 50:91–96
15. Carperter M, Hughes JR, Solomon LJ, Callas PW. 2004. Both smoking reduction and motivational advice increase future cessation among smokers not currently planning to quit. *J. Consult. Clin. Psychol.* 72(3):371–81
16. Cent. Dis. Control Prev. 2001. Cigarette smoking among adults—United States, 1999. *MMWR* 50:869–73
17. Cent. Dis. Control Prev. 2002. Use of FDA-approved pharmacologic treatments for tobacco dependence—United States, 1984–1998. *MMWR* 49:665–68
18. Cryan JF, Gasparini F, Van Heeke G, Markowu A. 2002. Non-nicotinic neuropharmacological strategies for nicotine dependence: beyond buproprion. *Drug Discovery Today* 8:1025–34
19. Cummings KM. 2002. In debate: Can capitalism advance the goals of tobacco control? *Addiction* 97:957–62
20. Cummings KM. 2002. Programs and policies to discourage the use of tobacco products. *Oncogene* 21:7349–64
21. Cummings KM, Biernbaum RM, Zevon MA, Deloughry T, Jaen CR. 1994. Use and effectiveness of transdermal nicotine

in primary care settings. *Arch. Fam. Med.* 3:682–89

22. Cummings KM, Hyland A, Giovino GA, Hastrup JL, Bauer JE, Bansal MA. 2004. Are smokers adequately informed about the health risks of smoking and medicinal nicotine? *Nicotine Tob. Res.* In press

23. Cummings KM, Hyland A, Ockene JK, Hymowitz N, Manley M. 1997. Use of the nicotine skin patch by smokers in 20 U.S. communities, 1992–1993. *Tob. Control* 6(Suppl. 2):S63–70

24. Curry SJ, Grothaus LC, McAfee T, Pabiniak C. 1998. Use and cost effectiveness smoking-cessation services under four insurance plans in a health maintenance organization. *N. Engl. J. Med.* 339: 673–79

25. Dale LC, Hurt RD, Offord KP, Lawson GM, Croghan IT, Schroeder DR. 1995. High-dose nicotine patch therapy. Percentage of replacement and smoking cessation. *JAMA* 274:1353–58

26. Dijkstra A, De Vries H. 2000. Subtypes of precontemplating smokers defined by different long-term plans to change their smoking behavior. *Health Educ. Res.* 15: 423–34

27. Dunn WL Jr. 1972. *Motives and Incentives in Cigarettes.* Richmond, VA: Philip Morris Res. Cent.

28. Etter JF, Laszlo E, Zellweger JP, Perrot C, Perneger TV. 2002. Nicotine replacement to reduce cigarette consumption in smokers who are unwilling to quit: a randomized trial. *J. Clin. Psychopharmacol.* 22:487–95

29. Etter JF, Perneger TV. 2001. Attitudes toward nicotine replacement therapy in smokers and ex-smokers in the general public. *Clin. Pharmacol. Ther.* 69:175–83

30. Farkas AJ. 1999. When does cigarette fading increase the likelihood of future cessation? *Ann. Behav. Med.* 21:71–76

31. Fiore MC, Bailey WC, Cohen SJ, Dorfman SF, Goldstein MG, Gritz ER, et al. 2000. *Treating Tobacco Use and Dependence. Clinical Practice Guideline.*

Rockville, MD: US Dep. Health Hum. Serv., Public Health Serv.

32. Fiore MC, Hatsukami DK, Baker T. 2002. Effective tobacco dependence treatment. *JAMA* 288:1768–70

33. Fiore MC, Novotny TE, Pierce JP, Giovino GA, Hatziandreu EJ, Newcomb PA, et al. 1990. Methods used to quit smoking in the United States. Do cessation programs help? *JAMA* 263:2760–65

34. Fiore MC, Thompson SA, Lawrence DL, Welsch S, Andrews K, Ziamik M, et al. 2000. Helping Wisconsin women quit smoking: a successful collaboration. *Wisc. Med. J.* April:68–72

35. Foulds J, Ramstrom L, Burke M, Fagerström K. 2003. Effect of smokeless tobacco (snus) on smoking and public health in Sweden. *Tob. Control* 12:349–59

36. Freedman AM. 1995. Philip Morris memo likens nicotine to drugs. *Wall Street J.* Dec. 8

37. George TO, O'Malley SS. 2004. Current pharmacological treatments for nicotine dependence. *Trends Pharmacol. Sci.* 25:42–48

38. Giardina TD, Hyland A, Bauer UE, Higbee C, Cummings KM. 2004. Which population-based interventions would motivate smokers to think seriously about stopping smoking? *Am. J. Health Prom.* 18:405–8

39. Gourlay SG, Forbes A, Marriner T, Pethica D, McNeil JJ. 1994. Prospective study of factors predicting outcome of transdermal nicotine treatment in smoking cessation. *BMJ* 309:842–46

40. Halpin Schauffler H, Barker DC, Orleans TC. 2001. Medicaid coverage for tobacco dependence treatments. *Health Aff.* 20:298–303

41. Henningfield JE, Cohen C, Pickworth WD. 1993. Psychopharmacology of nicotine. In *Nicotine Addiction. Principles and Management,* ed. CT Orleans, J Slade, pp. 24–45. New York: Oxford Univ. Press

42. Herrera N, Franco R, Herrera L, Partidas A, Roland R, Fagerstrom KO. 1995.

Nicotine gum, 2 and 4 mg, for nicotine dependence. A double-blind placebo-controlled trial within a behavior modification support program. *Chest* 108:447–51

43. Hieda Y, Keyler DE, VanDeVoort JT, Niedbala RS, Raphael DE, et al. 1999. Immunization of rats reduces nicotine distribution to brain. *Psychopharmacology* 143:150–57

44. Howell TM, Sweeney WR. 1998. Aerosol and a method and apparatus for generating an aerosol. Philip Morris Inc. Patent: US5743251, April 28

45. Hu T, Sung HY, Keeler TE, Marciniak M. 2000. Cigarette consumption and sales of nicotine replacement products. *Tob. Control* 9(Suppl. 2):S60–63

46. Hughes JR. Four beliefs that may impede progress in the treatment of smoking. *Tob. Control* 8:323–26

47. Hughes JR, Cummings KM, Hyland A. 1999. Ability of smokers to reduce their smoking and its association with future smoking cessation. *Addiction* 94:109–14

48. Hughes JR, Goldstein MG, Hurt RD, Shiffman S. 1999. Recent advances in the pharmacotherapy of smoking. *JAMA* 281: 72–76

49. Deleted in proof

50. Hughes JR, Shiffman S, Callas P, Zhang J. 2003. A meta-analysis of the efficacy of over-the-counter nicotine replacement. *Tob. Control* 12:21–27

51. Hurt RD, Robertson CR. 1998. Prying open the door to the cigarette industry's secrets about nicotine—the Minnesota Tobacco Trial. *JAMA* 280:1173–81

52. Hyland A, Levy D, Rezaishiraz H, Hughes J, Bauer JE, et al. 2005. Reduction in amount smoked predicts future cessation. *Psychol. Addict. Behav.* In press

53. Deleted in proof

54. Johnstone EC, Yudkin PL, Hey K, Roberts SJ, Welch SJ, Murphy MF, et al. 2004. Genetic variation in dopaminergic pathways and short-term effectiveness of the nicotine patch. *Pharmacogenetics* 14:83–90

55. Jorensby DE, Leischow SJ, Nides MA, Rennard SI, Johnston JA, et al. 1999. A controlled trial of sustained release buproprion, a nicotine patch, or both for smoking cessation. *N. Engl. J. Med.* 340:685–91

56. Kenford SL, Fiore MC, Jorenby DE, Smith SS, Wetter D, Baker TB. 1994. Predicting smoking cessation: who will quit with and without the nicotine patch. *JAMA* 271:589–94

57. Kozlowski LT, Strasser AA, Giovino GA, Erickson PA, Terza JV. 2001. Applying the risk/use equilibrium: use medicinal nicotine now for harm reduction. *Tob. Control* 10:201–3

58. MacLeod ZR, Charles MA, Arnaldi VC, Adams IM. 2003. Telephone counseling as an adjunct to nicotine patches in smoking cessation. A randomized controlled trial. *Med. J. Aust.* 179:349–52

59. Malin DH, Lake JR, Newlin-Maultsby P, Roberts LK, Lanier JG, et al. 1992. Rodent model of nicotine abstinence syndrome. *Pharmacol. Biochem. Behav.* 43: 779–84

60. Marks MJ, Burch JB, Collins AC. 1983. Effects of chronic nicotine infusion on tolerance development and nicotinic receptors. *J. Pharmacol. Exp. Ther.* 226:817–25

61. McNeill A. 2004. Harm reduction. *BMJ* 328:885–87

62. Deleted in proof

63. Park CR, Munday DL. 2002. Development and evaluation of a biphasic buccal adhesive tablet for nicotine replacement therapy. *Int. J. Pharm.* 237:215–26

64. Paul CL, Walsh RA, Girgis A. 2003. Nicotine replacement therapy products over the counter: real-life use in the Australian community. *Aust. N. Z. J. Public Health* 27:491–95

65. Pauly JL, Streck RJ, Cummings KM. 1995. US patents shed light on Eclipse and future cigarettes. *Tob. Control* 4:261–65

66. Perkins KA. 2001. Smoking cessation in women. Special considerations. *CNS Drugs* 15:391–411

67. Pidoplichko VI, DeBiasi M, Williams JT, Dani JA. 1997. Nicotine activates and desensitizes midbrain dopamine neurons. *Nature* 390:401–4

68. Pierce JP, Gilpin E, Farkas AJ. 1995. Nicotine patch use in the general population: results from the 1993 California Tobacco Survey. *J. Natl. Cancer Inst.* 87:87–93

69. Pierce JP, Gilpin EA. 2002. Impact of over-the-counter sales on effectiveness of pharmaceutical aids for smoking cessation. *JAMA* 288:1260–64

70. Pinney JM, Henningfield JE, Shiffman S. 2002. Two-stage transmucosal medicine delivery system for symptom relief. Pinney Assoc. Patent: US6358060, March 19

71. Pontieri FE, Tanda G, Orzi F, Di Chiara G. 1996. Effects of nicotine on the nucleus accumbens and similarity to those of addictive drugs. *Nature* 382:255–57

72. Richmond R, Zwar N. 2003. Review of bupropion for smoking cessation. *Drug Alcohol Rev.* 22:203–20

73. Role LW, Berg DK. 1996. Nicotinic receptors in the development and modulation of CNS synapses. *Neuron* 16:1077–85

74. Rose JE, Behm FM. 1995. There is more to smoking than the CNS effects of nicotine. In *Effects of Nicotine on Biological Systems II*, ed. PBS Clark, pp. 9–16. Basel: Burkhäuser Verlag

75. Rose JE, Behm FM, Levin ED. 1993. The role of nicotine dose and sensory cues in the regulation of smoke intake. *Pharmacol. Biochem. Behav.* 44:891–900

76. Rose JE, Levin ED. 1991. Interrelationships between conditioned and primary reinforcement in the maintenance of cigarette smoking. *Br. J. Addict.* 86:606–9

77. Schauffler HH, McMenammin S, Olson K, Boyce-Smith G, Rideout JA, Kamil J. 2001. Variations in treatment benefits influence smoking cessation: results of a randomized controlled trial. *Tob. Control* 10:175–80

78. Schuh KJ, Schuh LM, Henningfield JE. 1997. Nicotine nasal spray and vapor inhaler. Abuse liability assessment. *Psychopharmacology* 130:352–61

79. Seller EM, Kaplan HL, Tyndale RF. 2000. Inhibition of cytochrome P450 2A6 increases nicotine's oral bioavailability and decreases smoking. *Clin. Pharmacol. Ther.* 68:35–43

80. Shiffman S, Fant RV, Gitchell JG. 2003. Nicotine delivery systems: How far has technology come? *Am. J. Drug Deliv.* 1:112–24

81. Shiffman S, Gitchell J, Pinney JM. 1997. Public health benefit of over-the-counter nicotine medications. *Tob. Control* 6:306–10

82. Shiffman S, Hughes JR, DiMarino ME, Sweeney CT. 2003. Patterns of over-the-counter nicotine gum use: persistent use and concurrent smoking. *Addiction* 98:1747–53

83. Deleted in proof

84. Shiffman SA, Paty JA, Rohay JM, DiMarino ME, Gitchell JG. 2001. The efficacy of computer-tailored smoking cessation material as a supplement to nicotine patch therapy. *Drug Alcohol Depend.* 64:35–46

85. Silagy C, Lancaster T, Stead L, Mant D, Fowler G. 2002. Nicotine replacement therapy for smoking cessation. *Cochrane Database Syst. Rev.* 4:CD000146

86. Solomon LJ, Scharoun GM, Flynn BS, Secker-Walker RH, Sepinwall D. 2000. Free nicotine patches plus proactive telephone peer support to help low-income women stop smoking. *Prev. Med.* 31:68–74

87. Stratton K, Shetty P, Wallace R, Bondurant S, eds. 2001. *Clearing the Smoke: Assessing the Science Base for Tobacco Harm Reduction*. Washington, DC: Natl. Acad. Press

88. Sweanor D. 2000. Regulatory imbalance between medicinal and nonmedicinal nicotine. *Addiction* 95(Suppl.):S25–28

89. Thompson S. 2002. The nicotine vaccine. *Stop Mag.* 9:26–27

90. Thorndike A, Biener L, Rigotti NA. 2002. The impact on smoking cessation of switching nicotine replacement therapy to over-the-counter status. *Am. J. Public Health* 92:437–42

91. US Dep. Health Hum. Serv. 1988. *The Health Consequences of Smoking: Nicotine Addiction. A Report of the Surgeon General.* Rockville, MD: US Dep. Health Hum. Serv., Cent. Dis. Control, Off. Smok. Health

92. US Dep. Health Hum. Serv. 2000. *Reducing Tobacco Use: A Report of the Surgeon General.* Rockville, MD: U.S. Dep. Health Hum. Serv., Public Health Serv., Cent. Dis. Control Prev., Natl. Cent. Chronic Dis. Prev. Health Promot., Off. Smok. Health

93. Warner KE, Slade J, Sweanor DT. 1997. The emerging market for long-term nicotine maintenance. *JAMA* 278: 1087–92

94. Wennike P, Danielsson T, Landfeldt B, Westin A, Tønnesen P. 2003. Smoking reduction promotes smoking cessation: results from a double-blind, randomized, placebo-controlled trial of nicotine gum with a 2-year follow-up. *Addiction* 98:1395–402

95. West R, Hajek P, Nilsson F, Foulds J, May S, Meadows A. 2001. Individual differences in preferences for and responses to four nicotine replacement products. *Psychopharmacology* 153:225–30

96. Westman EC, Behm FM, Rose JE. 1996. Airway sensory replacement as a treatment for smoking cessation. *Drug Dev. Res.* 38:257–62

97. Westman EC, Behm FM, Rose JE. 1996. Dissociating the nicotine and airway sensory effects of smoking. *Pharmacol. Biochem. Behav.* 53:309–15

98. Deleted in press

99. Yudkin PL, Jones L, Lancaster T, Fowler GH. 1996. Which smokers are helped to give up smoking using transdermal nicotine patches? Results from a randomized, double-blinded, placebo-controlled trial. *Br. J. Gen. Pract.* 46:145–48

100. Zhu SH, Melcer T, Sun J, Rosbrook B, Pierce JP. 2000. Smoking cessation with and without assistance: a population-based analysis. *Am. J. Prev. Med.* 18:305–11

Subject Index

CUMULATIVE INDEXES

CONTRIBUTING AUTHORS, VOLUMES 17–26

CHAPTER TITLES, VOLUMES 17–26

Prefatory

Behavioral Aspects of Health

Environmental and Occupational Health

Health Services

Symposium: Cancers of Special Importance to Women

Symposium: Eating-Related Disorders

Symposium: Geographic Information Systems (GIS)

Symposium: Public Health Aspects of Ophthalmic Disease

Symposium: Public Health Genetics

Symposium: Public Health in the Twentieth Century

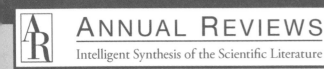

ANNUAL REVIEWS
Intelligent Synthesis of the Scientific Literature

Annual Reviews – Your Starting Point for Research Online
http://arjournals.annualreviews.org

- Over 900 Annual Reviews volumes—more than 25,000 critical, authoritative review articles in 31 disciplines spanning the Biomedical, Physical, and Social sciences—available online, including all Annual Reviews back volumes, dating to 1932

- Current individual subscriptions include seamless online access to full-text articles, PDFs, Reviews in Advance (as much as 6 months ahead of print publication), bibliographies, and other supplementary material in the current volume and the prior 4 years' volumes

- All articles are fully supplemented, searchable, and downloadable—see http://publhealth.annualreviews.org

- Access links to the reviewed references (when available online)

- Site features include customized alerting services, citation tracking, and saved searches

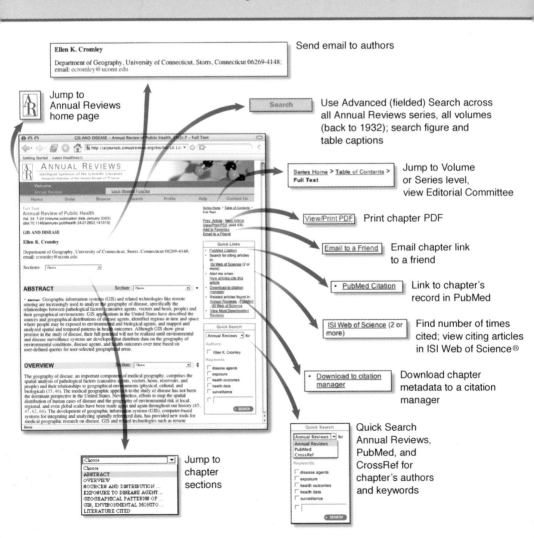